Cystic Fibrosis

Edited by
Marcus A. Mall and J. Stuart Elborn

Editor in Chief
Tobias Welte

This book is one in a series of *ERS Monographs*. Each individual issue provides a comprehensive overview of one specific clinical area of respiratory health, communicating information about the most advanced techniques and systems required for its investigation. It provides factual and useful scientific detail, drawing on specific case studies and looking into the diagnosis and management of individual patients. Previously published titles in this series are listed at the back of this *Monograph*.

ERS Monographs are available online at www.erspublications.com and print copies are available from www.ersbookshop.com

Continuing medical education (CME) credits are available through this issue of the *ERS Monograph*. Following evaluation, this book has been accredited by the European Board for Accreditation in Pneumology (EBAP) for 5 CME credits. To earn CME credits, read the book then complete the CME question form that is available at www.ers-education.org/e-learning/cme-tests.aspx

Editorial Board: Andrew Bush (London, UK), Peter Calverley (Liverpool, UK), Martin Kolb (Hamilton, ON, Canada), Kjell Larsson (Stockholm, Sweden)

Managing Editors: Rachel White and Catherine Pumphrey
European Respiratory Society, 442 Glossop Road, Sheffield, S10 2PX, UK
Tel: 44 114 2672860 | E-mail: Monograph@ersj.org.uk

Published by European Respiratory Society ©2014
June 2014
Print ISBN: 978-1-84984-050-7
Online ISBN: 978-1-84984-051-4
Print ISSN: 2312-508X
Online ISSN: 2312-5098
Printed by Charlesworth Press, Wakefield, UK

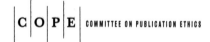

This journal is a member of and subscribes to the principles of the Committee on Publication Ethics.

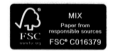

MIX
Paper from responsible sources
FSC® C016379

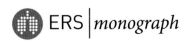

Contents

Cystic Fibrosis   Number 64
                                                                  June 2014

Preface   ix

Guest Editors   xi

Introduction   xiii

Pathophysiology

1. Pathophysiology of cystic fibrosis lung disease   1
    Marcus A. Mall and Richard C. Boucher

2. Airway inflammation in cystic fibrosis   14
    Cormac McCarthy, M. Emmet O'Brien, Kerstin Pohl, Emer P. Reeves and
    Noel Gerard McElvaney

3. Airway infection and the microbiome   32
    Jiangchao Zhao, J. Stuart Elborn and John J. LiPuma

4. Genetic and environmental modifiers of cystic fibrosis   47
    Burkhard Tümmler and Frauke Stanke

Diagnosis

5. Newborn screening for cystic fibrosis: opportunities and   65
    remaining challenges
    Anil Mehta, Olaf Sommerburg and Kevin W. Southern

6. Early cystic fibrosis lung disease   77
    Stephen M. Stick

7. Imaging the lungs in cystic fibrosis   88
    Harm A.W.M. Tiddens

8. End-points and biomarkers for clinical trials in cystic fibrosis   104
    Kris De Boeck, Isabelle Fajac and Felix Ratjen

Therapy

9. Correcting the basic ion transport defects in cystic fibrosis   116
    Emanuela Caci and Luis J.V. Galietta

10. Potentiating and correcting mutant CFTR in patients with cystic fibrosis 129
   Isabelle Sermet-Gaudelus, Jacques de Blic, Muriel LeBourgeois, Iwona Pranke, Aleksander Edelman and Bonnie W. Ramsey

11. New horizons for cystic fibrosis gene and cell therapy 150
   Uta Griesenbach, Rosanna F. Featherstone and Eric W.F.W. Alton

12. Improving airway clearance in cystic fibrosis lung disease 169
   Judy M. Bradley, Katherine O'Neill, Ruth Dentice and Mark Elkins

13. Antibiotic treatment of cystic fibrosis lung disease 188
   Christopher Orchard and Diana Bilton

14. Exercise in cystic fibrosis 203
   Helge Hebestreit

15. Extrapulmonary manifestations of cystic fibrosis 219
   Barry J. Plant and Michael D. Parkins

16. Lung transplantation for cystic fibrosis 236
   Jens Gottlieb and Mark Greer

Care

17. Standards of care for patients with cystic fibrosis 246
   Malena Cohen-Cymberknoh, David Shoseyov and Eitan Kerem

18. Using registries to improve cystic fibrosis care 262
   Edward F. McKone and Bruce C. Marshall

19. Transition from paediatric to adult cystic fibrosis care: a developmental framework 272
   Anjana S. Madan, Adrianne N. Alpern and Alexandra L. Quittner

20. Challenges of providing care to adults with cystic fibrosis 286
   Scott C. Bell and David W. Reid

21. Health-economic aspects of cystic fibrosis screening and therapy 304
   Jiří Klimeš, Tomáš Doležal, Kateřina Kubáčková, Marek Turnovec and Milan Macek Jr

Preface

Tobias Welte, Editor in Chief

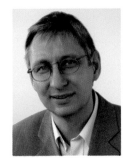

Although it is the most common genetic disease in Europe, cystic fibrosis (CF) is a rare disease. Nevertheless, it provides a good example of how a powerful patient organisation and dedicated researchers and doctors can help to arouse the interest of the public and the pharmaceutical industry in a disease. This was the key factor in maintaining continuous financial support to make translation from basic research into clinical practice possible.

The success in the treatment of CF patients has contributed to significant improvements in the care of other patient groups. Essential elements of CF therapy have been transferred into the management of non-CF bronchiectasis patients and have recently been approved in randomised controlled trials. The best examples are three major macrolide antibiotic trials that demonstrate impressive effects on exacerbations in non-CF bronchiectasis patients. The concept of inhaled antibiotic therapy to reduce microbiological burden, which was established in CF, has now been used in studies in long-term ventilated patients with Gram-negative pneumonia and could provide a new treatment option for these patients, who still suffer from high morbidity and mortality.

Along with pulmonary hypertension, CF is one of the few diseases where basic scientific findings have been translated into therapeutic concepts. The modification of the cystic fibrosis transmembrane conductance regulator (CFTR), even if it is possible only for particular mutations, represents a breakthrough in the development of new drugs. Through this, we have hopefully learned how dynamic basic research could be transferred into advanced therapies for other diseases, for example usual interstitial pneumonia, for which we do not have a convincing treatment option yet. Overall, CF research could be an excellent role model to stimulate research in respiratory medicine.

This issue of the *ERS Monograph* summarises the most important developments in CF diagnosis and treatment since the publication of the previous CF issue in 2006. I want to congratulate the Guest Editors, Marcus Mall and Stuart Elborn, for the tremendous work they have done in setting up this excellent

Monograph, which should be of interest to paediatric and adult CF physicians, basic researchers and people working in drug development. I hope this *Monograph* will stimulate joint research, leading to better understanding of and more successful therapy for respiratory diseases.

Guest Editors

Marcus A. Mall

Marcus A. Mall is Professor of Paediatrics and director of the Dept of Translational Pulmonology at the Heidelberg University Medical School, and head of the Division of Paediatric Pulmonology and Allergy and the Cystic Fibrosis Center at the Dept of Paediatrics, University Hospital Heidelberg, Heidelberg, Germany. In 2011, he was appointed director of the Translational Lung Research Center Heidelberg (TLRC) and member of the board of directors of the German Center for Lung Research (DZL). He is an active member of several professional societies, including the European Cystic Fibrosis Society (ECFS), the European Respiratory Society (ERS) and the American Thoracic Society (ATS). He serves on journal editorial boards and on the scientific committee of the ECFS.

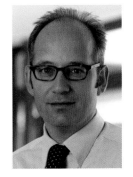

Marcus Mall qualified in medicine at the University of Freiburg, Freiburg, Germany, and received his clinical training at the Universities of Freiburg and Heidelberg, and his postdoctoral training at the University of North Carolina at Chapel Hill, NC, USA, where he was appointed Assistant Professor of Medicine. In 2005, he received a grant from the European Commission to establish a Marie Curie Excellence Team at the University of Heidelberg, and in 2009 he was awarded the prestigious Heisenberg Professorship by the German Research Foundation. He is board certified in paediatrics, paediatric pulmonology and infectious diseases.

Marcus Mall's research is focused on the cellular and molecular pathogenesis of CF and other airway diseases, and the development of novel diagnostic approaches and therapeutic strategies. His research programme has been funded by the German Research Foundation (DFG), the German Ministry for Education and Research (BMBF), the European Commission, and others, and he has received several research awards. He developed a mouse that overexpresses the epithelial sodium channel (βENaC), the first animal model with CF-like lung disease. He coordinates interdisciplinary translational research projects, integrating basic research with cohort studies and early phase clinical trials, to improve our understanding of CF lung disease and the translation of research results into the clinic.

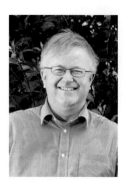

J. Stuart Elborn

J. Stuart Elborn is Dean of the School of Medicine, Dentistry and Biomedical Sciences (SMDBS), Queen's University Belfast, Belfast, UK. He was previously director of the Centre for Infection and Immunity in SMDBS and Professor of Respiratory Medicine. He is a consultant physician in Belfast City Hospital (Belfast, UK), where he started an adult CF programme that now has 300 patients, and he collaborates closely with his paediatric colleagues who provide care for 180 patients. Additionally, he is president of the ECFS and is a trustee of the UK CF Trust.

Stuart Elborn has led a number of clinical trials involving antibiotics, anti-inflammatory agents and cystic fibrosis trans-membrane conductance regulator (CFTR)-modulating drugs. He also leads a clinical trials programme in bronchiectasis. His team of pulmonary researchers has recently been selected as part of a Translational Research Partnership in the UK, which focuses on academics working with the pharmaceutical industry in pre-clinical and early clinical trials. His group is also part of the ECFS Clinical Trials Network. He is principal investigator on a number of early stage anti-inflammatory and potentially disease-modifying therapies in CF and other lung diseases.

Stuart Elborn has a major clinical and laboratory research programme in airways infection, funded jointly by the National Institutes of Health (Bethesda, MD, USA), the Research and Development Office in Northern Ireland, the UK Medical Research Council, the Science Foundation Ireland and the European Union Framework 7, investigating the clinical implications of bacterial diversity and, in particular, anaerobes in the CF airway. This involves clinical research and also a range of projects investigating the interaction between bacteria and the host innate immunity.

Introduction

Marcus A. Mall[1,2] and J. Stuart Elborn[3]

Twenty-five years ago, the sequencing of the cystic fibrosis transmembrane conductance regulator (*CFTR*) gene set the stage for unravelling the pathogenesis of cystic fibrosis (CF) and for development of therapies that target the basic defect of this common life-limiting hereditary disease. This scientific breakthrough brought hope that therapy of CF targeted at the dysfunction of the CFTR protein may be possible and has stimulated enormous multi-disciplinary research efforts towards this goal. In early studies, expression of wild-type and mutant CFTR in cell lines shed important light on normal CFTR function and the molecular defects that can cause CF. Further genetic studies predicted that CF may be caused by a large spectrum of *CFTR* mutations with different molecular consequences, indicating a need for mutation-specific therapies.

However, for many years, the drug discovery process for CF was slow and mostly limited to pre-clinical testing of individual compounds by academic investigators. These studies provided an important proof-of-concept that pharmacological rescue of mutant CFTR function is possible. However, therapeutic development was hampered by the limited efficacy and toxicity of candidate compounds that were identified by this cumbersome and inefficient approach. Nevertheless, the prospect of a therapy to treat the basic defect provided an important rationale for the optimisation of symptomatic therapies and establishment of specialised care centres for patients with CF, a development that has led to an improvement of survival and quality of life unprecedented for a fatal genetic disease.

In recent years, this landscape has been changed dramatically following a high-throughput screening programme for the discovery of CFTR "potentiator" and "corrector" drugs. In fewer than 10 years, this approach led to the development of the first mutation-specific therapy for CF, which has now become available for a subgroup of patients. With this important breakthrough, the CF field has clearly entered a new era of personalised/stratified medicine targeting the underlying genetic defect that may well serve as a model for other rare genetic lung diseases. Furthermore, widespread implementation of newborn screening has opened a window of opportunity for early or even preventive treatment with disease-modifying therapies of future generations of people with CF. Other examples of important progress include the generation of animal models for deciphering the complex *in vivo* pathogenesis of CF lung disease and pre-clinical testing of novel mucolytic, anti-inflammatory and antibacterial

[1]Dept of Translational Pulmonology, Translational Lung Research Center Heidelberg (TLRC), Heidelberg, Germany. [2]Division of Paediatric Pulmonology and Allergy and Cystic Fibrosis Center, Dept of Paediatrics, University of Heidelberg, Member of the German Center for Lung Research (DZL), Heidelberg, Germany. [3]Centre for Infection and Immunity, School of Medicine, Dentistry and Biomedical Sciences, Queen's University Belfast, Belfast, UK.

Correspondence: Marcus A. Mall, Dept of Translational Pulmonology, Translational Lung Research Center Heidelberg (TLRC), University of Heidelberg, Im Neuenheimer Feld 350, 69120 Heidelberg, Germany. E-mail: Marcus.Mall@med.uni-heidelberg.de

Copyright ERS 2014. Print ISBN: 978-1-84984-050-7. Online ISBN: 978-1-84984-051-4. Print ISSN: 2312-508X. Online ISSN: 2312-5098.

therapies, as well as progress in basic research on regenerative therapies that are needed to improve outcome of patients with irreversible lung damage.

Despite this enormous progress, important challenges remain that have to be solved in order to deliver disease-modifying treatment, ideally in all patients. These challenges range from the development of drugs that rescue a broader spectrum of CFTR mutations in the laboratory, including the most common mutation Phe508del, all the way to the training of a larger number of CF specialists, who are urgently needed in clinics for competent care of the rapidly growing population of patients with CF as they grow older.

This issue of the *ERS Monograph* provides an update on all aspects of CF lung disease, from infancy to adulthood, including current pathogenetic concepts of mucus plugging, chronic airway inflammation and polymicrobial infection, improvements in early diagnosis and monitoring, mutation-specific and other therapeutic approaches, and important issues related to further improvement of patient care. In state-of-the-art chapters, international experts in the field highlight important recent developments and discuss the next steps that will be required for further improvement of life expectancy and quality of life of patients with CF. As editors, it was a great pleasure to assemble this *Monograph* in the year of the 25th anniversary of the discovery of CFTR, and we trust that it will be a useful reference for basic and clinical scientists, and all members of the CF team.

Chapter 1

Pathophysiology of cystic fibrosis lung disease

Marcus A. Mall[1,2] and Richard C. Boucher[3]

Chronic obstructive lung disease starting in the first months of life remains the major cause of morbidity and mortality in patients with cystic fibrosis (CF). The discovery of the cystic fibrosis transmembrane conductance regulator (*CFTR*) gene 25 years ago paved the way for investigation of the molecular and cellular basis of CF lung disease, and the generation of animal models for *in vivo* studies of pathogenesis. In this chapter, we focus on major advances in the understanding of the link between mutations in CFTR and the predictable development of chronic mucus obstruction, inflammation and infection of CF airways. We discuss evidence from translational studies supporting the concept that increased mucus concentration (*i.e.* dehydration) and reduced pH of the airway surface layer are key abnormalities underlying impaired innate defence of the CF lung. Novel therapeutic strategies targeting these defects may be successful for the prevention and treatment of CF lung disease independent of the patient's CF genotype.

A progressive chronic obstructive lung disease, featuring early onset mucus plugging, chronic neutrophilic airway inflammation and polymicrobial infection, remains the major cause of morbidity and mortality in patients with CF [1, 2]. While the lungs of CF patients appear structurally normal at birth, *post mortem* studies performed in the 1940s of CF infants who died of meconium ileus reported heterogeneous mucus plugging in the small airways associated with air trapping, in the absence of histopathological evidence of infection or inflammation, as the earliest abnormality in the CF lung [3]. In the first months of life, airway mucus obstruction becomes associated with neutrophilic inflammation and airway wall thickening [3, 4].

The early onset of heterogeneous obstructive lung disease was recently confirmed in observational studies in infants and preschool children with CF. Using pulmonary function testing, chest imaging studies and bronchoalveolar lavage (BAL), these studies demonstrated a high prevalence of airflow limitation, ventilation inhomogeneity, air trapping, bronchiectasis, mucus plugging and neutrophilic inflammation with elevated levels of interleukin (IL)-8 and neutrophil elastase (NE) in infants with CF [5–10]. Of note, these abnormalities were detected as early as 3 months of age in both culture-positive and culture-negative CF patients and mostly in the absence of respiratory symptoms. With increasing age, patients expectorate mucus that is highly viscous and hyperconcentrated (*i.e.* has a reduced

[1]Dept of Translational Pulmonology, Translational Lung Research Center Heidelberg (TLRC), Heidelberg, Germany. [2]Division of Paediatric Pulmonology and Allergy and Cystic Fibrosis Center, Dept of Paediatrics, University of Heidelberg, Member of the German Center for Lung Research (DZL), Heidelberg, Germany. [3]Cystic Fibrosis/Pulmonary Research and Treatment Center, School of Medicine, The University of North Carolina at Chapel Hill, Chapel Hill, NC, USA.

Correspondence: Marcus A. Mall, Dept of Translational Pulmonology, Translational Lung Research Center Heidelberg (TLRC), University of Heidelberg, Im Neuenheimer Feld 350, 69120 Heidelberg, Germany. E-mail: Marcus.Mall@med.uni-heidelberg.de

Copyright ERS 2014. Print ISBN: 978-1-84984-050-7. Online ISBN: 978-1-84984-051-4. Print ISSN: 2312-508X. Online ISSN: 2312-5098.

water content) [11], exhibit reduced mucociliary clearance [12], and develop intermittent to chronic polymicrobial infection with *Staphylococcus aureus*, *Haemophilus influenzae*, *Pseudomonas aeruginosa* and other bacterial species [1]. Chronic infection is accompanied by persistent neutrophilic inflammation leading to progressive irreversible lung damage, including bronchiectasis and emphysema [13–15].

Based on the sequence of these clinical and histopathological findings, there is general agreement that the pathogenesis of this muco-obstructive lung disease reflects a defect of innate defence mechanisms of CF airway surfaces [1]. 25 years ago, the discovery that CF is caused by mutations in the cystic fibrosis transmembrane conductance regulator (*CFTR*) gene provided the tools to elucidate the molecular and cellular mechanisms that link mutant *CFTR* to the pathogenesis of CF lung disease [16–18]. Since then, diverse hypotheses have been put forward and debated in the CF community of how CFTR dysfunction may impair innate defence and produce chronic inflammation and infection of CF airways. These hypotheses include: impaired mucociliary clearance due to alterations in airway surface liquid (ASL) volume and/or composition that are caused by abnormal ion transport across the superficial airway epithelium and/or submucosal glands [19–21]; deficient antimicrobial activities in ASL [22]; reduced epithelial binding and clearance of *P. aeruginosa* [23]; impaired phagolysosomal function and intracellular bacterial killing by macrophages and neutrophils [24, 25]; altered ceramide metabolism [26]; and an intrinsically enhanced inflammatory response in CF airways [27]. However, all these hypotheses were largely based on *in vitro* studies and their *in vivo* validation was hampered for a long time because *CFTR* knockout mice failed to develop CF-like lung disease [28]. More recently, this hurdle was overcome by the generation of β-epithelial Na^+ channel-overexpressing (βENaC) transgenic mice and *CFTR*-deficient pigs that develop spontaneous lung diseases. Both models exhibit key features of CF in humans, including airway mucus plugging, neutrophilic inflammation and impaired bacterial killing [22, 29–32].

In this chapter, we will focus on recent translational studies in these animal models that link consequences of CFTR dysfunction in the airway epithelium to the *in vivo* pathogenesis of CF lung disease. The results obtained from these studies support the current concept that dehydration and reduced pH of the ASL are key abnormalities and probably disease-initiating events underlying impaired innate defence of the CF lung. Furthermore, these studies suggest that novel therapeutic strategies that target these fundamental defects may be successful in the prevention and treatment of lung disease in all patients with CF independent of their CF genotype.

CFTR dysfunction causes a basic ion transport defect in CF airways

The identification of the *CFTR* gene in 1989 set the stage for elucidating the molecular and cellular pathogenesis of CF lung disease [16–18]. Early studies demonstrated that CFTR is a multi-domain transmembrane protein belonging to the family of adenine nucleotide-binding cassette transporters [33], which functions as an anion channel regulated by cAMP-dependent phosphorylation that conducts Cl^- and bicarbonate [34, 35]. CFTR is expressed in many epithelia of the body, including airway surfaces and airway submucosal glands [36, 37]. Furthermore, *in vivo* measurements and studies in freshly excised native human airway tissues identified abnormal regulation of ENaC, which constitutes the limiting pathway for Na^+ and fluid absorption as a characteristic abnormality in CF airways [38–41]. ENaC is a multimeric transmembrane protein consisting of three homologous subunits (α, β and γ) that are probably arranged as a tetramer of two α, one β and one γ subunits all contributing to the central channel pore [42]. Following the cloning of the *ENaC* subunits [43], co-expression of CFTR and ENaC in heterologous cells demonstrated that cAMP-dependent activation of wild-type, but not mutant *CFTR*, results in inhibition of ENaC activity [44–46]. Taken together, these studies led to the hypothesis that CFTR dysfunction results in a basic defect of epithelial ion transport characterised by deficient cAMP-dependent anion secretion and abnormal ENaC-mediated Na$^+$ absorption across CF airway surfaces (fig. 1a and b) [47].

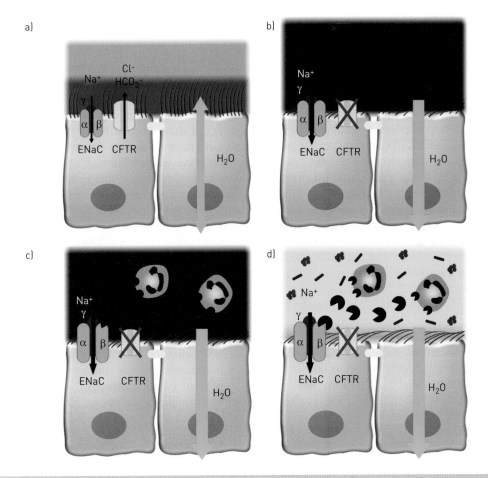

Figure 1. Consequences of cystic fibrosis transmembrane conductance regulator (CFTR) dysfunction on epithelial ion transport, airway surface hydration, mucociliary clearance and antibacterial host defence in cystic fibrosis (CF) airways. a) In normal airway epithelia, CFTR is expressed in the apical cell membrane where it functions as an anion channel that mediates secretion of Cl$^-$/HCO$_3^-$ and fluid, and controls the absorption of Na$^+$ and fluid mediated by the amiloride-sensitive epithelial Na$^+$ channel (ENaC). Coordinated secretion and absorption of salt and water is essential for proper hydration of airway surfaces (periciliary layer and overlying mucus gel) and normal mucus clearance. b) In CF airway epithelia, CFTR dysfunction due to various molecular mechanisms, including deficient synthesis, processing, gating, conductance or reduced stability of CFTR anion channels, causes dehydration of the periciliary and mucus layers leading to impaired mucus transport and airway mucus obstruction (dark blue area). c) Static, dehydrated mucus triggers airway inflammation and forms a nidus for bacterial infection. Once neutrophilic inflammation is established, the release of proteases, such as neutrophil elastase, augments ENaC activity by proteolytic cleavage and further aggravates airway surface dehydration and mucociliary dysfunction. d) Lack of CFTR-mediated HCO$_3^-$ secretion causes reduced airway surface liquid pH (yellow area), which renders antimicrobial peptides such as lysozyme and lactoferrin less effective and contributes to impaired defence against bacterial infection in CF airways.

The most common *CFTR* mutation, the deletion of phenylalanine (Phe508del) in nucleotide binding domain (NBD)-1, causes impaired protein folding, trafficking and stability and is present on at least one allele in ~90% of patients with CF [33]. However, CFTR dysfunction can result from over 1900 *CFTR* mutations causing different molecular defects ranging from defective protein synthesis, impaired channel gating or conductance to a reduced number of channels in the luminal plasma membrane. A common consequence of each mutational class is abnormal epithelial ion transport [48, 49].

Alternative Cl⁻ channels counteracting CFTR dysfunction

In addition to CFTR, it is well established that airway epithelia express alternative Ca^{2+}-activated Cl⁻ channels (CaCC) that mediate transient Cl⁻ secretion when intracellular Ca^{2+} levels are increased, *e.g.* following activation by extracellular nucleotides *via* purinergic ($P2Y_2$ receptor-mediated) signalling [50, 51]. Since the function of CaCC remains intact in CF airways and probably protects *CFTR* knockout mice from developing lung disease [28, 52], it has been hypothesised that more sustained activation of these alternative Cl⁻ channels may compensate for CFTR dysfunction in patients with CF. However, studies designed to test this notion were hampered for a long time because the molecular identity of CaCC was not known [53]. Important progress in this area was made by the identification of the transmembrane protein TMEM16A (also known as anoctamin-1) and demonstration that it functions as a Cl⁻ channel, which probably accounts for a major fraction of Ca^{2+}-induced Cl⁻ conductance in human and mouse airway epithelia [54, 55].

Emerging evidence suggests that SLC26A9, a member of the SLC26 family of anion transporters that is highly expressed in the lung [56], is also an alternative Cl⁻ channel relevant to CF [57, 58]. Recent studies in *SLC26A9* knockout mice showed that SLC26A9-mediated Cl⁻ secretion is increased in T-helper cell (Th) type 2-mediated airway inflammation and prevents mucus plugging in the presence of mucus hypersecretion [59, 60]. Interestingly, *SLC26A9* was identified as a modifier of meconium ileus in CF in a genome-wide association study (GWAS) [61], and *SLC26A9* variants were recently detected in patients with non-CF bronchiectasis [62]. While it is apparent that the endogenous activities of TMEM16A and SLC26A9 are not sufficient to prevent CF lung disease, their molecular identification, together with the availability of high throughput screens to identify potent activator compounds [63, 64], may facilitate therapeutic exploitation of these alternative Cl⁻ channels to counteract deficient Cl⁻ secretion in CF airways.

Modulation of basic CF ion transport defect by airway inflammation

A series of recent studies suggested that the CF ion transport defect can be aggravated by proteases secreted by inflammatory cells in chronic CF airway inflammation. First, it was shown that the serine protease NE, a major product of activated neutrophils, is a potent regulator of ENaC. NE has well described in the pathogenesis of chronic airway disease ranging from modulation of airway inflammation and mucus hypersecretion, bacterial killing to proteolytic lung damage [65–68]. Furthermore, recent data indicate that NE can activate near-silent ENaC channels in the apical membrane by proteolytic cleavage of the extracellular domains of its α- and γ-subunits to excise "inhibitory" peptide segments. This excision probably causes a conformational change that increases ENaC activity [69–71]. A similar activation was recently shown for proteolytic cleavage by the cysteine protease cathepsin S [72].

In the plasma membrane, ENaC appears to be associated with wild-type CFTR. The results from recent biochemical studies indicate that this interaction may protect ENaC from proteolytic cleavage and activation [73]. In contrast, co-expression of ENaC with Phe508del failed to inhibit proteolytic cleavage and activation in heterologous cells. Consistent with this observation, the fraction of cleaved ENaC subunits was increased in human CF compared with non-CF airway epithelial cultures [73].

Collectively, these results suggest that an increased susceptibility for proteolytic activation due to the lack of "protective" wild-type CFTR may contribute to increased Na^+ absorption in CF, and that Na^+ hyperabsorption may be further enhanced by elevated levels of free protease activity in inflamed airways (fig. 1c). A recent study also found that NE leads to degradation and loss of CFTR Cl^- channel function, probably through a pathway involving the activation of intracellular calpains [74]. Therefore, an imbalance between NE and protective anti-proteases in the extracellular fluid [70] may aggravate both CF Na^+ and Cl^- transport defects once chronic airway inflammation is established.

CF ion transport defects produce airway surface dehydration and mucostasis

Because the airways are lined by an epithelium that is relatively water permeable [75], the hydration of the ASL is determined by the mass of salt on airway surfaces. Transepithelial salt transport in airways is regulated by active Cl^- secretion mediated by CFTR and alternative Cl^- channels, and ENaC-mediated Na^+ absorption. Therefore, deficient Cl^- secretion and abnormal ENaC regulation, defined as the inability to respond (slow) to airway surface dehydration, were predicted to cause dehydration (i.e. ASL volume depletion) of airway surfaces in CF. However, due to the dimensions of the ASL ($\sim$7–50 µm), this hypothesis was difficult to test in patients. Consequently, for many years, the link between airway surface dehydration and the in vivo pathogenesis of CF lung disease remained elusive.

A major breakthrough in our current understanding of how the basic CF ion transport defect and related changes in airway surface hydration trigger CF lung disease resulted from studies in highly differentiated primary cultures of normal and CF airway epithelia that are grown at an air–liquid interface under near-physiological conditions. These cultures preserve the ion and mucus transport properties of native airway tissues and enable studies of regulation of ASL under the film conditions seen in vivo [20, 76]. The ASL consists of two layers, the mucus layer that entraps inhaled particles and pathogens, and the periciliary layer that facilitates ciliary beating and acts as a lubricant surface to promote mucus clearance [77]. By using confocal microscopy to image the ASL in this primary airway culture model, it became possible to show that normal airway epithelia have the capability to regulate ASL volume by responding to signals in ASL that regulate both Na^+ absorption and Cl^- secretion. In health, this regulation generates an ASL height of $\sim$7 µm, approximately corresponding to the length of extended cilia. In contrast, this periciliary layer auto-regulation fails in CF airway epithelia. Namely, the failure of Cl^- secretion produces reduced ASL volume, and the failure to regulate (i.e. inhibit) ENaC prevents a compensatory response. The consequences are that the periciliary layer height is substantially reduced and cilia are flattened/collapsed onto airway surfaces with reduced mucus transport rates in CF compared with normal airway cultures (fig. 1a and b) [20, 78, 79].

In the traditional "one-gel" mucus transport model, the periciliary layer was considered to be a mucin-free liquid layer providing a low viscosity space that facilitated ciliary beating and separated the mucus layer from the cell surface to prevent mucus adhesion [77]. However, with this model it was difficult to explain how the periciliary layer was protected from penetration by secreted mucins "smaller" than the inter-ciliary space under healthy conditions, and how reduced periciliary layer height impaired mucus transport in CF. This conceptual problem was recently solved in biophysical studies demonstrating that the periciliary layer is not a mucin-free fluid, but rather a membrane-tethered mucin gel (MUC1, MUC4 and MUC16) that is more densely packed than the overlaying mucus layer. In this revised "gel-on-brush" model, under conditions of normal airway surface hydration, the osmotic modulus (measure of "water-drawing power") generated by the tethered mucins in the periciliary layer exceeds the osmotic modulus of the mucus gel to maintain normal periciliary layer height and ciliary function [80]. However, when the ASL becomes dehydrated due to net hyperabsorptive ion transport phenotype (*i.e.* deficient Cl⁻ secretion and abnormal regulation of Na⁺ transport) in CF airways, the concentration of secreted mucins in the mucus gel increases and, above a critical threshold, the osmotic modulus of the dehydrated mucus layer exceeds the osmotic modulus of the periciliary layer. This imbalance leads to osmotic compression of the periciliary layer and cilia, with predictable mucus transport dysfunction on CF airway surfaces [80]. When viewed in combination with the ion transport studies in native CF airway tissues, these *in vitro* studies of mucus biophysics provide a quantitative link between the basic defect of ion and fluid transport and impaired mucus clearance in the airways of patients with CF.

Airway surface dehydration phenocopies CF lung disease in mice

Mice express little *CFTR* in the lower airways. Consequently, it is not surprising that *CFTR* knockout mice did not reproduce the basic CF ion transport defect in the lower airways and develop CF-like lung disease [52, 81, 82]. Consequently, the *in vivo* validation of the importance of airway surface dehydration in CF pathogenesis was hampered by the lack of an animal model. This limitation led to the development of mice with airway-specific overexpression of ENaC to recapitulate abnormally regulated ENaC-mediated Na⁺ absorption and test the *in vivo* consequences of an imbalance between secretion and absorption of salt and water on airway surface hydration, mucus clearance and lung health [29, 30]. Airway-specific overexpression of ENaC was achieved by using the club cell secretory protein (*CCSP*) promoter [83], targeting club cells that constitute the most abundant epithelial cell type in mouse airways (*i.e.* ~50% of epithelial cells in the trachea and up to ~80% in the small airways) and also express ENaC and CFTR endogenously [84, 85]. Because ENaC is composed of three subunits (α, β and γ), and heterologous expression studies indicated that co-expression of all three subunits is required for maximal Na⁺ channel activity [43], transgenic mouse lines were generated for all three ENaC subunits. Surprisingly, bioelectric studies in freshly excised tracheal tissues showed that overexpression of βENaC, but not αENaC or γENaC alone, was sufficient to produce increased amiloride-sensitive Na⁺ transport. Furthermore, transcript analyses demonstrated that endogenous βENaC is expressed at relatively low levels compared with the αENaC and γENaC subunits suggesting that βENaC is rate limiting for airway Na⁺ absorption in mouse airways [29, 30]. A series of studies in βENaC-overexpression (βENaC-Tg) mice validated the concept that a hyperabsorptive ion transport phenotype causes hyperconcentrated (*i.e.* dehydrated) mucus, reduced periciliary layer height, impaired mucus clearance, and CF-like lung disease *in vivo* (fig. 1a and b). Furthermore, these studies provided several important insights into the natural history of dehydration-induced mucus plugging and its relationship to chronic airway inflammation and infection [29–31, 86–89].

First, longitudinal studies in βENaC-Tg mice from neonatal to adult ages demonstrated that the lungs appear structurally normal at birth and identified mucus plugging in the first days of life as the earliest consequence of airway surface dehydration [29, 86]. Measurements of the percentage of mucus solids, as determined from wet-to-dry weights of mucus plugs extracted from neonatal βENaC-Tg mice, showed that the mucus was substantially dehydrated, with a solids content of ~20% compared to ~6% solids in wild-type littermates [29]. Of note, early mucus plugging occurred in the absence of goblet cell metaplasia, and the mRNA levels of important airway mucins such as MUC5ac, MUC5b and MUC4 were not different in neonatal βENaC-Tg *versus* wild-type mice [86, 90]. In addition, it was shown that genetic deletion of *CFTR*, *i.e.* removing the small amount of CFTR Cl⁻ secretion in mouse airways, exacerbated mucus plugging and associated mortality in βENaC-Tg mice [91, 92]. Importantly, early onset airway mucus plugging is also a consistent feature of *CFTR* knockout pigs and ferrets [32, 93]. While studies on mucus concentration/osmotic pressure and mucus clearance rates in these large animal models of CF lung disease are still pending, it was shown that fluid secretion from submucosal glands is deficient in *CFTR* knockout pigs [94]. Taken together, these studies indicate that an imbalance between CFTR-mediated anion secretion and ENaC-mediated Na$^+$ absorption, by the superficial airway epithelium and submucosal glands with subsequent airway surface dehydration, is sufficient to impede clearance of constitutively secreted mucus and produce mucus plugging in the absence of detectable mucin hypersecretion.

Secondly, studies in βENaC-Tg mice demonstrated that mucus plugging triggers chronic airway inflammation and constitutes a risk factor for bacterial infection *in vivo*. To determine if bacterial infection was a prerequisite for CF-like airway inflammation, βENaC-Tg mice were raised in an entirely germ-free environment [31]. Interestingly, even in the absence of bacteria in the vivarium, βENaC-Tg mice developed chronic airway inflammation characterised by airway neutrophilia and increased levels of macrophage inflammatory protein (MIP)-2 and keratinocyte chemoattractant (KC) (*i.e.* the IL-8 homologues in mice), which was already detectable in the neonatal period soon after the onset of airway mucus plugging [31]. Notably, CFTR is expressed normally and its function remains normal in βENaC-Tg mice [29, 91]. These results argue against intrinsic inflammation due to CFTR dysfunction and suggest that mucociliary dysfunction *per se*, probably due to entrapment and accumulation of inhaled particles and irritants triggering the release of proinflammatory chemokines such as IL-8/KC from inflammatory and epithelial cells, can cause airway inflammation in the absence of bacterial infection (fig. 1c) [29, 31].

Thirdly, studies in βENaC-Tg mice maintained in the presence of commensal and environmental bacteria demonstrated that neonatal βENaC-Tg mice developed spontaneous airway infection with microaerophilic Gram-positive, as well as Gram-negative, bacteria aspirated from the oropharynx [31]. Probably due to the development of innate and/or adaptive immune responses that enabled mice to eradicate bacteria even in mucostatic airways, this spontaneous infection is only intermittently observed in adult βENaC-Tg mice [29, 31]. The hypothesis that early spontaneous infection is efficiently eradicated by maturing innate immunity is supported by findings in βENaC-Tg mice deficient of the Toll-like receptor (TLR) adaptor protein myeloid differentiation factor 88 (MyD88), a key molecule involved in signalling of bacterial patterns that are recognised by TLRs at the epithelial surface [95]. In these studies, genetic deletion of MyD88 had no effect on airway mucus obstruction, but limited neutrophilic airway inflammation and caused chronic bacterial infection in βENaC-Tg mice [31].

Finally, recent studies in βENaC-Tg mice demonstrated that early improvement of airway surface hydration with different rehydration strategies is an effective approach to prevent CF-like mucus plugging. Specifically, preventive intrapulmonary treatment starting immediately after birth either with the osmolyte hypertonic saline (7%) or the classical ENaC blocker amiloride reduced intraluminal mucus to near-normal levels and led to a significant improvement of survival in this model of CF lung disease [89, 96, 97]. Furthermore, consistent with improved clearance of inhaled irritants that otherwise accumulate and trigger chronic airway inflammation in mucostatic airways, preventive amiloride treatment showed potent anti-inflammatory effects including a reduction of inflammatory cell counts and proinflammatory cytokines in BAL from βENaC-Tg mice [97].

When viewed in combination with early histopathology studies that found bland mucus plugs to be an early and invariant abnormality in the airways of CF infants who died of meconium ileus [3], and more recent data showing early airflow obstruction associated with neutrophilic inflammation in the absence or presence of bacteria in CF infants who were diagnosed by newborn screening [5–7, 98], these studies in βENaC-Tg mice support the concept that dehydration-induced mucus plugging is an early and disease promoting abnormality that causes airflow limitation, triggers airway inflammation and constitutes an important risk factor for bacterial infection in CF lung disease. Furthermore, these studies support the notion that rehydration therapies, especially when started early before the onset of irreversible structural lung damage, provide a rational and effective approach to prevent or at least delay mucus plugging and airway inflammation in CF.

Impaired bicarbonate secretion contributes to mucus hyperviscosity

In addition to its function as a cAMP-mediated Cl^- channel, CFTR also mediates epithelial HCO_3^- secretion and pH regulation of mucosal surfaces by conducting HCO_3^- itself and by providing the luminal Cl^- ions required for electroneutral HCO_3^- secretion effected by apical Cl^-/HCO_3^- exchangers [35]. Studies of the role of CFTR in HCO_3^- transport and pH regulation initially focused on the exocrine pancreas, where alkalinisation of the pancreatic fluid by CFTR-dependent HCO_3^- secretion in the pancreatic duct is essential for neutralising acidic gastric secretions and for proper activity of digestive enzymes after their secretion into the duodenum [99]. However, more recent studies demonstrated that CFTR dysfunction also causes impaired HCO_3^- secretion in the airways resulting in a reduced pH of the ASL in CF [100]. Interestingly, recent studies in the CF mouse intestine demonstrated that the presence of HCO_3^- on the luminal surface is important for normal unpacking, hydration and expansion of condensed mucin macromolecules when they are secreted from intracellular granules onto the intestinal surface [101, 102]. These results led to the hypothesis that defective HCO_3^- secretion, in addition to impaired Cl^--dependent fluid secretion, may also play a critical role in the formation of dehydrated and highly viscous mucus in the airways, and that this defect may contribute to mucociliary dysfunction and mucus plugging in CF [103].

Reduced airway surface pH impairs bacterial killing in CF airways

In addition, recent studies in *CFTR* knockout pigs demonstrated that reduced ASL pH due to deficient CFTR-mediated HCO_3^- secretion impairs bacterial killing on airway surfaces (fig. 1d). In addition to the development of CF-like mucus plugging, neutrophilic airway inflammation and bronchiectasis, neonatal CF pigs fail to eradicate commensal and environmental bacteria from their airways after birth and show delayed bacterial clearance when challenged with characteristic CF pathogens such as *S. aureus* [32]. Using a grid assay that enabled submerged linked bacteria into the ASL on airway surfaces *in vivo* and subsequently studied bacterial viability using a fluorescent live/dead strain, it was shown that normal ASL killed bacteria almost as effectively as ethanol, whereas bacterial killing was substantially reduced in ASL from CF pigs [22]. Reduced bacterial killing was associated with reduced pH in CF ASL, whereas the ionic strength (*i.e.* concentrations of Na^+, K^+ and Cl^-) and concentration of antimicrobial peptides including lysozyme and lactoferrin were not different in ASL from CF compared with wild-type pigs. However, it was found that reduced ASL pH in CF pigs rendered these anti-microbial peptides less effective and that bacterial killing can be improved by alkalinisation of CF airway surfaces by adding HCO_3^- as an aerosol [22]. Taken together, these studies in CF pigs indicate that reduced antimicrobial activity in more acidic ASL pH may contribute to reduced bacterial elimination of CF airways. The studies further suggest that re-alkalinisation of airway surfaces, *e.g.* by aerosolised HCO_3^- or rescue of mutant CFTR function, may restore anti-bacterial host defence and prevent chronic airway infection in CF lungs.

Conclusions

Data from basic and translational studies in primary human CF airway epithelial cultures, and in more recently developed small and large animal models of CF lung disease, have identified important mechanistic links between CF ion transport defects and the *in vivo* pathogenesis of CF lung disease. These studies demonstrated that airway surface dehydration, due to an imbalance between CFTR-dependent Cl^- secretion and ENaC-mediated Na^+ absorption, and reduced ASL pH, due to impaired HCO_3^- secretion caused by CFTR dysfunction, are key pathogenetic mechanisms that trigger mucus plugging, chronic inflammation and impaired anti-bacterial host defence in CF airways. These results provide a sound foundation for further elucidation of the steps involved in the progression of potentially reversible abnormalities to irreversible lung damage, and for further development of effective disease-modifying therapies that target these basic CF defects in all patients with CF irrespective of their *CFTR* genotypes and/or stage of lung disease.

References

1. Gibson RL, Burns JL, Ramsey BW. Pathophysiology and management of pulmonary infections in cystic fibrosis. *Am J Respir Crit Care Med* 2003; 168: 918–951.
2. Tunney MM, Field TR, Moriarty TF, *et al.* Detection of anaerobic bacteria in high numbers in sputum from patients with cystic fibrosis. *Am J Respir Crit Care Med* 2008; 177: 995–1001.
3. Zuelzer WW, Newton WA. The pathogenesis of fibrocystic disease of the pancreas: a study of 36 cases with special reference to the pulmonary lesions. *Pediatrics* 1949; 4: 53–69.
4. Andersen DH. Cystic fibrosis of the pancreas and its relation to celiac disease. *Am J Dis Child* 1938; 56: 344–399.
5. Belessis Y, Dixon B, Hawkins G, *et al.* Early cystic fibrosis lung disease detected by bronchoalveolar lavage and lung clearance index. *Am J Respir Crit Care Med* 2012; 185: 862–873.
6. Hoo AF, Thia LP, Nguyen TT, *et al.* Lung function is abnormal in 3-month-old infants with cystic fibrosis diagnosed by newborn screening. *Thorax* 2012; 67: 874–881.
7. Sly PD, Brennan S, Gangell C, *et al.* Lung disease at diagnosis in infants with cystic fibrosis detected by newborn screening. *Am J Respir Crit Care Med* 2009; 180: 146–152.
8. Sly PD, Gangell CL, Chen L, *et al.* Risk factors for bronchiectasis in children with cystic fibrosis. *N Engl J Med* 2013; 368: 1963–1970.
9. Stahl M, Joachim C, Blessing K, *et al.* Multiple breath washout is feasible in the clinical setting and detects abnormal lung function in infants and young children with cystic fibrosis. *Respiration* 2014 [In press DOI: 10.1159/000357075].

10. Wielputz MO, Puderbach M, Kopp-Schneider A, *et al.* Magnetic resonance imaging detects changes in structure and perfusion, and response to therapy in early cystic fibrosis lung disease. *Am J Respir Crit Care Med* 2014 [In press DOI: 10.1164/rccm.201309-1659OC].

11. Matthews LM, Spector S, Lemm J, *et al.* Studies on pulmonary secretions. *Am Rev Respir Dis* 1963; 88: 199–204.

12. Regnis JA, Robinson M, Bailey DL, *et al.* Mucociliary clearance in patients with cystic fibrosis and in normal subjects. *Am J Respir Crit Care Med* 1994; 150: 66–71.

13. de Jong PA, Nakano Y, Hop WC, *et al.* Changes in airway dimensions on computed tomography scans of children with cystic fibrosis. *Am J Respir Crit Care Med* 2005; 172: 218–224.

14. Esterly JR, Oppenheimer EH. Cystic fibrosis of the pancreas: structural changes in peripheral airways. *Thorax* 1968; 23: 670–675.

15. Wielputz MO, Weinheimer O, Eichinger M, *et al.* Pulmonary emphysema in cystic fibrosis detected by densitometry on chest multidetector computed tomography. *PLoS One* 2013; 8: e73142.

16. Rommens JM, Iannuzzi B-SK, Drumm ML, *et al.* Identification of the cystic fibrosis gene: chromosome walking and jumping. *Science* 1989; 245: 1059–1065.

17. Riordan JR, Rommens JM, Kerem B-S, *et al.* Identification of the cystic fibrosis gene: cloning and characterization of complementary DNA. *Science* 1989; 245: 1066–1072.

18. Kerem B, Rommens JM, Buchanan JA, *et al.* Identification of the cystic fibrosis gene: genetic analysis. *Science* 1989; 245: 1073–1080.

19. Smith JJ, Travis SM, Greenberg EP, *et al.* Cystic fibrosis airway epithelia fail to kill bacteria because of abnormal airway surface fluid. *Cell* 1996; 85: 229–236.

20. Matsui H, Grubb BR, Tarran R, *et al.* Evidence for periciliary liquid layer depletion, not abnormal ion composition, in the pathogenesis of cystic fibrosis airways disease. *Cell* 1998; 95: 1005–1015.

21. Verkman AS, Song Y, Thiagarajah JR. Role of airway surface liquid and submucosal glands in cystic fibrosis lung disease. *Am J Physiol Cell Physiol* 2003; 284: C2–C15.

22. Pezzulo AA, Tang XX, Hoegger MJ, *et al.* Reduced airway surface pH impairs bacterial killing in the porcine cystic fibrosis lung. *Nature* 2012; 487: 109–113.

23. Pier GB, Grout M, Zaidi TS. Cystic fibrosis transmembrane conductance regulator is an epithelial cell receptor for clearance of *Pseudomonas aeruginosa* from the lung. *Proc Natl Acad Sci USA* 1997; 94: 12088–12093.

24. Di A, Brown ME, Deriy LV, *et al.* CFTR regulates phagosome acidification in macrophages and alters bactericidal activity. *Nat Cell Biol* 2006; 8: 933–944.

25. Painter RG, Valentine VG, Lanson NA Jr, *et al.* CFTR Expression in human neutrophils and the phagolysosomal chlorination defect in cystic fibrosis. *Biochemistry* 2006; 45: 10260–10269.

26. Teichgraber V, Ulrich M, Endlich N, *et al.* Ceramide accumulation mediates inflammation, cell death and infection susceptibility in cystic fibrosis. *Nat Med* 2008; 14: 382–391.

27. Heeckeren A, Walenga R, Konstan MW, *et al.* Excessive inflammatory response of cystic fibrosis mice to bronchopulmonary infection with *Pseudomonas aeruginosa*. *J Clin Invest* 1997; 100: 2810–2815.

28. Grubb BR, Boucher RC. Pathophysiology of gene-targeted mouse models for cystic fibrosis. *Physiol Rev* 1999; 79: Suppl. 1, S193–S214.

29. Mall M, Grubb BR, Harkema JR, *et al.* Increased airway epithelial Na^+ absorption produces cystic fibrosis-like lung disease in mice. *Nat Med* 2004; 10: 487–493.

30. Zhou Z, Duerr J, Johannesson B, *et al.* The βENaC-overexpressing mouse as a model of cystic fibrosis lung disease. *J Cyst Fibros* 2011; 10: Suppl. 2, S172–S182.

31. Livraghi-Butrico A, Kelly EJ, Klem ER, *et al.* Mucus clearance, MyD88-dependent and MyD88-independent immunity modulate lung susceptibility to spontaneous bacterial infection and inflammation. *Mucosal Immunol* 2012; 5: 397–408.

32. Stoltz DA, Meyerholz DK, Pezzulo AA, *et al.* Cystic fibrosis pigs develop lung disease and exhibit defective bacterial eradication at birth. *Sci Transl Med* 2010; 2: 29–31.

33. Riordan JR. CFTR function and prospects for therapy. *Annu Rev Biochem* 2008; 77: 701–726.

34. Anderson MP, Gregory RJ, Thompson S, *et al.* Demonstration that CFTR is a chloride channel by alteration of its anion selectivity. *Science* 1991; 253: 202–205.

35. Smith JJ, Welsh MJ. cAMP stimulates bicarbonate secretion across normal, but not cystic fibrosis airway epithelia. *J Clin Invest* 1992; 89: 1148–1153.

36. Kreda SM, Mall M, Mengos A, *et al.* Characterization of wild-type and ΔF508 cystic fibrosis transmembrane regulator in human respiratory epithelia. *Mol Biol Cell* 2005; 16: 2154–2167.

37. Mall M, Kreda SM, Mengos A, *et al.* The ΔF508 mutation results in loss of CFTR function and mature protein in native human colon. *Gastroenterology* 2004; 126: 32–41.

38. Knowles MR, Gatzy JT, Boucher RC. Increased biolelectric potential difference across respiratory epithelia in cystic fibrosis. *N Engl J Med* 1981; 305: 1489–1495.

39. Boucher RC, Stutts MJ, Knowles MR, *et al.* Na^+ transport in cystic fibrosis respiratory epithelia. Abnormal basal rate and response to adenylate cyclase activation. *J Clin Invest* 1986; 78: 1245–1252.

40. Mall M, Bleich M, Greger R, *et al.* The amiloride inhibitable Na⁺ conductance is reduced by CFTR in normal but not in cystic fibrosis airways. *J Clin Invest* 1998; 102: 15–21.

41. Mall MA. Role of the amiloride-sensitive epithelial Na⁺ channel in the pathogenesis and as a therapeutic target for cystic fibrosis lung disease. *Exp Physiol* 2009; 94: 171–174.

42. Anantharam A, Palmer LG. Determination of epithelial Na⁺ channel subunit stoichiometry from single-channel conductances. *J Gen Physiol* 2007; 130: 55–70.

43. Canessa CM, Schild L, Buell G, *et al.* Amiloride-sensitive epithelial Na⁺ channel is made of three homologous subunits. *Nature* 1994; 367: 463–467.

44. Stutts MJ, Canessa CM, Olsen JC, *et al.* CFTR as a cAMP-dependent regulator of sodium channels. *Science* 1995; 269: 847–850.

45. Mall M, Hipper A, Greger R, *et al.* Wild type but not ΔF508 CFTR inhibits Na⁺ conductance when coexpressed in *Xenopus* oocytes. *FEBS Lett* 1996; 381: 47–52.

46. Hopf A, Schreiber R, Mall M, *et al.* Cystic fibrosis transmembrane conductance regulator inhibits epithelial Na⁺ channels carrying Liddle's syndrome mutations. *J Biol Chem* 1999; 274: 13894–13899.

47. Kunzelmann K, Mall M. Pharmacotherapy of the ion transport defect in cystic fibrosis. *Clin Exp Pharmacol Physiol* 2001; 28: 857–867.

48. Welsh MJ, Smith AE. Molecular mechanisms of CFTR chloride channel dysfunction in cystic fibrosis. *Cell* 1993; 73: 1251–1254.

49. Sosnay PR, Siklosi KR, Van Goor F, *et al.* Defining the disease liability of variants in the cystic fibrosis transmembrane conductance regulator gene. *Nat Genet* 2013; 45: 1160–1167.

50. Anderson MP, Welsh MJ. Calcium and cAMP activate different chloride channels in the apical membrane of normal and cystic fibrosis epithelia. *Proc Natl Acad Sci* 1991; 88: 6003–6007.

51. Knowles MR, Clarke LL, Boucher RC. Activation by extracellular nucleotides of chloride secretion in the airway epithelia of patients with cystic fibrosis. *N Engl J Med* 1991; 325: 533–538.

52. Clarke LL, Grubb BR, Yankaskas JR, *et al.* Relationship of a non-cystic fibrosis transmembrane conductance regulator-mediated chloride conductance to organ-level disease in *Cftr⁻/⁻* mice. *Proc Natl Acad Sci USA* 1994; 91: 479–483.

53. Mundhenk L, Johannesson B, Anagnostopoulou P, *et al.* mCLCA3 does not contribute to calcium-activated chloride conductance in murine airways. *Am J Respir Cell Mol Biol* 2012; 47: 87–93.

54. Caputo A, Caci E, Ferrera L, *et al.* TMEM16A, a membrane protein associated with calcium-dependent chloride channel activity. *Science* 2008; 322: 590–594.

55. Rock JR, O'Neal WK, Gabriel SE, *et al.* Transmembrane protein 16A (TMEM16A) is a Ca²⁺-regulated Cl⁻ secretory channel in mouse airways. *J Biol Chem* 2009; 284: 14875–14880.

56. Lohi H, Kujala M, Makela S, *et al.* Functional characterization of three novel tissue-specific anion exchangers SLC26A7, -A8, and -A9. *J Biol Chem* 2002; 277: 14246–14254.

57. Bertrand CA, Zhang R, Pilewski JM, *et al.* SLC26A9 is a constitutively active, CFTR-regulated anion conductance in human bronchial epithelia. *J Gen Physiol* 2009; 133: 421–438.

58. Loriol C, Dulong S, Avella M, *et al.* Characterization of SLC26A9, facilitation of Cl⁻ transport by bicarbonate. *Cell Physiol Biochem* 2008; 22: 15–30.

59. Anagnostopoulou P, Dai L, Schatterny J, *et al.* Allergic airway inflammation induces a pro-secretory epithelial ion transport phenotype in mice. *Eur Respir J* 2010; 36: 1436–1447.

60. Anagnostopoulou P, Riederer B, Duerr J, *et al.* SLC26A9-mediated chloride secretion prevents mucus obstruction in airway inflammation. *J Clin Invest* 2012; 122: 3629–3634.

61. Sun L, Rommens JM, Corvol H, *et al.* Multiple apical plasma membrane constituents are associated with susceptibility to meconium ileus in individuals with cystic fibrosis. *Nat Genet* 2012; 44: 562–569.

62. Bakouh N, Bienvenu T, Thomas A, *et al.* Characterization of SLC26A9 in patients with CF-like lung disease. *Hum Mutat* 2013; 34: 1404–1414.

63. Galietta LV, Jayaraman S, Verkman AS. Cell-based assay for high-throughput quantitative screening of CFTR chloride transport agonists. *Am J Physiol Cell Physiol* 2001; 281: C1734–C1742.

64. Van Goor F, Hadida S, Grootenhuis PD, *et al.* Rescue of CF airway epithelial cell function *in vitro* by a CFTR potentiator, VX-770. *Proc Natl Acad Sci USA* 2009; 106: 18825–18830.

65. Voynow JA, Fischer BM, Zheng S. Proteases and cystic fibrosis. *Int J Biochem Cell Biol* 2008; 40: 1238–1245.

66. Belaaouaj A, McCarthy R, Baumann M, *et al.* Mice lacking neutrophil elastase reveal impaired host defense against gram negative bacterial sepsis. *Nat Med* 1998; 4: 615–618.

67. Shapiro SD, Goldstein NM, Houghton AM, *et al.* Neutrophil elastase contributes to cigarette smoke-induced emphysema in mice. *Am J Pathol* 2003; 163: 2329–2335.

68. Hartl D, Latzin P, Hordijk P, *et al.* Cleavage of CXCR1 on neutrophils disables bacterial killing in cystic fibrosis lung disease. *Nat Med* 2007; 13: 1423–1430.

69. Caldwell RA, Boucher RC, Stutts MJ. Neutrophil elastase activates near-silent epithelial Na⁺ channels and increases airway epithelial Na⁺ transport. *Am J Physiol Lung Cell Mol Physiol* 2005; 288: L813–L819.

70. Gaillard EA, Kota P, Gentzsch M, *et al.* Regulation of the epithelial Na$^+$ channel and airway surface liquid volume by serine proteases. *Pflugers Arch* 2010; 460: 1–17.

71. Diakov A, Bera K, Mokrushina M, *et al.* Cleavage in the γ-subunit of the epithelial sodium channel (ENaC) plays an important role in the proteolytic activation of near-silent channels. *J Physiol* 2008; 586: 4587–4608.

72. Haerteis S, Krappitz M, Bertog M, *et al.* Proteolytic activation of the epithelial sodium channel (ENaC) by the cysteine protease cathepsin-S. *Pflugers Arch* 2012; 464: 353–365.

73. Gentzsch M, Dang H, Dang Y, *et al.* The cystic fibrosis transmembrane conductance regulator impedes proteolytic stimulation of the epithelial Na$_+$ channel. *J Biol Chem* 2010; 285: 32227–32232.

74. Le Gars M, Descamps D, Roussel D, *et al.* Neutrophil elastase degrades cystic fibrosis transmembrane conductance regulator *via* calpains and disables channel function *in vitro* and *in vivo*. *Am J Respir Crit Care Med* 2013; 187: 170–179.

75. Matsui H, Davis CW, Tarran R, *et al.* Osmotic water permeabilities of cultured, well-differentiated normal and cystic fibrosis airway epithelia. *J Clin Invest* 2000; 105: 1419–1427.

76. Tarran R, Boucher RC. Thin-film measurements of airway surface liquid volume/composition and mucus transport rates *in vitro*. *Methods Mol Med* 2002; 70: 479–492.

77. Wanner A, Salathe M, O'Riordan TG. Mucociliary clearance in the airways. *Am J Respir Crit Care Med* 1996; 154: 1868–1902.

78. Knowles MR, Boucher RC. Mucus clearance as a primary innate defense mechanism for mammalian airways. *J Clin Invest* 2002; 109: 571–577.

79. Mall MA. Role of cilia, mucus, and airway surface liquid in mucociliary dysfunction: lessons from mouse models. *J Aerosol Med Pulm Drug Deliv* 2008; 21: 13–24.

80. Button B, Cai LH, Ehre C, *et al.* A periciliary brush promotes the lung health by separating the mucus layer from airway epithelia. *Science* 2012; 337: 937–941.

81. Grubb BR, Paradiso AM, Boucher RC. Anomalies in ion transport in CF mouse tracheal epithelium. *Am J Physiol* 1994; 267: C293–C300.

82. Mall MA, Button B, Johannesson B, *et al.* Airway surface liquid volume regulation determines different airway phenotypes in liddle compared with βENaC-overexpressing mice. *J Biol Chem* 2010; 285: 26945–26955.

83. Hackett BP, Gitlin JD. Cell-specific expression of a Clara cell secretory protein-human growth hormone gene in the bronchiolar epithelium of transgenic mice. *Proc Natl Acad Sci USA* 1992; 89: 9079–9083.

84. Pack RJ, Al Ugaily LH, Morris G. The cells of the tracheobronchial epithelium of the mouse: a quantitative light and electron microscope study. *J Anat* 1981; 132: 71–84.

85. Van Scott MR, Hester S, Boucher RC. Ion transport by rabbit nonciliated bronchiolar epithelial cells (Clara cells) in culture. *Proc Natl Acad Sci USA* 1987; 84: 5496–5500.

86. Mall MA, Harkema JR, Trojanek JB, *et al.* Development of chronic bronchitis and emphysema in β-epithelial Na$^+$ channel-overexpressing mice. *Am J Respir Crit Care Med* 2008; 177: 730–742.

87. Livraghi A, Grubb BR, Hudson EJ, *et al.* Airway and lung pathology due to mucosal surface dehydration in β-epithelial Na$^+$ channel-overexpressing mice: role of TNF-α and IL-4Rα signaling, influence of neonatal development, and limited efficacy of glucocorticoid treatment. *J Immunol* 2009; 182: 4357–4367.

88. Wielpütz MO, Eichinger M, Zhou Z, *et al. In vivo* monitoring of cystic fibrosis-like lung disease in mice by volumetric computed tomography. *Eur Respir J* 2011; 38: 1060–1070.

89. Mall MA, Graeber SY, Stahl M, *et al.* Early cystic fibrosis lung disease: role of airway surface dehydration and lessons from preventive rehydration therapies in mice. *Int J Biochem Cell Biol* 2014 [In press DOI: 10.1016/j.biocel.2014.02.006].

90. Voynow JA, Gendler SJ, Rose MC. Regulation of mucin genes in chronic inflammatory airway diseases. *Am J Respir Cell Mol Biol* 2006; 34: 661–665.

91. Johannesson B, Hirtz S, Schatterny J, *et al.* CFTR regulates early pathogenesis of chronic obstructive lung disease in βENaC-overexpressing mice. *PLoS One* 2012; 7: e44059.

92. Livraghi-Butrico A, Kelly EJ, Wilkinson KJ, *et al.* Loss of CFTR function exacerbates the phenotype of Na$^+$ hyperabsorption in murine airways. *Am J Physiol Lung Cell Mol Physiol* 2013; 304: L469–L480.

93. Sun X, Olivier AK, Liang B, *et al.* Lung phenotype of juvenile and adult CFTR-knockout ferrets. *Am J Respir Cell Mol Biol* 2014; 50: 502–512.

94. Joo NS, Cho HJ, Khansaheb M, *et al.* Hyposecretion of fluid from tracheal submucosal glands of CFTR-deficient pigs. *J Clin Invest* 2010; 120: 3161–3166.

95. Hartl D, Gaggar A, Bruscia E, *et al.* Innate immunity in cystic fibrosis lung disease. *J Cyst Fibros* 2012; 11: 363–382.

96. Graeber SY, Zhou-Suckow Z, Schatterny J, *et al.* Hypertonic saline is effective in the prevention and treatment of mucus obstruction, but not airway inflammation, in mice with chronic obstructive lung disease. *Am J Respir Cell Mol Biol* 2013; 49: 410–417.

97. Zhou Z, Treis D, Schubert SC, *et al.* Preventive but not late amiloride therapy reduces morbidity and mortality of lung disease in βENaC-overexpressing mice. *Am J Respir Crit Care Med* 2008; 178: 1245–1256.

98. Grasemann H, Ratjen F. Early lung disease in cystic fibrosis. *Lancet Respir Med* 2013; 1: 148–157.

99. Hug MJ, Clarke LL, Gray MA. How to measure CFTR-dependent bicarbonate transport: from single channels to the intact epithelium. *Methods Mol Biol* 2011; 741: 489–509.

100. Coakley RD, Grubb BR, Paradiso AM, *et al.* Abnormal surface liquid pH regulation by cultured cystic fibrosis bronchial epithelium. *Proc Natl Acad Sci USA* 2003; 100: 16083–16088.

101. Garcia MA, Yang N, Quinton PM. Normal mouse intestinal mucus release requires cystic fibrosis transmembrane regulator-dependent bicarbonate secretion. *J Clin Invest* 2009; 119: 2613–2622.

102. Gustafsson JK, Ermund A, Ambort D, *et al.* Bicarbonate and functional CFTR channel are required for proper mucin secretion and link cystic fibrosis with its mucus phenotype. *J Exp Med* 2012; 209: 1263–1272.

103. Quinton PM. Cystic fibrosis: impaired bicarbonate secretion and mucoviscidosis. *Lancet* 2008; 372: 415–417.

Acknowledgements: We would like to thank S.Y. Graeber (Dept of Translational Pulmonology, Translational Lung Research Center (TLRC), Heidelberg, Germany) for excellent image design.

Disclosures: M.A. Mall has received grants from the German Research Foundation (DFG), the European Commission, Mukoviszidose e.V. and the German Ministry for Education and Research (BMBF). In addition, he has an issued patent filed by the University of North Carolina at Chapel Hill, Chapel Hill, NC, USA (United States Patent No. 7514593), and an issued patent filed by the University of Heidelberg, Heidelberg, Germany (European Patent No. 2114407 B1). R.C. Boucher has received funding from Parion Sciences and has a patent licensed to Parion Sciences.

Chapter 2

Airway inflammation in cystic fibrosis

Cormac McCarthy, M. Emmet O'Brien, Kerstin Pohl, Emer P. Reeves and Noel Gerard McElvaney

Cystic fibrosis (CF) is a multisystem disorder with significantly shortened life expectancy. The major cause of mortality and morbidity is lung disease. Inflammation is seen in the CF airways from a very early age and contributes significantly to symptoms and disease progression. It is unknown whether this inflammation is intrinsically driven by defective immune regulation or is a result of bacterial infection, but it is probably a combination of both. Abnormal cystic fibrosis transmembrane conductance regulator (CFTR) function affects elements of the innate immune system including neutrophils, monocytes/macrophages, lymphocytes and epithelial cells, and the interaction of these cells with bacteria, viruses and fungi, all of which contribute to the eventual parenchymal destruction that is the hallmark of this condition. There are numerous methods to measure the degree of airway inflammation; however, many are limited by either reliability or ease of use. Therapeutic interventions for CF have improved significantly in the last 20 years and now there are therapies targeted towards specific elements of inflammation, which may impact upon exacerbation frequency, symptoms and eventually mortality due to lung disease.

Cystic fibrosis (CF) is a multisystem inflammatory disorder in which the primary cause of morbidity and mortality is pulmonary destruction, characterised by chronic inflammation, bacterial colonisation and frequent exacerbations [1]. The aim of this chapter is to outline the mechanisms underlying the inflammation seen in the CF airways, discuss ways of measuring inflammation clinically, and to outline the therapeutics that target inflammation in CF.

Mechanisms: initial insult

It has long been established that the airway disease in CF is a complex inflammatory disorder. The initial process underlying the development of inflammation in the airways is still debated, namely whether abnormal cystic fibrosis transmembrane conductance regulator (CFTR) function itself leads to this inflammatory milieu or whether it is as a result of infection.

Respiratory Research Division, Royal College of Surgeons in Ireland, Beaumont Hospital, Dublin, Ireland.

Correspondence: Noel Gerard McElvaney, Education and Research Centre, Royal College of Surgeons in Ireland, Beaumont Hospital, Dublin 9, Ireland. E-mail: gmcelvaney@rcsi.ie

Copyright ERS 2014. Print ISBN: 978-1-84984-050-7. Online ISBN: 978-1-84984-051-4. Print ISSN: 2312-508X. Online ISSN: 2312-5098.

Children and infants with CF have high levels of neutrophils and pro-inflammatory cytokines in bronchoalveolar lavage (BAL), and this can occur in the absence of detectable infection [2]. Both increased levels of interleukin (IL)-8 and an excessive neutrophil burden can be seen in the CF airways, as early as 4 weeks after birth [3–5]. There is evidence of structural lung disease present in children with CF as young as 10 weeks old, with 50–70% of CF children having bronchiectasis identifiable on high-resolution computed tomography (HRCT) by 3–5 years, which is progressive in 75% of cases [6–10]. A recent study has shown that free neutrophil elastase (NE) activity is a good predictor of bronchiectasis development and ~25% of CF children are positive for free NE activity in BAL at 3 months of age [5]. In these studies, free NE activity was assessed in BAL samples and is a measure of the NE that is not bound to cell surfaces; thus, although it may be a good predictor of CF lung disease and its prognosis, it may, however, underestimate the true activity of NE in the lung, as NE can also be bound to cells and tissue.

Further understanding of the immune dysfunction and increased inflammatory response in CF can be inferred from animal models of CF. Many such models suggest that an intrinsic defect in immune regulation exists in CF regardless of bacterial infection. In CF mice raised in a pathogen-free environment, there are greater numbers of inflammatory cells in the airway [11], and this supports studies in human bronchial epithelial cells demonstrating increased IL-8 [12, 13] and lower levels of IL-10 in BAL [14]. Further evidence for the inflammatory predisposition of the CF airway has been shown where sterile CF airways were transplanted in severe combined immunodeficiency (SCID) mice, and higher IL-8 levels and neutrophil numbers were subsequently identified [15, 16]. Additionally, a mouse model overexpressing the epithelial sodium channel (ENaC) in the airways displays severe spontaneous lung disease similar to CF, caused by defective mucus transport, mucus obstruction and decreased clearance of bacteria [17]. In addition, the ENaC mouse demonstrates increased neutrophilic inflammation under sterile conditions, thus supporting the hypothesis that inflammation impairs the immune response in CF.

To further investigate the underlying mechanism of CF airway disease, the CF pig model has been developed as it may mirror the human disease more closely than mouse models. It has been shown that within months of birth, these pigs spontaneously develop lung disease with the classical CF features of inflammation, infection and mucus accumulation [18]. Similar to newborn infants, the newborn CF pig lacks significant airway inflammation but there is a reduced ability to eliminate bacteria; hence, this may be a catalyst for initiating the cycle of inflammation and infection in CF. A recent study in CF pigs demonstrated that prior to the onset of inflammation, infection or mucus plugging, there are structural changes including air trapping and airway obstruction [19]. Similarly, in humans, prenatal CF lungs show only slight morphological changes [20, 21], supporting the hypothesis that external stimuli can potentiate inflammation in the abnormal CF airways, which continues due to a dysregulated and dysfunctional immune system. In this regard, the cytokines IL-1 and tumour necrosis factor (TNF)-α stimulate CFTR-dependent secretion in the airways [22]; thus, if CFTR is abnormal, the response to bacterial infection may be dysregulated, leading to impaired bacterial eradication and increased inflammation. As CFTR also facilitates bicarbonate transport, its dysfunction in pigs leads to decreased airway surface liquid (ASL) pH, which affects the antimicrobial function of lactoferrin and lysozyme, thereby impairing bacterial clearance [23]. This functional defect may be corrected by elevating pH of the ASL using aerosolised sodium bicarbonate, with *Staphylococcus aureus* killing restored.

The dysfunctional immune system in the CF airway

CF bronchial epithelial cells in inflammation

The defence mechanisms afforded by airway epithelium go beyond its position as a mere physical barrier between the host and microbial pathogens. Bronchial epithelial cells play an important role in airway defence and immune regulation [24, 25] and these mechanisms may be defective in CF [26–29]. Such defects are exemplified by studies of Toll-like receptors (TLRs). Of relevance to CF, TLR5 plays a key role in primary recognition of flagellin of *Pseudomonas aeruginosa* [30] and inhibition of TLR5 signalling has a significant effect on inflammation in CF models [31]. Expression of TLR5 on neutrophils is significantly increased in CF, and enhances the phagocytic activity of neutrophils, *via* IL-8 secretion and CXCR1 signalling [32]. TLR4 is involved in initial detection of *P. aeruginosa* lipopolysaccharide (LPS). TLR4 is expressed on cell surfaces during bacterial infection; however, in the constantly challenged CF bronchial epithelium, TLR4 levels are decreased compared with healthy controls [33]. Indeed, reduced TLR4 response to *P. aeruginosa* has been proposed as a cause of chronic bacterial colonisation in the CF airways [34]. In females, during periods of high circulating oestrogen, a TLR hyporesponsive state occurs to a range of bacterial pathogens, leading to inhibition of IL-8 release. This is as a result, at least in part, of oestrogen receptor-β-mediated upregulation of secretory leukoprotease inhibitor (SLPI) [35], which in turn competitively inhibits nuclear factor (NF)-κB binding to DNA, thus inhibiting transcription of NF-κB-regulated genes such as *IL-8* [36]. As might be expected, this will vary over time and, indeed, increased activation of NF-κB has also been shown in CF epithelial cells, leading to elevated expression of cytokines such as IL-8 [37, 38] and others, including IL-6 (a promoter of inflammation), transforming growth factor-β (which contributes to airway remodelling) and granulocyte colony-stimulating factor (G-CSF) (which modulates the activation and survival of neutrophils). Moreover, CFTR-deficient airway epithelial cells demonstrate increased expression of the calcium release-activated calcium channel, ORAI1, leading to increased intracellular calcium and secretion of IL-8, an effect reversed by raising CFTR protein levels [39].

Epithelial cells also produce reactive oxygen species (ROS) including hydrogen peroxide and nitric oxide, the main sources of which are the dual oxidases DUOX1 and DUOX2 and the NADPH oxidase system. DUOX produce hydrogen peroxide that is used by lactoperoxidase to produce bactericidal hypothiocyanite anions, a reaction impaired in CF due to a lack of CFTR function [27]. Oxidants produced by neutrophils may also contribute to lung tissue damage. The normal protective agent against oxidant-modulated damage is the extracellular antioxidant glutathione, but this is significantly decreased in CF epithelial lining fluid [40–43]. Of major relevance is that CFTR has been linked to extracellular glutathione transport [44]. These findings have been borne out by paediatric studies showing extremely high levels of protein oxidation in the airways of children with CF [45].

The role of macrophages, neutrophils and lymphocytes in CF inflammation

In the CF airway, lymphocytes and eosinophils are present in very low numbers; in contrast to this, macrophages account for approximately 31% and neutrophils 61% of immune cells present in BAL fluid of adult patients with CF colonised by *P. aeruginosa* [46]. Key advances in our understanding of macrophage dysfunction in CF include identification of cell-associated CFTR. The presence of CFTR on human macrophages has been clearly demonstrated and dysfunctional CFTR leads to altered bactericidal capacity against

P. aeruginosa [47]. When comparing the killing ability of two cell types, it is imperative that the level of phagocytosis is similar. In this regard, a higher percentage of live bacteria was observed in macrophage colony-stimulating factor-differentiated macrophages from people with CF infected with *P. aeruginosa* compared with macrophages from healthy individuals, although the phagocytic activity was similar [48]. A further study has shown that CFTR function is required in monocytes for optimal CD11b expression and that the phagocytosis and intracellular killing of *P. aeruginosa* is reduced in CF monocytes [49]. Defects in lysosomal acidification as a result of lack of CFTR function has been one theory put forward for impaired macrophage-mediated bacterial killing [47], although the literature is currently contradictory [47, 48, 50–52]. Along the same lines of thought, however, it is of interest to observe that acidification of *Burkholderia cenocepacia*-containing vacuoles occurs in a lower percentage of CFTR-negative macrophages than CFTR-positive cells, supporting the theory that loss of CFTR function leads to enhanced bacterial survival [53]. Moreover, reduced levels of insulin-like growth factor 1 in CF has been linked to impaired alveolar macrophage function and decreased bacterial killing [54]. Macrophage dysregulation can impair resolution of inflammation. In this regard, analysis of BAL from CFTR$^{-/-}$ mice demonstrated significantly increased concentrations of macrophage-derived pro-inflammatory cytokines, including IL-1α, IL-6, G-CSF and keratinocyte chemoattractant (KC), compared with wild-type mice in response to LPS [55]. The TLR4 response to LPS in CF macrophages may be increased due to impaired negative regulation of TLR4 by the haem oxygenase-1/carbon monoxide pathway, thus posing a possible target for therapeutic intervention [56].

New mechanisms of neutrophil dysfunction have been described in CF, some of which are based on CFTR function [57]. Indeed, accumulating evidence supports CFTR protein expression on membranes and in secondary granules of neutrophils [58]. Of major relevance to neutrophil-mediated bacterial killing in CF, PAINTER *et al.* [58] reported defective intraphagolysosomal hypochlorous acid production directly caused by a lack of chloride influx into the phagosome due to defective CFTR. Subsequent studies illustrated recruitment of CFTR to the phagosomal membrane [59] and that impaired hypochlorous acid production affected chlorination of phagocytosed bacteria, resulting in reduced intravacuolar killing of *P. aeruginosa* [60]. Furthermore, COAKLEY *et al.* [61] reported defective regulation of cytosolic pH following phorbol 12-myristate 13-acetate stimulation, resulting in intensified acidification. This is especially interesting as an acidic pH is necessary for the release of primary granules containing NE and myeloperoxidase (MPO) [62]. Thus, impaired pH regulation may, in part, explain the reported excessive release of MPO [63] and NE [64] from primary granules in CF. NE is the most damaging serine protease released extracellularly by neutrophils and has the capacity to degrade structural proteins in the lung including elastin, collagen and fibronectin. NE has also been shown to promote IL-8 production by bronchial epithelial cells [65], to degrade antimicrobial peptides [66], to activate other proteases in the airways including matrix metalloprotease (MMP)-9, and to degrade antiproteases including α$_1$-antitrypsin (α$_1$-AT), SLPI [67] and elafin [68], leading to a protease/antiprotease imbalance [69]. In turn, MPO release from primary neutrophil granules is capable of enhancing oxidative damage to epithelial cells, due to the formation of hypochlorous acid [70, 71]. In line with this theory, a greater level of MPO-dependent activity and chloramine production by CF homozygote and asymptomatic heterozygote peripheral blood neutrophils was detected on the outside of the cell as compared with control cells, suggesting that the increased MPO activity seen in CF is constitutive, independent of infection and reflects altered pH regulation in CF neutrophils [72]. Further evidence that abnormal CFTR function contributes to impaired neutrophil killing in CF is in its role in affecting the activity of Rab27a, which regulates the release of antimicrobial proteins from secondary and tertiary granules. Rab27a is activated in a GTP-bound form and is stabilised by magnesium ions. CFTR inhibition or dysfunction reduces cytosolic magnesium levels, resulting in impaired Rab27a activity [73], ultimately reducing the CF neutrophils' ability to kill bacterial pathogens. Furthermore, prolonged neutrophil survival has been reported in people with CF independent of infection state and mutation type [74]. In support of this theory, MORICEAU and co-workers [75, 76] illustrated that neutrophils isolated from heterozygous asymptomatic parents of people with CF exhibited delayed apoptosis. Moreover, the expression of the apoptosis-inducing membrane receptor Fas and its ligand have been reported reduced on CF neutrophils [77] while, in addition, NE can degrade the phosphatidylserine receptor on macrophages, further delaying removal of apoptotic neutrophils in CF [78].

Support for the hypothesis that a genetic defect gives rise to dysregulated neutrophil responses in CF is given by a study demonstrating upregulation of genes coding for both chemokines and proteins involved in signal transduction in CF [79]. A recent study has demonstrated that CXCR1/CXCR2 haplotypes in CF modulate antibacterial neutrophil functions against *P. aeruginosa* [80]. In addition, CF circulating neutrophils display altered TLR expression when compared with blood neutrophils from healthy subjects, including reduced expression of TLR2 [81, 82]. A recently published study identified IFRD1, a transcriptional co-regulator, as a genetic modifier of CF disease severity. Neutrophils isolated from IFRD1-deficient mice exhibited impaired oxidative burst, bacterial clearance and cytokine production, leading to excessive bacterial burden and chronic infection of the lung [83]. Furthermore, levels of IFRD in bronchial epithelial cells with the Phe508del (formerly ΔF508) mutation were significantly reduced but could be rescued by treatment with glutathione, suggesting downregulation of IFRD1 expression in response to oxidative stress [84].

Despite the intrinsic nature of much of the neutrophil activity in CF, inflammation is also an important element. In contrast to normal ROS production by circulating neutrophils isolated from stable people with CF [85], CF neutrophils subjected to higher serum levels of pro-inflammatory cytokines following resolution of exacerbations spontaneously generated higher levels of ROS than healthy control cells [86]. Studies of impaired neutrophil function in the CF airway illustrate cleavage of neutrophil complement receptors and CXCR1 by proteases, thereby rendering the phagocytic properties of CF neutrophils inactive [87, 88]. Furthermore, neutrophils homing to the lung undergo critical changes as important receptors, including CD14 and CD16, both necessary for phagocytosis, are shed or cleaved, resulting in cellular inactivation [89]. In people with CF colonised with *P. aeruginosa*, there are increased numbers of neutrophils and higher levels of NE [67]. Bacterial biofilm formation can also impair neutrophil killing ability in the CF airways as the processes of degranulation and oxidative burst are diminished [90]. In addition, there is evidence regarding the role of Th17 lymphocyte signalling on neutrophil recruitment to the CF airway and the impact of IL-17 on airway epithelial cells resulting in IL-8 release [91, 92]. Elevated sputum levels of IL-17A, IL-17F and their upstream regulator IL-23 have been demonstrated in the sputum of people with CF during acute exacerbations [93], and IL-17 levels in BAL correlate with neutrophil counts in BAL [94]. IL-17 may also increase mucin gene expression through an IL-6 paracrine/autocrine loop and the ERK signalling pathway [95]. Whether or not IL-17 truly plays a major role in immune regulation in response to infection, its involvement in inflammation is unclear and is probably less important than innate cell immunity and requires further study.

What is evident in CF is that there is dysregulation of the immune system, not immunodeficiency; however, the primary sites of inflammation in CF remain the lung and gastrointestinal tract, providing further evidence of a role for abnormal mucus in pathogenesis. Overall, clinical and research studies have advanced our understanding of CF and altered our thinking on CF immune cells, in particular, the CF neutrophil, with impaired CFTR-related mechanisms described, thus providing the potential for therapeutic approaches in this area.

Clinical measurement of airway inflammation

Airway inflammation is present in CF and is the hallmark of CF lung disease. To measure the degree of airway inflammation is essential in both dictating treatment and predicting outcome in CF. There are many ways in which airway inflammation is measured and no single parameter is best, but a combination of several of these diagnostic tests often provides a picture of the general state of the inflammatory milieu in an individual's airway.

Chemical biomarkers: BAL, sputum and blood

Several candidate biomarkers of airway inflammation have been evaluated in CF. Direct quantification of biomarkers in BAL are valuable in research and clinical trials to demonstrate local anti-inflammatory efficacy of new treatments; however, in clinical practice, these are rarely employed due to their invasiveness [96]. BAL measurements include cell counts, cell differential counts and quantification of pro-inflammatory (IL-1β, IL-6, IL-8, IL-13, IL-17, TNF-α, leukotriene (LT)B$_4$ and C5a) and anti-inflammatory cytokines (IL-10). Cytokine gene expression and markers of neutrophil activation, including NE:α_1-AT complex and MPO, have also been evaluated in BAL [97, 98]. Some of these measurements of airway inflammation correlate with forced expiratory volume in 1 s (FEV1) and clinical disease but are difficult to obtain on an ongoing basis [96]. Noninvasive analysis of induced sputum or exhaled breath condensate can detect cytokine biomarkers as a direct measurement of airway inflammation in CF [99, 100]. Carbon monoxide, ethane and 8-isoprostane (by-products of oxidative stress and lipid peroxidation) are elevated [101] while nitric oxide levels are reduced in exhaled breath condensate [100]. Levels of MMP-9 measured in induced sputum have been shown to correlate with airway inflammation and lung function decline in children [102]. Markers of neutrophilic inflammation, IL-8 and LTB$_4$, are also increased in CF [103], and increased levels of neutrophils, NE, IL-8 [104] and IL-1β have been associated with lung function decline [105]. Furthermore, levels of desmosine in sputum, a marker of structural lung damage, correlate with inflammatory markers measured in sputum [106]. The increased production of bioactive eicosanoids through lipid peroxidation can also be detected in the urine of people with CF [107]. There are limitations to the use of these noninvasive markers of inflammation including lack of sensitivity, limited validation and significant variability between patients [108]. Additionally, the processing of sputum and subsequent laboratory analysis vary significantly between centres, with some methods actually interfering with biological measurements.

Blood biomarkers have long been employed for determining CF exacerbations, in particular white cell count and neutrophil differential count. C-reactive protein (CRP) levels may become elevated during pulmonary exacerbation, and CRP elevations can be used as a predictor of lung function decline but are nonspecific. Other blood biomarkers have been evaluated including, NE:α_1-AT complex, IL-6, MPO, lactoferrin and calprotectin [109]. The novel circulating biomarker α_1-AT:CD16B complex has been evaluated in people with CF and correlates well with inflammatory status during exacerbations [110]. The utility of these biomarkers in clinical practice is not established and no reliable biomarker has been identified to date, due to insufficient sensitivity and lack of standardisation and reproducibility [99, 100]. Longitudinal studies are needed to determine if they truly reflect CF airway inflammation [96].

Other measures of airway inflammation

The use of HRCT of the airways permits measurement of airway thickness, diameter and resultant air trapping. Changes in these parameters on HRCT correlate with spirometry and other inflammatory cytokine profiles [8, 111]. 2-fluoro-2-deoxy-D-glucose (FDG) positron emission tomography (PET) [112–114] and hyperpolarised helium-3 magnetic resonance imaging (^{3}He-MRI) have been shown to correlate with structural computed tomography (CT) abnormalities and improve following antimicrobial therapy, and ^{3}He-MRI may correlate better with spirometry than HRCT [115]. ^{3}He-MRI is in use in the evaluation of structural and functional pulmonary changes in a number of paediatric centres [116, 117], including those with normal lung function to detect early ventilatory changes [118]. However, the widespread employment of these imaging techniques is unlikely due to cost and the accessibility of all modalities. Furthermore, in the case of CT and FDG-PET, the increased cumulative exposure to ionising radiation is of concern [119].

Measurements of mucociliary clearance and sputum rheology have been used as surrogates for airway inflammation in research trials; however, *in vitro* improvements in sputum viscoelasticity do not always result in improved clinical outcomes [120]. Inert-gas washout techniques (lung clearance index (LCI)) have been evaluated as an indicator of lung function, particularly in young children and infants [121]. LCI may be a predictor of subsequent lung function abnormality in pre-school children [122] and may be a more sensitive indicator of response to intervention than FEV1 in a clinical trial setting [123]. The role of LCI is expanding and its use, in conjunction with other biomarkers, may be a useful outcome measure in early CF airway inflammation [124]. In specialised centres, accurate measurement of mucociliary clearance is possible using ventilation scans following inhalation of radiolabelled particles. This measurement technique has been used in a number of small clinical trials [125], but the lack of a standard operating procedure has prevented it from entering routine clinical practice [126].

Therapeutics for airway inflammation

CF lung disease is manifested in numerous ways and many specific therapies are available targeting different elements of the disease. Pulmonary exacerbations are common, and they predict lung function decline and mortality [127]; the use of systemic antibiotics to treat these is routine in CF, and it has been previously shown that early eradication of *P. aeruginosa* is beneficial to people with CF [128]. Numerous other treatments aimed at eradicating bacterial colonisation, improving mucus clearance, reducing exacerbation frequency and treating associated pulmonary symptoms have been developed. In this section, we will focus on the therapies available in CF that have beneficial effects on inflammation, both directly and indirectly. For a summary of the therapeutics covered in this section, see table 1.

Oral anti-inflammatory therapies

As CF is a multisystem disorder characterised by chronic inflammation, for many years, the intuitive use of traditional anti-inflammatory drugs has been employed in clinical practice. Several studies have reported the benefits of systemic corticosteroids in CF, most notably in children with mild lung disease [129]. The use of oral prednisolone at a dose of 1–2 mg·kg^{-1} on alternate days appears to slow the progression of lung disease [130], but this improvement is modest and must be weighed against the significant adverse effects of corticosteroids, such as growth retardation and impaired glucose tolerance [130]. Further evidence against the routine use of oral corticosteroids is the fact that their effect on slowing the progression of lung disease appears not to be sustained post-treatment [129].

Table 1. Summary of the therapies available to target airway inflammation in cystic fibrosis

Mechanism of action	Drug	Mechanism	Effect on inflammation	Clinical outcome
Anti-inflammatory	Corticosteroids	Inhibition of NF-κB activation	Decreased neutrophil migration [129]	Slow FEV1 decline [130]
	Ibuprofen	COX inhibition HSP70 inhibition [131]	Reduced prostaglandin synthesis	Slow FEV1 decline Improved BMI Reduced exacerbation frequency [132]
	Vitamin D	Inhibit pro-inflammatory cytokine production [133]	Reduced epithelial IL-6 and IL-8 secretion [134]	
Macrolide	Azithromycin	Attenuation of cytokine production [135]	Reduced neutrophil accumulation, adhesion, and apoptosis Reduced biofilm ormation [136]	Reduced exacerbations Improved health status Improved BMI [137]
Mucociliary clearance	Dornase alfa	Hydrolysis of sputum DNA aggregates	Improved mucociliary clearance [138]	Improved FEV1 [138] Reduced exacerbations [138]
	Hypertonic saline	Osmotic rehydration of the ASL Decrease IL-8 [139]	Improved mucociliary clearance [140] Decreased neutrophil burden [139]	Reduced exacerbations [140]
	Mannitol	Osmotic rehydration of the ASL	Improved sputum viscoelasticity [141]	Improved FEV1 and decreased pulmonary exacerbations [141]
Antioxidant	N-acetylcysteine Glutathione	Reduced cross-linking of disulfide to sulfhydryl bonds [142] Restoration of oxidative balance	Improved sputum viscoelasticity Decreased neutrophil burden [143] Decreased NE and IL-8 [143]	No significant clinical outcome improvements to date [144, 145]
Antiprotease	α$_1$-AT SLPI	Suppression of other protease activity, notably NE [146, 147]	Improved pseudomonal killing [148] Reduced neutrophil burden [149] Reduced IL-8 [149]	No significant clinical outcome improvements to date [148, 150]
	AZD9668	Inhibition of human NE [149]	Reduced urinary desmosine and sputum inflammatory biomarkers [149]	
Antipseudomonal	Tobramycin Colomycin Aztreonam Alginates$^{#}$	Antibacterial effects	Reduced Pseudomonas density [151, 152] Reduced biofilm formation [153]	Improved FEV1 [151, 152, 154] Reduced exacerbations [151, 152] Improved health status [153] Improved BMI
CFTR function	Ivacaftor Lumacaftor$^{#}$	Potentiation of CFTR opening [155] Improved trafficking of CFTR to the cell surface [155]	Reduced sweat chloride and NPD measurement [155]	Improved FEV1 [155] Improved BMI [155] Reduced exacerbations[155]
	Ataluren$^{#}$	Read through of premature stop codons [156]	Induces CFTR activity measured on nasal epithelium [156]	

CFTR: cystic fibrosis transmembrane conductance regulator; NF: nuclear factor; FEV1: forced expiratory volume in 1 s; COX: cyclo-oxygenase; HSP70: 70-kDa heat-shock protein; BMI: body mass index; IL: interleukin; ASL: airway surface liquid; NE: neutrophil elastase; α$_1$-AT: α$_1$-antitrypsin; SLPI: secretory leukoprotease inhibitor; NPD: nasal potential difference. $^{#}$: awaiting results of clinical trials.

The use of nonsteroidal anti-inflammatory drugs (NSAIDs) has also been evaluated in the treatment of CF lung disease. Ibuprofen has been shown *in vivo* to decrease neutrophil migration [157]; however, subtherapeutic levels of the drug may cause increased neutrophil migration. In animal models of CF, ibuprofen has been shown to reduce the inflammatory response to *P. aeruginosa* infection [157, 158]. In clinical trials, ibuprofen has been demonstrated to have a positive effect on pulmonary function in children, most notably in those with mild-to-moderate lung disease [132, 135]; this has also been shown in retrospective data collected from patient registries [133, 159]. In a 4-year trial, the use of ibuprofen, *versus* placebo, was shown to slow FEV1 decline, reduce frequency of exacerbations and improve weight, especially in younger people with CF with mild lung disease [132]. The safety profile of long-term ibuprofen remains an issue with the known side-effects of NSAIDs being a concern, particularly the increased incidence of gastritis, peptic ulcer disease and renal impairment. A recent Cochrane systemic review suggests that the benefit of NSAIDs may outweigh the risks; however, most of these studies were not powered to identify significant adverse events [160]. Thus, the possible beneficial use of NSAIDs must be measured against the potentially narrow therapeutic window of these medications.

Other oral anti-inflammatory medications include macrolide antibiotics, which are known to possess anti-inflammatory properties separate to their antimicrobial effect. Azithromycin is commonly used in CF lung disease and has been shown to improve lung function, increase body mass index and reduce the incidence of pulmonary exacerbations [137]. Azithromycin may also reduce biofilm formation in *P. aeruginosa* infection, hence reducing the overall inflammatory burden in the CF lung [136]. The recognised adverse effects of macrolide antibiotics, particularly development of resistance, hearing impairment and prolongation of the QT interval, have not proven problematic in CF. Vitamin D is another recognised anti-inflammatory and people with CF are often deficient in vitamin D, so dietary supplementation is often routine. Both 1,25-dihydroxycholecalciferol and other vitamin D receptor (VDR) agonists can significantly reduce the pro-inflammatory response seen in CF airway epithelial cells upon antigen presentation, leading to reduced IL-6 and IL-8 levels [134]. Vitamin D also has been shown to inhibit the production of IL-5 and IL-13 [161]. The anti-inflammatory effect of vitamin D requires active VDR to be present and, in people with CF colonised with *Aspergillus fumigatus*, there is significantly reduced VDR expression and increased levels of the fungal secondary metabolite, gliotoxin. Gliotoxin secreted by *A. fumigatus* downregulates VDR mRNA and protein expression and may thus increase IL-5 and IL-13 [162]. Treatment of *A. fumigatus* with itraconazole resulted in increased VDR expression and decreased IL-5 and IL-13 levels [162]. Significant systemic exposure to 1,25-dihydroxycholecalciferol can potentially lead to hypercalcaemia; however, newer VDR agonists have a decreased potential to do so, supporting their therapeutic potential as anti-inflammatories in CF following eradication of *A. fumigatus*. Another novel anti-inflammatory therapy is the use of CXCR2 antagonists, where a recent study demonstrated safety in 149 patients with CF and a trend for reduction in sputum inflammatory markers [163].

Nebulised antimicrobial therapies

Numerous aerosolised and inhaled anti·pseudomonal antibiotics are available or undergoing trials in CF. These include tobramycin, colomycin, aztreonam, amikacin, levofloxacin, ciprofloxacin and gentamicin [151, 152, 164–168]. They have shown significant improvements in FEV1, reductions in exacerbations [151, 168], reductions in *P. aeruginosa* density [152] and effective eradication of *P. aeruginosa* [169]. A promising nonantibiotic development is alginate lyase, which can reduce the viscoelasticity of CF sputum through the disruption of *P. aeruginosa* biofilms and promote antibiotic diffusion across the extracellular polysaccharide matrix [153]. The future use of oral alginate lyase in conjunction with antibiotic therapy may enhance the antimicrobial effect [170], and it may also be safely delivered to the lung by aerosolisation [171].

Mucociliary clearance-directed therapies

The thick viscous mucus found in the CF airway is an ideal environment for bacterial pathogens to colonise and then grow. Dehydration of the ASL may lead to infection and inflammation, and may be the initial catalyst resulting in CF airway inflammation. The use of several nebulised treatments has been shown to improve mucus clearance in CF; these include hypertonic saline (HTS) and dornase alfa (DNase).

HTS has been shown to have beneficial effects on the absolute change in lung function but not on the slope of FEV_1 change [140]. HTS has been shown to improve mucociliary clearance and reduce exacerbation frequency [140], and it may reduce the neutrophil burden in the CF airway [172]. HTS has also been shown to decrease IL-8 concentration in sputum of people with CF and does so by displacing IL-8 from negatively charged glycosaminoglycan matrices, allowing it to be degraded by proteases [139]. In addition, HTS may improve bacterial killing. LL-37, an antimicrobial peptide with activity against an array of bacteria, is also bound to glycosaminoglycans, which renders it inactive. HTS disrupts the electrostatic bonds between LL-37 and glycosaminoglycans, releasing LL-37 from its bound form; thus, HTS may directly impact upon the viability of bacteria within the CF airways [173, 174]. HTS has also been shown to increase antioxidant levels, including glutathione, in BAL [175] and to inhibit arachidonic acid- and LTB_4-induced priming of peripheral neutrophils [176]. All of these effects support the use of HTS in CF not only for improving mucociliary clearance but also for its anti-inflammatory properties. Mannitol has similar osmotic properties to HTS and may be a useful mucoactive therapy [177], and has been shown to improve FEV_1 marginally and reduce exacerbation frequency in two randomised controlled trials [141, 178]. As yet, mannitol has not been shown to have the anti-inflammatory effects of HTS.

DNA polymers contribute significantly to the dry weight and viscosity of CF mucus, and are involved in airway pathology. The use of dornase alfa, a recombinant human DNase, as an effective mucolytic significantly reduces exacerbation frequency and improves FEV_1 [138]. This is probably due to the direct effect of improving mucociliary clearance and, hence, it is an indirect modulator of airway inflammation. N-acetylcysteine (NAC) has been evaluated for its mucolytic properties in CF for many years, as it can break down mucin disulfide bonds [51] and improves sputum rheological properties. In recent years, additional beneficial effects of NAC have been explored. NAC is a prodrug of glutathione, which, as mentioned previously, is an antioxidant regulated by CFTR [44] with significantly decreased levels in CF [43]. High-dose oral NAC has been shown to decrease neutrophil burden, reduce NE activity and decrease IL-8 levels in the sputum of people with CF [143]. Despite being well tolerated, treatment with oral or inhaled NAC has not demonstrated a sustained improvement in FEV_1 or forced vital capacity (FVC) in any randomised controlled trial or meta-analysis [144]. A recent large randomised controlled trial of nebulised glutathione in CF did not show any benefits in lung function, exacerbation frequency or patient reported outcomes [145].

Nebulised antiproteases

As the inflammation in CF is primarily neutrophil driven and NE plays such a pivotal and destructive role, the use of antiproteases to counteract NE seems intuitive. The archetypal antiprotease against NE is α_1-AT, and early studies demonstrated that nebulised α_1-AT was well tolerated in CF, and could suppress NE activity and improve the neutrophilic killing of *P. aeruginosa* in the lung [146], at least in part by preventing the cleavage of neutrophil complement receptors by serine proteases, a previously reported adverse effect of NE [88]. Aerosolised α_1-AT may also prevent cleavage of CXCR1 by proteases [87], which, if it occurs unopposed, can disable effective bacterial killing in the CF lung. More recent studies have confirmed that nebulised α_1-AT may decrease NE activity and reduce *P. aeruginosa* colony counts *in vitro* [179]. Further studies in people with CF show marked decreases in NE activity, numbers of infiltrating neutrophils, pro-inflammatory cytokines and numbers of *P. aeruginosa* in sputum following treatment with α_1-AT, but no improvement in lung function was demonstrated [148].

SLPI is one of the major antiproteases in the lung [63]. The use of nebulised SLPI has been investigated in people with CF, demonstrating a reduction in active NE, reduced IL-8 levels and IL-8 gene expression, and decreased neutrophil numbers in the lung [147]. However, SLPI seems less effective than α_1-AT in its ability to inhibit NE *in vivo* in CF. Other serine protease inhibitors have also been studied with regard to their therapeutic potential in CF, including human monocyte/neutrophil elastase inhibitor (MNEI). Aerosolisation of recombinant MNEI in a rat model of chronic *P. aeruginosa* infection demonstrated enhanced bacterial killing, reduced inflammatory injury and increased clearance of *P. aeruginosa*, indicating its potential use as a nonantibiotic treatment in CF lung disease [180].

Newer synthetic compounds with anti-NE activity have been developed for both chronic obstructive pulmonary disease and CF, and have shown some promise as potential therapies. The compound AZD9668 has been shown in early trials to reduce inflammatory markers in sputum but had no effect on neutrophil burden, and further studies are needed on this and other synthetic anti-NE compounds [149]. Collectively, antiprotease therapies demonstrate anti-inflammatory properties and highlight the close relationship between neutrophil-mediated proteolysis and inflammation in CF lung disease.

Correction of CFTR function

The recent development of drugs to correct CFTR function, particularly ivacaftor, have shown significant improvements in lung function, reduction in exacerbation frequency and correction of CFTR dysfunction [155]. Recent work has shown that people with CF carrying the Gly551Asp (formerly G551D) mutation treated with ivacaftor have normalised Rab27a activity compared with untreated patients. This in turn corrects the degranulation of secondary and tertiary granules by CF neutrophils, improving bacterial killing [73]. Studies are ongoing to assess the potential of CFTR correctors and chaperone proteins to treat other mutations in people with CF [181].

Conclusion

It is evident from a very early stage in CF that there is significant inflammation in the lungs. What initiates the airway inflammation in CF is still debated, although it is probably a combination of intrinsic innate immune dysregulation and infection. With both early eradication of *P. aeruginosa* and specific inhibitors of inflammation, progressive CF lung disease may be abated. In addition, a promising development in the treatment of airway inflammation remains the correction of CFTR dysfunction. If CFTR dysfunction is corrected at a very early age, it is possible the issue of airway inflammation may be significantly curtailed in people with CF.

References

1. Ramsey BW. Management of pulmonary disease in patients with cystic fibrosis. *N Engl J Med* 1996; 335: 179–188.
2. Rosenfeld M, Gibson RL, McNamara S, *et al.* Early pulmonary infection, inflammation, and clinical outcomes in infants with cystic fibrosis. *Pediatr Pulmonol* 2001; 32: 356–366.
3. Khan TZ, Wagener JS, Bost T, *et al.* Early pulmonary inflammation in infants with cystic fibrosis. *Am J Respir Crit Care Med* 1995; 151: 1075–1082.
4. Armstrong DS, Grimwood K, Carzino R, *et al.* Lower respiratory infection and inflammation in infants with newly diagnosed cystic fibrosis. *BMJ* 1995; 310: 1571–1572.
5. Sly PD, Gangell CL, Chen L, *et al.* Risk factors for bronchiectasis in children with cystic fibrosis. *N Engl J Med* 2013; 368: 1963–1970.
6. Mott LS, Park J, Murray CP, *et al.* Progression of early structural lung disease in young children with cystic fibrosis assessed using CT. *Thorax* 2012; 67: 509–516.
7. Sly PD, Brennan S, Gangell C, *et al.* Lung disease at diagnosis in infants with cystic fibrosis detected by newborn screening. *Am J Respir Crit Care Med* 2009; 180: 146–152.
8. Davis SD, Fordham LA, Brody AS, *et al.* Computed tomography reflects lower airway inflammation and tracks changes in early cystic fibrosis. *Am J Respir Crit Care Med* 2007; 175: 943–950.
9. Wainwright CE, Vidmar S, Armstrong DS, *et al.* Effect of bronchoalveolar lavage-directed therapy on *Pseudomonas aeruginosa* infection and structural lung injury in children with cystic fibrosis: a randomized trial. *JAMA* 2011; 306: 163–171.
10. Stick SM, Brennan S, Murray C, *et al.* Bronchiectasis in infants and preschool children diagnosed with cystic fibrosis after newborn screening. *J Pediatr* 2009; 155: 623–628.
11. Zahm JM, Gaillard D, Dupuit F, *et al.* Early alterations in airway mucociliary clearance and inflammation of the lamina propria in CF mice. *Am J Physiol* 1997; 272: C853–C859.
12. Tabary O, Escotte S, Couetil JP, *et al.* High susceptibility for cystic fibrosis human airway gland cells to produce IL-8 through the IκB kinase α pathway in response to extracellular NaCl content. *J Immunol* 2000; 164: 3377–3384.
13. Tabary O, Zahm JM, Hinnrasky J, *et al.* Selective up-regulation of chemokine IL-8 expression in cystic fibrosis bronchial gland cells *in vivo* and *in vitro*. *Am J Pathol* 1998; 153: 921–930.
14. Bonfield TL, Konstan MW, Burfeind P, *et al.* Normal bronchial epithelial cells constitutively produce the anti-inflammatory cytokine interleukin-10, which is downregulated in cystic fibrosis. *Am J Respir Cell Mol Biol* 1995; 13: 257–261.
15. Tirouvanziam R, de Bentzmann S, Hubeau C, *et al.* Inflammation and infection in naive human cystic fibrosis airway grafts. *Am J Respir Cell Mol Biol* 2000; 23: 121–127.
16. Hubeau C, Lorenzato M, Couetil JP, *et al.* Quantitative analysis of inflammatory cells infiltrating the cystic fibrosis airway mucosa. *Clin Exp Immunol* 2001; 124: 69–76.
17. Mall M, Grubb BR, Harkema JR, *et al.* Increased airway epithelial Na$^+$ absorption produces cystic fibrosis-like lung disease in mice. *Nature Med* 2004; 10: 487–493.
18. Stoltz DA, Meyerholz DK, Pezzulo AA, *et al.* Cystic fibrosis pigs develop lung disease and exhibit defective bacterial eradication at birth. *Sci Transl Med* 2010; 2: 29–31.
19. Adam R, Abou-Alaiwa MH, Gross TJ, *et al.* Air trapping occurs prior to the onset of airway infection, inflammation, and mucus obstruction in CF pigs. *Pediatr Pulmonol* 2013; 48: 207–453.
20. Sturgess J, Imrie J. Quantitative evaluation of the development of tracheal submucosal glands in infants with cystic fibrosis and control infants. *Am J Pathol* 1982; 106: 303–311.
21. Chow CW, Landau LI, Taussig LM. Bronchial mucous glands in the newborn with cystic fibrosis. *Eur J Pediatr* 1982; 139: 240–243.
22. Baniak N, Luan X, Grunow A, *et al.* The cytokines interleukin-1β and tumor necrosis factor-α stimulate CFTR-mediated fluid secretion by swine airway submucosal glands. *Am J Physiol Lung Cell Mol Physiol* 2012; 303: L327–L333.
23. Pezzulo AA, Tang XX, Hoegger MJ, *et al.* Reduced airway surface pH impairs bacterial killing in the porcine cystic fibrosis lung. *Nature* 2012; 487: 109–113.
24. Greene CM, McElvaney NG. Toll-like receptor expression and function in airway epithelial cells. *Arch Immunol Ther Exp (Warsz)* 2005; 53: 418–427.

25. Ryu JH, Kim CH, Yoon JH. Innate immune responses of the airway epithelium. *Mol Cells* 2010; 30: 173–183.
26. Elizur A, Cannon CL, Ferkol TW. Airway inflammation in cystic fibrosis. *Chest* 2008; 133: 489–495.
27. Fischer H. Mechanisms and function of DUOX in epithelia of the lung. *Antioxid Redox Signal* 2009; 11: 2453–2465.
28. Jacquot J, Tabary O, Le Rouzic P, *et al.* Airway epithelial cell inflammatory signalling in cystic fibrosis. *Int J Biochem Cell Biol* 2008; 40: 1703–1715.
29. Terheggen-Lagro SW, Rijkers GT, van der Ent CK. The role of airway epithelium and blood neutrophils in the inflammatory response in cystic fibrosis. *J Cyst Fibros* 2005; 4: Suppl. 2, 15–23.
30. Morris AE, Liggitt HD, Hawn TR, *et al.* Role of Toll-like receptor 5 in the innate immune response to acute *P. aeruginosa* pneumonia. *Am J Physiol Lung Cell Mol Physiol* 2009; 297: L1112–L1119.
31. Blohmke CJ, Victor RE, Hirschfeld AF, *et al.* Innate immunity mediated by TLR5 as a novel antiinflammatory target for cystic fibrosis lung disease. *J Immunol* 2008; 180: 7764–7773.
32. Koller B, Kappler M, Latzin P, *et al.* TLR expression on neutrophils at the pulmonary site of infection: TLR1/TLR2-mediated up-regulation of TLR5 expression in cystic fibrosis lung disease. *J Immunol* 2008; 181: 2753–2763.
33. Hauber HP, Tulic MK, Tsicopoulos A, *et al.* Toll-like receptors 4 and 2 expression in the bronchial mucosa of patients with cystic fibrosis. *Can Respir J* 2005; 12: 13–18.
34. John G, Yildirim AO, Rubin BK, *et al.* TLR-4-mediated innate immunity is reduced in cystic fibrosis airway cells. *Am J Respir Cell Mol Biol* 2010; 42: 424–431.
35. Chotirmall SH, Greene CM, Oglesby IK, *et al.* 17β-estradiol inhibits IL-8 in cystic fibrosis by up-regulating secretory leucoprotease inhibitor. *Am J Respir Crit Care Med* 2010; 182: 62–72.
36. Taggart CC, Cryan SA, Weldon S, *et al.* Secretory leucoprotease inhibitor binds to NF-κB binding sites in monocytes and inhibits p65 binding. *J Exp Med* 2005; 202: 1659–1668.
37. Rottner M, Kunzelmann C, Mergey M, *et al.* Exaggerated apoptosis and NF-κB activation in pancreatic and tracheal cystic fibrosis cells. *FASEB J* 2007; 21: 2939–2948.
38. Venkatakrishnan A, Stecenko AA, King G, *et al.* Exaggerated activation of nuclear factor-κB and altered IκB-β processing in cystic fibrosis bronchial epithelial cells. *Am J Respir Cell Mol Biol* 2000; 23: 396–403.
39. Balghi H, Robert R, Rappaz B, *et al.* Enhanced Ca^{2+} entry due to ORAI1 plasma membrane insertion increases IL-8 secretion by cystic fibrosis airways. *FASEB J* 2011; 25: 4274–4791.
40. Galli F, Battistoni A, Gambari R, *et al.* Oxidative stress and antioxidant therapy in cystic fibrosis. *Biochim Biophys Acta* 2012; 1822: 690–713.
41. Griese M, Ramakers J, Krasselt A, *et al.* Improvement of alveolar glutathione and lung function but not oxidative state in cystic fibrosis. *Am J Respir Crit Care Med* 2004; 169: 822–828.
42. Roum JH, Borok Z, McElvaney NG, *et al.* Glutathione aerosol suppresses lung epithelial surface inflammatory cell-derived oxidants in cystic fibrosis. *J Appl Physiol (1985)* 1999; 87: 438–443.
43. Roum JH, Buhl R, McElvaney NG, *et al.* Systemic deficiency of glutathione in cystic fibrosis. *J Appl Physiol (1985)* 1993; 75: 2419–2424.
44. Linsdell P, Hanrahan JW. Glutathione permeability of CFTR. *Am J Physiol* 1998; 275: C323–C326.
45. Kettle AJ, Chan T, Osberg I, *et al.* Myeloperoxidase and protein oxidation in the airways of young children with cystic fibrosis. *Am J Respir Crit Care Med* 2004; 170: 1317–1323.
46. Hartl D, Griese M, Kappler M, *et al.* Pulmonary T_H2 response in *Pseudomonas aeruginosa*-infected patients with cystic fibrosis. *J Allergy Clin Immunol* 2006; 117: 204–211.
47. Di A, Brown ME, Deriy LV, *et al.* CFTR regulates phagosome acidification in macrophages and alters bactericidal activity. *Nat Cell Biol* 2006; 8: 933–944.
48. Del Porto P, Cifani N, Guarnieri S, *et al.* Dysfunctional CFTR alters the bactericidal activity of human macrophages against *Pseudomonas aeruginosa*. *PLoS One* 2011; 6: e19970.
49. Van de Weert-van Leeuwen PB, Van Meegen MA, Speirs JJ, *et al.* Optimal complement-mediated phagocytosis of *Pseudomonas aeruginosa* by monocytes is cystic fibrosis transmembrane conductance regulator-dependent. *Am J Respir Cell Mol Biol* 2013; 49: 463–470.
50. Barriere H, Bagdany M, Bossard F, *et al.* Revisiting the role of cystic fibrosis transmembrane conductance regulator and counterion permeability in the pH regulation of endocytic organelles. *Mol Biol Cell* 2009; 20: 3125–3141.
51. Haggie PM, Verkman AS. Cystic fibrosis transmembrane conductance regulator-independent phagosomal acidification in macrophages. *J Biol Chem* 2007; 282: 31422–31428.
52. Steinberg BE, Huynh KK, Brodovitch A, *et al.* A cation counterflux supports lysosomal acidification. *J Cell Biol* 2010; 189: 1171–1186.
53. Lamothe J, Valvano MA. *Burkholderia cenocepacia*-induced delay of acidification and phagolysosomal fusion in cystic fibrosis transmembrane conductance regulator (CFTR)-defective macrophages. *Microbiology* 2008; 154: 3825–3834.
54. Bessich JL, Nymon AB, Moulton LA, *et al.* Low levels of insulin-like growth factor-1 contribute to alveolar macrophage dysfunction in cystic fibrosis. *J Immunol* 2013; 191: 378–385.
55. Bruscia EM, Zhang PX, Ferreira E, *et al.* Macrophages directly contribute to the exaggerated inflammatory response in cystic fibrosis transmembrane conductance regulator$^{-/-}$ mice. *Am J Respir Cell Mol Biol* 2009; 40: 295–304.

56. Zhang PX, Murray TS, Villella VR, *et al.* Reduced caveolin-1 promotes hyperinflammation due to abnormal heme oxygenase-1 localization in lipopolysaccharide-challenged macrophages with dysfunctional cystic fibrosis transmembrane conductance regulator. *J Immunol* 2013; 190: 5196–5206.

57. Su X, Looney MR, Su HE, *et al.* Role of CFTR expressed by neutrophils in modulating acute lung inflammation and injury in mice. *Inflamm Res* 2011; 60: 619–632.

58. Painter RG, Valentine VG, Lanson NA Jr, *et al.* CFTR Expression in human neutrophils and the phagolysosomal chlorination defect in cystic fibrosis. *Biochemistry* 2006; 45: 10260–10269.

59. Zhou Y, Song K, Painter RG, *et al.* Cystic fibrosis transmembrane conductance regulator recruitment to phagosomes in neutrophils. *J Innate Immun* 2013; 5: 219–230.

60. Painter RG, Bonvillain RW, Valentine VG, *et al.* The role of chloride anion and CFTR in killing of *Pseudomonas aeruginosa* by normal and CF neutrophils. *J Leukoc Biol* 2008; 83: 1345–1353.

61. Coakley RJ, Taggart C, Canny G, *et al.* Altered intracellular pH regulation in neutrophils from patients with cystic fibrosis. *Am J Physiol Lung Cell Mol Physiol* 2000; 279: L66–L74.

62. Gewirtz AT, Seetoo KF, Simons ER. Neutrophil degranulation and phospholipase D activation are enhanced if the Na^+/H^+ antiport is blocked. *J Leukoc Biol* 1998; 64: 98–103.

63. Koller DY, Urbanek R, Gotz M. Increased degranulation of eosinophil and neutrophil granulocytes in cystic fibrosis. *Am J Respir Crit Care Med* 1995; 152: 629–633.

64. Taggart C, Coakley RJ, Greally P, *et al.* Increased elastase release by CF neutrophils is mediated by tumor necrosis factor-α and interleukin-8. *Am J Physiol Lung Cell Mol Physiol* 2000; 278: L33–L41.

65. Walsh DE, Greene CM, Carroll TP, *et al.* Interleukin-8 up-regulation by neutrophil elastase is mediated by MyD88/IRAK/TRAF-6 in human bronchial epithelium. *J Biol Chem* 2001; 276: 35494–35499.

66. Bergsson G, Reeves EP, McNally P, *et al.* LL-37 complexation with glycosaminoglycans in cystic fibrosis lungs inhibits antimicrobial activity, which can be restored by hypertonic saline. *J Immunol* 2009; 183: 543–551.

67. Weldon S, McNally P, McElvaney NG, *et al.* Decreased levels of secretory leucoprotease inhibitor in the *Pseudomonas*-infected cystic fibrosis lung are due to neutrophil elastase degradation. *J Immunol* 2009; 183: 8148–8156.

68. Guyot N, Butler MW, McNally P, *et al.* Elafin, an elastase-specific inhibitor, is cleaved by its cognate enzyme neutrophil elastase in sputum from individuals with cystic fibrosis. *J Biol Chem* 2008; 283: 32377–32385.

69. Birrer P, McElvaney NG, Rudeberg A, *et al.* Protease-antiprotease imbalance in the lungs of children with cystic fibrosis. *Am J Respir Crit Care Med* 1994; 150: 207–213.

70. Cantin A, Woods DE. Protection by antibiotics against myeloperoxidase-dependent cytotoxicity to lung epithelial cells *in vitro*. *J Clin Invest* 1993; 91: 38–45.

71. Cantin AM, North SL, Fells GA, *et al.* Oxidant-mediated epithelial cell injury in idiopathic pulmonary fibrosis. *J Clin Invest* 1987; 79: 1665–1673.

72. Witko-Sarsat V, Allen RC, Paulais M, *et al.* Disturbed myeloperoxidase-dependent activity of neutrophils in cystic fibrosis homozygotes and heterozygotes, and its correction by amiloride. *J Immunol* 1996; 157: 2728–2735.

73. Pohl K, Molloy K, Reeves EP, *et al.* Importance of CFTR function and effect of Kalydeco treatment on neutrophil activity in cystic fibrosis. *Pediatr Pulmonol* 2013; 48: 207–453.

74. McKeon DJ, Condliffe AM, Cowburn AS, *et al.* Prolonged survival of neutrophils from patients with ΔF508 CFTR mutations. *Thorax* 2008; 63: 660–661.

75. Moriceau S, Kantari C, Mocek J, *et al.* Coronin-1 is associated with neutrophil survival and is cleaved during apoptosis: potential implication in neutrophils from cystic fibrosis patients. *J Immunol* 2009; 182: 7254–7263.

76. Moriceau S, Lenoir G, Witko-Sarsat V. In cystic fibrosis homozygotes and heterozygotes, neutrophil apoptosis is delayed and modulated by diamide or roscovitine: evidence for an innate neutrophil disturbance. *J Innate Immun* 2010; 2: 260–266.

77. Downey DG, Brockbank S, Martin SL, *et al.* The effect of treatment of cystic fibrosis pulmonary exacerbations on airways and systemic inflammation. *Pediatr Pulmonol* 2007; 42: 729–735.

78. Vandivier RW, Fadok VA, Hoffmann PR, *et al.* Elastase-mediated phosphatidylserine receptor cleavage impairs apoptotic cell clearance in cystic fibrosis and bronchiectasis. *J Clin Invest* 2002; 109: 661–670.

79. Adib-Conquy M, Pedron T, Petit-Bertron AF, *et al.* Neutrophils in cystic fibrosis display a distinct gene expression pattern. *Mol Med* 2008; 14: 36–44.

80. Kormann MS, Hector A, Marcos V, *et al.* CXCR1 and CXCR2 haplotypes synergistically modulate cystic fibrosis lung disease. *Eur Respir J* 2012; 39: 1385–1390.

81. Jann NJ, Schmaler M, Ferracin F, *et al.* TLR2 enhances NADPH oxidase activity and killing of *Staphylococcus aureus* by PMN. *Immunol Lett* 2010; 135: 17–23.

82. Petit-Bertron AF, Tabary O, Corvol H, *et al.* Circulating and airway neutrophils in cystic fibrosis display different TLR expression and responsiveness to interleukin-10. *Cytokine* 2008; 41: 54–60.

83. Gu Y, Harley IT, Henderson LB, *et al.* Identification of *IFRD1* as a modifier gene for cystic fibrosis lung disease. *Nature* 2009; 458: 1039–1042.

84. Blanchard E, Marie S, Riffault L, *et al.* Reduced expression of Tis7/IFRD1 protein in murine and human cystic fibrosis airway epithelial cell models homozygous for the F508del-CFTR mutation. *Biochem Biophys Res Commun* 2011; 411: 471–476.

85. McKeon DJ, Cadwallader KA, Idris S, *et al.* Cystic fibrosis neutrophils have normal intrinsic reactive oxygen species generation. *Eur Respir J* 2010; 35: 1264–1272.

86. Brockbank S, Downey D, Elborn JS, *et al.* Effect of cystic fibrosis exacerbations on neutrophil function. *Int Immunopharmacol* 2005; 5: 601–608.

87. Hartl D, Latzin P, Hordijk P, *et al.* Cleavage of CXCR1 on neutrophils disables bacterial killing in cystic fibrosis lung disease. *Nat Med* 2007; 13: 1423–1430.

88. Berger M, Sorensen RU, Tosi MF, *et al.* Complement receptor expression on neutrophils at an inflammatory site, the *Pseudomonas*-infected lung in cystic fibrosis. *J Clin Invest* 1989; 84: 1302–1313.

89. Tirouvanziam R, Gernez Y, Conrad CK, *et al.* Profound functional and signaling changes in viable inflammatory neutrophils homing to cystic fibrosis airways. *Proc Natl Acad Sci USA* 2008; 105: 4335–4339.

90. Jesaitis AJ, Franklin MJ, Berglund D, *et al.* Compromised host defense on *Pseudomonas aeruginosa* biofilms: characterization of neutrophil and biofilm interactions. *J Immunol* 2003; 171: 4329–4339.

91. Laan M, Cui ZH, Hoshino H, *et al.* Neutrophil recruitment by human IL-17 *via* C-X-C chemokine release in the airways. *J Immunol* 1999; 162: 2347–2352.

92. Dubin PJ, McAllister F, Kolls JK. Is cystic fibrosis a TH17 disease? *Inflamm Res* 2007; 56: 221–227.

93. McAllister F, Henry A, Kreindler JL, *et al.* Role of IL-17A, IL-17F, and the IL-17 receptor in regulating growth-related oncogene-α and granulocyte colony-stimulating factor in bronchial epithelium: implications for airway inflammation in cystic fibrosis. *J Immunol* 2005; 175: 404–412.

94. Tan HL, Regamey N, Brown S, *et al.* The Th17 pathway in cystic fibrosis lung disease. *Am J Respir Crit Care Med* 2011; 184: 252–258.

95. Chen Y, Thai P, Zhao YH, *et al.* Stimulation of airway mucin gene expression by interleukin (IL)-17 through IL-6 paracrine/autocrine loop. *J Biol Chem* 2003; 278: 17036–17043.

96. Sagel SD, Chmiel JF, Konstan MW. Sputum biomarkers of inflammation in cystic fibrosis lung disease. *Proc Am Thorac Soc* 2007; 4: 406–417.

97. Konstan MW, Hilliard KA, Norvell TM, *et al.* Bronchoalveolar lavage findings in cystic fibrosis patients with stable, clinically mild lung disease suggest ongoing infection and inflammation. *Am J Respir Crit Care Med* 1994; 150: 448–454.

98. Kim JS, Okamoto K, Rubin BK. Pulmonary function is negatively correlated with sputum inflammatory markers and cough clearability in subjects with cystic fibrosis but not those with chronic bronchitis. *Chest* 2006; 129: 1148–1154.

99. Eickmeier O, Huebner M, Herrmann E, *et al.* Sputum biomarker profiles in cystic fibrosis (CF) and chronic obstructive pulmonary disease (COPD) and association between pulmonary function. *Cytokine* 2010; 50: 152–157.

100. Robroeks CM, Rosias PP, van Vliet D, *et al.* Biomarkers in exhaled breath condensate indicate presence and severity of cystic fibrosis in children. *Pediatr Allergy Immunol* 2008; 19: 652–659.

101. Paredi P, Kharitonov SA, Barnes PJ. Analysis of expired air for oxidation products. *Am J Respir Crit Care Med* 2002; 166: S31–S37.

102. Sagel SD, Kapsner RK, Osberg I. Induced sputum matrix metalloproteinase-9 correlates with lung function and airway inflammation in children with cystic fibrosis. *Pediatr Pulmonol* 2005; 39: 224–232.

103. Bodini A, D'Orazio C, Peroni D, *et al.* Biomarkers of neutrophilic inflammation in exhaled air of cystic fibrosis children with bacterial airway infections. *Pediatr Pulmonol* 2005; 40: 494–499.

104. Sagel SD, Sontag MK, Wagener JS, *et al.* Induced sputum inflammatory measures correlate with lung function in children with cystic fibrosis. *J Pediatr* 2002; 141: 811–887.

105. Sagel SD, Wagner BD, Anthony MM, *et al.* Sputum biomarkers of inflammation and lung function decline in children with cystic fibrosis. *Am J Respir Crit Care Med* 2012; 186: 857–865.

106. Laguna TA, Wagner BD, Luckey HK, *et al.* Sputum desmosine during hospital admission for pulmonary exacerbation in cystic fibrosis. *Chest* 2009; 136: 1561–1568.

107. Ciabattoni G, Davi G, Collura M, *et al. In vivo* lipid peroxidation and platelet activation in cystic fibrosis. *Am J Respir Crit Care Med* 2000; 162: 1195–1201.

108. Ordonez CL, Kartashov AI, Wohl ME. Variability of markers of inflammation and infection in induced sputum in children with cystic fibrosis. *J Pediatr* 2004; 145: 689–692.

109. Shoki AH, Mayer-Hamblett N, Wilcox PG, *et al.* Systematic review of blood biomarkers in cystic fibrosis pulmonary exacerbations. *Chest* 2013; 144: 1659–1570.

110. Reeves EP, Bergin DA, Fitzgerald S, *et al.* A novel neutrophil derived inflammatory biomarker of pulmonary exacerbation in cystic fibrosis. *J Cyst Fibros* 2012; 11: 100–107.

111. Judge EP, Dodd JD, Masterson JB, *et al.* Pulmonary abnormalities on high-resolution CT demonstrate more rapid decline than FEV1 in adults with cystic fibrosis. *Chest* 2006; 130: 1424–1432.

112. Klein M, Cohen-Cymberknoh M, Armoni S, *et al.* ^{18}F-fluorodeoxyglucose-PET/CT imaging of lungs in patients with cystic fibrosis. *Chest* 2009; 136: 1220–1228.

113. Amin R, Charron M, Grinblat L, *et al.* Cystic fibrosis: detecting changes in airway inflammation with FDG PET/CT. *Radiology* 2012; 264: 868–875.

114. Chen DL, Atkinson JJ, Ferkol TW. FDG PET imaging in cystic fibrosis. *Semin Nucl Med* 2013; 43: 412–419.

115. McMahon CJ, Dodd JD, Hill C, *et al.* Hyperpolarized ^{3}helium magnetic resonance ventilation imaging of the lung in cystic fibrosis: comparison with high resolution CT and spirometry. *Eur Radiol* 2006; 16: 2483–2490.

116. Eichinger M, Puderbach M, Fink C, *et al.* Contrast-enhanced 3D MRI of lung perfusion in children with cystic fibrosis – initial results. *Eur Radiol* 2006; 16: 2147–2152.

117. van Beek EJ, Hill C, Woodhouse N, *et al.* Assessment of lung disease in children with cystic fibrosis using hyperpolarized 3-helium MRI: comparison with Shwachman score, Chrispin-Norman score and spirometry. *Eur Radiol* 2007; 17: 1018–1024.

118. Bannier E, Cieslar K, Mosbah K, *et al.* Hyperpolarized ^{3}He MR for sensitive imaging of ventilation function and treatment efficiency in young cystic fibrosis patients with normal lung function. *Radiology* 2010; 255: 225–232.

119. O'Connell OJ, McWilliams S, McGarrigle A, *et al.* Radiologic imaging in cystic fibrosis: cumulative effective dose and changing trends over 2 decades. *Chest* 2012; 141: 1575–1583.

120. King M, Dasgupta B, Tomkiewicz RP, *et al.* Rheology of cystic fibrosis sputum after *in vitro* treatment with hypertonic saline alone and in combination with recombinant human deoxyribonuclease I. *Am J Respir Crit Care Med* 1997; 156: 173–177.

121. Davis SD, Brody AS, Emond MJ, *et al.* Endpoints for clinical trials in young children with cystic fibrosis. *Proc Am Thorac Soc* 2007; 4: 418–430.

122. Aurora P, Stanojevic S, Wade A, *et al.* Lung clearance index at 4 years predicts subsequent lung function in children with cystic fibrosis. *Am J Respir Crit Care Med* 2011; 183: 752–758.

123. Davies J, Sheridan H, Bell N, *et al.* Assessment of clinical response to ivacaftor with lung clearance index in cystic fibrosis patients with a G551D-*CFTR* mutation and preserved spirometry: a randomised controlled trial. *Lancet Respir Med* 2013; 1: 630–638.

124. Belessis Y, Dixon B, Hawkins G, *et al.* Early cystic fibrosis lung disease detected by bronchoalveolar lavage and lung clearance index. *Am J Respir Crit Care Med* 2012; 185: 862–873.

125. Robinson M, Daviskas E, Eberl S, *et al.* The effect of inhaled mannitol on bronchial mucus clearance in cystic fibrosis patients: a pilot study. *Eur Respir J* 1999; 14: 678–685.

126. Donaldson SH, Corcoran TE, Laube BL, *et al.* Mucociliary clearance as an outcome measure for cystic fibrosis clinical research. *Proc Am Thorac Soc* 2007; 4: 399–405.

127. McCarthy C, Dimitrov BD, Meurling IJ, *et al.* The CF-ABLE score: a novel clinical prediction rule for prognosis in patients with cystic fibrosis. *Chest* 2013; 143: 1358–1364.

128. Valerius NH, Koch C, Hoiby N. Prevention of chronic *Pseudomonas aeruginosa* colonisation in cystic fibrosis by early treatment. *Lancet* 1991; 338: 725–726.

129. Cheng K, Ashby D, Smyth RL. Oral steroids for long-term use in cystic fibrosis. *Cochrane Database Syst Rev* 2013; 6: CD000407.

130. Lai HC, FitzSimmons SC, Allen DB, *et al.* Risk of persistent growth impairment after alternate-day prednisone treatment in children with cystic fibrosis. *N Engl J Med* 2000; 342: 851–859.

131. Konstan MW, Davis PB. Pharmacological approaches for the discovery and development of new anti-inflammatory agents for the treatment of cystic fibrosis. *Adv Drug Deliv Rev* 2002; 54: 1409–1423.

132. Konstan MW, Byard PJ, Hoppel CL, *et al.* Effect of high-dose ibuprofen in patients with cystic fibrosis. *N Engl J Med* 1995; 332: 848–854.

133. Konstan MW. Ibuprofen therapy for cystic fibrosis lung disease: revisited. *Curr Opin Pulm Med* 2008; 14: 567–573.

134. McNally P, Coughlan C, Bergsson G, *et al.* Vitamin D receptor agonists inhibit pro-inflammatory cytokine production from the respiratory epithelium in cystic fibrosis. *J Cyst Fibros* 2011; 10: 428–434.

135. Lands LC, Milner R, Cantin AM, *et al.* High-dose ibuprofen in cystic fibrosis: Canadian safety and effectiveness trial. *J Pediatr* 2007; 151: 249–254.

136. Altenburg J, de Graaff CS, van der Werf TS, *et al.* Immunomodulatory effects of macrolide antibiotics - part 1: biological mechanisms. *Respiration* 2011; 81: 67–74.

137. Saiman L, Marshall BC, Mayer-Hamblett N, *et al.* Azithromycin in patients with cystic fibrosis chronically infected with *Pseudomonas aeruginosa*: a randomized controlled trial. *JAMA* 2003; 290: 1749–1756.

138. Fuchs HJ, Borowitz DS, Christiansen DH, *et al.* Effect of aerosolized recombinant human DNase on exacerbations of respiratory symptoms and on pulmonary function in patients with cystic fibrosis. The Pulmozyme Study Group. *N Engl J Med* 1994; 331: 637–642.

139. Reeves EP, Williamson M, O'Neill SJ, *et al.* Nebulized hypertonic saline decreases IL-8 in sputum of patients with cystic fibrosis. *Am J Respir Crit Care Med* 2011; 183: 1517–1523.

140. Elkins MR, Robinson M, Rose BR, *et al.* A controlled trial of long-term inhaled hypertonic saline in patients with cystic fibrosis. *N Engl J Med* 2006; 354: 229–2240.

141. Bilton D, Bellon G, Charlton B, *et al.* Pooled analysis of two large randomised phase III inhaled mannitol studies in cystic fibrosis. *J Cyst Fibros* 2013; 12: 367–376.

142. Sadowska AM, Manuel YKB, De Backer WA. Antioxidant and anti-inflammatory efficacy of NAC in the treatment of COPD: discordant *in vitro* and *in vivo* dose-effects: a review. *Pulm Pharmacol Ther* 2007; 20: 9–22.

143. Tirouvanziam R, Conrad CK, Bottiglieri T, *et al.* High-dose oral *N*-acetylcysteine, a glutathione prodrug, modulates inflammation in cystic fibrosis. *Proc Natl Acad Sci USA* 2006; 103: 4628–4633.

144. Tam J, Nash EF, Ratjen F, *et al.* Nebulized and oral thiol derivatives for pulmonary disease in cystic fibrosis. *Cochrane Database Syst Rev* 2013; 7: CD007168.

145. Griese M, Kappler M, Eismann C, *et al.* Inhalation treatment with glutathione in patients with cystic fibrosis. *a randomized clinical trial. Am J Respir Crit Care Med* 2013; 188: 83–89.

146. McElvaney NG, Hubbard RC, Birrer P, *et al.* Aerosol α1-antitrypsin treatment for cystic fibrosis. *Lancet* 1991; 337: 392–394.

147. McElvaney NG, Nakamura H, Birrer P, *et al.* Modulation of airway inflammation in cystic fibrosis. *In vivo* suppression of interleukin-8 levels on the respiratory epithelial surface by aerosolization of recombinant secretory leukoprotease inhibitor. *J Clin Invest* 1992; 90: 1296–1301.

148. Griese M, Latzin P, Kappler M, *et al.* α1-Antitrypsin inhalation reduces airway inflammation in cystic fibrosis patients. *Eur Respir J* 2007; 29: 240–250.

149. Elborn JS, Perrett J, Forsman-Semb K, *et al.* Efficacy, safety and effect on biomarkers of AZD9668 in cystic fibrosis. *Eur Respir J* 2012; 40: 969–976.

150. Martin SL, Downey D, Bilton D, *et al.* Safety and efficacy of recombinant α_1-antitrypsin therapy in cystic fibrosis. *Pediatr Pulmonol* 2006; 41: 177–183.

151. Ramsey BW, Pepe MS, Quan JM, *et al.* Intermittent administration of inhaled tobramycin in patients with cystic fibrosis. Cystic Fibrosis Inhaled Tobramycin Study Group. *N Engl J Med* 1999; 340: 23–30.

152. McCoy KS, Quittner AL, Oermann CM, *et al.* Inhaled aztreonam lysine for chronic airway *Pseudomonas aeruginosa* in cystic fibrosis. *Am J Respir Crit Care Med* 2008; 178: 921–928.

153. Hatch RA, Schiller NL. Alginate lyase promotes diffusion of aminoglycosides through the extracellular polysaccharide of mucoid *Pseudomonas aeruginosa. Antimicrob Agents Chemother* 1998; 42: 974–977.

154. Schuster A, Haliburn C, Doring G, *et al.* Safety, efficacy and convenience of colistimethate sodium dry powder for inhalation (Colobreathe DPI) in patients with cystic fibrosis: a randomised study. *Thorax* 2013; 68: 344–350.

155. Ramsey BW, Davies J, McElvaney NG, *et al.* A CFTR potentiator in patients with cystic fibrosis and the G551D mutation. *N Engl J Med* 2011; 365: 1663–1672.

156. Sermet-Gaudelus I, Boeck KD, Casimir GJ, *et al.* Ataluren (PTC124) induces cystic fibrosis transmembrane conductance regulator protein expression and activity in children with nonsense mutation cystic fibrosis. *Am J Respir Crit Care Med* 2010; 182: 1262–1272.

157. Konstan MW, Krenicky JE, Finney MR, *et al.* Effect of ibuprofen on neutrophil migration *in vivo* in cystic fibrosis and healthy subjects. *J Pharmaol Exp Ther* 2003; 306: 1086–1091.

158. Konstan MW, Vargo KM, Davis PB. Ibuprofen attenuates the inflammatory response to *Pseudomonas aeruginosa* in a rat model of chronic pulmonary infection. Implications for antiinflammatory therapy in cystic fibrosis. *Am Rev Respir Dis* 1990; 141: 186–192.

159. Konstan MW, Schluchter MD, Xue W, *et al.* Clinical use of ibuprofen is associated with slower FEV1 decline in children with cystic fibrosis. *Am J Respir Crit Care Med* 2007; 176: 1084–1089.

160. Lands LC, Stanojevic S. Oral non-steroidal anti-inflammatory drug therapy for lung disease in cystic fibrosis. *Cochrane Database Syst Rev* 2013; 6: CD001505.

161. Kreindler JL, Steele C, Nguyen N, *et al.* Vitamin D3 attenuates Th2 responses to *Aspergillus fumigatus* mounted by CD4[+] T cells from cystic fibrosis patients with allergic bronchopulmonary aspergillosis. *J Clin Invest* 2010; 120: 3242–3254.

162. Coughlan CA, Chotirmall SH, Renwick J, *et al.* The effect of *Aspergillus fumigatus* infection on vitamin D receptor expression in cystic fibrosis. *Am J Respir Crit Care Med* 2012; 186: 999–1007.

163. Moss RB, Mistry SJ, Konstan MW, *et al.* Safety and early treatment effects of the CXCR2 antagonist SB-656933 in patients with cystic fibrosis. *J Cyst Fibros* 2013; 12: 241–248.

164. Clancy JP, Dupont L, Konstan MW, *et al.* Phase II studies of nebulised Arikace in CF patients with *Pseudomonas aeruginosa* infection. *Thorax* 2013; 68: 818–825.

165. Geller DE, Flume PA, Staab D, *et al.* Levofloxacin inhalation solution (MP-376) in patients with cystic fibrosis with *Pseudomonas aeruginosa. Am J Respir Crit Care Med* 2011; 183: 1510–1516.

166. Adi H, Young PM, Chan HK, *et al.* Co-spray-dried mannitol-ciprofloxacin dry powder inhaler formulation for cystic fibrosis and chronic obstructive pulmonary disease. *Eur J Pharm Sci* 2010; 40: 239–247.

167. Aquino RP, Prota L, Auriemma G, *et al.* Dry powder inhalers of gentamicin and leucine: formulation parameters, aerosol performance and *in vitro* toxicity on CuFi1 cells. *Int J Pharm* 2012; 426: 100–107.

168. Konstan MW, Geller DE, Minic P, *et al.* Tobramycin inhalation powder for *P. aeruginosa* infection in cystic fibrosis: the EVOLVE trial. *Pediatr Pulmonol* 2011; 46: 230–238.

169. Hoiby N, Frederiksen B, Pressler T. Eradication of early *Pseudomonas aeruginosa* infection. *J Cyst Fibros* 2005; 4: Suppl. 2, 49–54.

170. Islan GA, Bosio VE, Castro GR. Alginate lyase and ciprofloxacin co-immobilization on biopolymeric microspheres for cystic fibrosis treatment. *Macromol Biosci* 2013; 13: 1238–1248.

171. Khan S, Tondervik A, Sletta H, *et al*. Overcoming drug resistance with alginate oligosaccharides able to potentiate the action of selected antibiotics. *Antimicrob Agents Chemother* 2012; 56: 5134–5141.

172. Aitken ML, Greene KE, Tonelli MR, *et al*. Analysis of sequential aliquots of hypertonic saline solution-induced sputum from clinically stable patients with cystic fibrosis. *Chest* 2003; 123: 792–799.

173. Bergsson G, Reeves EP, McNally P, *et al*. LL-37 complexation with glycosaminoglycans in cystic fibrosis lungs inhibits antimicrobial activity, which can be restored by hypertonic saline. *J Immunol* 2009; 183: 543–551.

174. Reeves EP, Bergin DA, Murray MA, *et al*. The involvement of glycosaminoglycans in airway disease associated with cystic fibrosis. *Sci World J* 2011; 11: 959–971.

175. Gould NS, Gauthier S, Kariya CT, *et al*. Hypertonic saline increases lung epithelial lining fluid glutathione and thiocyanate: two protective CFTR-dependent thiols against oxidative injury. *Respir Res* 2010; 11: 119.

176. Lee L, Kelher MR, Moore EE, *et al*. Hypertonic saline inhibits arachidonic acid priming of the human neutrophil oxidase. *J Surg Res* 2012; 174: 24–28.

177. Daviskas E, Anderson SD, Jaques A, *et al*. Inhaled mannitol improves the hydration and surface properties of sputum in patients with cystic fibrosis. *Chest* 2010; 137: 861–868.

178. Bilton D, Daviskas E, Anderson SD, *et al*. Phase 3 randomized study of the efficacy and safety of inhaled dry powder mannitol for the symptomatic treatment of non-cystic fibrosis bronchiectasis. *Chest* 2013; 144: 215–225.

179. Cantin AM, Woods DE. Aerosolized prolastin suppresses bacterial proliferation in a model of chronic *Pseudomonas aeruginosa* lung infection. *Am J Respir Crit Care Med* 1999; 160: 1130–1135.

180. Woods DE, Cantin A, Cooley J, *et al*. Aerosol treatment with MNEI suppresses bacterial proliferation in a model of chronic *Pseudomonas aeruginosa* lung infection. *Pediatr Pulmonol* 2005; 39: 141–149.

181. Vertex Pharmaceuticals Incorporated. Study of VX-661 Alone and in Combination With Ivacaftor in Subjects Homozygous or Heterozygous to the F508del-Cystic Fibrosis Transmembrane Conductance Regulator (CFTR) Mutation. http://clinicaltrials.gov/ct2/show/NCT01531673 Date last accessed: December 11, 2013. Date last updated: November 19, 2013.

Support statement: N.G. McElvaney acknowledges support from the US Cystic Fibrosis Foundation.

Disclosures: None declared.

Chapter 3 | 🔬

Airway infection and the microbiome

Jiangchao Zhao[1], J. Stuart Elborn[2] and John J. LiPuma[1]

The use of culture-independent microbiomic analyses is expanding our view of respiratory tract infection in cystic fibrosis (CF). Recent studies demonstrate that the airways of persons with CF harbour complex polymicrobial communities. Ongoing studies are assessing how the composition and dynamics of these communities relate to clinical states and lung disease progression. Interest is now also focusing on better understanding the network of microbe–microbe and microbe–host interactions inherent in these communities. This deeper appreciation of how microbial airway communities are structured and how they function has potential to drive advances in our management of lung infection in CF.

O ur understanding of the microbiology of lung infection in cystic fibrosis (CF) is undergoing significant change, driven by the advent of culture-independent methods to detect the presence of microorganisms. These methods allow us to identify, in unprecedented detail, the members of the polymicrobial communities typically inhabiting CF airways. This chapter will provide a succinct description of these methods and highlight what their use is teaching us about CF airway microbial communities, collectively referred to as the airway microbiome.

The term "microbiome" is reserved by some authors to describe the totality of microbes and their genomes in a defined environment (*i.e.* the gene complement of a microbial community) (table 1) [1]. The term "microbiota" refers to the microbes that inhabit a defined niche. For the purposes of this chapter, we will use these terms interchangeably. Furthermore, although microbiota refers to all microorganisms, including bacteria, viruses, fungi and protozoa, we will focus our review on bacteria; more specifically, we will refer to the bacterial microbiota that inhabit the airways as the airway or lung microbiome and/or the airway bacterial community.

In contrast to conventional wisdom, recent culture-independent studies suggest that the human lung is not sterile. Diverse microorganisms have been identified in healthy human lungs [2–4], although methodological challenges in sampling and analysing the healthy airway limit a complete understanding of the "normal" human lung microbiome at this time. It is unknown whether bacteria detected in healthy lungs reflect organisms in transit into or out of the lung or whether there may be a resident airway microbiome. What has become clear, however, is that unhealthy lungs harbour bacterial communities that vary with disease.

[1]Dept of Pediatrics and Communicable Diseases, University of Michigan, Ann Arbor, MI, USA. [2]Centre for Infection and Immunity, School of Medicine, Dentistry and Biomedical Sciences, Queen's University Belfast, Belfast, UK.

Correspondence: John J. LiPuma, Dept of Pediatrics and Communicable Diseases, 8323 MSRB III, 1150 W. Medical Center Drive, Ann Arbor, MI, 48109, USA. E-mail: jlipuma@umich.edu

ERS Monogr 2014; 64: 32–46. DOI: 10.1183/1025448x.10008713

Table 1. Terms and definitions

Term	Definition
Microbiome	The gene complement of a microbial community
Microbiota	The microorganisms that inhabit a defined niche
Metagenomics	A culture-independent, DNA-sequence-based approach to analysing the total genetic content of a given niche
Community structure	The composition of a community and the abundance of its members
Diversity	A measure of the degree of variety in a community; consists of richness and evenness
Richness	The number of types (e.g. species) in a community
Evenness	A measure of the distribution (i.e. relative abundance) of individuals across the different types in a community
Similarity	A measure of the relative richness and/or shared members, and sometimes the abundance of members, between two or more communities
Resistance	The ability of a community to resist change to its structure by an ecological challenge
Resilience	The ability of a community to recover to its native structure after a perturbation

The lungs of persons with asthma [5, 6], chronic obstructive pulmonary disease (COPD) [7–9], bronchiectasis [10, 11] and primary ciliary dyskinesia [12] typically harbour bacterial communities that include many more species than previously appreciated.

Several recent studies also indicate that the airways of persons with CF harbour complex bacterial communities [13–16]. The structure and activity of these communities, and how these features change relative to lung disease, are areas of considerable interest and active investigation.

Methods for studying the airway microbiome

Culture-dependent approaches

For several decades our understanding of bacterial infection in CF has relied on culture-based studies. Various bacterial species believed to contribute to lung disease in CF, including common human pathogens such as *Staphylococcus aureus* and *Haemophilus influenzae* and opportunistic pathogens such as *Pseudomonas aeruginosa*, are routinely cultured from CF respiratory samples. Other opportunists, including nosocomial pathogens such as *Stenotrophomonas maltophilia* and *Achromobacter xylosoxidans*, and species that are infrequently detected in other human infections, such as *Ralstonia* species, *Cupriavidus* species, *Pandoraea* species, *Burkholderia gladioli* and the species within the *Burkholderia cepacia* complex, are also recovered with routine culture methods [17].

Several types of respiratory samples, including spontaneously expectorated or induced sputum, bronchoalveolar lavage (BAL) fluid, cough swabs, cough plates and oropharyngeal swabs, have been used to assess CF airway microbiology. How well these samples represent bacteria present in the lower airways probably varies by specimen type and bacterial species. These issues and the use of culture-based methods to assess the airway microbiome in CF have been discussed in depth and are not a focus of this chapter [18]. It is of note, however, that by modification of routine culture methods with careful attention to media and incubation time, temperature and oxygen concentration, nearly all species detected by culture-independent methods can be recovered in culture [19]. It is also worth noting here that culture of bacteria *in vitro* is still required, to provide samples for comprehensive antimicrobial susceptibility testing of recovered species.

Culture-independent approaches

During the past decade, several culture-independent methods of bacterial detection have been used to assess the microbiology of CF airways. These methods rely on detecting bacterial DNA sequences that are specific for distinct species. Among the most commonly used species-specific sequences targeted by these methods is the gene encoding 16S ribosomal RNA (16S rRNA), a component of the 30S small subunit of bacterial ribosomes. This gene includes sequences that are highly conserved among bacteria and archaea, as well as sequences that are hypervariable and often species specific [20, 21]. This structure enables the use of universal primers targeting the conserved regions to amplify the intervening hypervariable segments by PCR. Analysis of the hypervariable regions provides a phylogenetically informative signature. The choice of which hypervariable regions to target is an important consideration in study design, however, since these regions differ with respect to the resolution they provide in identifying various taxa [22–24]. Three general approaches to exploiting the 16S rRNA gene (DNA fingerprinting, microarray analysis and direct sequencing) have been used to characterise the constituent members of polymicrobial bacterial communities in CF respiratory samples.

DNA fingerprinting techniques

These methods rely on the analysis of patterns formed by fragments of bacterial DNA that have been separated in a gel matrix. One such method, terminal restriction fragment length polymorphism (T-RFLP), was among the first culture-independent techniques to be applied to the study of CF airway microbiology. T-RFLP involves PCR amplification of the total 16S rRNA gene with a fluorescently labelled primer followed by restriction enzyme digestion. This generates fragments that differ in length due to the variation in the position of the first restriction endonuclease site in the hypervariable ribosomal sequences amplified from different bacterial species. The fragments are separated by gel electrophoresis or detected using a DNA sequencing machine, and their relative abundances are visualised as electropherograms. The pioneering studies by ROGERS and co-workers [25, 26] employed this method to characterise the lung microbiota in CF and to compare bacterial communities in the upper and lower airways. T-RFLP has also been used by SIBLEY et al. [27] to examine longitudinal changes in lung microbiota in persons with CF.

Denaturing gradient gel electrophoresis (DGGE) is another DNA fingerprinting technique that has been used to study the microbiome in CF. In this method, PCR-amplified 16S rRNA genes from a polymicrobial bacterial community are separated, based on differences in their GC content, on an acrylamide gel with an increasing denaturing gradient. Distinct DNA bands are visualised by staining and/or excised from the gel for sequencing, enabling species identification [28]. This technique has been used to compare the faecal microbiome of paediatric patients with CF and their healthy siblings [29].

Microarray hybridisation

In this approach, 16S rRNA genes, PCR amplified from a mixed bacterial community, are fragmented, biotin labelled and hybridised to a microarray chip that contains 16S-rRNA-based probes from thousands of known bacterial species [30, 31]. The intensity of fragment hybridisation to the array provides an approximation of the relative abundance of each species detected. This method has been used in several studies of the CF lung microbiome, including an important investigation by KLEPAC-CERAJ *et al.* [32] of the relationship between the lung microbiome and patient age and genotype, antibiotic use and *Pseudomonas* infection.

DNA-sequencing-based approaches

Several studies of the CF microbiome have relied on direct sequencing of phylogenetically informative DNA from bacterial communities to detect the member species. In an early approach, the 16S rRNA genes of a mixed bacterial community are PCR amplified, ligated to cloning vectors (plasmids) and transformed into *Escherichia coli* cells, which are then cultivated, thereby propagating the cloned DNA. Plasmids containing 16S rRNA inserts are purified from single *E. coli* colonies and sequenced *via* traditional Sanger sequencing. HARRIS *et al.* [33] characterised the lung microbiome in persons with CF and in healthy controls using this technique.

Currently, the most widely used approach to direct DNA sequencing for characterisation of bacterial communities involves so-called "next-generation sequencing". Here, the need for cloning and propagation of phylogenetically informative bacterial DNA before sequencing is circumvented by technology that provides high-throughput, massively parallel sequencing that produces millions of DNA sequences concurrently. In this approach, the 16S rRNA genes of the entire mixed bacterial community are PCR amplified using universal 16S rRNA primers and then this pool is subjected to deep sequencing. The sequencing platform that has been most widely used to date in studies of the CF microbiome is the Roche 454 GS FLX system (454 Life Sciences (a Roche company), Branford, CT, USA). This system employs pyrosequencing, which differs from Sanger sequencing in that it relies on synthesising a strand of DNA that is complementary to the target strand (*i.e.* the strand being sequenced). This "sequencing by synthesis" is based on the detection of pyrophosphate release as nucleosides are incorporated into the complementary strand [34–37]. The Roche 454 pyrosequencing platform recently has been discontinued, however, and is being replaced by other high-throughput sequencing technologies. One of these is the Illumina sequencing platform (Illumina, Inc., San Diego, CA, USA), which is also based on sequencing by synthesis and was compared to the Roche 454 system by MAUGHAN *et al.* [38] in an investigation of the CF lung microbiome. The Ion Torrent sequencing platform (Life Technologies, Carlsbad, CA, USA), which employs semiconductor technology to detect protons that are released when nucleotides are incorporated into the complementary DNA strand [39], was used by SALIPANTE *et al.* [40] to identify bacterial communities in CF lung.

A comprehensive description of the technical aspects of these methods is beyond the scope of this review. Suffice it to say that sequencing platforms differ with respect to several important variables that should be taken into account when considering study design. These differences, including sequencing depth, length and accuracy, as well as cost, have been discussed in detail elsewhere [34, 36, 37]. Furthermore, it is quite likely that high-throughput, next-generation sequencing technology will continue to develop and improve at a dizzying pace in the next several years.

Metagenomic analysis provides another approach to microbiomic analysis of mixed bacterial communities. In this strategy, the total gene complement of a given niche or sample is sequenced. Bioinformatic analysis of the resulting DNA sequences, albeit more rigorous than that needed for targeted (*e.g.* 16S rRNA) sequence data sets, has distinct advantages. For example, this approach obviates the need for PCR amplification of a specific target, thereby reducing biases inherent in this step. Furthermore, analysis of the entire gene complement of the sampled niche provides information not available in 16S rRNA sequence pools, such as detection of genes encoding metabolomic pathways, antibiotic resistance and virulence determinants. Importantly, metagenomic analyses theoretically provide for the detection of all microorganisms, including viruses and fungi, in a sample. A drawback of this approach in CF-related studies is the massive amount of human DNA sequenced from respiratory samples. Nevertheless, this approach has been used successfully by LIM and co-workers [41, 42] to characterise the CF airway microbiome.

As important as the emergence of new technologies for generating high-throughput DNA sequences has been to investigating complex bacterial communities, so too has the development of bioinformatic tools that provide an accessible means to analyse the resulting sequence data. Several open-source software packages and analytic pipelines are widely used. Among the most popular are mothur [43] and QIIME (quantitative insights into microbial ecology) [44], both of which bundle various algorithms for DNA sequence analysis. The analyses typically includes three steps: 1) cleaning the DNA sequence data to remove sequences with errors and sequence chimeras (artefact sequences composed of DNA from two or more species); 2) identification of individual bacterial taxa; and 3) calculation of the alpha and beta diversity of communities (see next section). After removing sequencing errors and chimeras, high quality sequence reads are binned into either operational taxonomic units (OTUs) or specific bacterial taxa (depending on the reliability of the taxon classification scheme used) for downstream ecological and statistical analyses. Because sequencing depth (the number of high quality reads produced) varies from sample to sample, the read number is often normalised to the smallest number by random subsampling in order to minimise bias introduced by sequencing depth.

Ecological and statistical analyses of bacterial communities

Assessment of the CF airway microbiome focuses on several clinically and scientifically relevant questions. In addition to determining the number of bacterial species present, it is often desirable to understand the degree of similarity between bacterial communities. Current investigations are also aimed at elucidating how bacterial communities change over time, particularly with respect to changes in the host's clinical state. Associations are being sought between bacterial community structure and function, and lung disease progression, which has the potential to significantly advance our understanding of CF pathophysiology.

Various ecological principles and statistical methods are employed to address these important questions. Again, definition of key terms is in order (table 1). Alpha diversity describes community diversity within a particular niche (*e.g.* within a single host). Beta diversity refers to the diversity between different niches (*e.g.* the difference in community structure between hosts). Diversity can be measured by several formulae. The commonly used Shannon index and Simpson index take community richness (the number of different types present) and evenness (the relative abundance of different types) into account, but do not consider membership (*i.e.* which specific types are present). Other indices, such as the Jaccard and unweighted UniFrac indices, consider the presence or absence of specific members, while still other metrics provide a measure of community structure by considering both membership and the relative abundance of each member. These latter metrics include the Bray-Curtis, Theta YC, Morisita-Horn and weighted UniFrac measures [45–50].

The relationships between microbial communities are often visualised by mathematical procedures that reduce high-dimension data sets (such as those generated by next-generation sequencing) into data sets whose relationships can be visualised in a simplified graphic plot. Among the most commonly used procedures is principal component analysis (PCA), which converts a set of observations of possibly correlated variables into a set of values of uncorrelated variables called principal components. The first principal component accounts for as much of the variability in the data set as possible, and each succeeding component accounts for the next greatest variability. Essentially, PCA and related procedures, such as principal coordinates analysis and nonmetric multidimensional scaling, provide a way of identifying patterns in high-dimension data sets. Typically, the data are visualised on a plot wherein each point represents the community structure of a different sample. The distances between points indicate the dissimilarities between the communities (fig. 1).

A variety of statistical methods and software packages are used to assess correlations between microbial communities and between these communities and various host-related parameters (*e.g.* clinical state, age, *etc.*). A comprehensive review of these methods is beyond the scope of this review [51–55]. However, a few specific methods are worth noting. Metastats uses a nonparametric t-test and Fisher's exact test to detect features that are differentially represented in metagenomic data sets [56]. This software is useful in detecting differences in microbial communities in samples collected from different disease conditions or during different types of therapy [56–59]. Linear discriminant analysis (LDA) effect size (LEfSe) is an algorithm developed by SEGATA *et al.* [60] to support high-dimensional comparisons of metagenomic data sets. LEfSe determines the features (OTUs, genes or functions) most likely to explain differences between groups by coupling standard tests for statistical significance with additional tests to assess whether these differences are consistent with respect to expected biological behaviour. As such, it is well suited to biomarker discovery. LEfSe has

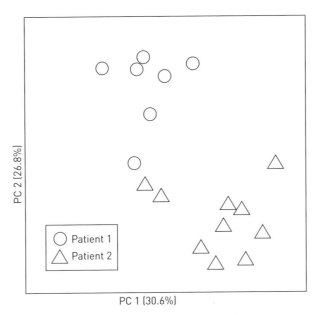

Figure 1. Representation of a principal component analysis plot. Each point represents the bacterial community composition in a different sputum sample from either patient 1 or patient 2. The communities occupy different positions in the ordination space, based on their relative similarity to each other. The first principal component (PC 1) accounts for the greatest variability (30.6%) between communities, while the second principal component (PC 2) accounts for the next greatest variability (26.8%) between communities.

been used, for example, to detect bacterial species associated with colorectal carcinoma [61] and inflammatory bowel disease [62], and to assess the effect of xenobiotics on the gut microbiome [63]. Random forests is a machine learning technique used to identify features that best predict different phenotypes [64–66]. This method has been applied in microbiome studies to identify bacterial genera associated with age and geography [67], bacterial taxa associated with colon tumorigenesis [68], and bacterial OTUs that predict the onset of pulmonary exacerbations in patients with CF [69].

Airway microbiome diversity and dynamics

Community diversity

Community richness

Culture-based approaches to studying the airway microbiota in CF typically focus on a very limited set of known CF opportunistic bacterial pathogens, including *Pseudomonas*, *Staphylococcus*, *Burkholderia*, *Achromobacter*, *Stenotrophomonas* and nontuberculous mycobacteria. In contrast, culture-independent methods offer far greater sensitivity in bacterial detection, providing a dramatically expanded view of airway bacterial community richness. It is important to note, however, that these methods vary with respect to sensitivity, thereby providing varying estimates of community richness in CF. Studies using T-RFLP and 16s rRNA gene cloning have relatively lower sensitivity, most often detecting a few dozen species [14, 26]. Analyses based on next-generation sequencing typically detect greater numbers of distinct taxa, while microarray-based studies may estimate that CF airway communities include many hundred taxa. For example, GUSS *et al.* [70] used pyrosequencing to detect >60 bacterial genera in a study of four CF patients. By using microarray analysis, KLEPAC-CERAJ *et al.* [32] detected a total of 2051 taxa in samples from a cohort of 45 CF patients; community richness ranged from 206 to 1329 OTUs per patient.

Community evenness

In considering diversity, the distribution of community members (or evenness of the community (table 1)) must be taken into account. This is most often expressed as the relative abundance of each of the members of the community. When next-generation sequencing is used to assess microbial communities, evenness is usually determined based on the relative number of DNA sequences (or "reads") specific for a given taxon. As with measures of community richness, a number of technical variables can have an impact on estimates of community evenness. For example, ZHAO *et al.* [71] demonstrated the significant impact that DNA extraction methods can have on measures of *Staphylococcus* relative abundance in CF sputum samples. DNA extraction method also has a profound effect on the detection and estimates of relative abundance of mycobacterial species in sputum (John J. LiPuma, unpublished observations). Other pre-analytical steps, such as the removal of dead bacteria [72, 73] and sample storage conditions [74], are further considerations that could affect measures of bacterial community structure.

Upper airway contamination

The conclusion that culture-independent analyses indicate that CF lower airways harbour complex bacterial communities is challenged by critics who claim that respiratory samples are highly contaminated by species present in the oropharynx. Although it is true that samples obtained through the mouth will reflect oropharyngeal inhabitants, several lines of evidence support that the species detected in CF respiratory specimens represent microbial presence in the lower airways. ROGERS *et al.* [75] showed that oral mouthwash samples contained distinct bacterial communities compared to sputum samples from the same individual. HARRIS *et al.* [33] found relatively high abundances of oral cavity-associated bacterial species in BAL fluid specimens. Collection of this sample type would be expected to bypass significant contamination by oral cavity inhabitants. FILKINS *et al.* [76] observed significant differences in the relative abundance of *Streptococcus* in sputum samples from outpatients with CF compared to samples from inpatients. Since contamination of expectorated sputum by oral cavity inhabitants such as *Streptococcus* would be expected to affect both sample sets equally, the finding of significant differences in abundance between these two patient groups indicates differences in lower airway community composition.

Community dynamics

Cross-sectional studies

Much of what has been learned about the population dynamics of CF airway bacterial communities has been derived from relatively small-scale, cross-sectional studies. These studies have demonstrated consistent correlations between community structure and certain clinical features. Specifically, a positive correlation has been observed between community diversity and lung function; lower diversity is generally found in persons with decreased lung function. Furthermore, a clear inverse relationship between diversity and patient age is found, at least in adolescents and young adults with CF [13, 14, 32, 77]. In contrast, scant data suggest that diversity increases with age in children [32, 77, 78]. Frequency of antibiotic therapy has also been found to correlate with decreasing diversity, but this metric is difficult to quantify in a patient population typically treated with chronic antibiotic therapy punctuated by highly variable and intermittent intensive courses of therapy [13, 79].

Longitudinal studies

A small number of longitudinal studies, where serial samples from specific individual patients are analysed, have begun to shed greater light on airway community dynamics at the individual level. These studies suggest that CF airway microbiomes are distinct between individuals (*i.e.* show greater inter-patient than intra-patient variation in serial samples), at least among young adults with intermediate lung disease, and are quite stable over periods of several months [13, 15, 16, 80]. Airway communities also demonstrate resilience after perturbation, such as that associated with antibiotic therapy; communities most often return to a pre-perturbation configuration suggesting a reassembly of taxa that is more ordered than stochastic.

In a study assessing community dynamics among six young adults with CF over the course of a decade, community diversity was found to decrease significantly coincident with a progressive decline in lung function, similar to the observations made in cross-sectional studies [13]. In this study, advanced lung disease was marked by a dramatic reduction in diversity such that communities in persons with end-stage disease were often dominated by a single species. Again, inter-patient variability in community structure exceeded intra-patient variability (*i.e.* among serial samples collected over several years from the same individual); however, this was observed only during the intermediate stages of lung disease. With advanced disease, community structures converged based on the dominant species present (*e.g.* communities markedly dominated by *Pseudomonas* were indistinguishable). This pattern was also observed by FODOR *et al.* [15], who described low-diversity communities dominated by *Pseudomonas* that were more similar to each other than to communities dominated by *Burkholderia*. Thus, the picture that has emerged suggests that airway community structure is relatively stable and distinct in persons with intermediate lung disease, but as disease progresses with advancing age and as antibiotic therapy intensifies, community diversity decreases, resulting in less distinct, markedly constricted communities in advanced stages of lung disease.

Community dynamics around exacerbations

The well described associations between pulmonary exacerbations and lung disease progression in CF have stimulated intense interest in gaining a better understanding of the pathophysiological underpinnings of these events. How airway bacterial community dynamics may be associated with exacerbation onset, severity and response to therapy is an area of active investigation.

A commonly held belief that exacerbations are associated with an increase in airway total bacterial density and/or an increase in community diversity has been dispelled by several studies that fail to show these associations. Although often limited by a lack of samples in the days immediately preceding exacerbation, several studies have shown no significant increases in total bacterial load or diversity when comparing communities in sample sets obtained from the same individuals at baseline and at exacerbation onset [13, 16, 69, 80, 81]. However, at least one study suggests that differences in diversity around exacerbation may be a function of the community's initial (baseline) structure [69]. In this same study, the relative abundance of *Gemella*, a facultative anaerobe, increased significantly in 83% of samples at exacerbation and was found to be the most discriminative genus between baseline and exacerbation communities. Whether these findings are confirmed by larger scale studies remains to be seen.

While culture-independent studies have begun to elucidate how changes in the composition of airway microbial communities relate to lung disease progression, the activities of these complex communities remain largely unexplored. It is conceivable that changes in overall community activity (*i.e.* with respect to inter-species interactions and host–microbe interactions) are disproportionately dynamic relative to changes in community structure. Studies employing metabolomic and/or transcriptomic approaches are needed to assess this possibility and to better understand how changes in community function relate to host clinical status. In a recent study, STRUSS *et al.* [82] reported the increased concentration of N-(3-oxododecanoyl)homoserine-L-lactone (3-oxo-C_{12}-HSL), a quorum sensing molecule known to regulate virulence gene expression and biofilm formation, at the onset of exacerbation. Studies such as this have great potential to provide us with a much deeper understanding of how airway community structure and function relate to lung disease progression and response to therapy.

The gut microbiome

The microbiome of the human gastrointestinal tract has been a major focus of the Human Microbiome Project supported by the National Institutes of Health (Bethesda, MD, USA) Common Fund. Rapidly emerging studies are describing the myriad ways in which the microbial inhabitants of the gut influence systemic health and illness. The functional contributions of the gut microbiota include digestion and harvest of otherwise inaccessible nutrients, the production of vitamins and metabolism of xenobiotics [1]. Of particular note are recent studies linking the gut microbiome to the integrity and activity of the human immune system [83–87]. To date, there have been very few reports pertaining to the gut microbiome in persons with CF. Nevertheless, these initial studies suggest that gut microbial communities may have a striking impact on airway microbiota, inflammation and possibly lung disease progression.

Dysbiosis of gut microbiota

DUYTSCHAEVER et al. [29] characterised the faecal microbiome in paediatric patients with CF and their healthy siblings by using both culture and culture-independent methods. Higher abundances of lactic acid bacteria, clostridia, *Bifidobacterium* spp., *Veillonella* spp. and *Bacteroides/Prevotella* spp. were observed in healthy siblings, whereas greater abundances of enterobacteria were found in CF patients. In a follow-on study, this research group used DGGE and real-time PCR to confirm the significantly lower abundances of *Bifidobacterium* spp. and *Clostridium* spp. in CF patients [88]. They further observed a higher prevalence of amoxicillin-resistant *Enterobacteriaceae* in the CF patients compared to healthy siblings [89]. By using microarray analyses, SCANLAN et al. [90] similarly found decreased relative abundances of *Bifidobacterium* spp. in CF patients, as well as overall decreased bacterial community richness, evenness and diversity compared to non-CF controls. HOFFMAN et al. [91] investigated the gut microbiome in very young children with and without CF using Roche 454 GS FLX pyrosequencing and Illumina HiSeq sequencing. They found significantly higher abundances of *E. coli* in young children with CF than in healthy controls. The higher abundance of *E. coli* was correlated with faecal measures of nutrient malabsorption and inflammation.

The dysbiosis of the gut microbiome noted in persons with CF is probably due to several factors, not the least of which are frequent administration of systemic antibiotics and cystic fibrosis transmembrane conductance regulator (CFTR) dysfunction in gut epithelial cells. The profound effects of antibiotics on the gut microbiome in persons without CF are well documented [92–96]. With respect to CFTR dysfunction, SCHIPPA et al. [97] recently demonstrated a correlation between CFTR variants and alterations in faecal microbiome by using temperature gradient gel electrophoresis (TGGE) and species-specific PCR.

The gut–lung axis

An emerging body of evidence is drawing links between gut microbial communities and airway inflammation [98]. These observations have raised the possibilities for gut microbiome manipulation strategies in the treatment of respiratory diseases. Several studies have explored the use of oral probiotic supplementation to regulate lung inflammation [98, 99]. In a prospective, randomised, placebo-controlled, cross-over study of 38 paediatric CF patients, BRUZZESE et al. [100] found that patients receiving oral *Lactobacillus* GG had a reduced frequency of pulmonary exacerbations and hospitalisations. MADAN et al. [78] recently characterised the parallel development of the gut and respiratory microbiomes in infants with CF. They found a high degree of concordance in the bacterial dynamics between the two compartments, with gut colonisation of seven genera presaging their appearance in the respiratory tract. They also observed that changes in diet led to altered respiratory microbiomes, further suggesting that nutrition and the gut microbiome play important roles in the development of the lung microbiome. This could present opportunities for early intervention in CF with dietary and/or gut probiotic strategies.

Implications for management and future research directions

The application of culture-independent techniques, particularly the use of next-generation DNA sequencing, has provided a greater appreciation of the complexity of the bacterial communities that inhabit the CF airways. Ongoing work focuses on deepening our understanding of how changes in these communities relate to fluctuations in clinical status and lung disease progression. Efforts to better understand how the activities of airway microbial communities have an impact on the host, and to better define the mechanisms underlying these complex interactions, are now underway.

It is unknown at present how these efforts may change our approach to clinical management of CF; however, several possible scenarios can be envisaged. Identifying community structures and/or changes in community structure or activity that track with clinical features of interest (*e.g.* impending exacerbation or lack of response to therapy) could provide useful biomarkers for anticipating these events. Finding correlations such as these would also certainly generate hypotheses regarding the pathological mechanisms underlying disease progression. From a diagnostic perspective, molecular identification of bacteria directly from sputum is an attractive proposition for clinical microbiology laboratories involved in CF sputum diagnostics. Technologies currently available allow rapid DNA sequencing, but the resulting data require curating and analysis by well-trained bioinformaticians. As analytical processes become more automated, it is likely that molecular diagnostics using next-generation sequencing will become part of the routine diagnostic pathway in sputum microbiology analysis.

A deeper understanding of the natural history of CF airway infection, based on longitudinal studies of large numbers of patients representing wide ranges of age, disease phenotype and lung function, would be expected to generate strategies to refine current approaches to therapy. We may find, for example, utility in employing a broader array of therapeutic approaches, ranging from use of intensive broad-spectrum antibiotic combinations to less aggressive, narrower spectrum therapy, or perhaps even probiotic strategies aimed at maintaining communities in "less harmful" configurations. As DNA sequencing technologies continue to advance, it is conceivable that monitoring of airway microbial communities will become routine and a critical component of a "personalised medicine" approach to CF care.

In this chapter, we have focused on bacterial communities. It is important to note that the inter-relationships between bacteria and other microbiota, such as fungi and viruses, are also largely unknown. Including nonbacterial microbes in future studies will be critical to a more complete understanding of the microbial ecology of the CF airway. It is also imperative that we better understand how the host epithelial and immune cell responses are modified by differences in these complex microbial communities. The integration of microbiomic analyses with other omics such as transcriptomics and metabolomics would be expected to advance our understanding of these processes. To do this effectively, longitudinal studies with deep phenotyping and genotyping of patients will be required.

References

1.   Turnbaugh PJ, Ley RE, Hamady M, *et al.* The human microbiome project. *Nature* 2007; 449: 804–810.
2.   Willner D, Haynes MR, Furlan M, *et al.* Spatial distribution of microbial communities in the cystic fibrosis lung. *ISME J* 2012; 6: 471–474.
3.   Charlson ES, Bittinger K, Haas AR, *et al.* Topographical continuity of bacterial populations in the healthy human respiratory tract. *Am J Respir Crit Care Med* 2011; 184: 957–963.
4.   Morris A, Beck JM, Schloss PD, *et al.* Comparison of the respiratory microbiome in healthy nonsmokers and smokers. *Am J Respir Crit Care Med* 2013; 187: 1067–1075.
5.   Hilty M, Burke C, Pedro H, *et al.* Disordered microbial communities in asthmatic airways. *PLoS One* 2010; 5: e8578.
6.   Goleva E, Jackson LP, Harris JK, *et al.* The effects of airway microbiome on corticosteroid responsiveness in asthma. *Am J Respir Crit Care Med* 2013; 188: 1193–1201.

7. Sze MA, Dimitriu PA, Hayashi S, *et al.* The lung tissue microbiome in chronic obstructive pulmonary disease. *Am J Respir Crit Care Med* 2012; 185: 1073–1080.

8. Molyneaux PL, Mallia P, Cox MJ, *et al.* Outgrowth of the bacterial airway microbiome after rhinovirus exacerbation of chronic obstructive pulmonary disease. *Am J Respir Crit Care Med* 2013; 188: 1224–1231.

9. Pragman AA, Kim HB, Reilly CS, *et al.* The lung microbiome in moderate and severe chronic obstructive pulmonary disease. *PLoS One* 2012; 7: e47305.

10. Rogers GB, van der Gast CJ, Cuthbertson L, *et al.* Clinical measures of disease in adult non-CF bronchiectasis correlate with airway microbiota composition. *Thorax* 2013; 68: 731–737.

11. Tunney MM, Einarsson GG, Wei L, *et al.* Lung microbiota and bacterial abundance in patients with bronchiectasis when clinically stable and during exacerbation. *Am J Respir Crit Care Med* 2013; 187: 1118–1126.

12. Rogers GB, Carroll MP, Zain NM, *et al.* Complexity, temporal stability, and clinical correlates of airway bacterial community composition in primary ciliary dyskinesia. *J Clin Microbiol* 2013; 51: 4029–4035.

13. Zhao J, Schloss PD, Kalikin LM, *et al.* Decade-long bacterial community dynamics in cystic fibrosis airways. *Proc Natl Acad Sci USA* 2012; 109: 5809–5814.

14. van der Gast CJ, Walker AW, Stressmann FA, *et al.* Partitioning core and satellite taxa from within cystic fibrosis lung bacterial communities. *ISME J* 2011; 5: 780–791.

15. Fodor AA, Klem ER, Gilpin DF, *et al.* The adult cystic fibrosis airway microbiota is stable over time and infection type, and highly resilient to antibiotic treatment of exacerbations. *PLoS One* 2012; 7: e45001.

16. Stressmann FA, Rogers GB, van der Gast CJ, *et al.* Long-term cultivation-independent microbial diversity analysis demonstrates that bacterial communities infecting the adult cystic fibrosis lung show stability and resilience. *Thorax* 2012; 67: 867–873.

17. LiPuma JJ. The changing microbial epidemiology in cystic fibrosis. *Clin Microbiol Rev* 2010; 23: 299–323.

18. Burns JL, Rolain JM. Culture-based diagnostic microbiology in cystic fibrosis: can we simplify the complexity? *J Cyst Fibros* 2014; 13: 1–9.

19. Sibley CD, Grinwis ME, Field TR, *et al.* Culture enriched molecular profiling of the cystic fibrosis airway microbiome. *PLoS One* 2011; 6: e22702.

20. Woese CR, Fox GE. Phylogenetic structure of the prokaryotic domain: the primary kingdoms. *Proc Natl Acad Sci USA* 1977; 74: 5088–5090.

21. Pace NR. A molecular view of microbial diversity and the biosphere. *Science* 1997; 276: 734–740.

22. Huse SM, Dethlefsen L, Huber JA, *et al.* Exploring microbial diversity and taxonomy using SSU rRNA hypervariable tag sequencing. *PLoS Genet* 2008; 4: e1000255.

23. Youssef N, Sheik CS, Krumholz LR, *et al.* Comparison of species richness estimates obtained using nearly complete fragments and simulated pyrosequencing-generated fragments in 16S rRNA gene-based environmental surveys. *Appl Environ Microbiol* 2009; 75: 5227–5236.

24. Schloss PD, Gevers D, Westcott SL. Reducing the effects of PCR amplification and sequencing artifacts on 16S rRNA-based studies. *PLoS One* 2011; 6: e27310.

25. Rogers GB, Hart CA, Mason JR, *et al.* Bacterial diversity in cases of lung infection in cystic fibrosis patients: 16S ribosomal DNA (rDNA) length heterogeneity PCR and 16S rDNA terminal restriction fragment length polymorphism profiling. *J Clin Microbiol* 2003; 41: 3548–3558.

26. Rogers GB, Carroll MP, Serisier DJ, *et al.* Characterization of bacterial community diversity in cystic fibrosis lung infections by use of 16s ribosomal DNA terminal restriction fragment length polymorphism profiling. *J Clin Microbiol* 2004; 42: 5176–5183.

27. Sibley CD, Parkins MD, Rabin HR, *et al.* A polymicrobial perspective of pulmonary infections exposes an enigmatic pathogen in cystic fibrosis patients. *Proc Natl Acad Sci USA* 2008; 105: 15070–15075.

28. Muyzer G, de Waal EC, Uitterlinden AG. Profiling of complex microbial populations by denaturing gradient gel electrophoresis analysis of polymerase chain reaction-amplified genes coding for 16S rRNA. *Appl Environ Microbiol* 1993; 59: 695–700.

29. Duytschaever G, Huys G, Bekaert M, *et al.* Cross-sectional and longitudinal comparisons of the predominant fecal microbiota compositions of a group of pediatric patients with cystic fibrosis and their healthy siblings. *Appl Environ Microbiol* 2011; 77: 8015–8024.

30. Brodie EL, Desantis TZ, Joyner DC, *et al.* Application of a high-density oligonucleotide microarray approach to study bacterial population dynamics during uranium reduction and reoxidation. *Appl Environ Microbiol* 2006; 72: 6288–6298.

31. DeSantis TZ, Brodie EL, Moberg JP, *et al.* High-density universal 16S rRNA microarray analysis reveals broader diversity than typical clone library when sampling the environment. *Microb Ecol* 2007; 53: 371–383.

32. Klepac-Ceraj V, Lemon KP, Martin TR, *et al.* Relationship between cystic fibrosis respiratory tract bacterial communities and age, genotype, antibiotics and *Pseudomonas aeruginosa*. *Environ Microbiol* 2010; 12: 1293–1303.

33. Harris JK, De Groote MA, Sagel SD, *et al.* Molecular identification of bacteria in bronchoalveolar lavage fluid from children with cystic fibrosis. *Proc Natl Acad Sci USA* 2007; 104: 20529–20533.

34. Mardis ER. Next-generation DNA sequencing methods. *Annu Rev Genomics Hum Genet* 2008; 9: 387–402.

35. Margulies M, Egholm M, Altman WE, *et al.* Genome sequencing in microfabricated high-density picolitre reactors. *Nature* 2005; 437: 376–380.

36. Metzker ML. Sequencing technologies – the next generation. *Nat Rev Genet* 2010; 11: 31–46.

37. Siqueira JF Jr, Fouad AF, Rocas IN. Pyrosequencing as a tool for better understanding of human microbiomes. *J Oral Microbiol* 2012; 4: 10743.

38. Maughan H, Wang PW, Diaz Caballero J, *et al.* Analysis of the cystic fibrosis lung microbiota *via* serial Illumina sequencing of bacterial 16S rRNA hypervariable regions. *PLoS One* 2012; 7: e45791.

39. Rothberg JM, Hinz W, Rearick TM, *et al.* An integrated semiconductor device enabling non-optical genome sequencing. *Nature* 2011; 475: 348–352.

40. Salipante SJ, Sengupta DJ, Rosenthal C, *et al.* Rapid 16S rRNA next-generation sequencing of polymicrobial clinical samples for diagnosis of complex bacterial infections. *PLoS One* 2013; 8: e65226.

41. Lim YW, Evangelista JS 3rd, Schmieder R, *et al.* Clinical insights from metagenomic analysis of sputum samples from patients with cystic fibrosis. *J Clin Microbiol* 2014; 52: 425–437.

42. Lim YW, Schmieder R, Haynes M, *et al.* Metagenomics and metatranscriptomics: windows on CF-associated viral and microbial communities. *J Cyst Fibros* 2013; 12: 154–164.

43. Schloss PD, Westcott SL, Ryabin T, *et al.* Introducing mothur: open-source, platform-independent, community-supported software for describing and comparing microbial communities. *Appl Environ Microbiol* 2009; 75: 7537–7541.

44. Caporaso JG, Kuczynski J, Stombaugh J, *et al.* QIIME allows analysis of high-throughput community sequencing data. *Nat Methods* 2010; 7: 335–336.

45. Koleff P, Gaston KJ, Lennon JJ. Measuring beta diversity for presence–absence data. *J Anim Ecol* 2003; 72: 367–382.

46. Legendre P, Legendre L. Numerical Ecology. 2nd Edn. Developments in Environmental Modelling 20. Amsterdam, Elsevier, 1998.

47. Bray JR, Curtis JT. An ordination of the upland forest communities of southern Wisconsin. *Ecol Monogr* 1957; 27: 325–349.

48. Lozupone C, Knight R. UniFrac: a new phylogenetic method for comparing microbial communities. *Appl Environ Microbiol* 2005; 71: 8228–8235.

49. Anderson MJ. A new method for non-parametric multivariate analysis of variance. *Austral Ecol* 2001; 26: 32–46.

50. Yue JC, Clayton MK. A similarity measure based on species proportions. *Commun Stat Theory Methods* 2005; 34: 2123–2131.

51. Gonzalez A, Knight R. Advancing analytical algorithms and pipelines for billions of microbial sequences. *Curr Opin Biotechnol* 2012; 23: 64–71.

52. Kuczynski J, Liu Z, Lozupone C, *et al.* Microbial community resemblance methods differ in their ability to detect biologically relevant patterns. *Nat Methods* 2010; 7: 813–819.

53. Ramette A. Multivariate analyses in microbial ecology. *FEMS Microbiol Ecol* 2007; 62: 142–160.

54. Prosser JI, Bohannan BJ, Curtis TP, *et al.* The role of ecological theory in microbial ecology. *Nat Rev Microbiol* 2007; 5: 384–392.

55. Kuczynski J, Lauber CL, Walters WA, *et al.* Experimental and analytical tools for studying the human microbiome. *Nat Rev Genet* 2012; 13: 47–58.

56. White JR, Nagarajan N, Pop M. Statistical methods for detecting differentially abundant features in clinical metagenomic samples. *PLoS Comput Biol* 2009; 5: e1000352.

57. Belda-Ferre P, Alcaraz LD, Cabrera-Rubio R, *et al.* The oral metagenome in health and disease. *ISME J* 2012; 6: 46–56.

58. Hsiao EY, McBride SW, Hsien S, *et al.* Microbiota modulate behavioral and physiological abnormalities associated with neurodevelopmental disorders. *Cell* 2013; 155: 1451–1463.

59. Robinson CJ, Young VB. Antibiotic administration alters the community structure of the gastrointestinal micobiota. *Gut Microbes* 2010; 1: 279–284.

60. Segata N, Izard J, Waldron L, *et al.* Metagenomic biomarker discovery and explanation. *Genome Biol* 2011; 12: R60.

61. Kostic AD, Gevers D, Pedamallu CS, *et al.* Genomic analysis identifies association of *Fusobacterium* with colorectal carcinoma. *Genome Res* 2012; 22: 292–298.

62. Morgan XC, Tickle TL, Sokol H, *et al.* Dysfunction of the intestinal microbiome in inflammatory bowel disease and treatment. *Genome Biol* 2012; 13: R79.

63. Maurice CF, Haiser HJ, Turnbaugh PJ. Xenobiotics shape the physiology and gene expression of the active human gut microbiome. *Cell* 2013; 152: 39–50.

64. Knights D, Costello EK, Knight R. Supervised classification of human microbiota. *FEMS Microbiol Rev* 2011; 35: 343–359.

65. Breiman L. Random Forests. *Mach Learn* 2001; 45: 5–32.

66. Cutler DR, Edwards TC Jr, Beard KH, *et al.* Random forests for classification in ecology. *Ecology* 2007; 88: 2783–2792.

67. Yatsunenko T, Rey FE, Manary MJ, *et al.* Human gut microbiome viewed across age and geography. *Nature* 2012; 486: 222–227.

68. Zackular JP, Baxter NT, Iverson KD, *et al.* The gut microbiome modulates colon tumorigenesis. *MBio* 2013; 4: e00692–13.

69. Carmody LA, Zhao J, Schloss PD, *et al.* Changes in cystic fibrosis airway microbiota at pulmonary exacerbation. *Ann Am Thorac Soc* 2013; 10: 179–187.

70. Guss AM, Roeselers G, Newton IL, *et al.* Phylogenetic and metabolic diversity of bacteria associated with cystic fibrosis. *ISME J* 2011; 5: 20–29.

71. Zhao J, Carmody LA, Kalikin LM, *et al.* Impact of enhanced *Staphylococcus* DNA extraction on microbial community measures in cystic fibrosis sputum. *PLoS One* 2012; 7: e33127.

72. Rogers GB, Cuthbertson L, Hoffman LR, *et al.* Reducing bias in bacterial community analysis of lower respiratory infections. *ISME J* 2013; 7: 697–706.

73. Rogers GB, Marsh P, Stressmann AF, *et al.* The exclusion of dead bacterial cells is essential for accurate molecular analysis of clinical samples. *Clin Microbiol Infect* 2010; 16: 1656–1658.

74. Zhao J, Li J, Schloss PD, *et al.* Effect of sample storage conditions on culture-independent bacterial community measures in cystic fibrosis sputum specimens. *J Clin Microbiol* 2011; 49: 3717–3718.

75. Rogers GB, Carroll MP, Serisier DJ, *et al.* Use of 16S rRNA gene profiling by terminal restriction fragment length polymorphism analysis to compare bacterial communities in sputum and mouthwash samples from patients with cystic fibrosis. *J Clin Microbiol* 2006; 44: 2601–2604.

76. Filkins LM, Hampton TH, Gifford AH, *et al.* Prevalence of streptococci and increased polymicrobial diversity associated with cystic fibrosis patient stability. *J Bacteriol* 2012; 194: 4709–4717.

77. Cox MJ, Allgaier M, Taylor B, *et al.* Airway microbiota and pathogen abundance in age-stratified cystic fibrosis patients. *PLoS One* 2010; 5: e11044.

78. Madan JC, Koestler DC, Stanton BA, *et al.* Serial analysis of the gut and respiratory microbiome in cystic fibrosis in infancy: interaction between intestinal and respiratory tracts and impact of nutritional exposures. *MBio* 2012; 3: e00251–12.

79. Zhao J, Murray S, LiPuma JJ. Modeling the impact of antibiotic exposure on human microbiota. *Sci Rep* 2014; 4: 4345.

80. Price KE, Hampton TH, Gifford AH, *et al.* Unique microbial communities persist in individual cystic fibrosis patients throughout a clinical exacerbation. *Microbiome* 2013; 1: 27.

81. Stressmann FA, Rogers GB, Marsh P, *et al.* Does bacterial density in cystic fibrosis sputum increase prior to pulmonary exacerbation? *J Cyst Fibros* 2011; 10: 357–365.

82. Struss AK, Nunes A, Waalen J, *et al.* Toward implementation of quorum sensing autoinducers as biomarkers for infectious disease states. *Anal Chem* 2013; 85: 3355–3362.

83. Hooper LV, Stappenbeck TS, Hong CV, *et al.* Angiogenins: a new class of microbicidal proteins involved in innate immunity. *Nat Immunol* 2003; 4: 269–273.

84. Kamada N, Seo SU, Chen GY, *et al.* Role of the gut microbiota in immunity and inflammatory disease. *Nat Rev Immunol* 2013; 13: 321–335.

85. Lee YK, Mazmanian SK. Has the microbiota played a critical role in the evolution of the adaptive immune system? *Science* 2010; 330: 1768–1773.

86. Mazmanian SK, Liu CH, Tzianabos AO, *et al.* An immunomodulatory molecule of symbiotic bacteria directs maturation of the host immune system. *Cell* 2005; 122: 107–118.

87. Nagalingam NA, Lynch SV. Role of the microbiota in inflammatory bowel diseases. *Inflamm Bowel Dis* 2012; 18: 968–984.

88. Duytschaever G, Huys G, Bekaert M, *et al.* Dysbiosis of bifidobacteria and *Clostridium* cluster XIVa in the cystic fibrosis fecal microbiota. *J Cyst Fibros* 2013; 12: 206–215.

89. Duytschaever G, Huys G, Boulanger L, *et al.* Amoxicillin-clavulanic acid resistance in fecal *Enterobacteriaceae* from patients with cystic fibrosis and healthy siblings. *J Cyst Fibros* 2013; 12: 780–783.

90. Scanlan PD, Buckling A, Kong W, *et al.* Gut dysbiosis in cystic fibrosis. *J Cyst Fibros* 2012; 11: 454–455.

91. Hoffman LR, Pope CE, Hayden HS, *et al.* *Escherichia coli* dysbiosis correlates with gastrointestinal dysfunction in children with cystic fibrosis. *Clin Infect Dis* 2014; 58: 396–399.

92. Dethlefsen L, Relman DA. Incomplete recovery and individualized responses of the human distal gut microbiota to repeated antibiotic perturbation. *Proc Natl Acad Sci USA* 2011; 108: Suppl. 1, 4554–4561.

93. Jernberg C, Lofmark S, Edlund C, *et al.* Long-term impacts of antibiotic exposure on the human intestinal microbiota. *Microbiology* 2010; 156: 3216–3223.

94. Jakobsson HE, Jernberg C, Andersson AF, *et al.* Short-term antibiotic treatment has differing long-term impacts on the human throat and gut microbiome. *PLoS One* 2010; 5: e9836.

95. Jernberg C, Lofmark S, Edlund C, *et al.* Long-term ecological impacts of antibiotic administration on the human intestinal microbiota. *ISME J* 2007; 1: 56–66.

96. Dethlefsen L, Huse S, Sogin ML, *et al.* The pervasive effects of an antibiotic on the human gut microbiota, as revealed by deep 16S rRNA sequencing. *PLoS Biol* 2008; 6: e280.

97. Schippa S, Iebba V, Santangelo F, *et al.* Cystic fibrosis transmembrane conductance regulator (CFTR) allelic variants relate to shifts in faecal microbiota of cystic fibrosis patients. *PLoS One* 2013; 8: e61176.

98. Nagalingam NA, Cope EK, Lynch SV. Probiotic strategies for treatment of respiratory diseases. *Trends Microbiol* 2013; 21: 485–492.

99. Fujimura KE, Demoor T, Rauch M, *et al.* House dust exposure mediates gut microbiome *Lactobacillus* enrichment and airway immune defense against allergens and virus infection. *Proc Natl Acad Sci USA* 2014; 111: 805–810.

100. Bruzzese E, Raia V, Spagnuolo MI, *et al.* Effect of *Lactobacillus* GG supplementation on pulmonary exacerbations in patients with cystic fibrosis: a pilot study. *Clin Nutr* 2007; 26: 322–328.

Disclosures: None declared.

Chapter 4

Genetic and environmental modifiers of cystic fibrosis

Burkhard Tümmler[1,2] and Frauke Stanke[1,2]

Contemporary cystic fibrosis (CF) has become a chronic disorder that is shaped by a complex network of cystic fibrosis transmembrane conductance regulator (*CFTR*) mutations, other genes and nongenetic influences. Environmental modifiers and non-*CFTR* genetic variants each account for about 50% of the pulmonary phenotypic variability in Phe508del homozygous CF patients. The organisation and funding of domestic healthcare systems, the access to and provision of qualified CF care, adherence to treatment and sex-related issues, such as body image and sex hormones, are major modifiers of CF disease outcomes. Climate and microbes are important environmental determinants of CF disease. The disease-causing *CFTR* mutations, the haplotype of the *CFTR* linkage group and non-*CFTR* genetic variants contribute to the inherited components of CF. Genome-wide and candidate gene approaches have identified genetic modifiers of the processing, trafficking and activity of mutant CFTR and have resolved inherited risk factors for meconium ileus, liver disease and CF-related diabetes mellitus (CFRD) that explain a substantial part of the variance of these clinical phenotypes.

Cystic fibrosis: a not-so-fatal disease.

Douglas Crozier, 1974 [1]

Starting as a Mendelian monogenetic disease at conception, cystic fibrosis (CF) soon becomes a complex disorder that is shaped by cystic fibrosis transmembrane conductance regulator (*CFTR*) mutation genotype, non-*CFTR* genetic variation and nongenetic influences [2–4]. The success of symptomatic treatment programmes, which within 50 years have transformed CF from a fatal disease with death in early childhood into a chronic disorder with a lifespan of currently more than 50 years, verifies Douglas Crozier's prophetic statement that at that time more narrow-minded peers appraised as a provocative delusion. In other words, over the years, our continuously improved understanding of the pathobiology of CF and its transformation into clinical management and treatment are the major non-CFTR modifiers of CF, at least in countries that allocate the necessary resources to CF care.

This chapter reports on our current knowledge of environmental modifiers of CF disease outcomes and critically reviews the attempts to resolve the genes other than *CFTR* that modify the basic defect and the clinical phenotypes of CF. Since a comprehensive review of the early modifier gene studies would be beyond the scope of this chapter, the reader is referred to published open-access reviews that comprehensively cover this topic [2, 3, 5–8].

[1]Clinical Research Group "Molecular Pathology of Cystic Fibrosis", Clinic for Paediatric Pneumology, Allergology and Neonatology, Hannover Medical School, Hannover Germany. [2]Biomedical Research in Endstage and Obstructive Lung Disease Hannover (BREATH), Member of the German Center for Lung Research, Hannover Medical School, Hannover, Germany.

Correspondence: Burkhard Tümmler, Clinical Research Group "Molecular Pathology of Cystic Fibrosis", Clinic for Paediatric Pneumology, Allergology and Neonatology, OE 6710, Hannover Medical School, Carl-Neuberg-Strasse 1, D-30625 Hannover, Germany. E-mail: tuemmler.burkhard@mh-hannover.de

Relative role of genetics and environment

The clinical phenotypes of CF are determined by variable contributions of *CFTR* mutation genotype, genetic modifiers and environmental influences [3, 4]. Heritability is close to one for ion transport abnormalities, male infertility [8], meconium ileus [9] and CF-related diabetes mellitus (CFRD) [10]. Male infertility and the salty sweat are determined by the underlying mutations in the two *CFTR* alleles [3, 8], and meconium ileus and CFRD, which are major complications of CF seen in a minority of patients, are predominantly determined by non-*CFTR* genetic variation [9, 10].

Weight-for-height and lung function are surrogate parameters for gastrointestinal and pulmonary CF disease. Data from two independent CF twin and sibling cohorts [11, 12] consistently demonstrated that inherited factors have a larger impact on the patient-to-patient variation in weight-for-height than on lung function (fig. 1). Non-*CFTR* genetic variants account for about 50% of the pulmonary phenotypic variability in CF patients with the same *CFTR* genotype (homozygous Phe508del) [12, 14].

Environmental factors that shape CF disease

Prenatal life

The comparison of lung function, weight and height between sibling pairs, dizygous and mono-zygous CF twins has revealed that dizygous twins are as concordant as monozygous twins in anthropometry, but differ in their lung function as if they were siblings from separate pregnancies.

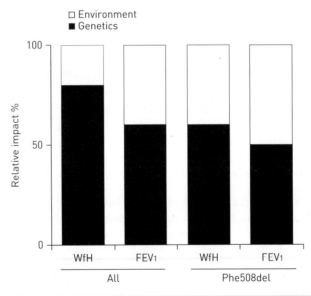

Figure 1. Relative impact of inherited and environmental factors on manifestation of cystic fibrosis (CF) disease as estimated by genetic modelling of monozygous CF twins, dizygous CF twins and CF sibling pairs. Covariance matrices of weight-for-height (WfH) % predicted and forced expiratory volume in 1 s (FEV1) % predicted were analysed by genetic modelling [13]. All CF pairs and the subgroup of Phe508del-*CFTR* (cystic fibrosis transmembrane conductance regulator) homozygotes were evaluated. Models were based on a linear combination of the four following factors: random environmental effects, shared environmental effects, and additive and dominant genetic effects. Reproduced and modified from [12] with permission from the publisher.

This data from the European CF Twin and Sibling Study (ECFTSS) [12, 15] indicates that life *in utero* strongly influences postnatal growth and anthropometry, whereas the course of lung disease is shaped after birth. Consistent with these findings from Europe, the CF Twin and Sibling Study conducted in the USA observed that active maternal smoking during pregnancy was associated with a significantly lower birthweight, as expected based on the well-established risk associated with smoking behaviour during pregnancy in the general population [16], but did not affect postnatal lung function [17].

Physical environment

Climate
When the parameters temperature, humidity and air pollution were studied, warmer ambient annual temperatures were shown to be significantly associated with a poorer lung function [18]. For example, an 18-year-old white male with CF (height 175 cm) with a forced expiratory volume in 1 s (FEV1) of 73.5% predicted living in a cold climate would be expected to have an FEV1 of 66.1% predicted had he resided in a 17°C warmer climate [18]. The prevalence of the lead pathogen *Pseudomonas aeruginosa* is also higher among individuals with CF who are living in a warmer climate [18].

Season plays a major role. In the northern hemisphere, lung function of a CF patient is better in cold January than in warm July [18]. In the temperate and continental climate zones, the environmental aquatic bacterium *P. aeruginosa* is more frequently acquired in summer and autumn than in winter and spring [19]. No seasonal difference, however, was observed in the rate of acquisition of the other major pathogen in CF, *Staphylococcus aureus*, which is reasonable because *S. aureus* resides in the human nares as its major habitat [19].

Environmental pollution
Outdoor air pollution influences the progression of CF lung disease. In a CF registry study, ozone exposure was associated with an increase in the number of pulmonary exacerbations, and particulate exposure was associated with both an increased number of pulmonary exacerbations and a decrease in FEV1 [4]. Similarly, second-hand smoke in the home adversely affects lung function in CF [17], as must be expected due to the well-characterised risks associated with exposure to second-hand smoke in the general population [20].

Exposure to the microbial world
The acquisition of infectious agents is the key environmental modifier that determines course and prognosis of most patients with CF. The major pathogens are (in alphabetical order) *Achromobacter xylosoxidans*, the *Burkholderia cepacia* complex (particularly *Burkholderia multivorans*, *Burkholderia cenocepacia*, and *Burkholderia dolosa*), *Haemophilus influenzae*, *Mycobacterium abscessus*, *Pandoraea* spp., *P. aeruginosa*, *Scedosporium* spp. and *S. aureus* (methicillin-sensitive and -resistant *S. aureus*). The CF host is compromised in bacterial clearance [21]; therefore, bacteria with low colonising capacity can take residence in the upper and lower CF airways. CF patients who are chronically infected with *B. multivorans*, *B. cenocepacia*, *B. dolosa*, *M. abscessus*, *Pandoraea* spp. or methicillin-resistant *S. aureus* experience a more rapid decline of lung function than their noncolonised CF peers.

The most prevalent bacterial species in CF airways are *S. aureus* and *P. aeruginosa*. Since 30–50% of the healthy population are colonised with *S. aureus* in their nares, the CF patient typically shares its clone with the non-CF family members [22]. *P. aeruginosa*, however, is

49

typically acquired from the aquatic inanimate environment and only by patient-to-patient spread in cases of highly transmissible lineages [23].

The species of the *B. cepacia* complex, particularly *B. multivorans* and *B. cenocepacia*, are especially problematic in CF because of the potential severity of respiratory infections, the easy patient-to-patient spread of the organisms and their innate resistance to a wide range of antimicrobial agents [24–26]. *Burkholderia* spp. preferentially inhabit the plant rhizosphere, and the risk of a CF patient acquiring a particular *Burkholderia* sp. depends on the local climate, plant and crop populations and the patient's activities and living conditions. *B. cenocepacia*, for example, was highly prevalent in the maize rhizosphere of fields with heavy use of pesticides, herbicides and fertilisers [26, 27].

Respiratory viral infections may be associated with the progression of CF airway disease, although this association is only well documented for the short term [4]. For example, the incidence rate of pulmonary exacerbations defined as treatment of a respiratory illness with intravenous antibiotics is increased by about 8% in the influenza season compared to the summer season [28].

Airway infections in CF are polymicrobial in nature [29]. The interaction of pathogens with commensals and nonpathogenic bystanders adds a further layer of complexity on the CF host: microbe interaction. Nonclassical members of the CF airway microbiome that are missed by standard conventional microbiology can contribute to disease either directly as pathogens or through synergy with conventional pathogens by triggering exacerbations [30]. Moreover, gut and airway microbiomes influence each other. The serial analysis of gut and respiratory microbiomes in CF infants demonstrated that colonisation of the respiratory tract by microbes is presaged by colonisation of the gut, and that changes in diet also result in altered respiratory microflora [31]. In other words, diet and the gut microbiome can modify the composition of the respiratory microbiome, which mediates the pulmonary damage in CF.

Sociodemographic, cultural and family context

Sociodemographic characteristics (ethnicity, sex, age and socioeconomic status) have important associations with CF disease outcome [4]. Social class, sex and region of residence are determinants of survival of patients with CF [32]. Moreover, personal and family function affect adherence and disease-management skills.

Socioeconomic status
Socioeconomic status is a strong modulator of the course and prognosis of CF. The risk of death was found to be 2.75 times higher for patients whose fathers had a manual *versus* non-manual occupation in the UK [32] and 3.65 times higher in Medicaid compared to non-Medicaid patients in the USA [33]. Survivors have significantly worse lung function and nutritional status.

Sex
The so-called "gender gap" in CF [34], which has been observed in many but not all studies, means that CF females have poorer survival, worse anthropometry and pulmonary function and are hospitalised more often [35] than age-matched CF males. This gap was consistent across a wide variety of national healthcare systems, suggesting a sex-specific effect on mortality [36]. CF males and CF females differ in their attitudes towards body image,

nutrition and exercise. Males desire a higher body size, exercise more regularly and eat better and more frequently, which are all favourable attitudes in the context of CF [37, 38].

Healthcare-related modifiers of CF

Therapy and management of CF have continuously improved since the 1950s. Healthcare-related modifiers strongly modulate CF disease, and show corresponding changes over recent decades.

Newborn screening

Newborn screening bears the potential to diagnose CF in the asymptomatic stage. Comparison of the CF registries in the USA and Australia revealed that patients benefit from newborn screening [39]. Children diagnosed after newborn screening had higher mean FEV1 and body mass index than children diagnosed clinically (absolute differences of 5.3% predicted and 0.26 kg·m^{-2}, respectively). Newborn screening is a beneficial modifier of CF disease.

Birth cohort

Thanks to the continuous refinement of the treatment of CF, the life expectancy of individuals with CF has dramatically increased over the last five decades. For example, in Germany, the median age at death was 9.3 years in 1980 and now is expected to be close to 50 years for the currently living patient cohort [40]. The date of birth is thus a major confounder of any study that aims to resolve genetic or environmental modifiers of CF. For example, a modifier detected in a CF population born in the 1970s may not be valid for those born in the 1990s. Conversely, a risk genotype identified in contemporary adolescents may be found significantly less frequently than expected in adults who were born in the 1960s. This depletion of risk genotypes at modifier loci will reduce the contrast that is detectable by genotyping and subsequent case–control comparisons between a CF case (severe) and a CF control (mild) population, leading the investigators to the false conclusion that the gene under study is not a modifier of CF disease because the test statistic returns a nonsignificant value. The survivor bias in the elder patient population may manifest in the deviation of genotype frequencies of modifiers from Hardy–Weinberg equilibrium or in a distortion of transmitted *versus* nontransmitted alleles when parent–offspring trios are considered.

Healthcare systems and access to care

The American and European CF societies have published consensus guidelines for the standards of care of CF [41, 42]. However, the access to and the quality of care still varies from country to country in Europe, reflecting the differential organisation of healthcare systems and the variable resources that are allocated to rare diseases such as CF.

The European Cystic Fibrosis Demographics Registry has uncovered demographic disparities between the CF patient populations in 12 European Union (EU) and 23 non-EU countries as per membership status in 2003 [43]. The median age of CF patients in EU and non-EU countries was 17.0 and 12.1 years, respectively, and the proportion of patients older than 40 years was higher in EU countries (5%) than in non-EU countries (2%). These differences persisted among the subgroup of Phe508del homozygotes. The CF population declines at an earlier age and with greater rapidity in non-EU countries than in EU countries.

The comparison of the organisation and funding of CF care gives a hint as to why survival still shows a large gradient in Europe. The spectrum ranges from the well-organised and well-funded CF care in Sweden to the absence of any special institution for CF care in some south-eastern and eastern European countries. In Sweden, where patients currently can expect the highest life expectancy, the support available to adults and children with disabilities is regulated by law. The county council and the municipality share responsibility for health and medical care, habilitation, rehabilitation and practical aids. In Germany, treatment is paid for by the 134 independent health insurance companies. The funding of a CF centre varies from centre to centre because the funding depends on the outcome of the individual negotiations of the CF centre with health insurance companies and the Kassenärztliche Vereinigung (Association of Statutory Health Insurance Physicians). Moreover, due to the limited interest of adult pneumologists at university hospitals for CF, CF centres for adults exist in only a few regions of the country. Spain belongs to the countries with no accredited CF centres according to European Cystic Fibrosis Society guidelines; however, specialised CF care is offered by approximately 70 hospitals. Albania has the highest frequency of CF. The sole CF clinic is run by specialist doctors. Most basic treatments are free, but there are regular shortages of drugs and supplies and some essential measures such as sputum tests must be paid for. CF care in Belarus and the Ukraine depends on the activity of a few enthusiastic doctors. There are no trained CF dieticians, CF nurses and CF physiotherapists and the access to some expensive medication is restricted to in-patient care.

In summary, the place of residence is (unfortunately) an important modifier of outcome in CF.

Diagnostic and treatment modalities

Although networks of CF centres with expertise in the treatment of CF have been set up in numerous countries, there is significant variation in disease outcomes among accredited CF centres [40, 41, 44]. According to registry studies, this variation reflects different modes of outpatient monitoring, drug prescription and implementation of guidelines. To battle these variations of effectiveness, quality improvement projects have been set up based upon the benchmarking procedure, learning from the best, and performing quality improvement work according to the plan–do–check–act cycle [45]. An instructive example is the German benchmarking project [45]. Best clinical practice was defined and marked by ranking and follow-up. Centres performing best were asked to define their specific strategy (more aggressive, earlier and more consistent antibiotic therapy and infection control, more individualised dietary counselling and follow-up). These points of best practice were then used by the other centres to feed a learning process and quality improvement procedure, and indeed improvement could be reached by several centres.

Disease outcome is not only modified by the practice of the local CF centre, but also by the quality of diagnostic services. Antimicrobial treatment is based on standard clinical microbiology testing of samples from the respiratory tract. Quality assessment uncovered a large gradient in the quality of CF microbiology service in Europe [46]. Rare or emerging pathogens were not detected or misclassified by many laboratories. The quartile with the largest number of mistakes was populated by laboratories located in southern, south-eastern or eastern Europe, each of which was a major reference laboratory for CF microbiology in their home country.

Adherence

Adherence to CF treatment recommendations is significantly associated with disease outcome. Adherence correlates with optimism, family function, disease knowledge and parental education [4]. In a recently published retrospective longitudinal study, the relation between medication adherence and health outcomes for people with CF was examined for the first time [47]. Patient pharmacy refill records were used to calculate a medication possession ratio (MPR), defined as the sum of all days of medication supply received, divided by the number of days the medication was prescribed for chronic use during the study period. The median composite MPR for all treatment was 63%. A lower composite MPR significantly predicted having one or more courses of *i.v.* antibiotics to treat a pulmonary exacerbation during the year. Lung function was maintained in those patients with adherence >80%, while those with <80% adherence experienced a loss in lung function. In summary, medication adherence in the treatment of CF is a highly relevant modifier.

Genetic factors that shape CF disease

Sex

Besides cultural sex-related issues that influence body image and physical activity (see above), sex as a biological entity is also a modifier of CF. The ECFTSS [15] investigated mixed-sex sibling pairs, who present the best group to resolve the impact of sex on disease outcome in CF. Girls had better body mass index (BMI) and lung function than boys until the age of 14 years, but worse anthropometry and pulmonary function during adolescence until the age of 20 years. Thereafter, no significant difference was seen between male and female CF siblings. Puberty seems to be the critical period that accounts for the "gender gap".

The underlying mechanisms are currently being resolved. The female sex hormone oestrogen affects key processes of CF pathophysiology, *i.e.* transepithelial ion transport, infection and inflammation [48, 49]. The most potent circulating oestrogen hormone, 17β-oestradiol, dehydrates the airway surface liquid in CF female bronchial epithelium [50, 51] and promotes the mucoid conversion of *P. aeruginosa* [52]. Circulating levels of 17β-oestradiol correlate with pulmonary exacerbations of menstruating females with CF. Exacerbations prominently occurred during the follicular phase, when oestradiol levels peak [52].

CFTR and neighbouring genes

The Mendelian monogenetic disease CF is caused by mutations in both *CFTR* alleles. However, *CFTR* is not only the primary cause of CF, but also one of its major modifiers. First, *CFTR* mutations can be sorted by severity and classified into "CF-causing mutation", "mutation of unknown significance" and "non-CF-causing mutation" [53, 54]. Secondly, the residual function of a CFTR mutant may be modified by intragenic polymorphisms and the *CFTR* haplotype. The following examples illustrate this argument.

The Met470Val variant is the most common missense polymorphism in the *CFTR* gene. The two variants differ in function. Met470 CFTR proteins mature more slowly and have a 1.7-fold increased intrinsic chloride channel activity compared with Val470 CFTR proteins [55], and correspondingly a CFTR mutant will have more residual activity on a Met470 than on a Val470 background. Please note that most sequence variants and CF mutations, including the major mutation Phe508del, are located on the ancestral Met470 allele [56].

Several *CFTR* mutations arose more than once on different genetic *CFTR* backgrounds, *i.e.* on different *CFTR* haplotypes. The clinically most relevant example is the Arg117His missense mutation, which is regularly associated with mild CF if it is linked with the T5 splice site allele in intron 8, and which, typically, is not disease causing if it is linked with the T7 splice site allele [57, 58].

Recombination is a further mechanism that can modify the phenotype of a CFTR mutant. Two major intragenic breakpoints are located distal of exon 13 in the *CFTR* gene [59]. If a mutation such as Phe508del occurred proximal to these breakpoints, the *CFTR* sequence distal to the breakpoint will differ between the original and the recombined alleles [59]. In case of Phe508del chromosomes, disease severity and basic defect of CF are significantly modified by the genetic background of the *CFTR* linkage group, which probably reflects genetic variation of cis-regulatory elements in the noncoding region of *CFTR* [12]. Moreover, the growth of Phe508del homozygous CF patients is associated with the genotype of markers located downstream of *CFTR* [60], and the so-called "extended B-haplotype" upstream of *CFTR*, which is in strong linkage disequilibrium with common CF mutations, is associated with extended postnatal female survival [61].

When disease-causing *CFTR* mutations are transmitted, the offspring will receive complete copies of the parental CF chromosomes if no recombination has occurred on chromosome 7. Starting in the *CFTR* gene, we have monitored the decay of parental allele sharing in the chromosome 7 of Phe508del homozygous sibling pairs who were either concordant or discordant in disease manifestation [62]. Concordant, but not discordant, CF sibling pairs shared a paternally imprinted locus about 20 Mb downstream of *CFTR*. In other words, the concordant sibling pairs shared a longer 3' segment of their paternal Phe508del chromosome than the discordant sibling pairs, whereby in the latter the meiotic recombination between non-CF and CF chromosome had occurred in the paternal germline in closer vicinity to the *CFTR* locus. Figure 2 visualises the principle of this generally applicable method to map imprinted modulators of disease in phenotypically informative sibling pairs.

Genetic modifiers in the genomic landscape

Approaches to identify genetic modifiers in the CF genome

The search for genetic modifiers of the Mendelian disease CF differs from the search for modifiers in non-Mendelian complex disorders such as asthma or chronic obstructive pulmonary disease [8]. CF is caused by mutations in the *CFTR* gene and any variants that influence the phenotype of a CFTR mutant are potentially more relevant than any *CFTR*-unrelated epistatic and gene–environment interactions.

Modifier studies in CF have been designed as case–control association and/or family-based (linkage) studies. The case–control approach has the advantage that it can more easily enrol a large number of affected subjects but the family-based sibling study can more properly control the impact of environmental confounders. To identify a modifier, researchers have pursued a candidate gene approach or have performed genome-wide association studies (GWASs) and linkage studies or (more recently) exome sequencing.

The choice of candidate genes is based on biological plausibility. In the early candidate gene modifier studies, few or even just one single-nucleotide polymorphism (SNP) in one candidate gene were tested (see table 1 in the review by WEILER and DRUMM [8]). This approach has the inherent flaw that any positive association signal may not be caused by the

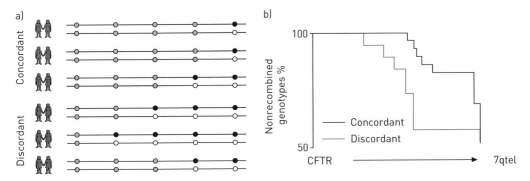

Figure 2. Differential decay of parent-of-origin-specific genomic sharing in cystic fibrosis (CF)-affected sibling pairs maps a paternally imprinted locus to 7q34. a) The principle of the assay is illustrated by three concordant sibling pairs and three discordant sibling pairs. Only one parental chromosome per sibling is shown next to the siblings. Alleles at five adjacent marker loci are visualised as circles, whereby grey colour for both siblings of a pair denotes a shared chromosomal segment, and black for one and white for the other sibling of a pair denotes an unshared genomic segment. b) The data was obtained from 29 clinically concordant and 19 clinically discordant Phe508del cystic fibrosis transmembrane conductance regulator (CFTR) homozygous sibling pairs at 11 loci spanning a 38-Mb genomic area from the *CFTR* gene on 7q32 to 7qtel. The decay of the proportion of nonrecombined and recombined paternal chromosomes was significantly different between concordant and discordant sibling pairs, indicating a paternally imprinted CF modifier gene on 7q34. Reproduced and modified from [62] with permission from the publisher.

queried SNP but by other sequence variants within this or neighbouring genes of the linkage group. The problem can be overcome in the context of a family-based study by haplotype-guided hierarchical fine mapping of the whole genomic region (fig. 3) [64]. Sequencing of the genomic fragment(s) for which contrasting phenotypes carry different haplotypes will finally identify the causal variant(s) by the base [64].

The major problem with a candidate gene approach is that it is a self-fulfilling hypothesis. Candidate genes are selected based on their possible role as a modifier, then the discovery of a significant association can lead to the conclusion that the choice of the candidate was correct. This has been a recurrent problem in association studies that have utilised candidate genes. The field has recognised that the solution to this problem is to insist upon independent replication. Functional studies based on the effect of the variant upon gene function can provide supportive information and if functional studies are extended to cell-based or animal model studies, a convincing argument can be made for a candidate gene playing a role as a modifier.

During the last decade, multi-array technology, which interrogates hundreds of thousands of SNPs for association at comparably low cost, has matured. Thus, unbiased GWASs that promise to identify gene modifiers not previously considered by heuristic reasoning have become possible. However, since population variants are tested with these commercial arrays, the effects at a particular locus are often low when there is substantial locus heterogeneity. To address this challenge, the hypothesis-driven GWAS (GWAS-HD) has recently been developed. A GWAS-HD exploits pre-existing knowledge about the pathobiology of CF to prioritise a set of genes (*e.g.* by ontology) [65] and, therefore, relies as strongly on the current perception of major disease determinants as a candidate gene approach.

Two consortia are currently conducting modifier studies in CF. The North American Cystic Fibrosis Gene Modifier Consortium (NACFGMC) [8, 66], which was recently joined by the French CF Modifier Gene Study, studies a large group of Phe508del homozygous patients

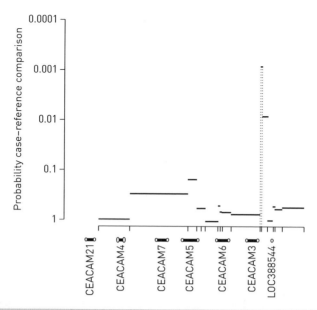

Figure 3. Haplotype-guided hierarchical fine mapping. Case–reference comparison of discordant and concordant sibling pairs from the European Cystic Fibrosis Twin and Sibling Study at 17 markers identified a 2.5-kb fragment in the intergenic region on 19q13 between carcinoembryonic antigen-related cell adhesion molecule (CEACAM)3 and the open reading frame LOC388544 (highlighted with dotted lines). After re-sequencing of carriers of contrasting haplotypes for this small genomic fragment, five single-nucleotide polymorphisms were identified that are responsible for the observed association. While this approach was not inspired by a candidate gene hypothesis but only by the markers' positions, the involvement of genes from the CEACAM family in host defence and innate immunity [63] designates these proteins as likely modifiers of cystic fibrosis, which is known for its cytokine imbalance and pro-inflammatory phenotype. Data from [64].

with mild or severe CF pulmonary disease, CF families with twins and siblings and a cohort of 70% of the patients from the Canadian CF population. The NACFGMC has pooled more than 5000 patient samples for genotyping to conduct GWASs of CF comorbidities and has set up two independent GWAS1 and GWAS2 cohorts. The ECFTSS [15, 67] has recruited Phe508del homozygous twin and sibling pairs from pre-selected European CF centres that are renowned for their high quality of care. By applying an age- and sex-adjusted disease severity algorithm [15], the extreme phenotypes of concordant mildly affected, concordant severely affected and clinically discordant sibling pairs were enrolled into the association study (fig. 4). Please note that discordant sibling pairs have the unique advantage of being able to identify modifiers that act in trans (fig. 5). The ECFTSS preferentially employs the pathophysiology of the basic defect rather than clinical variables such as pulmonary function [12].

Genetic modifiers of the basic defect

The ECFTSS has examined their Phe508del homozygous CF sibling cohort in the basic defect of impaired anion conductance by measurements of the transepithelial nasal potential difference (NPD) and the transepithelial ion transport in intestinal epithelium (intestinal current measurement (ICM)) [67]. Sequence variants in genes of the innate and adaptive immune systems were associated with residual Phe508del-*CFTR*-mediated current in respiratory and intestinal epithelium [12]. These unreplicated findings imply that genetic determinants of inflammation significantly influence residual ion flow in the CF epithelium. A cross-talk between epithelial ion transport and immune system already takes place at the level of the basic defect and not only secondary to infection.

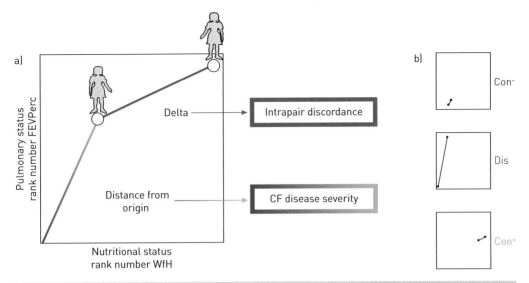

Figure 4. Extreme phenotypes for case–reference association studies in the European Cystic Fibrosis Twin and Sibling Study (ECFTSS). a) Definition of the composite parameter based on rank numbers for weight-for-height (WfH) % predicted and cystic fibrosis (CF) disease centiles for forced expiratory volume in 1 s % predicted (FEVPerc) [15]. Rank numbers were assigned for the entire study population of ECFTSS (318 pairs, individual patients ranked 1–636) and the most extreme phenotypes were selected for the association study based on delta and distance from origin. Note that the composite parameter delta is significantly lower for monozygous than for dizygous twins, while intrapair differences for WfH % predicted and FEVPerc are indistinguishable by zygosity. In other words, the composite parameter delta is more sensitive towards an inherited component than the individual parameters from which it is derived. b) Three examples of the same diagram for the extreme phenotypes. Con$^+$: concordant mildly affected; Con$^-$: concordant severely affected; Dis: discordant.

Lung disease

The NACFGMC identified and replicated significant association signals in a locus on chromosome 20q13.2 and on a chromosome 11p13 intergenic region near the *EHF* (Ets homologous factor) and *APIP* (apoptotic protease-activating factor 1-interacting protein) genes [66]. Two previously reported modifiers of CF lung disease, transforming growth factor (*TGF*)-*β1* [69] and interferon-related developmental regulator (*IFRD*)*1* [70], did not achieve genome-wide significance. EHF is an epithelia-specific Ets transcription factor and APIP is a known inhibitor of apoptosis. Selecting *EHF* as the likely candidate gene on 11p13, the ECFTSS has observed an association of rare *EHF* haplotypes among Phe508del homozygotes who exhibited CFTR-mediated residual chloride secretion in the ICM and an almost normal response to amiloride in the NPD [71]. The epithelial transcriptome of intestinal epithelial tissue derived from Phe508del homozygous carriers of two rare *EHF* alleles was enriched for genes that alter protein glycosylation and trafficking, both mechanisms being pivotal for the effective targeting of fully functional Phe508del CFTR to the apical membrane of epithelial cells. These data indicate that EHF modifies the CF phenotype by altering capabilities of the epithelial cell to correctly process the folding and trafficking of Phe508del-CFTR (fig. 6).

Chronic airway infections with *P. aeruginosa* represent a major comorbidity in CF. EMOND *et al.* [72] sequenced the whole coding region (exome) of the genomes of individuals with early age of onset of chronic *P. aeruginosa* infection and of the oldest individuals who had not reached chronic *P. aeruginosa* infection. Missense variants in a single gene, *DCTN4* (encoding dynactin 4) on chromosome 5q33.1, were found to modify the age-dependent risk of chronic airway acquisition of *P. aeruginosa*. Dynactin 4 is a component of the

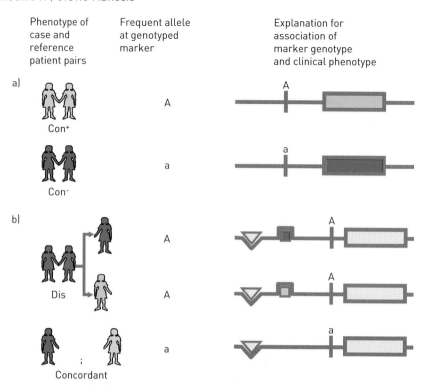

Figure 5. Mapping modifier genes in cystic fibrosis patient pairs by case–reference association studies in the European Cystic Fibrosis Twin and Sibling Study (ECFTSS). A genetic marker, here presenting alleles "A" and "a", can show an association with any of the extreme phenotypes: concordant mildly affected (Con⁺), concordant severely affected (Con⁻) or discordant (Dis). Genetic data in ECFTSS was evaluated by the software FAMHAP [68]. a) Mapping modifiers near the typed marker (in cis) by comparing Con⁺ and Con⁻ patient pairs. Association of the marker allele "A" with the phenotype Con⁺ can be explained if the targeted gene presents with a benign variant that occurs on the same haplotype as the marker allele "A" (green box). Analogously, if phenotype Con⁻ is associated with marker allele "a", the targeted candidate gene is likely to present as a risk allele on the same haplotype as the marker allele "a" (blue box). b) Mapping modifiers that are not near the typed marker (in trans) by comparing concordant and discordant patient pairs. An association of the marker allele "A" with the phenotype Dis cannot be explained by genetic variation close to the typed marker: two siblings of a Dis pair mostly share their alleles at the investigated loci, while their phenotype is dissimilar by designation. Consequently, their Dis phenotype cannot be based on the investigated sequence alone if these are shared by two Dis siblings. Instead, an observed allelic association with the Dis phenotype implies a regulatory element encoded in cis (not present among concordant chromosomes), which can be targeted by a DNA-binding protein encoded in trans (shown as blue/green boxes) or, alternatively, any similar gene–gene interaction at the transcriptional or post-transcriptional level. Functionally nonequivalent variants (blue or green) of these trans-acting factors can thus introduce discordance within sibling pairs, while concordant pairs who do not have this cis-responsive element are not sensitive to the allelic variants of the regulator.

dynein-dependent motor that moves autophagosomes along microtubules into lysosomes for degradation as part of the autophagy process. Autophagy seems to be essential for the clearance of *P. aeruginosa* in alveolar macrophages [73]. Therefore, one may hypothesise that the various isoforms of dynactin 4 are endowed with different efficacy to support the autophagy process.

Meconium ileus

Approximately 15% of newborns with CF experience meconium ileus. A family-based association analysis in a region of chromosome 8 that had previously shown linkage to meconium ileus [9] identified the methionine sulfoxide reductase A (*MSRA*) gene as a

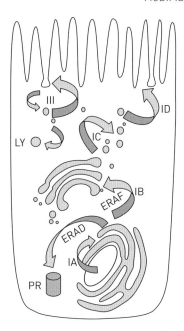

Figure 6. EHF (Ets homologous factor) regulates Phe508del-CFTR (cystic fibrosis transmembrane conductance regulator) biosynthesis, trafficking and post-translational modification. Mature, fully glycosylated and functional Phe508del-CFTR reaches the apical membrane through a complex trafficking pathway. These encompass biosynthesis and insertion into the lipid bilayer (IA), utilisation of the endoplasmic reticulum (ER)-associated folding (ERAF) pathway, passage through the ER, ERGIC (IB) and Golgi compartments, post-translational modifications and, finally, transport of mature Phe508del-CFTR to subapically localised vesicles (IC) and to the apical membrane (ID). In contrast, pathways that lead to degradation of Phe508del-CFTR are the ER-associated degradation (ERAD) pathway, which leads to degradation in the proteasome (PR), and the retrograde traffic of endosomes from the subapical compartment (III) toward the lysosome (LY). Reproduced and modified from [71] with permission from the publisher.

modifier of meconium ileus [74]. A causative role of *Msra* in meconium ileus could be inferred from studies in CF mice that demonstrated that the loss of Msra expression increased survival by reducing the rate of fatal intestinal obstruction [74]. An independent conventional GWAS identified SNPs in *SLC6A14* and *SLC26A9* to be significantly associated with meconium ileus, which accounted for less than 5% of the phenotypic variation [65]. A subsequent GWAS-HD single-SNP analysis identified the same SNPs in *SLC6A14* and *SLC26A9* as well as SNPs in *SLC9A3*, and GWAS-HD multi-SNP analysis spanning 155 genes provided evidence that multiple constituents of the apical plasma membrane are collectively associated with meconium ileus. These SNPs jointly explained a further ~17% of the meconium ileus variation in the North American sample [65]. The *SLC9A3* gene codes for a sodium-hydrogen exchanger, *SLC6A14* codes for a sodium- and chloride-dependent neutral and basic amino-acid transporter and *SLC26A9* encodes a chloride channel. The three genes are also expressed in the lungs. *SLC9A3* has been independently identified as a modifier of pulmonary function in CF [75] and SLC26A9-mediated chloride secretion is known to be essential for preventing mucus plugging in airways [76]. In other words, meconium ileus modifier genes also influence CF lung disease.

Diabetes mellitus

CFRD is highly prevalent among CF patients and is thought to result from the progressive destruction of islets of Langerhans by pancreatic fibrosis. Starting in the second decade of life, the prevalence continuously increases in a linear fashion. By the age of 35 years, 25% of the CF population is affected by CFRD [77]. Females are affected earlier than males. Compared with males, females have a 3.5 times higher risk for CFRD than males [77].

A GWAS identified *SLC26A9* as a genetic modifier of CFRD [78]. Thus, *SLC26A9* is a modifier of CFRD, meconium ileus [65] and probably also lung disease in CF. The fact that *SLC26A9* is recognised as a modifier for two disease manifestations with low phenotypic variability, as well as the more global outcome parameter lung function, suggests that SLC26A9 and CFTR share some functionalities, such as the direct response of ion transport in epithelial cells to inflammatory signals [12, 76]. A family history of type II diabetes triples the risk of CFRD, indicating that CFRD and type II diabetes may share common molecular determinants, and indeed BLACKMAN *et al.* [78] found significant associations for SNPs at the *TCF7L2*, *CDKN2A/B*, *CDKAL1* and *IGF2BP2* loci, the risk alleles being the same for type II diabetes and CFRD. When stratified by risk score for the five modifier alleles, the CFRD prevalence ranged from 11% in those with zero or one risk alleles to 40% in those with eight or more risk alleles [78].

Liver disease
The *SERPINA1* Z allele is a risk factor for severe liver disease in CF. Patients who carry the loss-of-function Z allele of the α_1-antitrypsin gene are at greater risk (odds ratio approximately 5) of developing severe liver disease with cirrhosis and portal hypertension [79].

Hindsight about the past and foresight for the future
Substantial progress in the identification of genetic modifiers of CF disease has been achieved in two areas: 1) the underlying genes and mechanisms that account for beneficial residual post-translational maturation, trafficking and activity of mutant CFTR activity in Phe508del homozygotes [12, 67, 71, 80–82]; and 2) genetic modifiers of CF comorbidities with a heritability of close to one (meconium ileus and CFRD) [65, 74–77].

Advances in the clinically most relevant field of CF lung disease are less impressive. *EHF*, which was identified in the GWAS of unrelated individuals as the only locus that significantly modulates lung disease [66], was later to be shown to be a global regulator of the processing of CFTR in epithelia [71]; hence, *EHF* is not a tissue-specific modifier but rather belongs to the aforementioned first area of progress.

Common sense and theoretical considerations readily explain the modest progress in the field of genetic modifiers of CF lung disease. First, in contrast to the two areas of progress already mentioned, heritability of lung disease is just 50% and we can envisage multiple epistatic and gene–environment interactions that are difficult to dissect. Secondly, more than a million variants can be simultaneously tested in GWASs. However, statistical penalties increase with the number of comparisons made [2, 8], thus making power a major limitation. To address this issue of power, we cannot deliberately increase the number of enrolled individuals as is possible for common diseases like asthma because 1) CF is a rare disease of small population size, and 2) the survivor bias and the differential quality of care in the global CF population will annihilate any gain of power theoretically obtainable from larger cohorts. A further bias is introduced by the commercial arrays that test common population variants. Relevant modifiers may be missed by locus heterogeneity, which may partly account for the low phenotypic variation that is explained by GWAS-identified modifiers. This is a major reason why we used an alternative approach to test candidate genomic regions in sibling pairs with extreme phenotypes [12, 64]. We typically first interrogate the region with a multi-allelic oligonucleotide repeat. Since these microsatellites show a higher mutation frequency than SNPs, any emergence of (rare) modifier variants during recent human evolution is more readily detectable with a microsatellite than with a phylogenetically ancient SNP. Haplotype-guided refined mapping in contrasting phenotypes will finally lead to the causal variant [64]. However, we have to admit that this procedure is slow, tedious and cannot be adopted as a high-throughput procedure because it has to be customised on a case-by-case basis. Fortunately, there are ongoing developments that may suit the needs of modifier studies in rare diseases.

The NACFGMC introduced GWAS-HD into the field [65]. The implementation of disease-specific knowledge into the evaluation of GWAS data will probably discover novel genetic modifiers of CF lung disease. Flagged genomic regions will then have to be scanned for the causal variant(s) by sequencing of many index cases. Conversely, one may first search for genetic modifiers by whole genome sequencing of selected individuals with extreme phenotypes and/or peculiar comorbidities and then test a promising set of variants in large patient cohorts [83]. The latter approach has the advantage that it directly identifies rare variants. Hot spots of rare variants are highly suggestive for clinically relevant susceptibility loci [84].

The genetic modifiers derived from GWASs and whole genome sequencing will not fully explain the phenotypic variation that is attributed to genomic variation. In the future we should consider the as yet unexplored (with one exception [62]) roles of imprinting and other epigenetic modifications on CF phenotype. The functional characterisation of causal variants and the transfer of knowledge to clinical care will be further important topics of the future agenda.

Conclusion

Contemporary CF has become a chronic disorder that is shaped by a complex network of *CFTR* mutations, other genes and nongenetic influences. We now appreciate the pivotal roles of domestic healthcare systems and of the individual quality of care and adherence for disease outcomes of CF. Cultural and biological causes of the "gender gap" are becoming clarified. Genetic modifier studies have contributed to our understanding of the pathobiology of Phe508del CFTR and have identified non-*CFTR* genetic variants that influence inherited complications of CF disease, such as meconium ileus and CFRD. The genotyping of validated risk alleles for liver disease and CFRD prior to clinical onset of symptoms could be tested in clinical studies or registries, to see whether it can improve management and disease outcomes.

CF disease is multifactorial. To wrap up the contents of the previous paragraphs into one conclusion, the major constitutional and man-made determinants of longevity of a life with CF are, listed in descending rank order: date of birth, (residual) activity of mutant CFTR in airway and intestinal epithelium, country of residence, CF team/CF physician in charge, individual socioeconomic status, airway microbiome, sex and non-*CFTR* genetic and epigenetic determinants of CF phenotypes.

References

1. Crozier DN. Cystic fibrosis: a not-so-fatal disease. *Pediatr Clin North Am* 1974; 21: 935–950.
2. Cutting GR. Modifier genes in Mendelian disorders: the example of cystic fibrosis. *Ann N Y Acad Sci* 2010; 1214: 57–69.
3. Drumm ML, Ziady AG, Davis PB. Genetic variation and clinical heterogeneity in cystic fibrosis. *Annu Rev Pathol* 2012; 7: 267–282.

4. Schechter MS. Nongenetic influences on cystic fibrosis outcomes. *Curr Opin Pulm Med* 2011; 17: 448–454.

5. Cutting GR. Modifier genetics: cystic fibrosis. *Annu Rev Genomics Hum Genet* 2005; 6: 237–260.

6. Knowles MR. Gene modifiers of lung disease. *Curr Opin Pulm Med* 2006; 12: 416–421.

7. Collaco JM, Cutting GR. Update on gene modifiers in cystic fibrosis. *Curr Opin Pulm Med* 2008; 14: 559–566.

8. Weiler CA, Drumm ML. Genetic influences on cystic fibrosis lung disease severity. *Front Pharmacol* 2013; 4: 40.

9. Blackman SM, Deering-Brose R, McWilliams R, *et al.* Relative contribution of genetic and nongenetic modifiers to intestinal obstruction in cystic fibrosis. *Gastroenterology* 2006; 131: 1030–1039.

10. Blackman SM, Hsu S, Vanscoy LL, *et al.* Genetic modifiers play a substantial role in diabetes complicating cystic fibrosis. *J Clin Endocrinol Metab* 2009; 94: 1302–1309.

11. Vanscoy LL, Blackman SM, Collaco JM, *et al.* Heritability of lung disease severity in cystic fibrosis. *Am J Respir Crit Care Med* 2007; 175: 1036–1043.

12. Stanke F, Becker T, Kumar V, *et al.* Genes that determine immunology and inflammation modify the basic defect of impaired ion conductance in cystic fibrosis epithelia. *J Med Genet* 2011; 48: 24–31.

13. Neale MC, Cardon LR, eds. Methodology for Genetic Studies of Twins and Families. Dordrecht, Kluwer Academic Publishers, 1992.

14. Collaco JM, Blackman SM, McGready J, *et al.* Quantification of the relative contribution of environmental and genetic factors to variation in cystic fibrosis lung function. *J Pediatr* 2010; 157: 802–807.

15. Mekus F, Ballmann M, Bronsveld I, *et al.* Categories of deltaF508 homozygous cystic fibrosis twin and sibling pairs with distinct phenotypic characteristics. *Twin Res* 2000; 3: 277–293.

16. Flower A, Shawe J, Stephenson J, *et al.* Pregnancy planning, smoking behaviour during pregnancy, and neonatal outcome: UK Millennium Cohort Study. *BMC Pregnancy Childbirth* 2013; 13: 238.

17. Collaco JM, Vanscoy L, Bremer L, *et al.* Interactions between secondhand smoke and genes that affect cystic fibrosis lung disease. *JAMA* 2008; 299: 417–424.

18. Collaco JM, McGready J, Green DM, *et al.* Effect of temperature on cystic fibrosis lung disease and infections: a replicated cohort study. *PLoS One* 2011; 6: e27784.

19. Psoter KJ, De Roos AJ, Wakefield J, *et al.* Season is associated with *Pseudomonas aeruginosa* acquisition in young children with cystic fibrosis. *Clin Microbiol Infect* 2013; 19: E483–E489.

20. Oberg M, Jaakkola MS, Woodward A, *et al.* Worldwide burden of disease from exposure to second-hand smoke: a retrospective analysis of data from 192 countries. *Lancet* 2011; 377: 139–146.

21. Pezzulo AA, Tang XX, Hoegger MJ, *et al.* Reduced airway surface pH impairs bacterial killing in the porcine cystic fibrosis lung. *Nature* 2012; 487: 109–113.

22. Goerke C, Kraning K, Stern M, *et al.* Molecular epidemiology of community-acquired *Staphylococcus aureus* in families with and without cystic fibrosis patients. *J Infect Dis* 2000; 181: 984–989.

23. Wiehlmann L, Cramer N, Ulrich J, *et al.* Effective prevention of *Pseudomonas aeruginosa* cross-infection at a cystic fibrosis centre – results of a 10-year prospective study. *Int J Med Microbiol* 2012; 302: 69–77.

24. Drevinek P, Mahenthiralingam E. *Burkholderia cenocepacia* in cystic fibrosis: epidemiology and molecular mechanisms of virulence. *Clin Microbiol Infect* 2010; 16: 821–830.

25. Lynch JP 3rd. *Burkholderia cepacia* complex: impact on the cystic fibrosis lung lesion. *Semin Respir Crit Care Med* 2009; 30: 596–610.

26. Vial L, Chapalain A, Groleau MC, *et al.* The various lifestyles of the *Burkholderia cepacia* complex species: a tribute to adaptation. *Environ Microbiol* 2011; 13: 1–12.

27. Fiore A, Laevens S, Bevivino A, *et al.* *Burkholderia cepacia* complex: distribution of genomovars among isolates from the maize rhizosphere in Italy. *Environ Microbiol* 2001; 3: 137–143.

28. Ortiz JR, Neuzil KM, Victor JC, *et al.* Influenza-associated cystic fibrosis pulmonary exacerbations. *Chest* 2010; 137: 852–860.

29. Rabin HR, Surette MG. The cystic fibrosis airway microbiome. *Curr Opin Pulm Med* 2012; 18: 622–627.

30. Sibley CD, Parkins MD, Rabin HR, *et al.* A polymicrobial perspective of pulmonary infections exposes an enigmatic pathogen in cystic fibrosis patients. *Proc Natl Acad Sci USA* 2008; 105: 15070–15075.

31. Madan JC, Koestler DC, Stanton BA, *et al.* Serial analysis of the gut and respiratory microbiome in cystic fibrosis in infancy: interaction between intestinal and respiratory tracts and impact of nutritional exposures. *MBio* 2012; 3: e00251–12.

32. Britton J. Effects of social class, sex, and region of residence on age at death from cystic fibrosis. *BMJ* 1989; 298: 483–487.

33. Schechter MS, Shelton BJ, Margolis PA, *et al.* The association of socioeconomic status with outcomes in cystic fibrosis patients in the United States. *Am J Respir Crit Care Med* 2001; 163: 1331–1337.

34. McIntyre K. Gender and survival in cystic fibrosis. *Curr Opin Pulm Med* 2013; 19: 692–697.

35. Stephenson A, Hux J, Tullis E, *et al.* Higher risk of hospitalization among females with cystic fibrosis. *J Cyst Fibros* 2011; 10: 93–99.

36. Fogarty A, Hubbard R, Britton J. International comparison of median age at death from cystic fibrosis. *Chest* 2000; 117: 1656–1660.

37. Willis E, Miller R, Wyn J. Gendered embodiment and survival for young people with cystic fibrosis. *Soc Sci Med* 2001; 53: 1163–1174.

38. Simon SL, Duncan CL, Horky SC, *et al.* Body satisfaction, nutritional adherence, and quality of life in youth with cystic fibrosis. *Pediatr Pulmonol* 2011; 46: 1085–1092.

39. Martin B, Schechter MS, Jaffe A, *et al.* Comparison of the US and Australian cystic fibrosis registries: the impact of newborn screening. *Pediatrics* 2012; 129: e348–e355.

40. Sens B, Stern M, eds. Qualitätssicherung Mukoviszidose [Quality Assurance in Cystic Fibrosis]. Bad Honnef, Hippocampus, 2012.

41. Cystic Fibrosis Foundation Patient Registry: Annual Data Report 2009. Bethesda, Cystic Fibrosis Foundation, 2011.

42. Kerem E, Conway S, Elborn S, *et al.* Standards of care for patients with cystic fibrosis: a European consensus. *J Cyst Fibros* 2005; 4: 7–26.

43. McCormick J, Mehta G, Olesen HV, *et al.* Comparative demographics of the European cystic fibrosis population: a cross-sectional database analysis. *Lancet* 2010; 375: 1007–1013.

44. Schechter MS. Demographic and center-related characteristics associated with low weight in pediatric CF patients. *Pediatr Pulmonol* 2002; 34: Suppl. 24, 331.

45. Stern M. The use of a cystic fibrosis patient registry to assess outcomes and improve cystic fibrosis care in Germany. *Curr Opin Pulm Med* 2011; 17: 473–477.

46. Hogardt M, Ulrich J, Riehn-Kopp H, *et al.* EuroCareCF quality assessment of diagnostic microbiology of cystic fibrosis isolates. *J Clin Microbiol* 2009; 47: 3435–3438.

47. Eakin MN, Bilderback A, Boyle MP, *et al.* Longitudinal association between medication adherence and lung health in people with cystic fibrosis. *J Cyst Fibros* 2011; 10: 258–264.

48. Sweezey NB, Ratjen F. The cystic fibrosis gender gap: potential roles of estrogen. *Pediatr Pulmonol* 2014; 49: 309–317.

49. Saint-Criq V, Harvey BJ. Estrogen and the cystic fibrosis gender gap. *Steroids* 2014; 81: 4–8.

50. Coakley RD, Sun H, Clunes LA, *et al.* 17β-Estradiol inhibits Ca^{2+}-dependent homeostasis of airway surface liquid volume in human cystic fibrosis airway epithelia. *J Clin Invest* 2008; 118: 4025–4035.

51. Saint-Criq V, Kim SH, Katzenellenbogen JA, *et al.* Non-genomic estrogen regulation of ion transport and airway surface liquid dynamics in cystic fibrosis bronchial epithelium. *PLoS One* 2013; 8: e78593.

52. Chotirmall SH, Smith SG, Gunaratnam C, *et al.* Effect of estrogen on *Pseudomonas* mucoidy and exacerbations in cystic fibrosis. *N Engl J Med* 2012; 366: 1978–1986.

53. The Clinical and Functional TRanslation of CFTR (CFTR2). www.cftr2.org Date last accessed: April 2, 2014. Date last updated: July 22, 2013.

54. Sosnay PR, Siklosi KR, Van Goor F, *et al.* Defining the disease liability of variants in the cystic fibrosis transmembrane conductance regulator gene. *Nat Genet* 2013; 45: 1160–1167.

55. Cuppens H, Lin W, Jaspers M, *et al.* Polyvariant mutant cystic fibrosis transmembrane conductance regulator genes. The polymorphic (Tg)m locus explains the partial penetrance of the T5 polymorphism as a disease mutation. *J Clin Invest* 1998; 101: 487–496.

56. Pompei F, Ciminelli BM, Bombieri C, *et al.* Haplotype block structure study of the *CFTR* gene. Most variants are associated with the M470 allele in several European populations. *Eur J Hum Genet* 2006; 14: 85–93.

57. Kiesewetter S, Macek M Jr, Davis C, *et al.* A mutation in *CFTR* produces different phenotypes depending on chromosomal background. *Nat Genet* 1993; 5: 274–278.

58. de Nooijer RA, Nobel JM, Arets HG, *et al.* Assessment of CFTR function in homozygous R117H-7T subjects. *J Cyst Fibros* 2011; 10: 326–332.

59. Dörk T, Neumann T, Wulbrand U, *et al.* Intra- and extragenic marker haplotypes of *CFTR* mutations in cystic fibrosis families. *Hum Genet* 1992; 88: 417–425.

60. Tümmler B, Aschendorff A, Darnedde T, *et al.* Marker haplotype association with growth in German cystic fibrosis patients. *Hum Genet* 1990; 84: 267–273.

61. Macek M Jr, Macek M Sr, Krebsová A, *et al.* Possible association of the allele status of the CS.7/HhaI polymorphism 5' of the *CFTR* gene with postnatal female survival. *Hum Genet* 1997; 99: 565–572.

62. Stanke F, Davenport C, Hedtfeld S, *et al.* Differential decay of parent-of-origin-specific genomic sharing in cystic fibrosis-affected sib pairs maps a paternally imprinted locus to 7q34. *Eur J Hum Genet* 2010; 18: 553–559.

63. Barnich N, Carvalho FA, Glasser AL, *et al.* CEACAM6 acts as a receptor for adherent-invasive E. coli, supporting ileal mucosa colonization in Crohn disease. *J Clin Invest* 2007; 117: 1566–1574.

64. Stanke F, Becker T, Hedtfeld S, *et al.* Hierarchical fine mapping of the cystic fibrosis modifier locus on 19q13 identifies an association with two elements near the genes *CEACAM3* and *CEACAM6*. *Hum Genet* 2010; 127: 383–394.

65. Sun L, Rommens JM, Corvol H, *et al.* Multiple apical plasma membrane constituents are associated with susceptibility to meconium ileus in individuals with cystic fibrosis. *Nat Genet* 2012; 44: 562–569.

66. Wright FA, Strug LJ, Doshi VK, *et al.* Genome-wide association and linkage identify modifier loci of lung disease severity in cystic fibrosis at 11p13 and 20q13.2. *Nat Genet* 2011; 43: 539–546.

67. Bronsveld I, Mekus F, Bijman J, *et al.* Chloride conductance and genetic background modulate the cystic fibrosis phenotype of Delta F508 homozygous twins and siblings. *J Clin Invest* 2001; 108: 1705–1715.

68. Herold C, Becker T. Genetic association analysis with FAMHAP: a major program update. *Bioinformatics* 2009; 25: 134–136.

69. Drumm ML, Konstan MW, Schluchter MD, *et al.* Genetic modifiers of lung disease in cystic fibrosis. *N Engl J Med* 2005; 353: 1443–1453.

70. Gu Y, Harley IT, Henderson LB, *et al.* Identification of *IFRD1* as a modifier gene for cystic fibrosis lung disease. *Nature* 2009; 458: 1039–1042.

71. Stanke F, van Barneveld A, Hedtfeld S, *et al.* The CF-modifying gene *EHF* promotes p.Phe508del-CFTR residual function by altering protein glycosylation and trafficking in epithelial cells. *Eur J Hum Genet* 2013 [In press DOI: 10.1038/ejhg.2013.209].

72. Emond MJ, Louie T, Emerson J, *et al.* Exome sequencing of extreme phenotypes identifies DCTN4 as a modifier of chronic *Pseudomonas aeruginosa* infection in cystic fibrosis. *Nat Genet* 2012; 44: 886–889.

73. Yuan K, Huang C, Fox J, *et al.* Autophagy plays an essential role in the clearance of *Pseudomonas aeruginosa* by alveolar macrophages. *J Cell Sci* 2012; 125: 507–515.

74. Henderson LB, Doshi VK, Blackman SM, *et al.* Variation in MSRA modifies risk of neonatal intestinal obstruction in cystic fibrosis. *PLoS Genet* 2012; 8: e1002580.

75. Dorfman R, Taylor C, Lin F, *et al.* Modulatory effect of the *SLC9A3* gene on susceptibility to infections and pulmonary function in children with cystic fibrosis. *Pediatr Pulmonol* 2011; 46: 385–392.

76. Anagnostopoulou P, Riederer B, Duerr J, *et al.* SLC26A9-mediated chloride secretion prevents mucus obstruction in airway inflammation. *J Clin Invest* 2012; 122: 3629–3634.

77. Scheuing N, Holl RW, Dockter G, *et al.* Diabetes in cystic fibrosis: multicenter screening results based on current guidelines. *PLoS One* 2013; 8: e81545.

78. Blackman SM, Commander CW, Watson C, *et al.* Genetic modifiers of cystic fibrosis-related diabetes. *Diabetes* 2013; 62: 3627–3635.

79. Bartlett JR, Friedman KJ, Ling SC, *et al.* Genetic modifiers of liver disease in cystic fibrosis. *JAMA* 2009; 302: 1076–1083.

80. Dupuit F, Kälin N, Brézillon S, *et al.* CFTR and differentiation markers expression in non-CF and ΔF508 homozygous CF nasal epithelium. *J Clin Invest* 1995; 96: 1601–1611.

81. Kälin N, Claass A, Sommer M, *et al.* ΔF508 CFTR protein expression in tissues from patients with cystic fibrosis. *J Clin Invest* 1999; 103: 1379–1389.

82. van Barneveld A, Stanke F, Tamm S, *et al.* Functional analysis of F508del CFTR in native human colon. *Biochim Biophys Acta* 2010; 1802: 1062–1069.

83. Guey LT, Kravic J, Melander O, *et al.* Power in the phenotypic extremes: a simulation study of power in discovery and replication of rare variants. *Genet Epidemiol* 2011; 35: 236–246.

84. Smirnova I, Mann N, Dols A, *et al.* Assay of locus-specific genetic load implicates rare Toll-like receptor 4 mutations in meningococcal susceptibility. *Proc Natl Acad Sci USA* 2003; 100: 6075–6080.

Acknowledgements: We would like to thank an anonymous reviewer for his instructive comments, particularly in the context of candidate gene modifier studies.

Support statement: Work in the authors' laboratory has been supported by grants from the BMBF (German Centre of Lung Research, Disease Area CF), DFG (SFB 621, C7), the Mukoviszidose e.V. and the Deutsche Fördergesellschaft für die Mukoviszidoseforschung.

Disclosures: None declared.

Chapter 5

Newborn screening for cystic fibrosis: opportunities and remaining challenges

Anil Mehta[1], Olaf Sommerburg[2] and Kevin W. Southern[3]

Newborn screening for cystic fibrosis (CF) is a reasonable public health strategy, when modified criteria for assessing such a programme are taken into account. A variety of protocols is employed, although all use measurement of immunoreactive trypsinogen (IRT) in the first week of life as a first step. Second-tier testing varies and there are insufficient data to critically compare strategies. In this chapter, we provide a subjective assessment of each protocol from the best available evidence, with the aim of highlighting how changes in protocol impact performance; for example, a strategy may improve specificity but at the expense of increased recognition of infants with an inconclusive diagnosis. Protocol selection is a matter of balancing priorities. Alternative strategies, such as measuring pancreatitis-associated protein (PAP), may improve performance, but further work is required to determine the optimal strategy. It is important that programmes continue to monitor performance against standards and aim to reduce unnecessary negative impact.

Evidence suggests that including cystic fibrosis (CF) in the panel of conditions for which newborn infants are screened results in an earlier diagnosis of this condition; however, it has been debated whether this has a significant impact on long-term health outcomes [1–3]. This has been one of the barriers to implementation of newborn screening in several countries across Europe. Other barriers have included political inertia and a lack of resources to support newborn screening or the appropriate processing of infants with a positive result.

When considering the validity of CF newborn screening, it is worth reflecting on the modified criteria developed by PETROS [4], who adapted and expanded the Wilson Junger criteria to provide a tool to rank newborn screening programmes. The expanded criteria take into account the mechanics of the programme, how the strategy integrates with existing public health resources and the impact on the family (table 1). By applying a scoring system to these modified criteria, PETROS [4] was able to provide a quantitative evaluation of newborn screening programmes, with excellent scores for established programmes such as phenylketonuria and congenital hypothyroidism, but poorer scores for other metabolic conditions.

[1]Medical Resarch Institute, Ninewells Hospital Medical School, University of Dundee, Dundee, UK. [2]Dept of Pediatric Oncology, Hematology, Immunology and Pulmonology, University Medical Center for Children and Adolescents, Angelika Lautenschläger Children's Hospital, Heidelberg, Germany. [3]Dept of Women's and Children's Health, University of Liverpool, Institute of Child Health, Alder Hey Children's Hospital, Liverpool, UK.

Correspondence: Anil Mehta, Medical Research Institute, Ninewells Hospital Medical School, University of Dundee, Dundee, DD1 9SY, UK. E-mail: a.mehta@dundee.ac.uk

Table 1. The revised criteria developed by PETROS [4] to evaluate the validity of a newborn screening programme

The test may be multiplexed or overlaid onto an existing structure or system
The "diagnostic odyssey" for the patient/family may be reduced or eliminated
Adverse outcome(s) are rare with a false-positive test
Treatment costs may be covered by third parties (either private or public)
Testing may be declined by parents/guardians
Adequate pre-testing information or counselling is available to parents/guardians
Screening in the newborn period is critical for prompt diagnosis and treatment
Public health infrastructure is in place to support all phases of the testing, diagnosis and
  interventions
If carriers are identified, genetic counselling is provided
Treatment risks and the impact of a false-positive test are explained to parents/guardians
The limitations of screening and the risks of a false-negative test are explained to parents/
  guardians

Each criterion is allocated a score, giving a quantitative assessment. Data from [4].

The CF programme scored well above the pre-determined threshold, supporting the validity of newborn screening as a strategy for early diagnosis and entry to appropriate care pathways.

However, the negative impact of this screening strategy on the population as a whole must be considered, most notably false-positive results, accidental recognition of carriers and "screen-positive" infants with an inconclusive diagnosis [5]. There is variability in the subjective appreciation of the importance of these, and to some degree, this has resulted in considerable variability across Europe with respect to protocol design and implementation. This is well illustrated by carrier recognition, considered negatively by some and positively by others (in that it may enable families to make informed reproductive decisions in future pregnancies).

The early diagnosis facilitated by a well-run screening programme removes the diagnostic odyssey that many families experience and has a positive impact on health outcomes, with a significantly reduced treatment burden [6, 7]. Most convincing have been the data from longer term epidemiological and cohort studies. One Australian study demonstrated a marked improvement in survival at 25 years in a screened cohort compared with a cohort diagnosed symptomatically immediately prior to the implementation of the newborn screening programme (fig. 1) [8]. This was an historical cohort study, performed before and after implementation of newborn screening in the region, meaning the screened infants may have been exposed to improved CF care; however, the length of the study makes the data compelling.

When designing a newborn screening protocol for CF, one is faced with a number of options and the choice of protocol may reflect opinion on the relative importance of avoiding negative outcomes. Strategies that improve the performance of a programme in one respect (*e.g.* timeliness) may have a negative impact on another aspect of the programme (*e.g.* incorporation of DNA testing improves timeliness but results in increased carrier recognition). The choice of protocol should also reflect the population characteristics of the region and, in some instances, the option to screen may not be valid if the prevalence of CF is very low or appropriate services are not available to properly care for these infants. In some poorly resourced countries, it has been recognised that implementation of newborn screening for CF may directly improve available services.

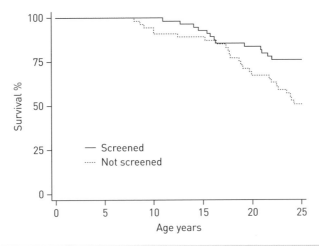

Figure 1. Kaplan–Meier plot of survival in two cohorts, one screened and one not screened. Reproduced and modified from [8] with permission from the publisher.

In this chapter, we will consider the dilemmas specific to CF screening, discuss the options available for screening newborns for CF, and balance the occurrence of negative impacts against the performance of the programme as demonstrated by good specificity (most positive newborn screening results identify an infant with CF), good sensitivity (minimal affected but not detected cases) and timeliness (prompt referral to a specialist CF team). These evaluations are based on available data, but for some strategies, more robust evidence is required and in these instances, we have made a subjective assessment based on available evidence.

Dilemmas specific to newborn screening

A national programme that embarks on newborn screening has to make a decision upfront as to whether the authorities consider that DNA analysis of the CF gene (the cystic fibrosis transmembrane conductance regulator (*CFTR*) gene) is, on balance, detrimental to the family or informative for future generations. If the developers of a particular programme decide that revealing this information is somehow different from any other kind of information about the infant, then an alternative strategy that does not involve any DNA analysis must be considered. The consequence of not incorporating DNA analysis (limited or extensive) is a significant increase in false-positive screening results, with impact on the family and on the health service (an increased number of sweat tests will need to be organised). At present there are two DNA-free strategies (described later), and it is possible that both strategies may result in a slightly reduced sensitivity, although more data are required to analyse this assertion [9, 10]. Incorporation of DNA analysis into a newborn screening protocol invariably has cost implications. In low-resource settings, DNA analysis may be seen as an alternative strategy to sweat testing, but this may lead to false-negative results and current guidelines support that sweat testing is an essential component of newborn screening for CF in order to confirm a diagnosis.

The inclusion of DNA analysis will result in increased carrier recognition and a rise in the number of infants with an inconclusive diagnosis. Some of these infants will have a condition that impacts negatively on their health at some point, but many will remain unaffected. The impact of this burden on families has not been studied at length, but is likely to be negative.

In the USA, infants with an unclear diagnosis following newborn screening are described as having *CFTR*-related metabolic syndrome (CRMS) [11]. The rationale behind this term is that it provides the family with a definitive end-point rather than leaving them "in limbo"; however, the reality is that this remains an unsatisfactory position for many families. It also facilitates inclusion of the infant into a health service, which requires a clear diagnosis. The European approach has been to avoid a definitive designation, and terms used to describe these infants such as "CF screen positive inconclusive diagnosis" have been advocated on the basis that they describe a fluid situation [12]. The recognition of infants with an unclear diagnosis is exacerbated by the inclusion of extended gene analysis in a newborn screening protocol. This is illustrated by data from California (USA), which showed that more infants with an unclear diagnosis (termed CRMS) were identified through their protocol than infants with a CF diagnosis [13]. To some degree, this also reflects the large Hispanic population in this region, and the choice of extended gene analysis for this protocol reflected a strategy to improve the positive predictive value (PPV) and sensitivity in this population with a relatively low prevalence of common CF causing mutations that affect northern European populations. This is not a problem that is unique to CF screening; in other monogenic disorders, such as metabolic enzyme defects, many more diagnoses are made than ever presented to clinicians, leaving metabolic clinics with uncertain diagnoses.

Identification of the CF gene when DNA analysis is added to the protocol remains a matter of discussion, with some arguing that the potential harms of carrier identification are so overwhelmingly bad that they call into question the use of DNA analysis in any newborn screening protocol. There are a number of issues that arise from the identification of a carrier: ongoing parental anxiety, induced depression, impaired bonding with the child, and treatment of the child thereafter as sickly or potentially sickly [14]. The quality of communication between the healthcare professionals and the patients has been criticised by both parents and the public health officials charged with implementing screening. Significant issues exist with the modes of communication between professionals and patients: use of jargon, a lack of assessment of the patient's understanding, an inability to organise a communication strategy, and a variable discussion of emotion as a hindrance to understanding (*i.e.* can recipients assimilate the information provided?). Healthcare professionals are aware of the need to include these aspects into the consultation when a carrier is identified, but are unable to access the relevant information as to the best application of that knowledge to improve the communication [15]. An important area for future research would be into a counselling approach that minimises misconceptions and takes into account the emotional distress of the subjects.

The internet as a positive tool

The issue of communication and its effects on the parents also applies to those who are falsely included in the initial screening test. In both instances (false positives and the identification of carriers), the parents views on the accuracy of the test, their child's future health and/or the implications of having a genetic mutation can lead to a sense of vulnerability in the emerging bond between the parents and the baby. Since it is common practice for parents to use the Internet, a good way forward would be for the best communication approaches to be laid out on an approved website with international agreement between different CF societies, and perhaps under the auspices of the World Health Organization, the European Union or some other international body. A place is needed for parents to access high-quality "curated" information safely and in a manner that can be regularly updated as techniques change over time.

The declining incidence

When a diagnosis of CF is made within the family context, the issue of termination of the pregnancy, whether it is the current pregnancy during an antenatal screening programme or a future pregnancy after newborn screening, is likely to arise. Experience shows that typically, the incidence of CF will decline by about 50% after an antenatal programme is instituted because parents chose to terminate the pregnancy [16]. For example, an antenatal screening programme performed around Edinburgh (UK) halved the number of diagnoses [17]. However, even in the Australian example, where newborn screening had existed for 20 years, and no antenatal programme was present, for every 5.5 diagnoses made by newborn screening, there was one termination of pregnancy [18]. The latter is more likely to have arisen because of the positive screening result in a previously affected child and a subsequent affected pregnancy being diagnosed by fetal sampling. As diagnostic science progresses, and maternal blood content of fetal DNA during pregnancy is now being analysed to examine the status of the baby *in utero*, it is likely that there will be increased opportunities for *in utero* diagnosis of CF. However, in some societies in which termination of pregnancy is unacceptable for religious or personal reasons, babies with CF will continue to be born, albeit perhaps at a lower frequency than today [19]. This issue has been brought sharply into focus with the possibility of new and expensive but potentially disease-arresting therapies targeted at the restoration of the ion transport functions of the CF protein and/or its relocation to its correct cellular position. Thus, today we sit at an interesting junction of new complex developments.

Mutations and admixture of populations

The previously discussed issues are compounded because the genetic mixture between races is increasing, particularly in the large cities of the world (one in 64 UK CF cases are from an ethnic minority, most from the Indian sub-continent). Traditionally felt to be a predominately Caucasian disease, CF will become a more racially diverse disease through genetic mixing. The net result is that the clinical validity of labelling a child as having "clear-cut CF" may become less certain as rarer genotypes enter the predominantly European gene pool. This will make genetic counselling an extremely difficult issue for future generations [20]. It is likely that registries with international standardisation of data are going to be most informative in our attempts to understand the outcomes that follow newborn screening. These issues have recently been reviewed and as these programmes evolve, robust procedures for auditing each programme must be put into place [21, 22].

FEREC and CUTTING [23] reviewed the disease liability of the mutations detected in the *CFTR* gene after screening. A cursory examination of the genetics of CF showed that in areas such as Israel, which has a high proportion of Ashkenazi Jews, the predominantly white northern European Caucasian mutation (Phe508del) is not the commonest genotype present in that population. However, should you live on the Faroe Islands of Denmark, the exact opposite is true. The Ashkenazi Jewish population commonly carry a stop mutation that causes the protein to be truncated at position 1281, near its C-terminus, which is not present in those indigenous to the Danish island. This finding encapsulates the difficulties of creating a uniform recommendation for CF screening that is applicable to every part of the globe. This argument may be flawed for a couple of principal reasons. Although in some countries, the uptake of selective termination for a CF-affected fetus is as high as 80% or 90%, this percentage varies dramatically between countries. In addition, the bioethics of the termination of pregnancy in a setting where new therapies might be disease-arresting poses new ethical dilemmas. Complexity increases further when this notion is coupled with concluding remarks from FEREC and CUTTING [23]: "Last but not least, it becomes more evident that the precise knowledge of the *CFTR* mutations will be a prerequisite for the rational basis for mutations-specific therapies that are now imminent". CF will not be the last such disease in which new therapies may point to the need to reconsider a termination as the solution of first choice in effected pregnancies. Principally these difficulties arise because of the uncertainty that lies between the genetic certainty that a mutation is present and the clinical validity of the argument that a particular mutation will lead to premature death for that particular baby in that particular family. As recently demonstrated, even the classification and placement of a patient into pancreatic-sufficient or pancreatic-insufficient groups is not a simple matter in the first year of life [24]. This is important because pancreatic status correlates with outcome in a number of studies. O'SULLIVAN *et al.* [24] point out that a grey zone exists between pancreatic sufficiency and insufficiency, and that patients may oscillate between the two states depending on the cut-off chosen for the pancreatic enzyme test level and dietary factors that may also influence the stimulation of the pancreas. Ultimately, it will be for countries to establish their own policies with respect to the decision on newborn screening.

Expansion of newborn screening across Europe has been steady but patchy, with a variety of factors impacting on implementation. In Germany, these factors have included DNA analysis concerns; a national German programme has not been established despite successful pilot studies in two regions [25]. In contrast, Switzerland successfully introduced a national programme in 2011 [26]. The programme received high satisfaction indices with a maximum of 11 refusals per year from >83 000 screened infants. RUEEGG *et al.* [27] tested the information given to the parents and their satisfaction index. The data showed that parents were highly satisfied with the information delivered either by telephone or at the specialist CF centre. The Swiss programme is interesting for a number of reasons. When a positive immunoreactive trypsinogen (IRT) test is found to be above the 99th percentile, seven common mutations are tested by DNA screening. Should both IRT and DNA mutation be present, a positive finding is reported to the CF centre nearest to where the child was born but the centre does not receive the genetic information, merely that the test was positive. It is only when a second dried blood spot sample is returned by the centre that further discussion takes place. This minimises the potential for harmful disclosure and prevents the parents focussing on the performance of the second test and a sweat test, giving rise to a holistic and later discussion. The maximum time taken for reporting back to the centre having obtained the first blood spot is 38 days, with a further maximum time of 63 days to gather all the information. The median time to a genetically confirmed, sweat test-positive diagnosis was 34 days (range 13–135 days).

Strategies to screen newborns

All currently available protocols rely on the measurement of IRT on the dried blood spot sample as a primary screening test (IRT-1) and on sweat test for confirmation or exclusion of CF diagnosis [28]. Intermediate tiers of testing are required to improve the specificity of the initial screening test. The intermediate tiers may consist of a second IRT test on a dried blood spot sample collected after 14 days (when this test is more specific because false-positive, *i.e.* non-CF infant, IRT values will have fallen), *CFTR* mutation analysis on the first blood spot sample, or a combination of these two. In addition, measurement of pancreatitis-associated protein (PAP) has been evaluated in the last decade as an alternative intermediate-tier test, with the potential of avoiding the need for DNA analysis. There are internationally agreed standards for the performance of a protocol: sensitivity >95% and PPV >0.3.

The first tier: IRT

The initial IRT cut-off has a great effect on newborn screening performance with regard to both sensitivity and specificity. Optimisation of the cut-off levels is important, should be ongoing and should be part of the quality control of every CF screening programme [28]. Early experience from the USA and Australia showed that good sensitivity can be achieved with IRT cut-offs higher than the 99th percentile [29]. Others reported that lower IRT cut-offs (~95–97th percentile) were appropriate [30, 31]. Further lowering of the IRT cut-off has little effect on sensitivity but dramatically reduces the specificity and the PPV, irrespective of the intermediate tier test.

There is variability with respect to the day of life on which the dried blood spot sample is obtained in different newborn screening programmes. In the USA, the first dried blood spot sample is taken on day 1 or 2 of life; in most European countries, it is taken on days 2 or 3; in some countries, it is even later (days 5–8) [3]. It is likely that the performance of the IRT assay will be affected by the day of life, and this may account for the variance in IRT-1 cut-off across the globe, with a lower cut-off tending to be used in countries that collect the dried blood spot sample earlier. The IRT assay may be influenced by seasonality (dried blood spots are generally posted to a newborn screening laboratory) and sometimes batch-to-batch variability has been described. For these reasons, a floating cut-off is recommended by some programmes to achieve a consistent number of referrals for intermediate testing [28]. A policy of replication in duplicate should be adopted for all samples with IRT above or slightly below the cut-off, to minimise the effects of volumetric variability of the punched discs, day-to-day variation in IRT assay calibration or contamination of the sample [1]. Nevertheless, it is important to assess false-negative cases to recognise whether the IRT cut-off is achieving a good PPV without reducing sensitivity. In reality, the majority of IRT-1 values in false-negative cases are well below the cut-off and this is an infrequent but well-recognised feature of this assay, even in infants with two classic CF-causing mutations such as Phe508del. Infants with meconium ileus have been reported to have an increased rate of false-negative newborn screening results (with low IRT-1), but as these infants are diagnosed clinically this does not result in a delayed diagnosis. In some protocols, these infants are referred directly for DNA analysis, with no IRT measurement undertaken.

Second- and third-tier tests

Second-tier tests can be either: 1) a repeated IRT from a second blood spot, taken at 3 weeks of age, 2) *CFTR* mutation analysis using the initial blood spot, or 3) PAP analysis using the initial blood spot. Third tier tests can be: 1) a repeated IRT from a second blood spot, or 2) extended *CFTR* gene mutation analysis (extended gene analysis).

Second sample IRT assay
The IRT concentration in blood declines much faster in infants who do not have CF than in those who do [32]. Therefore, a raised IRT at about 3–4 weeks of age is supportive of a CF diagnosis. Although the rate of decline of IRT in infants with CF is variable, most CF newborn screening programmes that rely on IRT/IRT protocols select a lower IRT cut-off for the second sample compared with the first tier test.

CFTR *mutation analysis*

Many CF newborn screening programmes around the world rely on *CFTR* mutation analysis as a second- or third-tier test. In most of the protocols, a limited panel of well-known population-specific CF-causing mutations is analysed on samples with a raised IRT [33]. If one or two mutations are identified, a confirmatory sweat test has to be performed before the CF diagnosis can be made. The great advantage of an IRT/DNA protocol compared with an IRT/IRT protocol is the short time to diagnosis, meaning the therapeutic management for the infant with CF can be initiated within the first 3 weeks of life. In some protocols, infants carrying only one identified *CFTR* mutation are recalled for a second IRT test, in order to try to distinguish CF patients from carriers before the sweat test is performed [1].

The majority of IRT/DNA protocols achieve good sensitivity and specificity. However, the use of population-based molecular genetic screening has raised some ethical concerns [34]. Depending on the *CFTR* mutation panel, a substantial portion of the newborns who initially tested positive are healthy carriers. The communication of these results may require extensive genetic counselling of the families, contradicting the general goals of newborn screening. In this context, the current trend to increase the panel of tested *CFTR* mutations in countries with a large ethnic diversity will further increase the number of newborns known as CF carriers and thus increase the demand for genetic counselling. Another potential disadvantage of genetic CF newborn screening is the detection of CF patients with an equivocal diagnosis who are not the target of CF newborn screening.

In a number of CF newborn screening protocols, extended *CFTR* mutation analysis is used as a third tier test. The rationale of extended gene analysis is to improve sensitivity by recognising unusual *CFTR* gene mutations and to reduce the need for sweat testing, hence improving the PPV of the test. The precise nature of extended gene analysis can be variable, ranging from full sequencing to next-generation sequencing of specific areas of the *CFTR* gene, known to be regularly affected by mutations. This strategy will result in the recognition of infants with *CFTR* mutations, the consequences of which are not clear. When these infants have a normal or intermediate sweat test, the long-term consequence to the child and family is not clear. As discussed earlier, the approaches to this situation in Europe and the USA are somewhat different and more research is needed to fully appreciate the impact of this on families and children. Some relatively common *CFTR* mutations, such as R117H and D1152H, are associated with a milder phenotype and there is debate as to the appropriateness of including these mutations in a newborn screening panel. It is probably not appropriate to include them in the first level of testing.

PAP analysis

The use of PAP as an intermediate tier test was first investigated by SARLES *et al.* [10], and the feasibility of this biochemical approach has since been evaluated by a number of groups [9, 35]. An IRT/PAP protocol avoids the issues raised by *CFTR* mutation analysis. Another advantage of PAP is that, in contrast to an IRT/IRT protocol, PAP can be measured from the first dried blood spot sample. Published studies have not been performed in large populations, but suggest that IRT/PAP protocols can reach acceptable sensitivities [9]. The IRT/PAP strategy results in a considerable reduction in the recognition of carriers and a significant reduction in the recognition of infants with an inconclusive diagnosis, albeit at the expense of a reduction in PPV, with 10 or more sweat tests required to recognise one infant with CF. To improve specificity, VERNOOIJ-VAN LANGEN *et al.* [9] combined the original IRT/PAP protocol with an extensive genetic analysis as the third tier. This approach seems to combine the mentioned positive properties of an IRT/PAP protocol with the improved specificity of extended gene analysis. This does, however, counterbalance some of the earlier benefits achieved with respect to the recognition of carriers and infants with an inconclusive diagnosis. The Dutch national programme will continue to monitor the progress of this protocol over the next 5 years.

Safety net strategies

To improve sensitivity (particularly when screening a culturally diverse population), a number of programmes have employed a safety net strategy [1]. When the first IRT sample is very high but the intermediate tier test (DNA analysis or PAP) is negative, then the result is not classed as negative, but further testing is organised. The further testing is either a repeat IRT sample at 21 days of age or calling the family for a sweat test. This strategy will have a negative impact on specificity with a reduction in PPV.

The decision to use a safety net strategy should be reviewed as populations change and mutation panels become more specific. For example, in a study performed in Massachusetts (USA), the safety net protocol could be stopped after more CFTR mutations were included into the screening panel [30]. Experience with IRT/PAP protocols is low compared with IRT/ DNA. Most of the studies published used IRT/PAP protocols without a safety net. However, there is evidence from recent regional studies that the sensitivity of IRT/PAP protocols without a safety net is insufficient [35].

Balancing the advantages and disadvantages of different strategies

A CF newborn screening programme has to meet political and ethical requirements as well as the financial resources of a country. In a few countries, ethical concerns about genetic testing and legislative issues impede the implementation of CF newborn screening programmes using CFTR mutation analysis. In other countries, the use of genetic testing is not considered affordable.

Figure 2 presents a decision-making algorithm, beginning with IRT-1 and then considering the feasibility of DNA analysis. If DNA analysis is precluded, a protocol based on biochemical tests is advocated with the measurement of a repeated IRT or PAP as a second-tier test. If CFTR mutation analysis is possible, an IRT/DNA protocol may be considered and then a further question is presented: is the detection of a high number of healthy carriers and infants with an inconclusive diagnosis is acceptable? If so, than DNA testing should be considered as a second tier test. If not, DNA analysis should be considered as a third tier test, and a biochemical parameter (repeated IRT from a second blood spot or PAP) as the second tier test.

The decision about which biochemical measure should be used as a second-tier test depends on the feasibility of obtaining a second dried blood spot sample. If this is possible, then a repeated IRT test from a second blood spot should be considered. In contrast, PAP as second-tier test can be performed from the initial blood spot, which is an important issue with regard to the time until CF diagnosis can be made. However, data from Australia suggest that the sensitivity of PAP as a second tier test is low if initial blood sampling was performed before day 2 of life, as is currently the case in parts of Australia and a number of states in the USA (E. Ranieri, Dept of Genetics, Adelaide Women's and Children's Hospital, Adelaide, Australia; personal communication).

The combination of a two-tier protocol with a third tier might improve performance under certain conditions. In cases of an IRT/DNA protocol, combination with extended gene

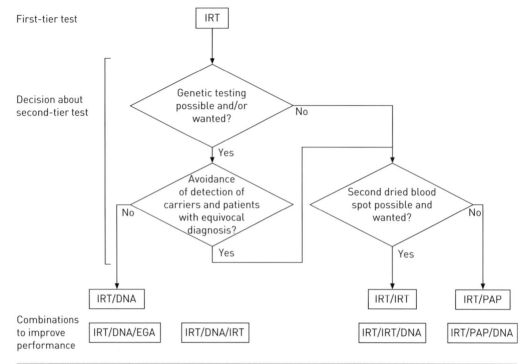

Figure 2. Proposed algorithm to guide decision making with respect to protocol choice. IRT: immunoreactive trypsinogen; PAP: pancreatitis-associated protein; EGA: extended gene analysis (sequencing).

analysis or repeated IRT from a second blood spot will improve the specificity of the whole protocol resulting in a lower recall rate for sweat tests. Extended gene analysis can also be performed using the initial blood spot and does not usually require a second blood spot. An IRT/DNA/extended gene analysis protocol offers a high sensitivity, a high specificity as well as a high PPV. However, the value of such a protocol has to be balanced against the costs, which are higher than those of an IRT/DNA protocol, with a limited *CFTR* mutation panel, and increased recognition of carriers and inconclusive diagnosis.

Both biochemical protocols, IRT/IRT and IRT/PAP, can be combined with DNA testing as a third tier. These combinations retain the advantages (reduced detection of healthy carriers and CF patients with equivocal diagnosis) but also the disadvantage (less sensitivity) of the respective biochemical CF screening protocol. However, genetic testing as a third tier will improve the performance of these protocols towards a better specificity and a better PPV.

Conclusion

In summary, there are several strategies available to screen infants for CF from the dried blood spot obtained in the first week of life. An algorithm is presented with the various options available, but to a significant degree the choice of protocol reflects a subjective appreciation of the relative importance of negative impacts, such as carrier recognition and the desire of a health service to reduce these (table 2). A considerable amount of research is required to provide the robust data required to clarify the best strategy for improving the health of these infants in the most cost-effective manner.

Table 2. Protocol options for screening newborns for cystic fibrosis, scored according to their performance, taking into account the positive and negative impact on families

Protocol	Sensitivity	Specificity	PPV	Avoiding detection of patients with equivocal diagnosis	Avoiding carrier detection
IRT/IRT	++	+		+++	+++
IRT/DNA limited panel	++	+++		++	++
IRT/DNA extended panel	+++	+++		+	+
IRT/DNA/EGA	+++	++++		-	-
IRT/DNA/IRT	+++	+++		++	+++
IRT/IRT/DNA	+	+++		+	+
IRT/PAP	++	-		+++	+++
IRT/PAP/DNA	++	+++		++	++
IRT/PAP/DNA/EGA	++	++++		+	++

Performance has been ranked subjectively by the authors after review of the available data. -: weakness in the protocol; +: adequate performance; ++: average; +++: strength in the protocol; ++++: could not be better. Sensitivity: programme's ability not to miss affected cases (relates to the false-negative rate); specificity: programme's ability to recognise affected cases without false-positive screening results (a programme with a poor positive predictive value (PPV) will require more sweat tests on unaffected infants to identify cystic fibrosis cases). IRT: immunoreactive trypsinogen; EGA: extended gene analysis; PAP: pancreatitis-associated protein.

References

1. Castellani C, Southern KW, Brownlee K, *et al.* European best practice guidelines for cystic fibrosis neonatal screening. *J Cyst Fibros* 2009; 8: 153–173.
2. Farrell PM. Is newborn screening for cystic fibrosis a basic human right? *J Cyst Fibros* 2008; 7: 262–265.
3. Southern KW, Munck A, Pollitt R, *et al.* A survey of newborn screening for cystic fibrosis in Europe. *J Cyst Fibros* 2007; 6: 57–65.
4. Petros M. Revisiting the Wilson-Jungner criteria: how can supplemental criteria guide public health in the era of genetic screening? *Genet Med* 2012; 14: 129–134.
5. Southern KW. Newborn screening for cystic fibrosis: the practical implications. *J R Soc Med* 2004; 97: Suppl. 44, 57–59.
6. Southern KW, Merelle MM, Dankert-Roelse JE, *et al.* Newborn screening for cystic fibrosis. *Cochrane Database Syst Rev* 2009; 1: CD001402.
7. Sims EJ, Mugford M, Clark A, *et al.* Economic implications of newborn screening for cystic fibrosis: a cost of illness retrospective cohort study. *Lancet* 2007; 369: 1187–1195.
8. Dijk FN, McKay K, Barzi F, *et al.* Improved survival in cystic fibrosis patients diagnosed by newborn screening compared to a historical cohort from the same centre. *Arch Dis Child* 2011; 96: 1118–1123.
9. Vernooij-van Langen AM, Loeber JG, Elvers B, *et al.* Novel strategies in newborn screening for cystic fibrosis: a prospective controlled study. *Thorax* 2012; 67: 289–295.
10. Sarles J, Berthezene P, Le Louarn C, *et al.* Combining immunoreactive trypsinogen and pancreatitis-associated protein assays, a method of newborn screening for cystic fibrosis that avoids DNA analysis. *J Pediatr* 2005; 147: 302–305.
11. Borowitz D, Parad RB, Sharp JK, *et al.* Cystic Fibrosis Foundation practice guidelines for the management of infants with cystic fibrosis transmembrane conductance regulator-related metabolic syndrome during the first two years of life and beyond. *J Pediatr* 2009; 155: Suppl. 6, S106–S116.
12. Mayell SJ, Munck A, Craig JV, *et al.* A European consensus for the evaluation and management of infants with an equivocal diagnosis following newborn screening for cystic fibrosis. *J Cyst Fibros* 2009; 8: 71–78.
13. Kharazi M, Prach L, Lessing S, *et al.* Results of including a DNA sequencing step into a CF IRT/DNA newborn screening model. *Pediatr Pulmonol* 2013; 48: Suppl. 36, 384.
14. Farrell MH, Christopher SA, Tluczek A, *et al.* Improving communication between doctors and parents after newborn screening. *WMJ* 2011; 110: 221–227.
15. Kai J, Ulph F, Cullinan T, *et al.* Communication of carrier status information following universal newborn screening for sickle cell disorders and cystic fibrosis: qualitative study of experience and practice. *Health Technol Assess* 2009; 13: 1–82.

16. Castellani C, Picci L, Tamanini A, *et al.* Association between carrier screening and incidence of cystic fibrosis. *JAMA* 2009; 302: 2573–2579.
17. Livingstone J, Axton RA, Gilfillan A, *et al.* Antenatal screening for cystic fibrosis: a trial of the couple model. *BMJ* 1994; 308: 1459–1462.
18. Massie RJ, Curnow L, Glazner J, *et al.* Lessons learned from 20 years of newborn screening for cystic fibrosis. *Med J Aust* 2012; 196: 67–70.
19. Massie J, Castellani C, Grody WW. Carrier screening for cystic fibrosis in the new era of medications that restore CFTR function. *Lancet* 2014; 383: 923–925.
20. Kleyn MJ, Langbo C, Abdulhamid I, *et al.* Evaluation of genetic counseling among cystic fibrosis carriers, Michigan Newborn Screening. *Pediatr Pulmonol* 2013; 48: 123–129.
21. Martin B, Schechter MS, Jaffe A, *et al.* Comparison of the US and Australian cystic fibrosis registries: the impact of newborn screening. *Pediatrics* 2012; 129: e348–e355.
22. Mehta A. The how (and why) of disease registers. *Early Hum Dev* 2010; 86: 723–728.
23. Ferec C, Cutting GR. Assessing the disease-liability of mutations in CFTR. *Cold Spring Harb Perspect Med* 2012; 2: a009480.
24. O'Sullivan BP, Baker D, Leung KG, *et al.* Evolution of pancreatic function during the first year in infants with cystic fibrosis. *J Pediatr* 2013; 162: 808–812.
25. Nahrlich L, Zimmer KP. Neonatal cystic fibrosis screening – time to begin!. *Dtsch Arztebl Int* 2013; 110: 354–355.
26. Torresani T, Fingerhut R, Rueegg CS, *et al.* Newborn screening for cystic fibrosis in Switzerland – consequences after analysis of a 4 months pilot study. *J Cyst Fibros* 2013; 12: 667–674.
27. Rueegg CS, Kuehni CE, Gallati S, *et al.* One-year evaluation of a neonatal screening program for cystic fibrosis in Switzerland. *Dtsch Arztebl Int* 2013; 110: 356–363.
28. Therrell BL Jr, Hannon WH, Hoffman G, *et al.* Immunoreactive trypsinogen (IRT) as a biomarker for cystic fibrosis: challenges in newborn dried blood spot screening. *Mol Genet Metab* 2012; 106: 1–6.
29. Wilcken B, Wiley V, Sherry G, *et al.* Neonatal screening for cystic fibrosis: a comparison of two strategies for case detection in 1.2 million babies. *J Pediatr* 1995; 127: 965–970.
30. Comeau AM, Parad RB, Dorkin HL, *et al.* Population-based newborn screening for genetic disorders when multiple mutation DNA testing is incorporated: a cystic fibrosis newborn screening model demonstrating increased sensitivity but more carrier detections. *Pediatrics* 2004; 113: 1573–1581.
31. Wagener JS, Zemanick ET, Sontag MK. Newborn screening for cystic fibrosis. *Curr Opin Pediatr* 2012; 24: 329–335.
32. Wilcken B, Brown AR, Urwin R, *et al.* Cystic fibrosis screening by dried blood spot trypsin assay: results in 75,000 newborn infants. *J Pediatr* 1983; 102: 383–387.
33. Dequeker E, Stuhrmann M, Morris MA, *et al.* Best practice guidelines for molecular genetic diagnosis of cystic fibrosis and CFTR-related disorders–updated European recommendations. *Eur J Hum Genet* 2009; 17: 51–65.
34. Wilfond B, Rothenberg LS. Ethical issues in cystic fibrosis newborn screening: from data to public health policy. *Curr Opin Pulm Med* 2002; 8: 529–534.
35. Sommerburg O, Krulisova V, Hammermann J, *et al.* Comparison of different IRT-PAP protocols to screen newborns for cystic fibrosis in three central European populations. *J Cyst Fibros* 2014; 13: 15–23.

Disclosures: None declared.

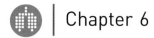
Early cystic fibrosis lung disease

Stephen M. Stick

Lung disease was recognised as an early component of cystic fibrosis (CF) when it was first described as a syndrome. However, until midway through the 20th century, when the generalised mucous abnormality was identified, it was considered secondary to low vitamin A due to malabsorption of fat. Improved nutrition resulting from pancreatic enzyme replacement and comprehensive care in specialist clinics has resulted in improved survival, and lung disease is now the major determinant of morbidity and mortality. Early surveillance studies have demonstrated the very early onset of lung disease associated with neutrophilic airway inflammation and indicate potential strategies to prevent or slow the onset of structural lung disease.

The first definitive description of the condition we refer to as cystic fibrosis (CF), by Dorothy Andersen in 1938 [1], included pulmonary disease. As survival beyond early childhood was rare at this time, it was self-evident that lung disease is an early feature of the disease. However, Andersen and others considered the lung disease to be secondary to infection due to vitamin A deficiency [2]. This view was widely held at the time; however, in 1943, Farber recognised the contribution of thickened mucous to both pancreatic duct and airway obstruction [3].

With the introduction of pancreatic enzyme supplementation and the establishment of specialist clinics in a number of centres around the world, the outlook for infants born with CF improved and the focus shifted somewhat from the gastroenterological/nutritional consequences to the pulmonary aspects of the disease and methods to monitor disease progression.

The first attempts to quantify the nature and severity of chest disease used radiography. Attwood reported the first radiological features of lung disease in 1942 in a series of four case histories of children who died before the age of 2 years [4]. Gas trapping and atelectasis were both evident as early as 3 months. In 1958, Shwachman and Kulczycki proposed a clinical scoring system that included a rudimentary chest radiograph score [5], but it was not until 1974 that Chrispin and Norman published a systematic method of assessing and scoring the chest radiograph in CF [6, 7]. A version of this system, published in 1982 by van der Put and colleagues [8], was used for the first longitudinal assessment of early lung changes in CF. Although changes that could be interpreted as being due to bronchiectasis were unusual

Telethon Kids Institute, School of Paediatrics and Child Health, University of Western Australia, Princess Margaret Hospital for Children, Perth, Australia.

Correspondence: Stephen M. Stick, Dept of Respiratory Medicine, Princess Margaret Hospital for Children, Roberts Road, Subiaco 6008, Perth, Australia. E-mail: stephen.stick@health.wa.gov.au before the age of 3 years, gas trapping was evident even in the first year of life and was thought to be due to mucus plugging in small peripheral airways.

At about the same time, there was intense interest in defining the physiological consequences and mechanisms of early lung abnormalities. Phelan and colleagues were pioneers in this field [9]. In 1969, using lung function tests adapted from those used in adults, they reported that infants who presented with meconium ileus without respiratory symptoms had raised thoracic gas volume, suggesting that gas trapping occurred in the first months of life in apparently asymptomatic children [9]. In 1978, Godfrey and colleagues published longitudinal measurements of lung function in children with CF obtained in infancy and at 5 years of age [10]. In this study, airways obstruction and hyperinflation were evident in the more severely affected children but functional effects were even detected in children with minimal symptoms. None of the functional indices improved with time and these authors concluded that the lungs of infants with CF are likely to be physiologically normal at birth but that disturbances develop even in the absence of clinical symptoms.

Further developments in infant lung function testing allowed better characterisation of airway disease. These included the tidal compression technique and the raised volume rapid thoraco-abdominal compression (RVRTC) technique to assess forced expiratory flows. Tepper and colleagues [11] reported longitudinal outcomes during infancy from clinical diagnosis. Using the tidal compression technique, these authors reported tracking of forced expiratory flows in early life and lower flows in symptomatic children than asymptomatic children [11]. In 1994, Turner and colleagues [12] reported that the RVRTC technique was a more sensitive test to detect abnormal lung function in CF than the tidal breathing technique; and, in 2001, a London-wide CF collaboration (UK) reported their early results using a modification of this technique. Ranganathan and colleagues [13] observed that forced expiratory flows were significantly diminished in infants with CF even in the absence of clinically recognised lower respiratory illness.

There was clearly accumulating evidence that significant lung abnormalities could occur early in life, even in the absence of clinical pulmonary disease. However, there was little to indicate whether these early disturbances were reversible or whether the functional outcomes reflected irreversible structural disease.

Two important studies used chest computed tomography (CT) to assess lung disease in young children. In 1999, Helbich and colleagues [14] reported the evolution of chest CT changes in CF. The authors observed bronchiectasis during the first year of life and that the severity of abnormalities was associated with the duration of follow-up. In 2004, Long and colleagues [15] reported increased airway/vessel ratios in young children with CF. These studies suggested that bronchiectasis, the major cause of morbidity and mortality in CF, develops early in life and, as a consequence, some of the observed early functional deficits might not be reversible. The implication of these observations is that early intervention to prevent lung disease was likely to be the best strategy to improve long-term morbidity and mortality.

The Wisconsin randomised controlled study of newborn screening for CF demonstrated that early interventions can improve outcomes [16]. Better results in the newborn screening group were most notable for nutrition and growth; these results were probably due to earlier intervention with effective therapies, *i.e.* pancreatic enzyme replacement and diet. However, there are few specific early interventions to prevent lung disease and, therefore, the pulmonary benefits resulting from newborn screening were less obvious. In the meantime, widespread adoption of newborn screening has provided opportunities to investigate the early pathobiology of CF lung disease with a view to developing effective early intervention strategies. For example, in Melbourne in 1997, Armstrong and colleagues [17] reported that newly diagnosed infants with CF and without infection had bronchoalveolar lavage (BAL) inflammatory profiles comparable with control subjects while those with a lower respiratory infection had evidence of airway inflammation. Thus BAL was established as an effective means to investigate the roles of lung inflammation and infection following diagnosis.

By the start of the 21st century, the outlook for children born with CF had improved significantly from the condition described by Andersen in 1938 [1]. Median survival had increased from ~4 years to >30 years, newborn screening was being implemented in many countries, and the use of infant lung function testing and techniques such as BAL and chest CT were providing new insights into the development of early lung disease. Thus, the scene was set for longitudinal assessments of disease ontogeny using multiple modalities, with a view to identifying suitable targets for early intervention and determining the best outcome measures for patient management and clinical trials.

The nature and progress of early CF lung disease

Data from various national registries confirm that whilst the median age of survival and age-adjusted lung function have improved in successive cohorts [18], most of those improvements can be attributed to better outcomes in children, particularly in those <6 years of age (fig. 1) [19]. Furthermore, the rate of decline in lung function appears to have been unchanged for several decades.

NIXON et al. [19] reported the first cross-sectional data from a study of infants performed soon after diagnosis following newborn screening. The subjects were investigated using a combination of BAL and infant lung function. Perhaps surprisingly, the presence of symptoms and bacterial airway infection was independently associated with lower lung function measured using the RVRTC technique, whereas airway inflammation was not. These data indicated complex relationships between markers of disease activity and clinical and physiological outcomes. Furthermore, in light of data from other subjects, the issue of

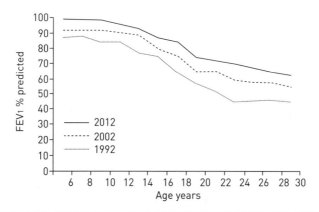

Figure 1. Forced expiratory volume in 1 s (FEV1) *versus* age for three cohorts obtained in 1992, 2002 and 2012. Most of the overall change in lung function can be attributed to better outcomes in children <6 years of age. The rate of decline in FEV1 has been virtually unchanged for two decades. Data from [19].

whether the RVRTC outcomes are sensitive early indicators of disease was raised. Although forced expiratory volume in 1 s (FEV1) is in the healthy range for school-aged children with CF, there are persuasive data that this measure poorly reflects the presence and severity of lung disease [20]. Therefore, the Australian Early Surveillance Team for Cystic Fibrosis (AREST CF; www.arestcf.org), and later the London Cystic Fibrosis Collaboration (LCFC), commenced systematic investigations of children with CF soon after diagnosis following newborn screening, using combinations of techniques that included infant/pre-school lung function, BAL and chest CT. Whereas most of the data regarding early lung disease had previously been obtained from cohorts of children with CF diagnosed clinically and were therefore not necessarily relevant to the current standards of care, these studies provide comprehensive longitudinal data in children diagnosed following newborn screening.

The AREST CF surveillance programme provided the first snapshot of the earliest pathobiological changes in the lung associated with CF and the significant factors that contribute to structural lung disease, notably bronchiectasis.

The initial cross-sectional analyses established that structural lung disease (including bronchiectasis) occurs soon after birth, is common in the first years of life and is associated with inflammation and infection [21, 22]. Limited (three-slice) chest CT and BAL were performed annually in children from approximately 2 months of age to 6 years of age. Scans were analysed for the presence and extent of abnormalities. Bronchial dilatation was detected in nearly 20% of children between 2 and 5 months of age and overall nearly 80% of children at this age had evidence of pulmonary disease manifest by infection, inflammation or radiological changes [21, 22]. In children up to the age of 6 years, the overall prevalence of bronchiectasis was 22% and increased with age (p=0.001), reaching 70% by 6 years of age [22]. Factors associated with bronchiectasis included: absolute neutrophil count (p=0.03), neutrophil elastase concentration (p=0.001), and *Pseudomonas aeruginosa* infection (p=0.03). These prevalence data have been confirmed in other cohorts [23].

Early lung function data using the RVRTC technique suggested that the mean FEV0.5 z-score did not differ between infants with CF and healthy control subjects <6 months of age (-0.06 and 0.02, respectively; p=0.87) but the mean FEV0.5 z-score was 1.15 lower in infants with CF who were >6 months of age compared with healthy infants (p<0.001) [24]. However, more recent data from the LCFC using contemporaneous age-matched, healthy controls demonstrated that up to 35% of infants at 3 months of age had abnormal lung function [25].

Early reports suggest that in the first 2 years of life there is a decline in lung function assessed using the RVRTC technique [26]. Infants with free neutrophil elastase detected in the BAL had lower forced vital capacity (FVC) and FEV0.5 z-scores than children in whom neutrophil elastase was undetectable. A significantly greater decline in FEV0.5 z-scores occurred in those infected with *Staphylococcus aureus* (p=0.018) or *P. aeruginosa* (p=0.021), detected in BAL, compared to children who were uninfected. More recent reports from the LCFC showed that despite identification of lung function abnormalities in approximately one-third of infants who underwent newborn screening by 3 months of age, no subsequent deterioration was observed during the first year of life in either ventilation inhomogeneity (lung clearance index (LCI)) or plethysmographic measures of hyperinflation, and there were significant improvements in FEV0.5 over this time-period [27]. Inclusion of contemporaneous healthy controls in the LCFC study might, at least partially, explain these differences.

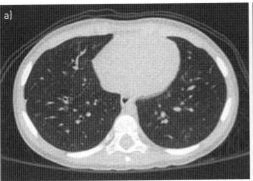 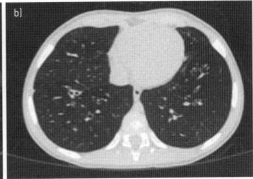

Figure 2. Computed tomography scans assessing the progression of bronchiectasis from a) a 2-year-old child and b) a 4-year-old child.

The impact of early infection has been emphasised in a study by MOTT *et al.* [28]. The authors reported an analysis of 301 paired, three-slice limited CT scans obtained 1 year apart in children whose first scan was at the age of 1–3 years. Bronchiectasis was never present in 74 (25%) pairs, and was detected at either the initial or subsequent scan in 227 (75%) pairs. Bronchiectasis was detected at the initial scan in 133 (44%) scan pairs and persisted at the subsequent scan in 98 (74%) pairs. Air-trapping present at the initial scan persisted in >80% of subsequent scans. The extent of bronchiectasis and air trapping increased over 1 year in 63% and 47% of scans, respectively. Radiological progression of bronchiectasis (fig. 2) and air trapping (fig. 3) was associated with severe cystic fibrosis transmembrane conductance regulator (CFTR) genotype, pulmonary infection and worsening neutrophilic inflammation.

Early inflammation and infection

Inflammation in the lower airways can be identified in children around the time of diagnosis following newborn screening [19, 21]. Furthermore, neutrophil elastase detected in BAL is a predictor of the development of bronchiectasis [29] and is associated with accelerated decline in infant lung function [26].

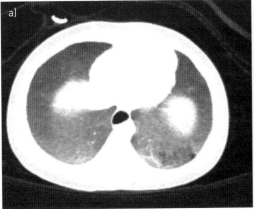 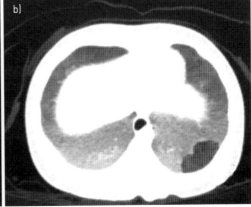

Figure 3. Computed tomography scans assessing the progression of gas trapping from a) a child aged 3 months and b) a 1-year-old child.

Neutrophil elastase is a serine protease mainly found in the azurophil granules in neutrophil cytoplasm [30]. It is capable of degrading bacterial outer membrane proteins as well as proteins in the extracellular matrix. Anti-proteases, including α_1-antitrypsin (α_1-AT), are important inactivators of neutrophil elastase [30]. When neutrophil elastase levels exceed the anti-protease activity of the lung, it can be measured in BAL fluid as free neutrophil elastase activity. Neutrophil elastase in BAL fluid at 3 months of age was associated with persistent bronchiectasis (present on two or more sequential scans), with the odds seven-times as high at 12 months of age and four-times as high at 3 years of age [29].

Although early colonisation with pathogenic bacteria has long been thought to be the major factor driving early inflammatory lung disease [17], the relationships between inflammation and bacterial infection are complex. For example, there are children in the AREST CF programme who have neutrophil elastatse present in BAL in the first years of life with no overt bacterial infection detectable using standard sampling and microbiological culture techniques. Possible explanations for such apparently inconsistent observations include: insensitive sampling and detection techniques for identifying bacterial infection; complex temporal associations between the acquisition of pathogens and the development of inflammation; triggers of inflammation other than bacteria (*e.g.* viruses) [31]; gastro-oesophageal reflux [32]; airway surface liquid dehydration and macrophage activation [33]; and a pro-inflammatory microenvironment resulting from the intrinsic epithelial gene defect [34]. Regardless of the initial trigger, there appear to be clear associations between lower airway infection with a range of pathogens and the severity of airway inflammation at any given time. Individual organisms such as *Haemophilus influenzae*, *S. aureus*, *P. aeruginosa*, *Streptococcus pneumoniae* and *Aspergillus fumigatus* appear to be particularly associated with airway inflammation [35].

Furthermore, infection with multiple organisms is associated with greater levels of inflammation than infection with single organisms [36]. Most of the organisms that have been associated with inflammation or with disease severity can be detected in children very soon after diagnosis (table 1). However, the most common organisms that are detected in the early years are *S. aureus* and *H. influenzae*, with *P. aeruginosa* being relatively uncommon until school age [23]. Importantly, early recognition and eradication of *P. aeruginosa* before the age of 5 years does not result in a decrease in the prevalence of bronchiectasis at school age [23]. This begs the question: what are the most significant early pathogens in CF?

Table 1. Pathogens detected in bronchoalveolar lavage at 3 months of age in the AREST CF cohort

Pathogen	Age first detected	Genotype	Anti-*Staphylococcus* prophylaxis
Pseudomonas aeruginosa	13 weeks	Phe508del/Lys447ArgfsX2	Yes
Staphylococcus aureus	24 days	Phe508del/Phe508del	No
Haemophilus influenzae	11 weeks	Gly542X/Gly542X	No
Aspergillus fumigatus	8 weeks	Phe508del/Asn1303Lys	Yes
Moraxella catarrhalis	11 weeks	Gly542X/Gly542X	No
Stenotrophomonas maltophilia	8 weeks	Phe508del/Gly551Asp	No
Candida albicans	7 weeks	Phe508del/Phe508del	Yes

Unpublished data from the Australian Early Surveillance Team for Cystic Fibrosis (AREST CF).

Recent metagenomic studies have demonstrated that, even in health, the lung is not a sterile environment and that different disease states can influence the bacterial microenvironment of the lung [37, 38]. As we learn more about the complexity of lung bacterial microbiota, we will gain a greater insight into the factors that can result in a pro-inflammatory microenviron-ment and the potential interventions that might be possible to maintain a "healthy" microbiome in the lung.

The data from AREST CF [29], which demonstrate the strong association between neutrophil elastase and later development of structural lung disease, and observations in the CF pig that the airway pH is critical in the defence against bacteria [39], suggest that antimicrobial therapy alone might not be sufficient to prevent lung disease. The development of combinations of therapies that aim to restore a healthy airway micro-environment and reduce inflammation could be a successful strategy for preventing lung damage until such time as more definitive treatments become available for the majority of children with CF [40].

Monitoring early disease

Critical to the establishment of new intervention strategies to prevent lung disease is the development of robust outcome measures for clinical trials, which reflect important aspects of early pulmonary disease and which are responsive to small clinically relevant changes in what is generally a mild disease over short time-periods. The current status of various outcome measures proposed for clinical trials was discussed at a recent European Respiratory Society research seminar (Rotterdam, the Netherlands) and recently published [41]. In summary, two methodologies were specifically highlighted: 1) chest CT to assess structural damage of the lung; and 2) multiple-breath washout (MBW) as a technique to quantify ventilation inhomogeneity (e.g. LCI).

Emerging technology allows high-quality, volumetric inspiratory and expiratory chest CT images to be obtained at very low radiation doses approaching those of traditional chest radiographs. However, whilst image quality is not a significant issue, even at very low radiation doses, image analysis is more problematic. A commonly used CF CT score [42] assesses abnormalities, such as bronchiectasis, using a lobar score of 0–3 based on whether 0%, ⩽50% or >50% of the lobe is affected. As in early lung disease there is often <50% of only one or two lobes affected, the overall outcome is dichotomous for a given abnormality. Such an analysis strategy does not account for the heterogeneity of early disease that usually affects a small proportion of the lung and is often mild and, therefore, prone to increased interobserver variability [43]. Consequently, in order to see the effects of an intervention, larger study numbers are required than for a continuous outcome measure, which is less likely to be subject to between-observer error and better reflects disease heterogeneity than a crude, discrete score with low resolution. With these issues in mind, the PRAGMA (Perth–Rotterdam Annotated Morphometric Analysis) score has been developed [44]. Preliminary data suggest that the sensitivity of this analysis technique to mild disease affecting, for example, <5% of the lungs appears to be better than the CF CT scoring method. New fast scanning technology means that young children can be investigated without the need for sedation (although the impact of not controlling for lung volume needs to be assessed further) [45], and radiation doses well below 0.1 mSv can be easily achieved for combined inspiratory and expiratory volumetric images. Therefore, CT is a useful technique that can be used effectively as an end-point in clinical trials of interventions intended to prevent or halt the development of structural disease. However, for clinical monitoring of disease, where more frequent assessments might be needed than for clinical trials, additional tools are required that are relatively noninvasive and do not expose young children to radiation.

A number of studies have shown that early in the course of lung disease, marked abnormalities may be present in the uniformity of ventilation distribution in CF measured using the MBW technique [46, 47]. An increased LCI is associated with concurrent structural lung damage on CT scans in schoolchildren [48], and abnormal pre-school LCI predicts subsequent lung function abnormalities several years later [49]. However, the relationships between LCI and irreversible structural changes are less clear in younger children [50]. Although the MBW is a simple test, uncooperative young children probably still need to be asleep, usually achieved with sedation, for reliable results to be obtained. Despite these reservations, the feasibility of using LCI for clinical trials in young children has recently been reported [51]. However, this technique has been largely limited to centres with access to mass spectroscopy that is not suitable for routine clinical surveillance. Although new commercial devices based on nitrogen washout have been released, these have yet to be validated for use in children <5 years of age.

Surveillance to understand early disease: what are the gold standards?

The emerging data suggest complex associations between CF gene mutations, airway microenvironment, inflammation and infection. These associations have been identified by relating observations obtained from direct sampling of the lower airway using BAL, to surrogate clinicometric outcomes such as CT and lung function.

Relatively noninvasive markers of lower airway inflammation, such as metabolomic profiles in exhaled breath condensate [52], might be feasible and informative in the future and these tools are in development. However, although non-BAL samples might provide useful information regarding lower airway inflammation, the available evidence suggests that upper airway samples do not adequately reflect the relationships between lower airway infection and inflammation [36], nor are they a substitute for direct samples when investigating the topography and ontogeny of lung microbiota. Therefore, BAL remains the gold standard for evaluating the airway microenvironment in CF. There are obvious limitations with such a strategy, including the need for anaesthesia and the frequency of observations that can be made. However, by combining procedures such as BAL and CT it is possible to gain maximum information from a single anaesthetic. Furthermore, since lower airway pathogens can only be specifically identified using BAL, an annual anaesthetic can be justified on clinical grounds. In a clinical setting, the development of non-BAL techniques might ultimately help guide antibiotic treatment where it is important to balance the risk of over-treating children who have upper airway colonisation without lung infection against the risk of failing to halt irreversible lung damage due to infection. However, in the current state of knowledge, BAL remains the gold standard for the investigation of the pathogenic role of organisms and their contributions to an abnormal pulmonary microenvironment in CF.

Whilst the MBW (LCI) appears sensitive to early lung disease and is likely to have an important role as an outcome measure in early intervention studies [46, 47], it is not a substitute for CT but can provide complimentary information for investigating the evolution of early structural lung disease [53] and impact on respiratory function.

Finally, the early surveillance strategies suggested here are time-consuming and can be onerous for families. Encouragingly, early data from the LCFC suggest that parents have a positive attitude to early surveillance [54]. However, any centre employing such a programme should consider the psychosocial impact on participants and balance this against perceived and actual benefits [55]. These relationships are likely to be dependent upon local factors and the manner of implementation of any comprehensive surveillance programme.

Conclusion

There is a consensus developing that intervening at diagnosis to prevent irreversible lung damage in childhood will reduce adult mortality. Furthermore, outcome measures need to be defined that reflect the early onset, progression and heterogeneity of lung disease to enable clinical trials with potential disease-modifying agents to be performed [56, 57]. The emerging data suggest that early intervention to reduce neutrophilic inflammation and mitigate neutrophil protease activity should be priorities for futher investigation.

References

1. Andersen DH. Cystic fibrosis of the pancreas and its relation to celiac disease: a clinical and pathological study. *Am J Dis Child* 1938; 56: 344–399.
2. Andersen D. Cystic fibrosis of the pancreas, vitamin A deficiency and bronchiectasis. *J Pediatr* 1939; 15: 763–771.
3. Farber S. Pancreatic insufficiency and the celiac syndrome. *N Engl J Med* 1943; 229: 653–657.
4. Attwood CJ, Sargent WMH. Cystic fibrosis of the pancreas with observations on the roentgen appearance of the associated pulmonary lesions. *Radiology* 1942; 39: 417–425.
5. Shwachman H, Kulczycki LL. Long-term study of one hundred five patients with cystic fibrosis; studies made over a five- to fourteen-year period. *AMA J Dis Child* 1958; 96: 6–15.
6. Chrispin AR, Norman AP. The systematic evaluation of the chest radiograph in cystic fibrosis. *Pediatr Radiol* 1974; 2: 101–105.
7. Matthew DJ, Warner JO, Chrispin AR, *et al.* The relationship between chest radiographic scores and respiratory function tests in children with cystic fibrosis. *Pediatr Radiol* 1977; 5: 198–200.
8. van der Put JM, Meradji M, Danoesastro D, *et al.* Chest radiographs in cystic fibrosis. A follow-up study with application of a quantitative system. *Pediatr Radiol* 1982; 12: 57–61.
9. Phelan PD, Gracey M, Williams HE, *et al.* Ventilatory function in infants with cystic fibrosis. Physiological assessment of halation therapy. *Arch Dis Child* 1969; 44: 393–400.
10. Godfrey S, Mearns M, Howlett G. Serial lung function studies in cystic fibrosis in the first 5 years of life. *Arch Dis Child* 1978; 53: 83–85.
11. Tepper RS, Montgomery GL, Ackerman V, *et al.* Longitudinal evaluation of pulmonary function in infants and very young children with cystic fibrosis. *Pediatr Pulmonol* 1993; 16: 96–100.
12. Turner DJ, Lanteri CJ, LeSouef PN, *et al.* Improved detection of abnormal respiratory function using forced expiration from raised lung volume in infants with cystic fibrosis. *Eur Respir J* 1994; 7: 1995–1999.
13. Ranganathan SC, Dezateux C, Bush A, *et al.* Airway function in infants newly diagnosed with cystic fibrosis. *Lancet* 2001; 358: 1964–1965.
14. Helbich TH, Heinz-Peer G, Eichler I, *et al.* Cystic fibrosis: CT assessment of lung involvement in children and adults. *Radiology* 1999; 213: 537–544.
15. Long FR, Williams RS, Castile RG. Structural airway abnormalities in infants and young children with cystic fibrosis. *J Pediatr* 2004; 144: 154–161.
16. Jadin SA, Wu GS, Zhang Z, *et al.* Growth and pulmonary outcomes during the first 2 y of life of breastfed and formula-fed infants diagnosed with cystic fibrosis through the Wisconsin Routine Newborn Screening Program. *Am J Clin Nutr* 2011; 93: 1038–1047.
17. Armstrong D, Grimwood K, Carlin JB, *et al.* Lower airway inflammation in infants and young children with cystic fibrosis. *Am J Respir Crit Care Med* 1997; 156: 1197–1204.
18. Dodge JA, Lewis PA, Stanton M, *et al.* Cystic fibrosis mortality and survival in the UK: 1947–2003. *Eur Respir J* 2007; 29: 522–526.
19. Nixon GM, Armstrong DS, Carzino R, *et al.* Early airway infection, inflammation, and lung function in cystic fibrosis. *Arch Dis Child* 2002; 87: 306–311.
20. de Jong PA, Lindblad A, Rubin L, *et al.* Progression of lung disease on computed tomography and pulmonary function tests in children and adults with cystic fibrosis. *Thorax* 2006; 61: 80–85.

21. Sly PD, Brennan S, Gangell C, *et al.* Lung disease at diagnosis in infants with cystic fibrosis detected by newborn screening. *Am J Respir Crit Care Med* 2009; 180: 146–152.

22. Stick SM, Brennan S, Murray C, *et al.* Bronchiectasis in infants and preschool children diagnosed with cystic fibrosis after newborn screening. *J Pediatr* 2009; 155: 623–628.

23. Wainwright CE, Vidmar S, Armstrong DS, *et al.* Effect of bronchoalveolar lavage-directed therapy on *Pseudomonas aeruginosa* infection and structural lung injury in children with cystic fibrosis: a randomized trial. *JAMA* 2011; 306: 163–171.

24. Linnane B, Hall G, Nolan G, *et al.* Lung function in infants with cystic fibrosis diagnosed by newborn screening. *Am J Respir Crit Care Med* 2008; 178: 1238–1244.

25. Hoo AF, Thia LP, Nguyen TT, *et al.* Lung function is abnormal in 3-month-old infants with cystic fibrosis diagnosed by newborn screening. *Thorax* 2012; 67: 874–881.

26. Pillarisetti N, Williamson E, Linnane B, *et al.* Infection, inflammation, and lung function decline in infants with cystic fibrosis. *Am J Respir Crit Care Med* 2011; 184: 75–81.

27. Nguyen TT, Thia LP, Hoo AF, *et al.* Evolution of lung function during the first year of life in newborn screened cystic fibrosis infants. *Thorax* 2013 [In press DOI: 10.1136/thoraxjnl-2013-204023].

28. Mott LS, Park J, Murray CP, *et al.* Progression of early structural lung disease in young children with cystic fibrosis assessed using CT. *Thorax* 2012; 67: 509–516.

29. Sly PD, Gangell CL, Chen L, *et al.* Risk factors for bronchiectasis in children with cystic fibrosis. *N Engl J Med* 2013; 368: 1963–1970.

30. Griese M, Kappler M, Gaggar A, *et al.* Inhibition of airway proteases in cystic fibrosis lung disease. *Eur Respir J* 2008; 32: 783–795.

31. Sutanto EN, Kicic A, Foo CJ, *et al.* Innate inflammatory responses of pediatric cystic fibrosis airway epithelial cells: effects of nonviral and viral stimulation. *Am J Respir Cell Mol Biol* 2011; 44: 761–767.

32. McNally P, Ervine E, Shields MD, *et al.* High concentrations of pepsin in bronchoalveolar lavage fluid from children with cystic fibrosis are associated with high interleukin-8 concentrations. *Thorax* 2011; 66: 140–143.

33. Boucher RC. Evidence for airway surface dehydration as the initiating event in CF airway disease. *J Intern Med* 2007; 261: 5–16.

34. Miele L, Cordella-Miele E, Xing M, *et al.* Cystic fibrosis gene mutation (deltaF508) is associated with an intrinsic abnormality in Ca^{2+}-induced arachidonic acid release by epithelial cells. *DNA Cell Biol* 1997; 16: 749–759.

35. Gangell C, Gard S, Douglas T, *et al.* Inflammatory responses to individual microorganisms in the lungs of children with cystic fibrosis. *Clin Infect Dis* 2011; 53: 425–432.

36. Sagel SD, Gibson RL, Emerson J, *et al.* Impact of *Pseudomonas* and *Staphylococcus* infection on inflammation and clinical status in young children with cystic fibrosis. *J Pediatr* 2009; 154: 183–188.

37. Dickson RP, Erb-Downward JR, Huffnagle GB. The role of the bacterial microbiome in lung disease. *Expert Rev Respir Med* 2013; 7: 245–257.

38. Molyneaux PL, Mallia P, Cox MJ, *et al.* Outgrowth of the bacterial airway microbiome after rhinovirus exacerbation of chronic obstructive pulmonary disease. *Am J Respir Crit Care Med* 2013; 188: 1224–1231.

39. Pezzulo AA, Tang XX, Hoegger MJ, *et al.* Reduced airway surface pH impairs bacterial killing in the porcine cystic fibrosis lung. *Nature* 2012; 487: 109–113.

40. Ramsey BW, Davies J, McElvaney NG, *et al.* A CFTR potentiator in patients with cystic fibrosis and the G551D mutation. *N Engl J Med* 2013; 365: 1663–1672.

41. Stick S, Tiddens H, Aurora P, *et al.* Early intervention studies in infants and preschool children with cystic fibrosis: are we ready? *Eur Respir J* 2013; 42: 527–538.

42. Brody AS, Kosorok MR, Li Z, *et al.* Reproducibility of a scoring system for computed tomography scanning in cystic fibrosis. *J Thorac Imaging* 2006; 21: 14–21.

43. Thia LP, Calder A, Stocks J, *et al.* Is chest CT useful in newborn screened infants with cystic fibrosis at 1 year of age? *Thorax* 2014; 69: 320–327.

44. Rosenow T. Quantitation of chest CT abnormalities in early life CF: back to the basics. *Pediatr Pulmonol* 2013; 48: 372A.

45. Mott LS, Graniel KG, Park J, *et al.* Assessment of early bronchiectasis in young children with cystic fibrosis is dependent on lung volume. *Chest* 2013; 144: 1193–1198.

46. Belessis Y, Dixon B, Hawkins G, *et al.* Early cystic fibrosis lung disease detected by bronchoalveolar lavage and lung clearance index. *Am J Respir Crit Care Med* 2012; 185: 862–873.

47. Lum S, Gustafsson P, Ljungberg H, *et al.* Early detection of cystic fibrosis lung disease: multiple-breath washout *versus* raised volume tests. *Thorax* 2007; 62: 341–347.

48. Gustafsson PM, De Jong PA, Tiddens HA, *et al.* Multiple-breath inert gas washout and spirometry *versus* structural lung disease in cystic fibrosis. *Thorax* 2008; 63: 129–134.

49. Aurora P, Stanojevic S, Wade A, *et al.* Lung clearance index at 4 years predicts subsequent lung function in children with cystic fibrosis. *Am J Respir Crit Care Med* 2010; 183: 752–758.

50. Hall GL, Logie KM, Parsons F, *et al.* Air trapping on chest CT is associated with worse ventilation distribution in infants with cystic fibrosis diagnosed following newborn screening. *PLoS One* 2011; 6: e23932.

51. Amin R, Subbarao P, Jabar A, *et al.* Hypertonic saline improves the LCI in paediatric patients with CF with normal lung function. *Thorax* 2010; 65: 379–383.

52. Patel K, Davis SD, Johnson R, *et al.* Exhaled breath condensate purines correlate with lung function in infants and preschoolers. *Pediatr Pulmonol* 2012; 48: 182–187.

53. Owens CM, Aurora P, Stanojevic S, *et al.* Lung clearance index and HRCT are complementary markers of lung abnormalities in young children with CF. *Thorax* 2013; 66: 481–488.

54. Chudleigh J, Hoo AF, Ahmed D, *et al.* Positive parental attitudes to participating in research involving newborn screened infants with CF. *J Cyst Fibros* 2013; 12: 234–240.

55. Branch-Smith CA, Pooley J, Shields L, *et al.* WS2.2 What do parents experience and how do they cope with the AREST CF early surveillance program for infants and children with cystic fibrosis? *J Cyst Fibros* 2013; 12: Suppl. 1, S3.

56. Sly PD, Ware RS, de Klerk N, *et al.* Randomised controlled trials in cystic fibrosis: what, when and how? *Eur Respir J* 2011; 37: 991–993.

57. Stick SM, Sly PD. Exciting new clinical trials in cystic fibrosis: infants need not apply. *Am J Respir Crit Care Med* 2012; 183: 1577–1578.

Disclosures: None declared.

Chapter 7 |

Imaging the lungs in cystic fibrosis

Harm A.W.M. Tiddens[1,2]

Cystic fibrosis (CF) lung disease starts early in life and is characterised by chronic lung inflammation and infection that persists throughout life. Both inflammation and infection lead to early irreversible structural lung damage. The most important pathological changes are bronchiectasis and bronchiolitis obliterans-like changes of the small airways. The course of disease and spectrum of the structural changes vary widely between patients due to genotypic and environmental differences.

The primary aim of CF therapy is to prevent any structural damage and to conserve lung function. Adequate monitoring of CF lung disease is paramount to tailoring treatment to a patient's need. Imaging techniques are needed to visualise the structural changes related to CF lung disease. Chest computed tomography (CT) is currently the best validated and most sensitive imaging modality to detect and monitor structural lung abnormalities. Magnetic resonance imaging (MRI) is a promising technique that is of specific interest for studying dynamic aspects of the lung.

In most children with cystic fibrosis (CF), progressive lung disease starts in infancy and progresses throughout life [1, 2]. Multiple modalities are used in parallel to monitor CF lung disease, each with their strengths and weaknesses. The most important imaging techniques used to evaluate structural changes related to CF lung disease are chest radiography, chest computed tomography (CT) and chest magnetic resonance imaging (MRI). Of these modalities, chest CT is currently the most systematically validated and, in most clinics, is the most feasible modality to diagnose and monitor bronchiectasis and trapped air. For this reason, this chapter will primarily focus on the role and technique of chest CT in the monitoring and treatment of CF lung disease. In addition, the role of chest MRI and chest radiography will be briefly discussed.

The most important components of CF lung disease are bronchiectasis, which is an irreversible widening of bronchi, and trapped air reflecting small airways disease [3]. CT has been recognised as the gold standard for the detection of bronchiectasis since the mid-1990s [4, 5]. Bronchiectasis, as detected on inspiratory chest CT scans, has been well validated as a clinical outcome measure in recent decades [6–8]. In more recent years, it has become clear that trapped air is an early and important feature of CF lung disease [2]. Trapped air can be detected on expiratory CT scans (fig. 1) [8]. Other structural findings that can be observed on

---

[1]Dept of Paediatric Pulmonology and Allergology, Erasmus Medical Centre Sophia Children's Hospital, Rotterdam, The Netherlands. [2]Dept of Radiology, Erasmus Medical Centre Sophia Children's Hospital, Rotterdam, The Netherlands.

Correspondence: Harm A.W.M. Tiddens, Dept of Paediatric Pulmonology and Allergology, Erasmus Medical Centre Sophia Children's Hospital, Wytemaweg 80, 3015 CN, Rotterdam, The Netherlands. E-mail: h.tiddens@erasmusmc.nl

Copyright ERS 2014. Print ISBN: 978-1-84984-050-7. Online ISBN: 978-1-84984-051-4. Print ISSN: 2312-508X. Online ISSN: 2312-5098.

ERS Monogr 2014; 64: 88–103. DOI: 10.1183/1025448x.10009213

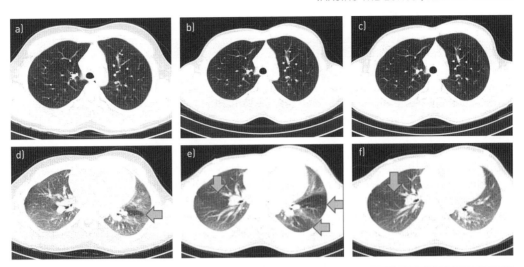

Figure 1. Routine spirometry-controlled inspiratory and expiratory chest computed tomography scans obtained within a biennial period. No structural abnormalities are seen in the inspiratory images (a–c); however, the three expiratory images show evidence of small airways disease (d–f). d) The baseline image shows minor trapped air in the left lung (arrow). e) At follow-up 2 years later, major trapped air can be seen in the left and right lungs (arrows). f) At the next follow-up (biennial within 4 years), resolved trapped air can be seen in the left lung while trapped air in the right lung persisted.

chest CT in CF are airway wall thickness, mucus impaction, atelectasis/consolidation, alveolar consolidation, sacculations/abscesses, bullae and thickening of septa [9–11].

Newborn screening for CF has been introduced in many countries. Important aims of early diagnosis are the prevention of irreversible structural damage, such as bronchiectasis and trapped air, and the reduction of the progression of CF lung disease to a minimum. Unfortunately, the course of CF lung disease varies widely between patients and cannot be adequately predicted for the individual patient based on genotype alone. Hence, therapy must be guided using sensitive monitoring modalities to tailor treatment to the individual patient's needs. In addition, the desirability of therapy should be weighed against negative aspects associated with CF therapy such as interference with regular life, toxicity and costs [12]. Pulmonary function tests (PFTs) such as spirometry are an important tool for closely monitoring CF lung disease on a day-to-day basis. However, PFTs are only an indirect measure of lung structure and are insensitive to localised or early damage [13–15]. To monitor lung structure more directly, many CF centres use chest radiography. Unfortunately, chest radiographs are insensitive to the detection of early disease [16], the technique is variable and correct interpretation of the nature of the structural abnormalities is difficult. Chest CT emerged in the early 1990s to become the gold standard of bronchiectasis diagnosis [5, 17, 18]. It was found to be superior to chest radiography in monitoring lung structure in CF patients [19–23]. In more recent years, chest MRI has been studied as a radiation-free imaging alternative for chest CT. Although promising, chest MRI is currently not sensitive enough to replace chest CT. However, chest MRI should be considered as a monitoring tool for specific clinical and research questions.

Structural lung abnormalities

As a result of the chronic airway inflammation and infection, sputum and bronchoalveolar lavage (BAL) fluid of even young CF patients contains large quantities of aggressive enzymes, such as free neutrophil elastase (NE) [7, 24, 25]. This chronic airway inflammation and infection leads to early changes in the architecture of the lung. The morphological features of CF lungs obtained at autopsy, lobectomy or lung transplant have been described previously in a number of studies [9, 26–28]. These studies showed extensive inflammation of the bronchial wall and airway wall thickening, especially of the small airways and to a lesser extent the large airways. Indeed, airway wall thickening of the small airways in CF patients with end-stage lung disease is as severe as in asthmatics who die from an asthma attack [9, 29].

Using chest CT imaging we have learned more about the development of the above-mentioned small and large airways abnormalities. Notably, the lungs of CF patients show extreme inhomogeneity of pathological changes within the lung (fig. 2) [30]. Large areas of normal lung tissue can be adjacent to areas with localised end-stage structural changes [11, 15, 31, 32]. The small airways cannot be directly observed on CT scans since they are too small for the resolution of chest CT. However, small airways disease can be identified indirectly as areas of low attenuation, especially on expiratory chest CT (figs 1–5) [33]. Areas of low attenuation on inspiratory scans are thought to be the result of hypo-perfusion. Mosaic perfusion is the terminology used when areas of normal and increased density are observed with patchy areas of low attenuation. On expiratory scans, these areas of low attenuation are more visible as they result from a combination of hypoperfusion and trapped air. Such areas contrast clearly with the adjacent healthier deflated, normal or hyperperfused denser parenchyma [33, 34]. The contrast between areas of low attenuation and normal lung tissue can be maximised using a spirometry-controlled chest CT protocol [35]. Areas of low attenuation can be observed in the early stages of disease, in line with the idea that small airways are involved early in the disease process [2, 25, 32]. Airway wall thickening of more central airways can also be observed in young children with CF [31, 36].

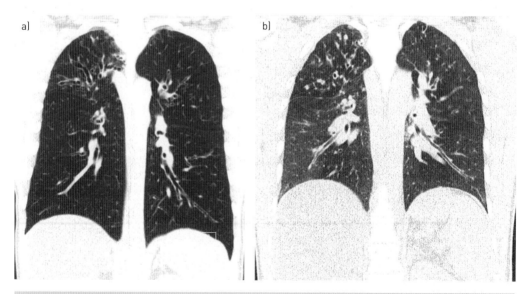

Figure 2. A routine spirometry-controlled a) inspiratory and b) expiratory chest computed tomography scan. Note the inhomogeneity of cystic fibrosis lung disease. The right upper lobe shows localised end-stage lung disease with major diffuse bronchiectasis, while the other lobes are less affected. Trapped air on the expiratory scan (b) is more prominent in the left lung relative to the right lung.

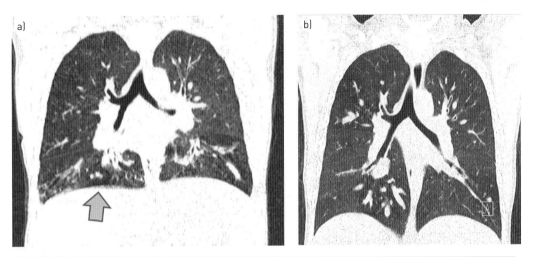

Figure 3. a) A baseline chest computed tomography (CT) scan of 2-year-old girl with cystic fibrosis obtained while she was free breathing. The image was obtained using a very fast CT scanner (Somatom Definition Flash; Siemens, Erlangen, Germany). Extensive bronchiectasis is present, as well as large hypodense areas with trapped air (arrow). b) The CT scan was repeated 2 years later using a lung function technician-coached protocol. Mucus plugging is reduced and trapped air is substantially less. The severity and extent of bronchiectasis remained stable; however, not all anatomical structures are visible in the same plane.

In addition to small airways disease, bronchiectasis is another important feature of CF lung disease. Bronchiectatic airways are airways that are widened, most often as a result of chronic inflammation and infection. In the first year of life it can be observed in 20% of patients. Bronchiectasis is progressive in early childhood [2]. In early school age, it is prevalent in up to 76% of CF patients [10, 25, 31, 37]. Bronchiectatic airways are reservoirs of large quantities of bacteria, inflammatory mediators and DNA released from the nuclei of decomposed neutrophils. Bronchiectasis is likely to damage adjacent healthy regions of the lung. The presence of bronchiectasis is a highly relevant clinical finding. First, it represents an irreversible change of lung structure that is progressive, as has been shown in several longitudinal cohort studies [2, 14]. Secondly, it is a strong predictor of respiratory tract exacerbations, independent of spirometry measurements [38, 39]. Thirdly, its presence is associated with a lower quality of life (QoL) [40]. Fourthly, it is an important component of end-stage lung disease, which is characterised by massive bronchiectasis that can involve 60% of the total lung volume [3, 41]. Finally, its severity in end-stage lung disease is an independent predictor of mortality while on the waiting list for a lung transplant [41].

Mucus plugging is another structural abnormality that can be frequently observed on chest CT scans of CF patients. Mucus plugging is prevalent in up to 79% of CF patients [10]. This is the result of the abnormal mucociliary clearance caused by the abnormal composition of the epithelial lining fluid, high DNA content of the mucus, and interruptions of the mucociliary escalator by bronchiectasis and epithelial damage [9, 42, 43]. Other structural abnormalities that can be observed on CT scans are atelectasis/consolidation (51%), alveolar consolidation (42%), sacculations/abscesses (11%), bullae (8%) and thickening of septa (4%) [10].

In summary, the most relevant structural changes occurring in CF lungs, such as trapped air, bronchiectasis, airway wall thickening and mucus plugging, can be detected using CT.

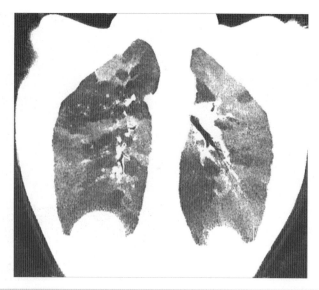

Figure 4. Minimal intensity projection of a spirometer-controlled expiratory computed tomography scan. This post-processing technique is helpful to visualise trapped air by increasing the contrast between the normal density of deflated normally perfused lung tissue and that of hypodense, non-deflated hypoperfused lung regions, reflecting small airways disease.

Chest CT protocol

In general, the CT protocol for CF includes an inspiratory CT scan to evaluate structural changes, especially bronchiectasis, and an expiratory CT scan to evaluate trapped air. In the late 1990s, high-resolution CT (HRCT) was used, *i.e.* incremental 1-mm slices were acquired every 10–20 mm. A disadvantage of limited-slice HRCT is that it underestimates the severity of structural abnormalities, and differentiation between blood vessels and occluded airways is often difficult [44]. Hence, in more recent years, inspiratory volumetric data sets have become routine, using modern, fast multi-slice CT scanners. From these data sets, continuous slices of different thicknesses can be reconstructed in different planes. Anatomical structures of the lungs and abnormal structural changes, such as bronchiectasis, can be easily recognised. This greatly facilitates the longitudinal follow-up of CF lung disease, as perfect slice-per-slice matching at identical anatomical positions can be obtained (fig. 1). An expiratory scan is needed to diagnose and monitor small airways disease, which presents on chest CT as an area of low attenuation. One slice every 30 mm is probably sufficient to establish the severity of small airways disease [45]. However, a volumetric expiratory low-dose CT scan is currently preferred to establish severity, distribution and extent of trapped air. For these expiratory scans, a very low radiation dose is sufficient since there is great contrast between normally deflated dense lung parenchyma and the hypodense parenchyma containing trapped air. Furthermore, on these volumetric expiratory scans it is possible to diagnose tracheal and bronchial malacia, which is frequently observed in CF and the diagnosis of which is highly relevant to the personalisation of physiotherapy treatment [46].

Lung volume control

For optimal image quality and standardisation, lung volume control during CT scanning is of key importance [47, 48]. For children <4 years of age, two different methods can be used.

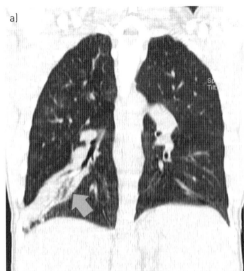
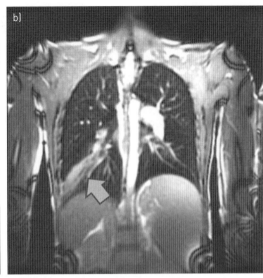

Figure 5. a) A routine spirometer-controlled expiratory chest computed tomography scan. Note the atelectasis in the right lower lobe and areas of trapped air (arrow). b) A routine spirometer-controlled expiratory chest magnetic resonance image 1 year later. Atelectasis can still be observed. Regions of trapped air are more difficult to identify on the chest magnetic resonance image compared to the chest computed tomography scan.

The first method is a pressure-controlled protocol using general anaesthesia or sedation [49–52]. An important condition for this protocol is that it should be executed by a well-trained anaesthesiology team. In anaesthetised children, atelectasis can develop within minutes, making proper evaluation of the chest CT difficult. After intubation and prior to scanning, the lung should be inflated at least five times up to a transpulmonary pressure of 40 cmH$_2$O to recruit atelectatic lung regions. Next, an inspiratory CT scan is performed at a volume level near total lung capacity (TLC) by inflating the lung to a transpulmonary pressure of 25 cmH$_2$O. This is followed by an expiratory scan at a transpulmonary pressure of 0 cmH$_2$O, hence at a volume level near functional residual capacity (FRC).

The second method of acquiring a chest CT in young children is during spontaneous quiet breathing. This method requires the availability of the latest generation of ultra-fast scanners, which allow acquisition of images that are almost free of motion artefacts (fig. 3). A great advantage of this method is that sedation/anaesthesia and its associated risks can be avoided. The volume level of such scans will be near FRC. For children aged $\geqslant 4$ years, the chest CT can be performed without sedation or anaesthesia. It is important that the patient is trained by a lung function technician 30–60 min prior to the CT scan on how to execute the required breath-hold manoeuvres [53]. The same technician will then join the patient in the CT room to provide breathing instructions during the scan. This has the advantage that the radiographer can focus on operating the CT scanner while the lung function technician focuses on the patient's breathing manoeuvres. The lung function technician indicates to the CT technician when the CT acquisition can start, taking into account the delay (1–4 s) between pushing the start button on the CT scanner and the start of the actual acquisition. Lung function technician-coached chest CT scans result in a substantially better standardisation of inspiratory and expiratory volume levels and a minimisation of movement artefacts, thus improving the diagnostic yield of the scans considerably. It is recognised that breath-hold instructions given by a radiographer often result in suboptimal volume levels. The average volume level of inspiratory scans using a voluntary breath-hold is in the range of

80% of TLC [11]. The average volume level of expiratory scans using a voluntary breath-hold is near FRC, hence well above residual volume. For lung function technician-coached chest CT scans, the aim is to achieve inspiratory and expiratory scans that are >95% of the maximal inspiratory vital capacity and >95% of the maximal expiratory vital capacity, respectively. For children aged between 4 and 6 years, the breath-hold manoeuvres can be taught prior to undergoing the CT scan without the use of a spirometer while in the supine position. For more cooperative children aged ⩾6 years, when feasible, a spirometer should be used for the training and chest CT. In order to use a spirometer in the CT scanner, the spirometer used by the patient is connected *via* an extension wire to a monitor positioned in front of the window of the CT control room (fig. 6) [53].

Chest CT and radiation

The challenge of monitoring structural lung disease with biennial chest CT is the selection of a protocol that enables the acquisition of images of sufficient quality using a radiation dose that is "as low as reasonably achievable" (ALARA principle; www.eu-alara.net/index.php/newsletters-mainmenu-37/77-newsletter-31/289-development-and-dissemination-of-alara-culture.html). Using a biennial inspiratory and expiratory CT scan in the follow-up of CF-related lung disease exposes the patient to an amount of radiation comparable to 3–12 months of natural background radiation in a low radiation dose region. In a computational model it was shown that routine lifelong biennial chest CT carries a low risk of radiation-induced mortality in CF [54, 55]. These data suggest that lifelong serial imaging strategies can be used as long as cumulative radiation exposure remains below acceptable risk levels. Technical improvements in scanner technology and software have allowed a 10-fold reduction in the radiation dose of a chest CT scan over the past 10 years. More recently, new, powerful reconstruction algorithms have been developed that allow further reduction in the radiation dose, by ~30%, without loss in image quality [56, 57]. It is highly likely that in the near future the radiation dose can be reduced further due to ongoing technological innovations in hardware and software. In addition, at some point chest MRI may become sensitive enough to replace chest CT and thus eliminate the radiation risk altogether.

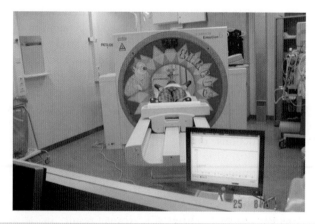

Figure 6. Performance of a spirometer-controlled computed tomography (CT) scan. The patient is placed in the supine position into the scanner with the spirometer. The spirometer is connected *via* an extension wire to the monitor, which is positioned in front of the window of the CT control room. The lung function technician observes the patient's breathing manoeuvres in response to their comments on the monitor. When a breath-hold at full inflation or deflation level is obtained, the scan can be performed.

Therefore, it is likely that current computational models overestimate the risks related to current CT monitoring strategies. Clearly, the use of additional chest CT scans in addition to the routine biennial chest CT scans should be avoided as much as possible. If imaging is needed between routine CT scans (for example, because of unexplained deterioration of the pulmonary condition), a chest radiograph, chest MRI or an ultra-low dose expiratory chest CT should be considered. Findings of these examinations can be compared to the latest routine chest CT scan.

Storage and transfer of data

After a CT scan has been obtained, data are saved in a raw format that requires substantial disk storage space. From this raw data-set, routine reconstructions in the axial, coronal and sagittal plane are made and stored in DICOM (digital imaging and communication in medicine) format on a PACS (picture archiving and communication system) system. In addition, more sophisticated post-processing techniques can be used to generate images that facilitate identification of the lung pathology. For example, minimal intensity projection facilitates visualisation of hypodense regions related to small airways disease (fig. 4). A three-dimensional reconstruction of the bronchial tree can be used to visualise bronchiectasis. It is important to complete post-processing in the days following the CT examination, since raw data are usually deleted from the CT scanner workstation after several weeks. Hence, in chest CT protocols for CF it is important to define all relevant series that must be stored in the PACS system. Such protocols should include reconstruction planes (axial, coronal and sagittal), slice thickness (*e.g.* 5 mm, 3 mm and 1 mm) and reconstruction kernels. It is advisable to store at least one series of thin slices ($\leqslant$1 mm) in the axial plane using an appropriate reconstruction kernel. These thin slices allow additional post-processing when needed. For example, such series can be used to generate three-dimensional reconstructions that facilitate the understanding of anatomical relationships and that are often needed for image analysis purposes using commercially available image analysis software.

Image analysis

For clinical use, possible progression of structural lung changes on chest CT scans of a CF patient can best be examined by comparing, in the axial or other plane, the baseline examination to the follow-up examination slice by slice. Most PACS viewers allow coupling of two examinations in a single window and scrolling through the lung from the lung top to the lung base. These comparisons should be performed for the inspiratory as well as for the expiratory CT scan. Doing so allows conclusions to be drawn as to whether observed structural changes on the baseline CT scan have progressed, are stable or have improved on the follow-up CT, or whether new abnormalities have developed. Unfortunately, this comparison is subjective and does not generate numerical values that can be used for follow-up.

Ideally, the diagnosis and monitoring of the most relevant structural changes on chest CT should be quantified. The most important structural changes to quantify are bronchiectasis and trapped air. For chest CT in CF, the method of choice to date has been scoring. A CT scoring system is a tool to express the severity of the most relevant structural changes in a semi-quantitative way. Several scoring systems have been developed [10]. Important abnormalities that are included in most of the scoring systems are bronchiectasis, mucus plugging, airway wall thickening and parenchymal opacities. Other abnormalities, such as small nodules, mosaic attenuation, sacculations and air trapping on expiratory images, are included in only some of the systems. An advantage of scoring systems is that they are relatively insensitive to the CT scanner and protocol being used. Previously, the Brody-II scoring system was most often used [10]. More recently, the CF CT scoring system was developed, which is an upgraded version of the Brody-II system. The CF CT scoring training module includes clear definitions and reference images for the structural abnormalities that are to be scored. The CF CT score has been used successfully in a number of studies [37, 39, 40]. Scoring systems for chest MRI have been described; however, they are still in an early phase of validation [58, 59]. Using these scoring systems, it has been shown that the sensitivity of MRI to detect mild bronchiectasis is inferior to that of chest CT scoring systems [58].

To date, there are no automated validated image analysis systems available for CF lung disease to quantify bronchiectasis and trapped air on chest CT scans. It is likely that in the near future commercially available (semi-)automated systems will come to market and replace visual scoring. The use of such systems requires standardisation of lung volume during CT acquisition and standardisation of CT protocols. Semi-automated systems to compare airway/artery ratios have been used in CF studies [11]. In addition, software to segment the lung parenchyma and the bronchial tree has been developed. These systems can be used in the near future to detect and quantify bronchiectasis, even in early CF lung disease. Furthermore, systems have been developed to visualise and quantify trapped air [33, 60]. Ideally, such systems should be able to compute the volume of trapped air, expressed as a percentage of total lung volume.

Chest CT and long-term clinical management

Most centres that routinely use chest CT to monitor CF lung disease perform HRCT every other year at the time of the annual check-up in combination with PFTs [14]. A few centres perform a CT scan every third year [1]. This routine is considered useful to determine the long-term efficacy of therapy and monitoring. CT images provide a more sensitive and accurate estimate of the severity and progression of CF lung disease compared with PFTs. The contribution of chest CT to clinical decision making in the management of CF lung disease is difficult to establish. In clinical practice, a multitude of modalities, including PFTs, are used to monitor CF lung disease; each of these modalities contributes to clinical decision making [61]. It is generally accepted that PFTs are not sufficient to monitor CF lung disease, considering that 50% of patient discordance is observed between PFTs and chest CT data [1, 14, 15, 40]. In addition, multiple studies have shown that the severity of bronchiectasis is an independent risk factor from PFTs for respiratory tract exacerbations [38, 39] and mortality [41]. Whether or not progression of bronchiectasis on CT scans can be observed should have an important impact on determining a treatment strategy for the 2 years following the CT scan. It has been well recognised that progression of disease should be prevented, but that the treatment burden to accomplish this has reached a near unacceptable level. Hence, robust data are needed to step up treatment intensity, to keep therapy unchanged, or even to step down treatment intensity [12].

A gap of 2 years between CT scans is considered to be too long between assessments of lung structural changes. Other modalities such as PFTs, physical examinations and symptom scores are all needed to monitor the progression of CF lung disease in the period between CT scans. When a more sensitive monitoring protocol of lung structure for a high-risk patient is needed, one can consider alternating routine biennial chest CT with biennial chest MRI or with ultra-low dose expiratory CT [62]. Further reductions in radiation dose will reduce the risks related to routine use of chest CT.

Chest CT and short-term clinical management

In general, chest CT is not used to monitor the short-term effect of therapeutic interventions, due to the risks of ionising radiation. However, there are a number of acute indications for chest CT in CF patients. First, when there is a strong suspicion of pneumothorax that is not visible on a chest radiograph. It can be difficult to rule out a pneumothorax based on a chest radiograph, especially in advanced disease, due to air trapping preventing the collapse of the lung [63]. In addition, in the case of severe haemoptoe, a CT angiogram can be considered to identify the vessels that need to be embolised.

In several interventional studies, CT-related outcome measures have been used as end-points. In a small 100-day placebo-controlled study, dornase alfa had a positive effect on the CT score [64]. In another small 12-month placebo-controlled study, a positive effect of dornase alfa on mucus impaction was observed, especially in the small airways [65]. However, this effect was only significant when measurements of air trapping were combined with PFT parameters related to the condition of the small airways. In a sub-study of the Pulmozyme Early Intervention Trial (PEIT), no effect of dornase alfa on CT score could be detected [38, 66]. However, this study was underpowered to detect changes in the CT score. In a pooled data analysis, the number of exacerbations correlated with the severity of the CT abnormalities.

CT was also used to evaluate the effect of the treatment of exacerbations with antibiotics [30, 67, 68]. Theoretically, the use of antibiotics should reduce infection and thus inflammation and the amount of free DNA. In a small study, it was shown that mucus plugging was less severe after CF patients were treated for their exacerbation [34]. In another study, treatment of exacerbation improved the air–fluid content of bronchiectasis, mucus and airway wall thickening [68–70]. CT has also been used to monitor the side-effects of gene therapy [71].

As discussed previously, anecdotal studies suggest that the short-term effect of therapy can be visualised using chest CT. Chest MRI might be an interesting alternative method to image changes related to therapeutic interventions, such as mucociliary clearance techniques [72].

Chest MRI

Pulmonary proton MRI sequences have been developed as a radiation-free alternative to chest CT to visualise bronchiectasis, mucus plugging, air fluid levels, consolidation and segmental/lobar destruction [72, 73]. It has been shown that large airways and large bronchiectasis are well visualised on MRI. However, bronchi smaller than the third to fourth generation are poorly visualised [74]. Hence, sensitivity to detect bronchiectasis at an early stage and in the smaller airways is considered poor [58, 75, 76]. Mucus plugging is well visualised by MRI, even down to the small airways, due to the high T2 signal related to its high water content. This makes MRI an interesting modality to study the effects of interventions, for example mucolytic therapy. Furthermore, large pulmonary consolidations, such as atelectasis, can be detected on MRI and CT with a similar appearance (fig. 5). However, in general, the ability of MRI to evaluate lung structure is considered inferior to that of CT [58, 73, 75–77].

The major strength of MRI is the ability to assess functional aspects of the lung, such as perfusion, pulmonary haemodynamics, central airway dynamics and ventilation [78, 79].

Furthermore, chest MRI is an interesting research tool for evaluating short-term changes in response to therapies [72, 78].

To date, a wide variety of chest MRI protocols have been used in CF-related studies. Standardisation of chest MRI protocols and identification and validation of clinically relevant outcome measures from chest MRI images are needed to position its role relative to other routinely used monitoring modalities [61]. It has been advocated that chest MRI should be used to increase the time between chest CT scans [76]. For this reason, my centre has been alternating biennial chest CT with that of biennial chest MRI since 2007.

Volume control during acquisition of MRI images is even more important than when performing CT scans [80]. An important reason for this is that breath-hold times are substantially longer than for CT (up to 15 s) and the impact of movement artefacts during acquisition is critical. Furthermore, expiratory images near residual volume are, in general, more informative than the inspiratory images, since the signal of the denser lung tissue is higher. However, a long breath-hold in expiration is a challenge for many children, in addition to the challenging MRI scanner environment (fig. 7). However, most children aged ⩾8 years can perform spirometer-controlled MRI after adequate training and preparation. The availability of wide bore MRI scanners is likely to improve acceptability for younger children. An intravenously administered contrast agent is needed to study lung perfusion, which increases the burden and risks related to the procedure.

Protocols for combined study of lung structure and function are available and are relatively easy to implement on most MRI scanners that are currently in use. The average examination time for a CF MRI protocol is ~20 min. Unfortunately, in most hospitals MRI time is very competitive and the costs are substantially higher than chest CT.

In summary, currently MRI cannot surpass HRCT in terms of speed, image contrast, content and spatial resolution. It has even been stated that, due to its inherent limitations, MRI may never replace HRCT for diagnosis and monitoring of lung disease [77]. However, the ability

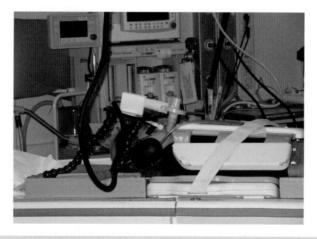

Figure 7. Routine spirometer-controlled magnetic resonance imaging. A spirometer is positioned in the child's mouth, hearing protection covers the ears, and a receiver coil is placed on the chest. The child's arms are positioned alongside the thorax, which is suboptimal as it increases artefacts. This positioning and preparation is required in order to reduce discomfort due to the time spent in the magnetic resonance imaging scanner (15–20 min).

of chest MRI to evaluate various functional characteristics is very interesting and promising. Further standardisation and longitudinal validation studies of reproducible outcome measures are needed to further establish the role of MRI in multi-modality monitoring of CF lung disease.

Chest radiographs

There is a limited role for chest radiographs in the sensitive monitoring of the most important components of CF lung disease, such as bronchiectasis and trapped air. The reason for this is that chest radiographs give a two-dimensional representation of the complex three-dimensional lung structure. Hence, all lung structures are superimposed. For this reason, when increased markings are observed on a chest radiograph it is not often possible to determine the nature of these abnormalities with certainty. This limits the usefulness of chest radiographs in clinical practice, as it is important to understand with certainty the exact nature of the increased markings on chest radiographs in order to adjust or start treatment. Another important reason for the low sensitivity of chest radiographs is that almost one-third of the lung cannot be examined since the tissue is hidden behind the diaphragm or mediastinum [16].

Scoring systems to quantify the structural abnormalities on chest radiographs are available and have been used in clinical studies to track disease progression [81–83]. Using these composite systems, progression of scores with age can be observed. In a cross-sectional study it was shown that chest radiograph scores correlate to CT scores [84]. This is not a surprise, as in cross-sectional studies outcome measures related to CF lung disease will mostly correlate as long as a wide variety of disease severities are included. Overall, the sensitivity of a chest radiograph to detect early bronchiectasis and monitor disease progression is considered poor compared to chest CT. In centres that routinely use chest CT to monitor progression of CF lung disease, the role of chest radiographs is nowadays mostly restricted to diagnosing and monitoring pneumothorax or major atelectasis. There are centres that perform a chest radiograph at each exacerbation. The rationale for this strategy has not been systematically studied.

Tomosynthesis

Tomosynthesis has been developed over the past decade as an alternative to chest radiography and chest CT [85]. Tomosynthesis has better contrast resolution compared to chest radiography and provides coronal lung images that aren't obscured by overlapping anatomy. Hence, it allows substantially better identification of structural abnormalities relative to chest radiography. The radiation dose of this technique is double that of conventional chest radiography and approximately 25% of that of an inspiratory and expiratory low-dose chest CT protocol [86]. A scoring system for tomosynthesis has been previously described [85].

It is unlikely that tomosynthesis will play an important role in monitoring CF lung disease in the near future. First, it has not been systematically validated as only very limited studies in CF have been performed. Secondly, the technique requires a breath-hold of ~10 s and is only considered feasible in children ⩾8 years of age [85]. Hence, it cannot be used for monitoring CF lung disease in young children. Thirdly, tomosynthesis is currently not widely distributed. Finally, the difference in radiation dose between tomosynthesis and state-of-the-art chest CT is very small [86].

In summary, tomosynthesis has clear advantages over chest radiography; however, its advantages over state-of-the-art chest CT are questionable.

Conclusions

CF lung disease is monitored by using multiple modalities in parallel, each with their strengths and weaknesses. Chest CT is the current gold standard for diagnosis of bronchiectasis, which is a highly clinically relevant feature of CF lung disease. Routine biennial chest CT helps us to monitor the severity and progression of CF-related lung disease with extreme precision. It allows the CF team to tailor treatment to the nature of the structural changes and to the patient's disease severity. When adequate low-dose protocols are used, the risk related to ionising radiation exposure is considered to be low. Technical improvements are expected to reduce radiation dose even further in the near future. Chest MRI is in development as a radiation-free alternative for the detection and monitoring of CF lung disease. However, its sensitivity is currently still inferior to that of chest CT and further standardisation of MRI protocols is needed. The role of chest radiography for monitoring CF lung disease is limited. It can be used for the detection of pneumothorax and for the diagnosis of atelectasis.

References

1. de Jong PA, Lindblad A, Rubin L, *et al.* Progression of lung disease on computed tomography and pulmonary function tests in children and adults with cystic fibrosis. *Thorax* 2006; 61: 80–85.
2. Mott LS, Park J, Murray CP, *et al.* Progression of early structural lung disease in young children with cystic fibrosis assessed using CT. *Thorax* 2012; 67: 509–516.
3. Loeve M, van Hal PT, Robinson P, *et al.* The spectrum of structural abnormalities on CT scans from patients with CF with severe advanced lung disease. *Thorax* 2009; 64: 876–882.
4. Kang EY, Miller RR, Muller NL. Bronchiectasis: comparison of preoperative thin-section CT and pathologic findings in resected specimens. *Radiology* 1995; 195: 649–654.
5. Hansell DM. Bronchiectasis. *Radiol Clin North Am* 1998; 36: 107–128.
6. Stick S, Tiddens H, Aurora P, *et al.* Early intervention studies in infants and preschool children with cystic fibrosis: are we ready? *Eur Respir J* 2013; 42: 527–538.
7. Sly PD, Gangell CL, Chen L, *et al.* Risk factors for bronchiectasis in children with cystic fibrosis. *N Engl J Med* 2013; 368: 1963–1970.
8. Loeve M, Krestin GP, Rosenfeld M, *et al.* Chest computed tomography: a validated surrogate endpoint of cystic fibrosis lung disease? *Eur Respir J* 2013; 42: 844–857.
9. Tiddens HA, Koopman LP, Lambert RK, *et al.* Cartilaginous airway wall dimensions and airway resistance in cystic fibrosis lungs. *Eur Respir J* 2000; 15: 735–742.
10. de Jong PA, Ottink MD, Robben SGF, *et al.* Pulmonary disease assessment in cystic fibrosis: comparison of CT scoring systems and value of bronchial and arterial dimension measurements. *Radiology* 2004; 231: 434–439.
11. de Jong PA, Nakano Y, Hop WC, *et al.* Changes in airway dimensions on computed tomography scans of children with cystic fibrosis. *Am J Respir Crit Care Med* 2005; 172: 218–224.
12. Sawicki GS, Tiddens H. Managing treatment complexity in cystic fibrosis: challenges and opportunities. *Pediatr Pulmonol* 2012; 47: 523–533.
13. Tiddens HA. Detecting early structural lung damage in cystic fibrosis. *Pediatr Pulmonol* 2002; 34: 228–231.
14. de Jong PA, Nakano Y, Lequin MH, *et al.* Progressive damage on high-resolution computed tomography despite stable lung function in cystic fibrosis. *Eur Respir J* 2004; 23: 93–97.
15. Owens CM, Aurora P, Stanojevic S, *et al.* Lung Clearance Index and HRCT are complementary markers of lung abnormalities in young children with CF. *Thorax* 2011; 66: 481–488.
16. Bennett TI. Discussion on the stethoscope *versus* x-rays. *Proc R Soc Med* 1945; 355: 7–9.
17. Munro NC, Cooke JC, Currie DC, *et al.* Comparison of thin section computed tomography with bronchography for identifying bronchiectatic segments in patients with chronic sputum production. *Thorax* 1990; 45: 135–139.
18. Young K, Aspestrand F, Kolbenstvedt A. High resolution CT and bronchography in the asssessment of bronchiectasis. *Acta Radiologica* 1991; 32: 439–441.
19. Bhalla M, Turcios N, Aponte V, *et al.* Cystic fibrosis: scoring system with thin-section CT. *Radiology* 1991; 179: 783–788.

20. Maffessanti M, Candusso M, Brizzi F, *et al.* Cystic fibrosis in children: HRCT findings and distribution of disease. *J Thorac Imaging* 1996; 11: 27–38.

21. Nathanson I, Conboy K, Murphy S, *et al.* Ultrafast computerized tomography of the chest in cystic fibrosis: a new scoring system. *Pediatr Pulmonol* 1991; 11: 81–86.

22. Santamaria F, Grillo G, Guidi G, *et al.* Cystic fibrosis: when should high-resolution computed tomography of the chest be obtained? *Pediatrics* 1998; 101: 908–913.

23. Shale DJ. Chest radiology in cystic fibrosis: is scoring useful. *Thorax* 1994; 49: 847.

24. Meyer KC, Sharma A. Regional variability of lung inflammation in cystic fibrosis. *Am J Respir Crit Care Med* 1997; 156: 1536–1540.

25. Stick SM, Brennan S, Murray C, *et al.* Bronchiectasis in infants and preschool children diagnosed with cystic fibrosis after newborn screening. *J Pediatr* 2009; 155: 623–628.

26. Bedrossian CWM, Greenberg SD, Singer DB, *et al.* The lung in cystic fibrosis: a quantitative study including prevalence of pathologic findings among different age groups. *Human Pathology* 1976; 7: 195–204.

27. Tomashefski JF, Bruce M, Goldberg HI, *et al.* Regional distribution of macroscopic lung disease in cystic fibrosis. *Am Rev Respir Dis* 1986; 133: 535–540.

28. Hamutcu R, Rowland JM, Horn MV, *et al.* Clinical findings and lung pathology in children with cystic fibrosis. *Am J Respir Crit Care Med* 2002; 165: 1172–1175.

29. Kuwano K, Bosken CH, Pare PD, *et al.* Small airways dimensions in asthma and chronic obstructive pulmonary disease. *Am J Respir Crit Care Med* 1993; 148: 1220–1225.

30. Davis S, Fordham LA, Brody AS, *et al.* Computed tomography reflects lower airway inflammation and tracks changes in early cystic fibrosis. *Am J Respir Crit Care Med* 2007; 175: 943–950.

31. Long FR, Williams RS, Castile RG. Structural airway abnormalities in infants and young children with cystic fibrosis. *J Pediatr* 2004; 144: 154–161.

32. Tiddens HAWM, Donaldson SH, Rosenfeld M, *et al.* Cystic fibrosis lung disease starts in the small airways: can we treat it more effectively? *Pediatr Pulmonol* 2010; 45: 107–117.

33. Goris ML, Zhu HJ, Blankenberg F, *et al.* An automated approach to quantitative air trapping measurements in mild cystic fibrosis. *Chest* 2003; 123: 1655–1663.

34. Robinson TE, Leung AN, Northway WH, *et al.* Spirometer-triggered high-resolution computed tomography and pulmonary function measurements during an acute exacerbation in patients with cystic fibrosis. *J Pediatr* 2001; 138: 553–559.

35. Robinson TE, Leung AN, Moss RB, *et al.* Standardized high-resolution CT of the lung using a spirometer-triggered electron beam CT scanner. *Am J Roentgenol AJR* 1999; 172: 1636–1638.

36. Martinez TM, Llapur CJ, Williams TH, *et al.* High resolution computed tomography imaging of airway disease in infants with cystic fibrosis. *Am J Respir Crit Care Med* 2005; 172: 1133–1138.

37. Wainwright CE, Vidmar S, Armstrong DS, *et al.* Effect of bronchoalveolar lavage-directed therapy on *Pseudomonas aeruginosa* infection and structural lung injury in children with cystic fibrosis: a randomized trial. *JAMA* 2011; 306: 163–171.

38. Brody AS, Sucharew H, Campbell JD, *et al.* Computed tomography correlates with pulmonary exacerbations in children with cystic fibrosis. *Am J Respir Crit Care Med* 2005; 172: 1128–1132.

39. Loeve M, Gerbrands K, Hop WC, *et al.* Bronchiectasis and pulmonary exacerbations in children and young adults with cystic fibrosis. *Chest* 2010; 140: 178–185.

40. Tepper LA, Utens E, Caudri D, *et al.* Impact of bronchiectasis and trapped air on quality of life and exacerbations in cystic fibrosis. *Eur Respir J* 2013; 42: 371–379.

41. Loeve M, Hop WC, de Bruijne M, *et al.* Chest computed tomography scores are predictive of survival in patients with cystic fibrosis awaiting lung transplantation. *Am J Respir Crit Care Med* 2012; 185: 1096–1103.

42. Paul K, Rietschel E, Ballmann M, *et al.* Effect of treatment with dornase alpha on airway inflammation in patients with cystic fibrosis. *Am J Respir Crit Care Med* 2004; 169: 719–725.

43. Ratjen F. Restoring airway surface liquid in cystic fibrosis. *N Engl J Med* 2006; 354: 291–293.

44. de Jong PA, Nakano Y, Lequin MH, *et al.* Dose reduction for CT in children with cystic fibrosis: is it feasible to reduce the number of images per scan. *Pediatr Radiol* 2005; 36: 50–53.

45. Loeve M, de Bruijne M, Hartmann IC, *et al.* Three-section expiratory CT: insufficient for trapped air assessment in patients with cystic fibrosis? *Radiology* 2012; 262: 969–976.

46. McDermott S, Barry SC, Judge EE, *et al.* Tracheomalacia in adults with cystic fibrosis: determination of prevalence and severity with dynamic cine CT. *Radiology* 2009; 252: 577–586.

47. Mueller KS, Long FR, Flucke RL, *et al.* Volume-monitored chest CT: a simplified method for obtaining motion-free images near full inspiratory and end expiratory lung volumes. *Pediatr Radiol* 2010; 40: 1663–1669.

48. Kongstad T, Buchvald FF, Green K, *et al.* Improved air trapping evaluation in chest computed tomography in children with cystic fibrosis using real-time spirometric monitoring and biofeedback. *J Cyst Fibros* 2013; 12: 559–566.

49. Long FR, Castile RG. Technique and clinical applications of full-inflation and end-exhalation controlled-ventilation chest CT in infants and young children. *Pediatr Radiol* 2001; 31: 413–422.

50. Long FR, Castile RG, Brody AS, *et al.* Lungs in infants and young children: improved thin-section CT with a noninvasive controlled-ventilation technique–initial experience. *Radiology* 1999; 212: 588–593.

51. Long FR, Williams RS, Adler BH, *et al.* Comparison of quiet breathing and controlled ventilation in the high-resolution CT assessment of airway disease in infants with cystic fibrosis. *Pediatr Radiol* 2005; 35: 1075–1080.

52. Long FR, Williams RS, Castile RG. Inspiratory and expiratory CT lung density in infants and young children. *Pediatr Radiol* 2005; 35: 677–683.

53. Lever S, van der Wiel EC, Koch A, *et al.* Feasibility of spirometry controlled chest CT in children. *Eur Respir J* 2009; 34: Suppl. 53, 36s.

54. de Jong PA, Mayo JR, Golmohammadi K, *et al.* Estimation of cancer mortality associated with repetitive computed tomography scanning (CT) scanning in cystic fibrosis. *Am J Respir Crit Care Med* 2005; 173: 199–203.

55. Huda W. Radiation doses and risks in chest computed tomography examinations. *Proc Am Thorac Soc* 2007; 4: 316–320.

56. Singh S, Kalra MK, Shenoy-Bhangle AS, *et al.* Radiation dose reduction with hybrid iterative reconstruction for pediatric CT. *Radiology* 2012; 263: 537–546.

57. Willemink MJ, de Jong PA. Pediatric chest computed tomography at a radiation dose approaching a chest radiograph. *Am J Respir Crit Care Med* 2013; 188: 626–627.

58. Failo R, Wielopolski PA, Tiddens HA, *et al.* Lung morphology assessment using MRI: a robust ultra-short TR/TE 2D steady state free precession sequence used in cystic fibrosis patients. *Magn Reson Med* 2009; 61: 299–306.

59. Eichinger M, Optazaite DE, Kopp-Schneider A, *et al.* Morphologic and functional scoring of cystic fibrosis lung disease using MRI. *Eur J Radiol* 2012; 81: 1321–1329.

60. Bonnel AS, Song SM, Kesavarju K, *et al.* Quantitative air-trapping analysis in children with mild cystic fibrosis lung disease. *Pediatr Pulmonol* 2004; 38: 396–405.

61. Tiddens HA, Stick SM, Davis S. Multi-modality monitoring of cystic fibrosis lung disease: the role of chest computed tomography. *Paediatr Respir Rev* 2014; 15: 92–97.

62. Loeve M, Lequin MH, de Bruijne M, *et al.* Cystic fibrosis: are volumetric ultra-low-dose expiratory CT scans sufficient for monitoring related loung disease? *Radiology* 2009; 253: 223–229.

63. Phillips GD, Trotman-Dickenson B, Hodson ME, *et al.* Role of CT in the management of pneumothorax in patients with complex cystic lung disease. *Chest* 1997; 112: 275–278.

64. Nasr SZ, Kuhns LR, Brown RW, *et al.* Use of computerized tomography and chest x-rays in evaluating efficacy of aerosolized recombinant human DNase in cystic fibrosis patients younger than age 5 years: a preliminary study. *Pediatr Pulmonol* 2001; 31: 377–382.

65. Robinson TE, Leung AN, Northway WH, *et al.* Composite spirometric-computed tomography outcome measure in early cystic fibrosis lung disease. *Am J Respir Crit Care Med* 2003; 168: 588–593.

66. Quan JM, Tiddens HAWM, Sy J, *et al.* A two-year randomized, placebo controlled trial of dornase alfa in young cystic fibrosis patients with mild lung function abnormalities. *J Pediatr* 2001; 139: 813–820.

67. Amin R, Charron M, Grinblat L, *et al.* Cystic fibrosis: detecting changes in airway inflammation with FDG PET/CT. *Radiology* 2012; 264: 868–875.

68. Horsley AR, Davies JC, Gray RD, *et al.* Changes in physiological, functional and structural markers of cystic fibrosis lung disease with treatment of a pulmonary exacerbation. *Thorax* 2013; 68: 532–539.

69. Shah RM, Sexauer W, Ostrum BJ, *et al.* High-resolution CT in the acute exacerbation of cystic fibrosis: evaluation of acute findings, reversibility of those findings, and clinical correlation. *Am J Roentgenol AJR* 1997; 169: 375–380.

70. Brody AS, Molina PL, Klein JS, *et al.* High-resolution computed tomography of the chest in children with cystic fibrosis: support for use as an outcome surrogate. *Pediatr Radiol* 1999; 29: 731–735.

71. Joseph PM, O'Sullivan BP, Lapey A, *et al.* Aerosol and lobar administration of a recombinant adenovirus to individuals with cystic fibrosis. I. Methods, safety, and clinical implications. *Hum Gene Ther* 2001; 12: 1369–1382.

72. Woodhouse N, Wild JM, van Beek EJ, *et al.* Assessment of hyperpolarized [3]He lung MRI for regional evaluation of interventional therapy: a pilot study in pediatric cystic fibrosis. *J Magn Reson Imaging* 2009; 30: 981–988.

73. Eichinger M, Heussel CP, Kauczor HU, *et al.* Computed tomography and magnetic resonance imaging in cystic fibrosis lung disease. *J Magn Reson Imaging* 2010; 32: 1370–1378.

74. Puderbach M, Eichinger M, Gahr J, *et al.* Proton MRI appearance of cystic fibrosis: comparison to CT. *Eur Radiol* 2007; 17: 716–724.

75. Ciet P, Serra G, Bertolo S, *et al.* Comparison of chest-MRI to chest-CT to monitor cystic fibrosis lung disease. *Pediatric Pulmonology*, 2010: Suppl. 33, 362.

76. Sileo C, Corvol H, Boelle PY, *et al.* HRCT and MRI of the lung in children with cystic fibrosis: comparison of different scoring systems. *J Cyst Fibros* 2014; 13: 198–204.

77. Washko GR, Parraga G, Coxson HO. Quantitative pulmonary imaging using computed tomography and magnetic resonance imaging. *Respirology* 2012; 17: 432–444.

78. Ley-Zaporozhan J, Molinari F, Risse F, *et al.* Repeatability and reproducibility of quantitative whole-lung perfusion magnetic resonance imaging. *J Thorac Imaging* 2011; 26: 230–239.

79. Ciet P, Wielopolski P, Manniesing R, *et al.* Spirometer controlled cine-magnetic resonance imaging to diagnose tracheobronchomalacia in pediatric patients. *Eur Respir J* 2014; 43: 115–124.

80. Eichinger M, Puderbach M, Smith HJ, *et al.* Magnetic resonance-compatible-spirometry: principle, technical evaluation and application. *Eur Respir J* 2007; 30: 972–979.

81. Rosenfeld M, Farrell PM, Kloster M, *et al.* Association of lung function, chest radiographs and clinical features in infants with cystic fibrosis. *Eur Respir J* 2013; 42: 1545–1552.

82. Terheggen-Lagro S, Truijens N, van Poppel N, *et al.* Correlation of six different cystic fibrosis chest radiograph scoring systems with clinical parameters. *Pediatr Pulmonol* 2003; 35: 441–445.

83. Terheggen-Lagro SW, Arets HG, van der Laag J, *et al.* Radiological and functional changes over 3 years in young children with cystic fibrosis. *Eur Respir J* 2007; 30: 279–285.

84. Sanders DB, Li Z, Brody AS, *et al.* Chest computed tomography scores of severity are associated with future lung disease progression in children with cystic fibrosis. *Am J Respir Crit Care Med* 2011; 184: 816–821.

85. Vult von Steyern K, Bjorkman-Burtscher I, Geijer M. Tomosynthesis in pulmonary cystic fibrosis with comparison to radiography and computed tomography: a pictorial review. *Insights Imaging* 2012; 3: 81–89.

86. Vult von Steyern K, Bjorkman-Burtscher IM, Weber L, *et al.* Effective dose from chest tomosynthesis in children. *Radiat Prot Dosimetry* 2014; 158: 290–298.

Acknowledgements: I would like to thank Tim Rosenow (Telethon Institute for Child Health Research and School of Paediatrics and Child Health Research, University of Western Australia, Perth, Australia, and Dept of Paediatric Pulmonology, Erasmus Medical Centre Sophia Children's Hospital, Rotterdam, The Netherlands) for critical reading of the manuscript as a native speaker, as well as an expert on the topic.

Disclosures: In the past 4 years H.A.W.M. Tiddens has acted as consultant for the BV Kindergeneeskunde of the Sophia Children's Hospital (Rotterdam, the Netherlands), and on advisory boards for Gilead Sciences, Novartis Pharmaceuticals, Pharmaxis Pharmaceuticals, Insmed and Vertex. He has received fees for symposia from Roche and Pharmaxis Pharmaceuticals. In addition, the BV Kindergeneeskunde received speaker fees for presentations by H.A.W.M. Tiddens from Chiesi, Gilead, Novartis, Forest and Roche; he does not own any stock. The BV Kindergeneeskunde received unconditional research grants from Roche, Chiesi and Gilead for research supervised by H.A.W.M. Tiddens. He is the founder and director of LungAnalysis, a core laboratory for image analysis of the Erasmus Medical Centre (Rotterdam) under the supervision of the research bureaus of the Depts of Pediatrics and Radiology (Erasmus Medical Centre) for which he has received funding from CFF. He also has a licenced patent funded by ActivAero.

Chapter 8

End-points and biomarkers for clinical trials in cystic fibrosis

Kris De Boeck[1], Isabelle Fajac[2,3] and Felix Ratjen[4]

The development of new treatments for patients with cystic fibrosis (CF) was paralleled by a renewed interest in the development and critical evaluation of new and existing end-points. The improved outcome of patients was the main reason why mortality, and even forced expiratory volume in 1 s (FEV1) could no longer be used as sensitive outcome measures.

In this chapter, we review the pros and cons of commonly used outcome measures in clinical trials, as well as the factors that determine the choice of end-points in a specific trial. We then "put the theory into practice" by elaborating on scenarios for CF clinical trials addressing different aspects of CF lung disease.

Since CF is a rare disorder, phase III clinical trials require multicentre cooperation. The development of clinical trial networks and task forces striving for rigorous standardisation and agreement on detailed standard operating procedures for outcome measures are other important steps in bridging the gap between drug discovery and robust evaluation of drug benefit.

In recent years, several reviews have been written about the utility of specific end-points for clinical trials in cystic fibrosis (CF). Therefore, we will not duplicate this work but refer to these reviews for details on individual outcome parameters. The approach in this chapter is to discuss the classification of end-points used in clinical research, to list the major advantages and disadvantages of end-points commonly used in CF clinical trials and to discuss which factors influence the choice of a particular end-point. We will then "put the theory into practice" by elaborating on a few scenarios for CF clinical trials addressing different aspects of CF lung disease.

Classification of end-points into categories

There are in essence three types of outcome measures (table 1) [1, 2].

Clinical end-points

Clinical end-points reflect how a patient feels, functions or survives. Clinical end-points are supposed to detect a tangible benefit for the patient. Indeed, any intervention in a patient is

[1]Paediatric Pulmonology, Dept of Pediatrics, University of Leuven, Leuven, Belgium. [2]Paris Descartes University, Sorbonne Paris Cité, Paris, France. [3]Physiology Dept, Cochin Hospital, AP-HP, Paris, France. [4]Dept of Pediatrics, University of Toronto, Toronto, ON, Canada.

Correspondence: Kris De Boeck, Paediatric Pulmonology, Dept of Pediatrics, University Hospital Leuven, Herestraat 49, 3000 Leuven, Belgium. E-mail: Christiane.deboeck@uzleuven.be

Copyright ERS 2014. Print ISBN: 978-1-84984-050-7. Online ISBN: 978-1-84984-051-4. Print ISSN: 2312-508X. Online ISSN: 2312-5098.

Table 1. Monitoring success in clinical trials: categories of outcome parameters

Category	Definition	Example in CF
Clinical end-point	Reflects how a patient feels, functions, survives	Survival Rate of pulmonary exacerbations Quality of life Nutritional status
Surrogate end-point	Lab measure as substitute for above Predicts efficacy of therapy	FEV1
Biomarker	Objective indicator of a process	Sweat chloride Sputum neutrophil elastase Sputum *Pseudomonas aeruginosa* density

supposed to make their life better, either in duration or in quality. With the improved life expectancy in CF, survival has become an impossible end-point for use in clinical trials. Therefore, intermediate clinical efficacy measures, such as frequency of pulmonary exacerbations have been used more often [3]. Quality of life (QoL) measures such as the Cystic Fibrosis Questionnaire Revised (CFQ-R) are another accepted clinical end-point that quantifies the treatment benefit in patients with CF [4].

Surrogate end-points

A surrogate end-point is a laboratory measure that can be used as a substitute for a clinical end-point. A laboratory measure can only have the status of surrogate end-point if it reliably reflects the clinical efficacy of therapy and is linked to survival or long-term prognosis. Until recently, only forced expiratory volume in 1 s (FEV1) was considered as an acceptable surrogate end-point by health authorities.

Biomarkers

A biomarker is a characteristic that is objectively measured and evaluated as an indicator of a normal biological process, a pathological process or a pharmacological response to a therapeutic intervention. Thus, biomarkers are mainly used to test the "proof of concept" of a specific compound in phase I and phase II clinical trials.

When clinical benefit must be proven in phase III trials, an outcome measure of the first two categories must be chosen. Of course, adding a biomarker as a secondary outcome measure in phase III trials has the advantage to gain more insight on the correlation between change in biomarker and clinical benefit, so that the evidence base for promoting this biomarker to the status of surrogate end-point can be increased.

Main advantages and disadvantages of some commonly used outcome measures

For detailed information on specific outcome measures for use in CF clinical trials, we refer to recent reviews on cystic fibrosis transmembrane conductance receptor (CFTR) biomarkers [5], lung clearance index (LCI) [6, 7], markers of inflammation in bronchoalveolar lavage (BAL) fluid

[8] and sputum and chest imaging [9]. Additionally, we refer to recent overviews on outcome measures in CF with a specific focus on emerging end-points such as pulmonary magnetic resonance imaging (MRI) scans [10–12] and to a document on the European Medicines Agency website providing answers to questions about specific outcome measures, the latter document being the combined work of CF specialists, regulators and participants from the pharmaceutical industry [13].

In table 2 we list commonly used end-points in CF clinical trials and highlight their main advantages and disadvantages. For conciseness only a few key references are included.

An additional point of attention and ongoing discussion for all biomarkers listed in table 2, is the need for rigorous standardisation and agreement on detailed standard operating procedures from acquisition of data all the way through to analysis of test result. This is very important in multicentre trials and a prerequisite for building a consistent and useful evidence base about a specific end-point. Furthermore, it should be known what change in biomarker corresponds with a relevant change in clinical benefit for the patient. However, whereas the minimal clinically important difference has been derived for the QoL measure CFQ-R [4], there is no such agreement for what represents the minimal clinically important change in FEV1.

Factors that drive the choice of outcome measure

Scientific rationale and duration of the study

Many clinical or surrogate end-points and biomarkers are available as possible outcome measures when designing a clinical trial in CF. The decision will mainly be based on the scientific rationale and the physiological/pathogenic process that the outcome measure needs to reflect. Obviously, the relevant biomarkers will be very different if the scientific question is to verify the proof of concept of an anti-inflammatory agent or of a CFTR modifying drug. Once the type of outcome measures is chosen, key questions are how much the outcome measure is expected to change in response to the intervention and how long it will take to see the expected change [26]. The magnitude of the expected change must be within the range of detection and it must occur within the duration of the study.

Phase of study

Phase I and II studies about a new medicinal product usually aim at gaining information about short-term safety and tolerability and at providing pharmacodynamic and pharmacokinetic information to choose a suitable dosage range [27]. Phase II studies are also often proof-of-concept studies to confirm the mechanism of action of a potential drug. Biomarkers that are "indicators of normal biologic processes, pathogenic processes, or pharmacologic responses to a therapeutic intervention" are the main choices for outcome measures in those phase II trials [2].

Aside from gaining further information on drug safety and tolerability, phase III studies aim to demonstrate/confirm a drug's therapeutic benefit. Thus, the primary end-point in a phase III trial should be a clinical end-point or a surrogate end-point. FEV1 has been the most used surrogate end-point in CF clinical trials. This was because FEV1 was shown to be related to mortality [28–30]. Other end-points used in phase III trials are time to exacerbation or the number of exacerbations during the treatment period; although there is still no uniform agreement about exacerbation definition [3]. To some extent, phase III randomised controlled

Table 2. Commonly used end-points

Outcome parameter	Advantages	Disadvantages
Clinical end-points		
Pulmonary exacerbations	Relevant to patient Drive lung function decline [17]	No uniform definition [3] Difficult to standardise between physicians Rare in mild disease [18] Large number needed in phase III trials
QoL scores	"Quantification" of patient well-being Information directly from patient/parent	Patients don't like completing questionnaires Ceiling effect in mild disease
Surrogate end-points		
FEV1	Correlates with mortality Noninvasive Very well standardised Widely available Large evidence base	Insensitive in mild or early disease
Biomarkers moving towards surrogate end-point status		
LCI [6]	Sensitive to early or mild lung disease Emerging data on correlation with long-term evolution [19, 20]	Not widely available Long-term significance not entirely clear Unclear which size of improvement corresponds with a significant change
Chest CT scores for bronchiectasis [9, 14, 15]	Quantify structural lung disease Correlate with long-term outcome	Radiation exposure Standardisation between imaging centres is complex Long timeline needed to assess structural changes
Biomarkers		
CFTR biomarkers [16] Sweat chloride NPD measurements Intestinal current measurements	Quantification of CFTR function in different organs	Relative sensitivity of different organs to changes in CFTR function is not known and may differ between CFTR modulators Test reproducibility of NPD is not optimal [21] No linear correlation between CFTR function improvement and FEV1 improvement
Biomarkers of inflammation in BAL fluid [8] and sputum	In infants, BAL inflammation parameters are predictive of subsequent structural lung disease [15, 22] Change in sputum elastase and neutrophil count correlates with change in FEV1 [23, 24]	BAL is invasive Many patients do not expectorate, not even after sputum induction Poor feasibility in phase III trials

Table 2. Continued

Outcome parameter	Advantages	Disadvantages
Bacterial culture results of throat swab, sputum or BAL fluid	Natural history in CF relatively well known Relevant short-term information	Natural history complex and variable Difficult to standardise and quantify Throat swab has low PPV for presence of lower airway pathogens Long timeline needed to assess significant changes New paradigms are developing since data on complexity of lung microbiota are emerging [25]

QoL: quality of life; FEV1: forced expiratory volume in 1 s; LCI: lung clearance index; CT: computed tomography; CFTR: cystic fibrosis transmembrane conductance regulator; NPD: nasal potential difference; BAL: bronchoalveolar lavage; CF: cystic fibrosis; PPV: positive predictive value.

trials can also be used as observational trials: extensively phenotyping patients at baseline allows the running of subgroup analyses to develop prediction models for efficacy.

Post-marketing studies

Post-marketing studies are studies conducted after a product has been approved by regulatory agencies for marketing. They allow gathering of additional information about a product's safety, efficacy or optimal use. They are usually studies required by regulatory agencies and agreed to by a sponsor. They might be interventional trials with the usual safety and efficacy outcome measures to evaluate long-term effectiveness or durability of response. They are more often observational pharmaco-epidemiological studies for which existing registries can be used or specifically designed. The choice of end-points will be guided by the scientific rationale, which can be estimating the risk of a serious adverse event or toxicity associated with use of a drug, identifying risk factors (*e.g.* patient characteristics, duration of drug use) or assessing pregnancy incidence or outcomes and/or child outcomes after patient drug exposure [31].

Observational studies

In an observational study, investigators assess health outcomes in groups of participants according to a protocol or research plan. The main difference to a clinical trial is that participants are not assigned to specific interventions by the investigator. Participants may receive interventions, such as drugs or procedures, as long as those interventions are part of their routine medical care. Therefore, the outcome measures need to be captured as part of routine medical care. For example, if the aim is to monitor the long-term effect on health economics of a marketed CFTR corrector, the numbers of days of hospitalisation or the numbers of days out of school/work could be monitored in an observational study.

Industry-sponsored *versus* investigator-driven studies

In all studies, the choice of the outcome measures is based on scientific rationale. However, an industry-sponsored study usually aims at gaining a license for marketing. Therefore, the sponsor is bound by the regulatory agencies' guidelines. In those guidelines, the gold standard as a surrogate end-point for most pulmonary indications is FEV1 [32]. Advances in CF care have resulted in higher mean FEV1 levels and lower mean rates of decline in consecutive CF cohorts [33]. Therefore, FEV1 is no longer a very sensitive measurement. FEV1 will also not detect a subtle improvement of a baseline subnormal lung function induced by a drug. The need for new and more sensitive surrogate end-points has been the topic of discussions in articles [16] and at a workshop hosted by the European Medicines Agency with representatives of all stakeholders in September 2012 [13]. Due to their sensitivity in detecting early or mild disease and growing evidence that they are linked to established clinical outcomes, the evaluation of LCI [6, 7] and of chest computed tomography (CT) scan [9, 14] as possible future agencies-approved surrogate end-points is ongoing.

Paediatric subjects

Outcome measures for studies in infants and young children will differ from those in older patients for a number of reasons. First, traditional lung function tests require cooperation and are not feasible in this age group. In preschool children, incentive spirometry has been utilised in observational studies, but interventional trials using preschool spirometry as an outcome measure are lacking. FEV0.75 is considered to be the equivalent of FEV1 in this age group due to the fact that a forced expiration lasts for a shorter time period. Tracking over time is therefore difficult for this lung function parameter in studies bridging the age between preschool and school age children. In infants, FEV0.5 has been utilised and one interventional study has demonstrated a treatment effect for hypertonic saline in CF infants [34]. However, these tests require expensive equipment, skilled personnel and sedation of study subjects; therefore, it is unlikely that this will reach widespread applicability. Multiple-breath washout (MBW) tests are currently being explored as a potential outcome measure that can overcome some of these hurdles. The test assesses ventilation inhomogeneity, has been shown to have a higher sensitivity to detect early abnormalities and requires minimal cooperation; thus is feasible without sedation beyond infancy. One recent study has demonstrated a treatment effect of hypertonic saline in children younger than 6 years of age and further studies are currently planned [6].

Alternatively, symptoms scores or assessment of the number or time to next exacerbation could be used in young children. However, with newborn screening and early aggressive management, most young CF children are now symptom free and symptoms are largely driven by viral infections. Viral infections do not vary in frequency between CF and non-CF children and are thus unlikely to be influenced in their rate by any treatment intervention. This is supported by a recent interventional trial in which no differences were seen in the rate of pulmonary exacerbations between hypertonic and isotonic saline treated children whereas measurements of infant lung function [34] or LCI [6] were able to demonstrate treatment effects. The definition of rate of pulmonary exacerbations was the events per person per year of treatment with oral, inhaled or intravenous antibiotics for one or more pre-specified signs or symptoms within the period 3 days prior to the antibiotic start date.

Alternatively or in addition to functional tests, lung imaging has been proposed as a potential end-point for clinical trials. While there is currently one study ongoing to assess the effect of early intervention therapy with azithromycin on the development of bronchiectasis assessed by CT scans, so far lung imaging data are limited to shorter trials with dornase alfa in which air trapping has been used to quantify a treatment effect [35]. Future studies will link functional and structural measures of lung disease and will help to delineate which test is best suited as an end-point for clinical trials in young children.

Size of study population

CF, while being the most common monogenetic disease in Caucasians, is overall relatively rare, limiting the number of subjects that can be recruited for clinical trials. Despite this, studies in CF have been remarkably successful which reflects the excellent collaboration between centres across the world and an impressive commitment by patients and families to participate in interventional studies. Due to the limited number of subjects and the marked improvement in survival, mortality is not a suitable outcome measure for any CF trial and biomarkers that have either been predictive of survival or are linked to established measures of lung disease are usually used as proxies to demonstrate treatment effects. In patients with established lung disease, these include measures of lung function as there is room for improvement that can be quantified within a reasonable time frame. However, not every intervention is expected to have immediate beneficial effects on lung function; f.i. agents that modulate inflammation may require a longer observation period and the effect may be better reflected in demonstrating differences in rate of decline of lung function. The latter is also a more suitable parameter for studies in subjects with preserved lung function. As lung function decline is low in CF patients, these studies require a long observation period, a very large sample size or both [36]. Estimating effect sizes of therapies are important considerations in determining sample sizes and are easier for studies where sufficient prior experience exists such as for antibiotic therapies to treat chronic *Pseudomonas aeruginosa* infection. Realistic estimations are crucial to ensure that a study can actually be successful in recruiting study subjects in a reasonable time frame; a problem that has plagued many investigator-driven studies.

Mono-centre and multicentre studies

Proof-of-concept studies are more likely to be feasible with a small sample size in a single or a small number of centres. Outcome measures in these trials are not necessarily aiming to provide definitive proof for the efficacy of the intervention, but rather evidence that the "drug does what it is supposed to do". This could mean improved chloride conductance in the nasal epithelium for CFTR pharmacotherapy, reduction of bacterial density for an antibiotic or reducing neutrophil elastase burden for an anti-inflammatory drug. More definitive studies require more established outcome measures, such as FEV_1 or pulmonary exacerbations and can only be performed in a multicentre setting. These studies require a higher level of funding that is more likely to be available for industry-sponsored than investigator-driven trials. The complexity and infrastructure requirements for these studies are also much higher and thus require a well-organised clinical trial network that can oversee these studies as well as detailed standardisation of the outcome measures used. While in the past this was available for only a few measures, recent efforts have broadened the spectrum of tests that can be reliably performed in a multicentre setting. Including these outcome measures in clinical trials will not only improve the ability to detect treatment effects but also help to better understand the utility of these outcome measures in later phase studies.

Invasiveness of outcome measures

Another important consideration for an outcome measure to be used in a clinical trial is the risk–benefit ratio of a given test. This is less of an issue for simple measures of lung function such as spirometry, but other tests do have potential downsides. Imaging techniques often require ionised radiation and, while the doses have been largely reduced in recent years [37], this continues to be a concern, particularly if these tests need to be performed repeatedly. The "gold standard" to quantify inflammation is BAL, but the test is invasive and associated with potential morbidity. Thus, while its use may be justified in a proof-of-concept study, less invasive biomarkers may replace BAL in subsequent studies to limit the burden and maximise the safety for patients. While ideally one biomarker will fulfil all needs by being noninvasive without side-effects and strongly linked to hard outcomes such as mortality, it is more likely that a battery of tests will be required which are tailored to each individual study [14]. In the subsequent section we will thus provide some examples how a spectrum of biomarkers could be used in drug development for compounds with different modes of action.

Specific scenarios

Evaluating the efficacy of a new anti-inflammatory drug

Inflammation is a hallmark of CF lung disease and dominated by neutrophils and their products. Drugs addressing inflammation should decrease neutrophil influx into the airways, reduce neutrophilic products that are thought to be detrimental for lung health, such as proteases, or both. To detect a change in markers of inflammation may require longer time than for studies involving a mucolytic or antibiotic in which the intervention is expected to be associated with benefits in lung function within a time frame of days to a few weeks. The time frame for a response in lung function is less well defined and the only anti-inflammatory drug that has entered clinical care (ibuprofen) has had no immediate effect on lung function, but rather impacted on lung function decline in longer term studies [38, 39]. While a phase II study of an anti-inflammatory drug would likely include FEV1 as an outcome measure, treatment effects are more likely to be seen in markers of inflammation. BAL would be the gold standard to quantify this in an early phase study. Sputum markers of inflammation such as absolute neutrophil counts or neutrophil elastase and interleukin (IL)-8 are potential alternatives, but markers of inflammation are highly variable both within and between individuals [24]. Serum markers of inflammation may be a potential option and a recent study has demonstrated significant treatment effects for azithromycin within 4 weeks for absolute neutrophil count in blood and neutrophil products, such as calprotectin, even in patients with mild lung disease [40]. Therefore, a phase II study could include both serum and sputum markers as measures of proof of concept. A phase III study would then likely use pulmonary exacerbation as a primary outcome measure because a drug reducing inflammation would likely reduce the number of and time to next pulmonary exacerbation as well. Since rate of pulmonary exacerbations requires a large sample size, chest CT could also be an appropriate end-point to study the efficacy of an anti-inflammatory drug as it is thought to reduce airway wall thickening, development and progression of bronchiectasis. Measures of lung function could be used as secondary outcome measure, but may not show a signal unless the study is conducted over multiple years.

Evaluating the efficacy of a new inhaled antibiotic

Lung damage secondary to chronic infection is the main cause of death in CF. When managing CF-associated chronic lung infection, the main objective is to maintain CF patients' lung function over extended periods of time in the presence of the persistent pathogen in the airways. When antibacterial agents are designed for CF lung disease, it usually consists in developing an aerosol formulation of a well-known antibiotic with a long proven antimicrobiological efficacy in systemic administration. Therefore, showing the local microbiological effect of such an inhaled antibiotic is not the main aim and it might even prove difficult. Obtaining microbiological samples particularly in children is not easy, sputum is not homogenous and the result depends to a large extent on the sample-taking procedure. Therefore, it is expected that phase II and phase III clinical trials on inhaled antibacterial agents in patients with CF demonstrate that FEV1 is improved or maintained [13, 32]. Change of sputum *P. aeruginosa* density was the primary end-point in a recent phase II study on levofloxacin inhalation solution [41]. Alternatively, most phase II studies and all phase III studies chose change in FEV1 as the primary end-point and microbiological criteria as secondary end-points [42–44]. The differences in the phase II and III trials would not be in the choice of the outcome measures, but rather in the study design and duration: for example, a placebo-controlled study over a month for a phase II trial and an active comparator over 6–12 months for a phase III trial.

However, the majority of chronically infected patients are no longer treatment naïve and improved symptomatic treatment options result in preservation of good lung function over prolonged period of life with the majority of (young) children having FEV1 values within the normal range. Thus, the change in FEV1 might not reach the desired magnitude for a phase II placebo-controlled trial or might not be better than the standard-of-care comparator in a phase III trial. In the latter, non-inferiority trials are usually chosen but need careful consideration when selecting the non-inferiority margin [45]. Other clinical end-points are also often considered as secondary end-points: number and time to exacerbation which needs a (not yet available) clear definition of exacerbation, proportion of patients with decreased number or time to exacerbations, number of hospitalisations, number of intravenous treatments, duration of hospitalisation, patient-reported outcomes (PRO). While chronic infection with *P. aeruginosa* has been associated with faster rate of FEV1 decline [46, 47], antibiotic therapy initiated shortly after a new detection of *P. aeruginosa* was shown to be effective in preventing or delaying the onset of chronic infection [48–50]. This strategy might also be applied to other bacteria associated with CF. Finding the best eradication regimen with marketed inhaled antibiotics has been/is the aim of several trials, some of them investigator initiated [51, 52]. In that case, microbiological end-points are the first outcome measures and negative cultures for the bacteria of interest are the usual end-point. However, there is still much debate about sample-taking procedures, microbiological techniques and timelines.

Evaluating the efficacy of CFTR modulators

CFTR modulators are small molecules that aim at increasing the amount or function of CFTR protein at the cell membrane. In phase II studies, the obvious biomarker of choice is an end-point that reflects CFTR function. Sweat chloride measurement, nasal potential difference (NPD) measurement and intestinal current measurement (ICM) assess the CFTR function in different organs. We do not know whether CFTR modulators improve CFTR function in different organs to the same extent, nor whether the relative improvement in different organs differs between compounds. In studies performed with the CFTR potentiator ivacaftor, sweat chloride was more responsive to changes in CFTR function than parameters derived from NPD [53]. However, the advantage of NPD in trials with CFTR modulators is that it measures CFTR and also epithelial sodium channel function in the respiratory tract, the organ of major concern in CF [21]. Less data are available for ICM, which seems quite responsive to relatively small changes in CFTR function [5]. In the past year, another *ex vivo* end-point has been developed, *i.e.* intestinal organoids [54]. *Ex vivo* biomarkers can facilitate functional studies with new CFTR modulators and have potential for personalised drug development in patients with rare mutations.

In phase III trials, the clinical benefit will have to been proven. Therefore the surrogate end-point FEV_1 is the first choice and/or possibly improvement in LCI in subjects with mild or early lung disease. As an alternative, changes in CT-related outcome measures can be considered. Since these will mainly be studies to gain marketing authorisation, it will be essential to follow regulatory agencies' guidelines. Many end-points can be used as secondary outcomes: time or number of pulmonary exacerbations, QoL measures, lung imaging, markers of inflammation and improved nutritional state (since this therapy is given systemically). To assess the full benefit of treatment with CFTR modulators, a longer timeline is needed, possibly as part of a post-marketing programme or as investigator-initiated trials; decreased acquisition of new respiratory pathogens, change in the rate of decline in FEV_1, change in the progression of bronchiectasis and trapped air on CT imaging, lower occurrence of CF complications, such as allergic bronchopulmonary aspergillosis (ABPA) and CF-related diabetes mellitus (CFRD). Given these drugs' current high cost, an assessment from a health-technology point of view is also needed.

Conclusion

The development of new treatments for patients with CF was paralleled by a renewed interest in the development and critical evaluation of new and existing end-points. The improved outcome of patients was the main cause that mortality and even FEV_1 could no longer be used as sensitive outcome measures. The evidence base showing that changes in biomarkers, such as lung imaging and LCI, reflect long-term patient evolution is increasing. They are thus moving closer to the status of surrogate outcome measure and might replace or complement FEV_1 in future trials.

In this chapter, we have reviewed the pros and cons of commonly used outcome measures in clinical trials as well as the factors that determine the choice of end-points in a specific trial.

Since CF is a rare disorder, phase III clinical trials require multicentre cooperation. The development of clinical trial networks and task forces to strive for rigorous standardisation and agreement on detailed standard operating procedures for outcome measures are other important steps in bridging the gap between drug discovery and robust evaluation of drug benefit.

References

1. De Gruttola VG, Clax P, DeMets DL, et al. Considerations in the evaluation of surrogate end-points in clinical trials. Summary of a National Institutes of Health workshop. *Control Clin Trials* 2001; 22: 485–502.
2. Atkinson A, Colburn W, De Gruttola V, et al. Biomarkers and surrogate end-points: preferred definitions and conceptual framework. *Clin Pharmacol Ther* 2001; 69: 89–95.
3. Bilton D, Canny G, Conway S, et al. Pulmonary exacerbation: towards a definition for use in clinical trials. Report from the EuroCareCF Working Group on outcome parameters in clinical trials. *J Cyst Fibros* 2011; 10: Suppl. 2, S79–S81.
4. Quittner AL, Modi AC, Wainwright C, et al. Determination of the minimal clinically important difference scores for the Cystic Fibrosis Questionnaire-Revised respiratory symptom scale in two populations of patients with cystic fibrosis and chronic *Pseudomonas aeruginosa* airway infection. *Chest* 2009; 135: 1610–1618.
5. De Boeck K, Kent L, Davies J, et al. CFTR biomarkers: time for promotion to surrogate end-point. *Eur Respir J* 2013; 41: 203–216.
6. Subbarao P, Stanojevic S, Brown M, et al. Lung clearance index as an outcome measure for clinical trials in young children with cystic fibrosis. A pilot study using inhaled hypertonic saline. *Am J Respir Crit Care Med* 2013; 188: 456–460.

7. Kent L, Reix P, Innes JA, *et al.* Lung clearance index: evidence for use in clinical trials in cystic fibrosis. *J Cyst Fibros* 2014; 13: 123–138.

8. Fayon M, Kent L, Bui S, *et al.* Clinimetric properties of bronchoalveolar lavage inflammatory markers in cystic fibrosis. *Eur Respir J* 2014; 43: 610–626.

9. Loeve M, Krestin GP, Rosenfeld M, *et al.* Chest computed tomography: a validated surrogate end-point of cystic fibrosis lung disease? *Eur Respir J* 2013; 42: 844–857.

10. Stick S, Tiddens H, Aurora P, *et al.* Early intervention studies in infants and preschool children with cystic fibrosis: are we ready? *Eur Respir J* 2013; 42: 527–538.

11. Simpson SJ, Mott LS, Esther CR Jr, *et al.* Novel end points for clinical trials in young children with cystic fibrosis. *Expert Rev Respir Med* 2013; 7: 231–243.

12. Amin R, Ratjen F. Cystic fibrosis. *In:* Kolb M, Vogelmeier CF. eds. Outcomes in Clinical Trials. *ERS Monogr* 2013; 62: 54–69.

13. EMA. Workshop on end-points for cystic fibrosis clinical trials. www.ema.europa.eu/ema/index.jsp?curl=pages/news_and_events/events/2012/07/event_detail_000609.jsp&mid=WC0b01ac058004d5c3 Date last updated: 2012. Date last accessed: November 22, 2013.

14. Tiddens HA, Stick SM, Davis S. Multi-modality monitoring of cystic fibrosis lung disease: the role of chest computed tomography. *Paediatr Respir Rev* 2014; 15: 92–97.

15. Mott LS, Park J, Murray CP, *et al.* Progression of early structural lung disease in young children with cystic fibrosis assessed using CT. *Thorax* 2012; 67: 509–516.

16. De Boeck K. Trying to find a cure for cystic fibrosis: CFTR biomarkers as outcomes. *Eur Respir J* 2013; 42: 1156–1157.

17. Waters V, Stanojevic S, Atenafu EG, *et al.* Effect of pulmonary exacerbations on long-term lung function decline in cystic fibrosis. *Eur Respir J* 2012; 40: 61–66.

18. Goss CH, Burns JL. Exacerbations in cystic fibrosis. 1: Epidemiology and pathogenesis. *Thorax* 2007; 62: 360–367.

19. Aurora P, Stanojevic S, Wade A, *et al.* Lung clearance index at 4 years predicts subsequent lung function in children with cystic fibrosis. *Am J Respir Crit Care Med* 2010; 183: 752–758.

20. Vermeulen F, Proesmans M, Boon M, *et al.* Lung clearance index predicts pulmonary exacerbations in young patients with cystic fibrosis. *Thorax* 2014; 69: 39–45.

21. Rowe SM, Liu B, Hill A, *et al.* Optimizing nasal potential difference analysis for CFTR modulator development: assessment of ivacaftor in CF subjects with the G551D-CFTR mutation. *PLoS One* 2013; 8: e66955.

22. Sly PD, Gangell CL, Chen L, *et al.* Risk factors for bronchiectasis in children with cystic fibrosis. *N Engl J Med* 2013; 368: 1963–1670.

23. Sagel SD, Wagner BD, Anthony MM, *et al.* Sputum biomarkers of inflammation and lung function decline in children with cystic fibrosis. *Am J Respir Crit Care Med* 2012; 186: 857–865.

24. Mayer-Hamblett N, Aitken ML, Accurso FJ, *et al.* Association between pulmonary function and sputum biomarkers in cystic fibrosis. *Am J Respir Crit Care Med* 2007; 175: 822–828.

25. Lynch SV, Bruce KD. The cystic fibrosis airway microbiome. *Cold Spring Harb Perspect Med* 2013; 3: a009738.

26. Mayer-Hamblett N, Ramsey BW, Kronmal RA. Advancing outcome measures for the new era of drug development in cystic fibrosis. *Proc Am Thorac Soc* 2007; 4: 370–377.

27. EMA. ICH Topic E 8 - General Considerations for Clinical Trials. www.ema.europa.eu/docs/en_GB/document_library/Scientific_guideline/2009/09/WC500002877.pdf Date last updated: 2006. Date last accessed: March 25, 2014.

28. Kerem E, Reisman J, Corey M, *et al.* Prediction of mortality in patients with cystic fibrosis. *N Engl J Med* 1992; 326: 1187–1191.

29. Huang NN, Schidlow DV, Szatrowski TH, *et al.* Clinical features, survival rate, and prognostic factors in young adults with cystic fibrosis. *Am J Med* 1987; 82: 871–879.

30. Corey M, McLaughlin FJ, Williams M, *et al.* A comparison of survival, growth, and pulmonary function in patients with cystic fibrosis in Boston and Toronto. *J Clin Epidemiol* 1988; 41: 583–591.

31. Postmarketing Studies and Clinical Trials: Implementation of Section 505(o)(3) of the Federal Food, Drug, and Cosmetic Act. www.fda.gov/downloads/Drugs/GuidanceComplianceRegulatoryInformation/Guidances/UCM172001.pdf Date last updated: 2011. Date last accessed: November 22, 2013.

32. Guideline on the clinical development of medicinal products for the treatment of cystic fibrosis. www.ema.europa.eu/docs/en_GB/document_library/Scientific_guideline/2009/12/WC500017055.pdf Date last updated: 2009. Date last accessed: November 22, 2013.

33. Que C, Cullinan P, Geddes D. Improving rate of decline of FEV1 in young adults with cystic fibrosis. *Thorax* 2006; 61: 155–157.

34. Rosenfeld M, Ratjen F, Brumback L, *et al.* Inhaled hypertonic saline in infants and children younger than 6 years with cystic fibrosis: the ISIS randomized controlled trial. *JAMA* 2012; 307: 2269–2277.

35. Robinson TE, Goris ML, Zhu HJ, *et al.* Dornase alfa reduces air trapping in children with mild cystic fibrosis lung disease: a quantitative analysis. *Chest* 2005; 128: 2327–2335.

36. Konstan MW, Wagener JS, Yegin A, *et al.* Design and powering of cystic fibrosis clinical trials using rate of FEV1 decline as an efficacy end-point. *J Cyst Fibros* 2010; 9: 332–338.

37. Willemink MJ, de Jong PA. Pediatric chest computed tomography at a radiation dose approaching a chest radiograph. *Am J Respir Crit Care Med* 2013; 188: 626–627.
38. Konstan MW, Byard PJ, Hoppel CL, *et al.* Effect of high-dose ibuprofen in patients with cystic fibrosis. *N Engl J Med* 1995; 332: 848–854.
39. Konstan MW, Schluchter MD, Xue W, *et al.* Clinical use of Ibuprofen is associated with slower FEV1 decline in children with cystic fibrosis. *Am J Respir Crit Care Med* 2007; 176: 1084–1089.
40. Ratjen F, Saiman L, Mayer-Hamblett N, *et al.* Effect of azithromycin on systemic markers of inflammation in patients with cystic fibrosis uninfected with *Pseudomonas aeruginosa. Chest* 2012; 142: 1259–1266.
41. Geller DE, Flume PA, Staab D, *et al.* Levofloxacin inhalation solution (MP-376) in patients with cystic fibrosis with *Pseudomonas aeruginosa. Am J Respir Crit Care Med* 2011; 183: 1510–1516.
42. Clancy JP, Dupont L, Konstan MW, *et al.* Phase II studies of nebulised Arikace in CF patients with *Pseudomonas aeruginosa* infection. *Thorax* 2013; 68: 818–825.
43. Trapnell BC, McColley SA, Kissner DG, *et al.* Fosfomycin/tobramycin for inhalation in patients with cystic fibrosis with pseudomonas airway infection. *Am J Respir Crit Care Med* 2011; 185: 171–178.
44. Maiz L, Giron RM, Olveira C, *et al.* Inhaled antibiotics for the treatment of chronic bronchopulmonary *Pseudomonas aeruginosa* infection in cystic fibrosis: systematic review of randomised controlled trials. *Expert Opin Pharmacother* 2013; 14: 1135–1149.
45. Fleming TR, Odem-Davis K, Rothmann MD, *et al.* Some essential considerations in the design and conduct of non-inferiority trials. *Clin Trials* 2011; 8: 432–439.
46. Ballmann M, Rabsch P, von der Hardt H. Long-term follow up of changes in FEV1 and treatment intensity during *Pseudomonas aeruginosa* colonisation in patients with cystic fibrosis. *Thorax* 1998; 53: 732–737.
47. Taylor-Robinson D, Whitehead M, Diderichsen F, *et al.* Understanding the natural progression in % FEV1 decline in patients with cystic fibrosis: a longitudinal study. *Thorax* 2012; 67: 860–866.
48. Littlewood JM, Miller MG, Ghoneim AT, *et al.* Nebulised colomycin for early pseudomonas colonisation in cystic fibrosis. *Lancet* 1985; 1: 865.
49. Valerius NH, Koch C, Hoiby N. Prevention of chronic *Pseudomonas aeruginosa* colonisation in cystic fibrosis by early treatment. *Lancet* 1991; 338: 725–726.
50. Ratjen F, Doring G, Nikolaizik WH. Effect of inhaled tobramycin on early *Pseudomonas aeruginosa* colonisation in patients with cystic fibrosis. *Lancet* 2001; 358: 983–984.
51. Ratjen F, Munck A, Kho P, *et al.* Treatment of early *Pseudomonas aeruginosa* infection in patients with cystic fibrosis: the ELITE trial. *Thorax* 2010; 65: 286–291.
52. Taccetti G, Bianchini E, Cariani L, *et al.* Early antibiotic treatment for *Pseudomonas aeruginosa* eradication in patients with cystic fibrosis: a randomised multicentre study comparing two different protocols. *Thorax* 2012; 67: 853–859.
53. Accurso FJ, Rowe SM, Clancy JP, *et al.* Effect of VX-770 in persons with cystic fibrosis and the G551D-CFTR mutation. *N Engl J Med* 2010; 363: 1991–2003.
54. Dekkers JF, Wiegerinck CL, de Jonge HR, *et al.* A functional CFTR assay using primary cystic fibrosis intestinal organoids. *Nat Med* 2013; 19: 939–945.

Disclosures: K. De Boeck is a member of the steering committee/advisory board for Vertex, Aptalis and Pharmaxis, and has been a principal investigator for studies by Vertex, Gilead, Pharmaxis and PTC Therapeutics. She has also received fees for consultancy from Ablynx, Galapagos, Gilead and PTC Therapeutics. I. Fajac reports personal fees outside the submitted work from Actelion, Boehringer, GSK, Insmed, Mpex, Novartis, Pfizer, PTC Therapeutics and Vertex Pharmaceuticals. F. Ratjen has acted as a consultant for Vertex, Novartis, Bayer, Talecris, CSL Behring, Roche, Gilead, Aptalis and Insmed. He is the principal investigator for a grant pending from Novartis, and has had travel expenses sponsored by Pari.

Chapter 9 |

Correcting the basic ion transport defects in cystic fibrosis

Emanuela Caci and Luis J.V. Galietta

The basic defect in cystic fibrosis (CF) is the loss of function of the cystic fibrosis transmembrane conductance regulator (CFTR), a cAMP-activated ion channel permeable to chloride and bicarbonate. Correction of the basic defect may be obtained by rescuing the mutant CFTR proteins with drugs that specifically target the alterations caused by CF mutations. For example, small molecules known as "potentiators" are able to improve the activity of CFTR proteins with channel gating mutations. Instead, "correctors" may contrast the destabilising effects that the Phe508del mutation, the most frequent among CF patients, causes to CFTR protein. Recent studies suggest the possibility that a high extent of Phe508del-CFTR rescue may only be obtained by a combination of correctors having different mechanisms of action. Alternative strategies to correct the CF ion-transport defect are based on the stimulation of alternative chloride channels, such as TMEM16A or SLC26A9, or the improvement of airway surface hydration using osmotically active agents.

In cystic fibrosis (CF), mutations in the cystic fibrosis transmembrane conductance regulator (CFTR) gene impair the transport of chloride and bicarbonate across the apical membrane of different types of epithelial cells [1]. The *CFTR* gene codes for a membrane protein that, similarly to many other members of the ATP-binding cassette (ABC) transporters superfamily, is composed of two homologous halves, each one consisting of a membrane-spanning domain (MSD) and a nucleotide-binding domain (NBD) (fig. 1a) [2]. The two halves are connected by a "regulatory" region (R domain).

The two MSDs (MSD1 and MSD2), each one composed of six transmembrane segments, contribute to the formation of the CFTR pore; however, the sixth and twelfth segments have a more direct interaction with the flowing anions [3]. Anions move through the CFTR pore passively. This means that the intensity and direction of the net flow is determined by differences in anion concentration between the two sides of the membrane and by the transmembrane electrical potential. The two NBDs (NBD1 and NBD2), which are exposed to the cytosolic environment, form a dimer that is important for the control of CFTR channel gating [2]. Indeed, CFTR channel opening requires the binding of two molecules of ATP at the NBD1/NBD2 interface. Cycles of binding and hydrolysis of ATP at the NBDs cause changes in conformation that are transmitted to the MSDs. Additional control of CFTR

U.O.C. Genetica Medica, Istituto Giannina Gaslini, Genova, Italy.

Correspondence: Luis J.V. Galietta, U.O.C. Genetica Medica, Istituto Giannina Gaslini, via Gerolamo Gaslini 5, 16147 Genova, Italy. E-mail: galietta@unige.it

ERS Monogr 2014; 64: 116–128. DOI: 10.1183/1025448x.10009413

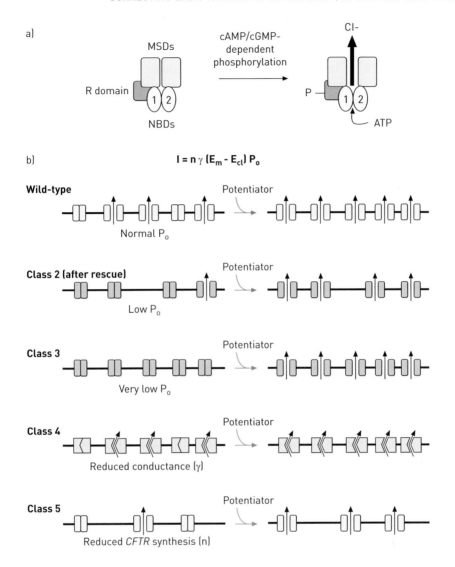

Figure 1. a) Structure and function of cystic fibrosis transmembrane conductance regulator (CFTR). CFTR is composed of two membrane-spanning domains (MSDs), each one with six transmembrane segments and two nucleotide-binding domains (NBD), NBD1 and NBD2. In addition, CFTR has a regulatory domain, which has multiple sites for phosphorylation by the cAMP-dependent protein kinase A or by the cGMP-dependent protein kinase 2. The opening of the CFTR channel requires phosphorylation of the R domain and the concurrent binding and hydrolysis of ATP at the interface between the NBDs. b) Mechanisms of action for potentiators on wild-type and mutant CFTR. The net transport of chloride through CFTR channels in a cell is determined by the formula: $I = n \gamma (E_m - E_{Cl}) P_o$, where I is the total chloride current, n is the number of CFTR channels in the membrane, γ is the single channel conductance, $(E_m - E_{Cl})$ is the difference between the membrane potential and the equilibrium (Nernst) potential for chloride (i.e. the driving force), and P_o is the open channel probability (i.e. the fraction of the time that is spent by CFTR in the open configuration). Active (phosphorylated) CFTR normally oscillates between the closed and open state. In general, potentiators act by increasing P_o. This is particularly important for class 3 mutations in which CFTR channels are always permanently closed (very low P_o). Potentiators may also be beneficial for Phe508del-CFTR. When rescued to the plasma membrane by correctors, Phe508del-CFTR shows a channel-gating defect; although less severe than that of class 3 mutations. Potentiators could also be used for class 4 and class 5 mutations, even if these mutations do not cause a channel gating defect. The increase in P_o may compensate for the reduced single-channel anion conductance γ (class 4 mutations) or the reduced number of channels in the membrane n (class 5 mutations).

activity occurs at the R domain. Phosphorylation of this domain by the cAMP-dependent or cGMP-dependent protein kinases is required for CFTR channel opening [2, 4].

Regulation of CFTR at the apical membrane of epithelial cells is also dependent on a sophisticated system of proteins (G-protein coupled receptors, adenylyl cyclases, phospho-diesterases, protein kinases and scaffolding proteins), which allow compartmentalised and precisely controlled cAMP signalling [5–7].

Although CF is a multi-organ disease, the majority of the novel therapeutic approaches under investigation are focused on the respiratory system. The correction of the ion transport defect in CF airways is believed to be highly beneficial to patients [1]. Stimulation of chloride and bicarbonate transport through mutant CFTR or through other alternative pathways could improve mucociliary clearance and restore innate antimicrobial activity.

CFTR as a drug target

CFTR potentiators

CF mutations cause CFTR loss of function through a variety of mechanisms, which can be grouped into five main classes: 1) truncation of CFTR protein by nonsense mutations, *e.g.* Gly542X and Trp1282X; 2) impaired protein maturation caused by mutations that destabilise CFTR, *e.g.* Phe508del; 3) drastically reduced channel activity, *e.g.* Gly551Asp, Gly1349Asp and Gly970Arg; 4) partial decrease in ion transport ability due to an altered channel pore, *e.g.* Arg117His and Arg347Pro; and 5) reduced CFTR synthesis due to, in most cases, altered splicing of CFTR mRNA, *e.g.* 3849+10kbC>T [8].

Interestingly, in many cases the activity of mutant CFTR is not irreversibly lost but can be rescued by specific treatments. In the early 1990s, just a few years after the discovery of the *CFTR* gene in 1989, it was found that CFTR protein activity can be stimulated by various pharmacological compounds such as genistein, apigenin, xanthines and benzimidazolones [9–11]. In particular, at micromolar concentrations these compounds, generically called potentiators, are able to dramatically increase the activity of several class 3 mutations, particularly of Gly551Asp-CFTR (fig. 1b). This mutation has a severe channel gating defect [12]. Even if maximally stimulated by cAMP, it spends only 1% of the time in the open configuration. However, in the presence of a potentiator, channel activity increases more than 10-fold [9, 13]. The discovery of the effect of genistein and other compounds was an important proof of principle in favour of drug discovery projects.

To discover novel potentiators with strongly enhanced potency and specificity, the chosen strategy was to screen large numbers of chemical compounds with a cell-based functional assay. In this way, various classes of potentiators with novel chemical scaffolds have been discovered [14–18]. The most successful molecule is ivacaftor (former name VX-770, brand name Kalydeco) developed by Vertex Pharmaceuticals Inc. (Boston, MA, USA) [19]. This compound has obtained positive results when administered orally to Gly551Asp patients. The phase III clinical trial (48 weeks) demonstrated a rapid and sustained improvement of respiratory function and of other clinically relevant parameters [20]. Because of these results, ivacaftor has been approved by the US Food and Drug Administration (FDA) and the European Medicines Agency (EMA) for the treatment of CF patients with at least one copy of the Gly551Asp mutation. Clinical trials are also in progress to demonstrate the efficacy of ivacaftor on other class 3 mutations. Such trials are based on reported *in vitro* studies that have proved the general ability of potentiators to correct a variety of mutations associated with channel gating defect [21, 22].

Ivacaftor is also tested on patients with residual CFTR function, *i.e.* with class 4 and class 5 mutations (fig. 1b). The rationale for such trials is that potentiators stimulate channel activity even if applied to wild-type CFTR or to CFTR mutants without channel gating defects [23]. In particular this may occur under conditions of partial CFTR phosphorylation. Therefore, potentiators could boost CFTR-dependent anion transport and, thus, partially compensate for the decreased function (decreased single-channel conductance for class 4 mutations and decreased number of CFTR channels in the plasma membrane for class 5 mutations).

CFTR correctors

The most frequent mutation in CF, Phe508del, is responsible for multiple defects of the CFTR protein. In particular, the lack of phenylalanine 508, a highly conserved amino acid residue among ABC proteins, causes intrinsic instability of NBD1 and impaired docking of this domain to the cytosolic side of MSD2 [2]. Cells have a multiplicity of quality control systems to detect unstable and misfolded membrane proteins. Quality control systems in the endoplasmic reticulum (ER) detect Phe508del-CFTR as a defective protein even before its translation is completed [2, 24–26]. The consequent tagging with ubiquitin targets CFTR for degradation by the proteasome system. A small fraction of Phe508del-CFTR actually escapes from the ER and traffics to the plasma membrane [27]. However, additional checkpoints at the cell periphery remove mutant CFTR from the plasma membrane and cause its elimination in the lysosome [28–30].

The Phe508del misfolding and trafficking defect is also correctable (fig. 2). It was found that incubation of cells for several hours at low temperature [31] or with high concentrations of the chemical chaperone glycerol [32] rescues the mutant protein from the ER. These findings paved the way for the search of pharmacological compounds, named Phe508del correctors that have the same effect of low temperature or chemical chaperones. The identification of Phe508del correctors was attempted with high-throughput screenings as carried out for potentiators. In the past 10 years, several hundreds of thousands of chemical compounds, including natural substances, have been screened by academic laboratories or by pharmaceutical industries. The search has identified a series of active compounds such as VRT-325, VRT-640, corr-4a, sildenafil analogs, glafenine, latonduine and VX-809 [17, 33–37]. The ideal goal of high-throughput screenings was to find correctors possibly acting as pharmacological chaperones, *i.e.* by directly stabilising Phe508del-CFTR protein. However, since the screenings were based on functional assays, the resulting correctors could also work indirectly by interacting with other proteins. These interactions could protect Phe508del-CFTR from degradation, favour its export from ER, and/or prevent its internalisation from the plasma membrane. Importantly, all Phe508del correctors discovered to date show partial efficacy. Incubation of cells with these compounds never results in total rescue of the mutant protein. In fact, the percentage of correction *in vitro* is 10–25% at maximum.

An explanation for the partial efficacy of correctors arises from various studies, particularly from those based on the use of suppressing mutations. Such mutations are artificial changes in the CFTR amino acid sequence that are introduced to suppress the effect of the Phe508del mutation [38, 39]. It has been found that Phe508del effects can be suppressed by two classes of mutations. Mutations introduced into NBD1 (*e.g.* Gly550Glu) can correct the instability caused by the phenylalanine 508 deletion [38]. Instead mutations like Arg1070Trp can

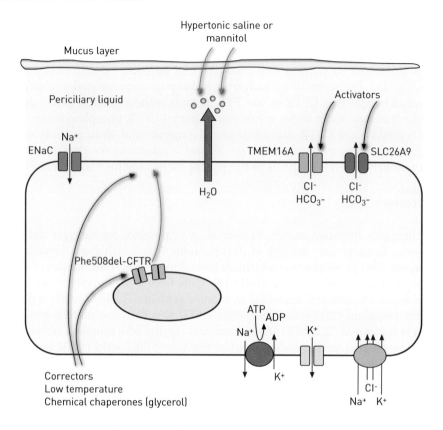

Figure 2. Strategies to correct the cystic fibrosis (CF) basic defect. The transepithelial transport of anions in the epithelium is determined by the concerted action of channels in the apical membrane and co-transporters, channels and pumps in the basolateral membrane. The misfolding and trafficking defect caused by Phe508del can be targeted by correctors, i.e. small molecules that: 1) improve Phe508del-cystic fibrosis transmembrane conductance regulator (CFTR) stability and folding; 2) protect Phe508del-CFTR from degradation; and 3) stabilise Phe508del-CFTR on the cell surface. Similar effects can be achieved (in vitro) by incubating the cells at low temperature or with high concentrations of chemical chaperones (e.g. glycerol). Alternatively, the ion transport defect can be corrected by stimulating other channels (e.g. TMEM16A or SLC26A9) or by using osmotically active agents (e.g. mannitol and high sodium chloride solution) to draw water on the airway surface. For simplicity, TMEM16A and SLC26A9 are depicted within the same cell type expressing CFTR. However, it is possible that these proteins are differentially expressed in the cell types of the airway epithelium. ENaC: epithelial sodium channel.

improve the interaction between NBD1 and MSD2 [40]. Interestingly, it has been found that both types of mutations are needed to rescue Phe508del-CFTR to near wild-type levels [41, 42]. These studies indicate that both types of defects, intra-domain and inter-domain defects, have to be targeted by correctors. Recently, a study has demonstrated that correctors discovered to date, act with different mechanisms of action [43]. For example, the corrector lumacaftor (formerly known as VX-809) developed by Vertex Pharmaceuticals Inc., mimics the effect of the Arg1070Trp mutation, improving the NBD1/MSD2 interaction. Other correctors like corr-4a act with a separate mechanism, probably involving NBD2. Intriguingly, the stabilisation of NBD1 can only be obtained with chemical chaperones like glycerol but not with known correctors. Only combinations of two or three compounds were able to rescue Phe508del-CFTR to very high levels [43]. This study proves an important concept: patients may require combinations of correctors to show a high clinical benefit.

So far, two Phe508del correctors are being tested in clinical trials on CF patients with the Phe508del mutation: VX-809 and VX-661. The initial studies with VX-809 have not been very satisfactory [44]. However, a better outcome is expected from phase III clinical trials in which VX-809 is tested at higher concentrations and in combination with the potentiator VX-770. This combination is justified because Phe508del-CFTR has also a channel gating defect although less severe than that of pure class 3 mutations like Gly551Asp (fig. 1b).

While waiting for the results from clinical trials, additional correctors are being searched. In particular, correctors that stabilise NBD1 are highly anticipated [43]. As suggested by results obtained with chemical chaperones, these types of correctors could produce the highest effect on Phe508del-CFTR, particularly in combination with other molecules [43].

A promising strategy to find correctors is to exploit the increasing knowledge on CFTR structure. In particular, structural information on NBD1 is being used to perform screenings of chemical compounds *in silico*. With this approach, novel correctors, possibly acting as pharmacological chaperones, have been discovered [45].

Additional strategies to find correctors may benefit from the investigation of the CFTR interactome. By finding the proteins that are responsible for Phe508del mis-trafficking and degradation it could be possible to design approaches that contrast their activity. For example, it has been found that the interaction of Phe508del-CFTR with the protein CAL, which leads to protein degradation, can be weakened by treating the cells with insulin-like growth factor 1 [46]. Furthermore, it has been shown that stabilisation of Phe508del-CFTR at the cell periphery may be obtained by stimulating the GTPase Rac1 with the hepatocyte growth factor [47]. More extensive effects on CFTR interactome could be obtained by hitting at multiple sites using compounds with a large effect on cell proteome and transcriptome. For example, it has been proposed that histone deacetylase inhibitors could work as correctors by creating a proteostasis environment more benign for Phe508del [48].

Read-through drugs for premature stop codons

CF mutations belonging to class 1 cause premature termination of CFTR protein translation by the insertion of a nonsense codon in the CFTR coding sequence. Because of the total loss of CFTR function, these mutations are typically associated with a severe phenotype. However, the effect of premature stop codons can be suppressed with drug-like small molecules called read-through agents. It was found that aminoglycosides such as gentamycin can correct these mutations, probably by forcing the ribosome to introduce an amino acid instead of stopping the protein translation. The result is a protein of correct length but with an amino acid change. This change may cause minor functional effects compared to that of a truncated protein. Topical application of gentamycin to the nasal mucosa of CF patients with a nonsense mutation resulted in restoration of CFTR protein expression and increased chloride secretion [49]. However, aminoglycosides cannot be used systemically at the concentrations needed for read-through activity because of serious toxic effects. Therefore, other read-through drugs were searched for to provide a safer alternative to gentamycin. A strategy based on the high-throughput screening of a large collection of chemical compounds identified PTC-124, also known as ataluren (PTC Therapeutics, South Plainfield, NJ, USA) [50]. Interestingly, experiments *in vitro* demonstrated that PTC-124 does not affect the normal stop codons present at the end of all coding sequences in a cell, but is specific for nonsense codon mutations [50]. Clinical studies have demonstrated that treatment with ataluren elicits a significant rescue of CFTR function and expression, as demonstrated with nasal electrical potential and immunofluorescence experiments [51, 52]. A trend toward improvement in pulmonary function was also observed [52].

Further studies are needed to assess the efficacy of read-through strategies for class 1 CF mutations [53]. It is important to note that the treatment of these mutations is significantly affected by a biological process known as nonsense-mediated mRNA decay (NMD) [54]. This is a quality control mechanism that causes early degradation of mRNAs carrying stop codon mutations. Therefore, NMD may seriously limit the efficacy of read-through drugs.

Alternative strategies for the CF basic defect

CFTR role in the airways

The alternative to pharmacological treatments, which are aimed at rescuing the mutant CFTR (*i.e.* with potentiators, correctors and read-trough drugs), is to correct the CF ion transport defect and/or its consequences by acting on other targets. Most of these alternative strategies are focused on the respiratory system because they are based on specific mechanisms that are organ specific. In the lungs, the goal is to restore mucociliary clearance and to increase antimicrobial activity on the airway surface [1].

The airway epithelium is covered by a thin layer of fluid known as the periciliary liquid (PCL). The PCL is in turn covered by a mucus layer. The beating of cilia by airway epithelial cells propels the mucus layer towards the oropharynx. In the absence of CFTR, impaired electrolyte/fluid secretion causes the dehydration of the PCL and of the mucus layer [55]. This phenomenon seriously impairs the process of mucociliary transport. The accumulation of dense and sticky mucus creates a favourable niche for bacterial survival and proliferation.

Mucus accumulation in the airways may also be caused by a more direct involvement of CFTR. Mucins are highly condensed within the secretory granules of goblet cells, despite the electrostatic repulsion that results from the high density of negative charges on mucin molecules. To allow mucin condensation, the negative charges are neutralised by high concentrations of protons and calcium ions. It has been found that mucin release and expansion requires the concurrent secretion of bicarbonate through CFTR [56, 57]. Bicarbonate neutralises the acidic pH and removes the interaction of calcium with mucins, thus favouring their expansion. In agreement with this model, direct bicarbonate delivery to CF epithelia resulted in improved mucus fluidity and detachment [56, 57].

CFTR-dependent bicarbonate transport may also be required for antibacterial activity. In a recent study, bacteria immobilised on a grid were placed for a short time on the airway surface of normal and CF pigs [58]. After recovery of the grids, it was found that CF airways showed impaired bacterial killing. This alteration appeared to be directly linked to bicarbonate transport. Direct delivery of a high bicarbonate concentration to airway surface restored bactericidal activity on CF epithelia [58].

Osmotic agents

Several strategies have been designed to improve hydration of the airway surface and to mobilise mucus. One of the most direct approaches is the delivery of high osmolarity solutions or osmotically active substances into the airways. The goal is to draw water into the airway lumen to improve the fluidity of mucus secretions. Inhalation by aerosol of a hypertonic solution containing a high concentration of sodium chloride is a current approach. Hypertonic saline has been shown to greatly reduce the frequency of pulmonary exacerbations and to improve lung function [59]. An alternative to hypertonic saline is the inhalation of a mannitol dry powder. Mannitol, a relatively inert and safe osmolyte, has been shown to improve mucociliary clearance in CF patients [60–62]. The results of a recent phase III clinical trial with mannitol revealed a difference in sputum weight that appeared to be due to increased use of antibiotics in the placebo group [63]. Further studies are needed to understand if mannitol reduces pulmonary exacerbations and antibiotic need in CF patients.

Alternative chloride channels

Airway epithelial cells have other chloride channels besides CFTR. In particular, these cells express at least one type of calcium-activated chloride channel (CaCC). The stimulation of airway epithelial cells with calcium-elevating agents, such as purinergic receptor agonists (ATP or UTP), triggers a rapid and transient increase in chloride secretion [64]. Since calcium-activated chloride secretion is preserved in CF epithelia, its modulation with pharmacological agents could be a way to bypass the primary CF defect.

Denufosol, a UTP analog more resistant to nucleotidases, was developed to stimulate CaCC in the airways of CF patients. Patients were treated with denufosol by inhalation. Despite initial promising results [65], the completion of a phase III clinical trial did not succeed in demonstrating a benefit on respiratory function [66].

The interest on CaCC as a drug target for CF was reinvigorated by the discovery, in 2008, of the TMEM16A protein [67–69]. TMEM16A, which belongs to a family of orphan membrane proteins with unknown function, was found to function as a CaCC. TMEM16A is expressed in the airway epithelium [70], as well as in submucosal glands of the airways [71]. It is activated by cytosolic calcium concentrations in the high nanomolar range and by membrane depolarisation [67–69]. The mechanism of activation seems to be mediated by direct binding of calcium to a cytosolic region of TMEM16A [72]. An additional mechanism of regulation may involve calmodulin binding to the N-terminal [73, 74]. Interestingly, in one of the studies on calmodulin, it was found that cytosolic calcium, in addition to channel gating, also affects TMEM16A anion permeability. At high micromolar calcium concentrations, TMEM16A was converted to a CaCC highly permeable to bicarbonate [74].

Interestingly, TMEM16A is upregulated by T-helper cell (Th) type 2 cytokines *in vitro*. Treatment of bronchial epithelial cells with interleukin (IL)-4 or IL-13 causes a strong increase in TMEM16A expression and function [69]. These cytokines induce mucus metaplasia, *i.e.* a large increase in the number of goblet cells, which resembles what happens *in vivo* in asthmatic patients. Intriguingly, TMEM16A upregulation by Th2 cytokines mainly occurs in goblet cells [75, 76]. TMEM16A expression in goblet cells was confirmed in the airways of asthmatic patients [75]. This cell localisation suggests a specific role of TMEM16A in mucin release. Secretion of chloride and, particularly, bicarbonate through TMEM16A on the membrane of goblet cells could be important for the expansion of mucins. In contrast to TMEM16A, CFTR is specifically expressed in ciliated cells [76]. Therefore, it is not clear if TMEM16A and CFTR have overlapping or different functions.

The identification of TMEM16A paves the way for the search for selective pharmacological modulators. In fact, TMEM16A activators have already been identified by screening chemical libraries with a functional assay [77]. Such molecules do not increase intracellular calcium but may directly activate TMEM16A protein. TMEM16A activators could be utilised to stimulate chloride/bicarbonate secretion in the airways of CF patients. However, several issues need to be clarified. It needs to be shown that TMEM16A activation really compensates for CFTR dysfunction by improving the hydration of airway surface, the fluidity of mucus secretion, and/or the antimicrobial activity in PCL.

Recent studies have added further interest on the role of TMEM16A in the airways. It has been found that CFTR loss of function causes an increased release of IL-8, a pro-inflammatory cytokine, from airway epithelial cells [78]. Stimulation of TMEM16A-dependent chloride transport inhibited IL-8 release [78]. Therefore, targeting of TMEM16A with activators could also result in anti-inflammatory effects. In another study, a TMEM16 protein expressed in *Drosophila melanogaster* appeared to be important for host defence activity against the pathogenic bacterium *Serratia marcescens* [79]. This could suggest that a similar role could be played by TMEM16A in human airways.

The design of pharmacological strategies to modulate TMEM16A in the airway epithelium needs to consider that this protein is also expressed in airway smooth muscle cells. TMEM16A, as a CaCC, participates in the process of smooth muscle contraction [70, 75]. Accordingly, TMEM16A activators could potentially cause bronchoconstriction as an undesired side-effect. Further studies are needed to explore the possibility to develop pharmacological modulators of TMEM16A with a selective effect on airway epithelial cells.

Epithelial cells also have another chloride channel, SLC26A9, which may serve as a therapeutic target in CF. This protein belongs to a family of membrane proteins different from that of CFTR and TMEM16A [80]. The SLC26 family includes electroneutral transporters as well as chloride channels. Interestingly, SLC26A9 is expressed in the airway epithelium and, similarly to TMEM16A, is upregulated by Th2 cytokines [81]. SLC26A9-dependent anion transport, which is required to prevent airway obstruction by mucus [81], is linked to CFTR function, an association that may imply direct physical interaction between the two proteins [82, 83]. The relevance of SLC26A9 as a drug target in CF is further supported by the finding of patients carrying mutations in the *SLC26A9* gene [84]. Such patients display a CF-like pulmonary disease. These results indicate that SLC26A9 also contributes to the mucociliary function and innate defence mechanisms. Therefore, pharmacological stimulation of SLC26A9 function, independently from CFTR, could be a way to treat the ion transport defect in CF. However, the druggability of SLC26A9 needs to be demonstrated.

Conclusions

The success of ivacaftor in the treatment of CF patients with the Gly551Asp mutation has strongly increased the interest towards a pharmacological approach to CF basic defect. The clinical efficacy of correctors for the rescue of the Phe508del mutant needs to be demonstrated. However, the increasing knowledge on this mutation and the results obtained *in vitro* with a combination of correctors indicate that rescue to a large extent can also be obtained *in vivo*. High efficacy correctors or combinations of correctors will be particularly important for patients with only one copy of the Phe508del mutation. In these cases, correctors with partial efficacy could not rescue a sufficient number of channels to obtain clinical benefit.

Despite the success of potentiators and correctors, a significant number of patients carrying "untreatable" mutations, could remain without a treatment. For these patients, it could be important to develop alternative strategies based on the stimulation of other types of channels or on the normalisation of PCL properties.

References

1. Clunes MT, Boucher RC. Cystic fibrosis: the mechanisms of pathogenesis of an inherited lung disorder. *Drug Discov Today Dis Mech* 2007; 4: 63–72.
2. Riordan JR. CFTR function and prospects for therapy. *Annu Rev Biochem* 2008; 77: 701–726.
3. Linsdell P. Functional architecture of the CFTR chloride channel. *Mol Membr Biol* 2014; 31: 1–16.
4. Vaandrager AB, Smolenski A, Tilly BC, *et al.* Membrane targeting of cGMP-dependent protein kinase is required for cystic fibrosis transmembrane conductance regulator Cl⁻ channel activation. *Proc Natl Acad Sci USA* 1998; 95: 1466–1471.
5. Huang P, Lazarowski ER, Tarran R, *et al.* Compartmentalized autocrine signaling to cystic fibrosis transmembrane conductance regulator at the apical membrane of airway epithelial cells. *Proc Natl Acad Sci USA* 2001; 98: 14120–14125.
6. Penmatsa H, Zhang W, Yarlagadda S, *et al.* Compartmentalized cyclic adenosine 3′,5′-monophosphate at the plasma membrane clusters PDE3A and cystic fibrosis transmembrane conductance regulator into microdomains. *Mol Biol Cell* 2010; 21: 1097–1110.
7. Monterisi S, Casavola V, Zaccolo M. Local modulation of cystic fibrosis conductance regulator: cytoskeleton and compartmentalized cAMP signalling. *Br J Pharmacol* 2013; 169: 1–9.
8. Welsh MJ, Smith AE. Molecular mechanisms of CFTR chloride channel dysfunction in cystic fibrosis. *Cell* 1993; 73: 1251–1254.
9. Illek B, Zhang L, Lewis NC, *et al.* Defective function of the cystic fibrosis-causing missense mutation G551D is recovered by genistein. *Am J Physiol* 1999; 277: C833–C839.
10. Haws CM, Nepomuceno IB, Krouse ME, *et al.* DeltaF508-CFTR channels: kinetics, activation by forskolin, and potentiation by xanthines. *Am J Physiol* 1996; 270: C1544–C1555.
11. Dérand R, Bulteau-Pignoux L, Becq F. Comparative pharmacology of the activity of wild-type and G551D mutated CFTR chloride channel: effect of the benzimidazolone derivative NS004. *J Membr Biol* 2003; 194: 109–117.
12. Bompadre SG, Sohma Y, Li M, *et al.* G551D and G1349D, two CF-associated mutations in the signature sequences of CFTR, exhibit distinct gating defects. *J Gen Physiol* 2007; 129: 285–298.
13. Zegarra-Moran O, Romio L, Folli C, *et al.* Correction of G551D-CFTR transport defect in epithelial monolayers by genistein but not by CPX or MPB-07. *Br J Pharmacol* 2002; 137: 504–512.
14. Becq F, Mettey Y, Gray MA, *et al.* Development of substituted Benzo[c]quinolizinium compounds as novel activators of the cystic fibrosis chloride channel. *J Biol Chem* 1999; 274: 27415–27425.
15. Ma T, Vetrivel L, Yang H, *et al.* High-affinity activators of cystic fibrosis transmembrane conductance regulator (CFTR) chloride conductance identified by high-throughput screening. *J Biol Chem* 2002; 277: 37235–37241.
16. Yang H, Shelat AA, Guy RK, *et al.* Nanomolar affinity small molecule correctors of defective ΔF508-CFTR chloride channel gating. *J Biol Chem* 2003; 278: 35079–35085.
17. Van Goor F, Straley KS, Cao D, *et al.* Rescue of ΔF508-CFTR trafficking and gating in human cystic fibrosis airway primary cultures by small molecules. *Am J Physiol* 2006; 290: L1117–L1130.
18. Pedemonte N, Diena T, Caci E, *et al.* Antihypertensive 1,4-dihydropyridines as correctors of the cystic fibrosis transmembrane conductance regulator channel gating defect caused by cystic fibrosis mutations. *Mol Pharmacol* 2005; 68: 1736–1746.
19. Van Goor F, Hadida S, Grootenhuis PD, *et al.* Rescue of CF airway epithelial cell function *in vitro* by a CFTR potentiator, VX-770. *Proc Natl Acad Sci USA* 2009; 106: 18825–18830.
20. Ramsey BW, Davies J, McElvaney NG, *et al.* A CFTR potentiator in patients with cystic fibrosis and the G551D mutation. *N Engl J Med* 2011; 365: 1663–1672.
21. Caputo A, Hinzpeter A, Caci E, *et al.* Mutation-specific potency and efficacy of cystic fibrosis transmembrane conductance regulator chloride channel potentiators. *J Pharmacol Exp Ther* 2009; 330: 783–791.
22. Yu H, Burton B, Huang CJ, *et al.* Ivacaftor potentiation of multiple CFTR channels with gating mutations. *J Cyst Fibros* 2012; 11: 237–245.
23. Van Goor F, Yu H, Burton B, *et al.* Effect of ivacaftor on CFTR forms with missense mutations associated with defects in protein processing or function. *J Cyst Fibros* 2014; 13: 29–36.
24. Kim SJ, Skach WR. Mechanisms of CFTR folding at the endoplasmic reticulum. *Front Pharmacol* 2012; 3: 201.

25. Younger JM, Chen L, Ren HY, *et al.* Sequential quality-control checkpoints triage misfolded cystic fibrosis transmembrane conductance regulator. *Cell* 2006; 126: 571–582.

26. Farinha CM, Amaral MD. Most F508del-CFTR is targeted to degradation at an early folding checkpoint and independently of calnexin. *Mol Cell Biol* 2005; 25: 5242–5252.

27. Penque D, Mendes F, Beck S, *et al.* Cystic fibrosis F508del patients have apically localized CFTR in a reduced number of airway cells. *Lab Invest* 2000; 80: 857–868.

28. Lukacs GL, Chang XB, Bear C, *et al.* The ΔF508 mutation decreases the stability of cystic fibrosis transmembrane conductance regulator in the plasma membrane. Determination of functional half-lives on transfected cells. *J Biol Chem* 1993; 268: 21592–21598.

29. Sharma M, Pampinella F, Nemes C, *et al.* Misfolding diverts CFTR from recycling to degradation: quality control at early endosomes. *J Cell Biol* 2004; 164: 923–933.

30. Okiyoneda T, Barrière H, Bagdány M, *et al.* Peripheral protein quality control removes unfolded CFTR from the plasma membrane. *Science* 2010; 329: 805–810.

31. Denning GM, Anderson MP, Amara JF, *et al.* Processing of mutant cystic fibrosis transmembrane conductance regulator is temperature-sensitive. *Nature* 1992; 358: 761–764.

32. Sato S, Ward CL, Krouse ME, *et al.* Glycerol reverses the misfolding phenotype of the most common cystic fibrosis mutation. *J Biol Chem* 1996; 271: 635–638.

33. Pedemonte N, Lukacs GL, Du K, *et al.* Small-molecule correctors of defective ΔF508-CFTR cellular processing identified by high-throughput screening. *J Clin Invest* 2005; 115: 2564–2571.

34. Robert R, Carlile GW, Pavel C, *et al.* Structural analog of sildenafil identified as a novel corrector of the F508del-CFTR trafficking defect. *Mol Pharmacol* 2008; 73: 478–489.

35. Robert R, Carlile GW, Liao J, *et al.* Correction of the ΔPhe508 cystic fibrosis transmembrane conductance regulator trafficking defect by the bioavailable compound glafenine. *Mol Pharmacol* 2010; 77: 922–930.

36. Carlile GW, Keyzers RA, Teske KA, *et al.* Correction of F508del-CFTR trafficking by the sponge alkaloid latonduine is modulated by interaction with PARP. *Chem Biol* 2012; 19: 1288–1299.

37. Van Goor F, Hadida S, Grootenhuis PD, *et al.* Correction of the F508del-CFTR protein processing defect *in vitro* by the investigational drug VX-809. *Proc Natl Acad Sci USA* 2011; 108: 18843–18848.

38. Roxo-Rosa M, Xu Z, Schmidt A, *et al.* Revertant mutants G550E and 4RK rescue cystic fibrosis mutants in the first nucleotide-binding domain of CFTR by different mechanisms. *Proc Natl Acad Sci USA* 2006; 103: 17891–17896.

39. DeCarvalho AC, Gansheroff LJ, Teem JL. Mutations in the nucleotide binding domain 1 signature motif region rescue processing and functional defects of cystic fibrosis transmembrane conductance regulator ΔF508. *J Biol Chem* 2002; 277: 35896–35905.

40. Thibodeau PH, Richardson JM 3rd, Wang W, *et al.* The cystic fibrosis-causing mutation ΔF508 affects multiple steps in cystic fibrosis transmembrane conductance regulator biogenesis. *J Biol Chem* 2010; 285: 35825–35835.

41. Mendoza JL, Schmidt A, Li Q, *et al.* Requirements for efficient correction of ΔF508 CFTR revealed by analyses of evolved sequences. *Cell* 2012; 148: 164–174.

42. Rabeh WM, Bossard F, Xu H, *et al.* Correction of both NBD1 energetics and domain interface is required to restore ΔF508 CFTR folding and function. *Cell* 2012; 148: 150–163.

43. Okiyoneda T, Veit G, Dekkers JF, *et al.* Mechanism-based corrector combination restores ΔF508-CFTR folding and function. *Nat Chem Biol* 2013; 9: 444–454.

44. Clancy JP, Rowe SM, Accurso FJ, *et al.* Results of a phase IIa study of VX-809, an investigational CFTR corrector compound, in subjects with cystic fibrosis homozygous for the F508del-CFTR mutation. *Thorax* 2012; 67: 12–18.

45. Odolczyk N, Fritsch J, Norez C, *et al.* Discovery of novel potent ΔF508-CFTR correctors that target the nucleotide binding domain. *EMBO Mol Med* 2013; 5: 1484–1501.

46. Lee HW, Cheng J, Kovbasnjuk O, *et al.* Insulin-like growth factor 1 (IGF-1) enhances the protein expression of CFTR. *PLoS One* 2013; 8: e59992.

47. Moniz S, Sousa M, Moraes BJ, *et al.* HGF stimulation of Rac1 signaling enhances pharmacological correction of the most prevalent cystic fibrosis mutant F508del-CFTR. *ACS Chem Biol* 2013; 8: 432–442.

48. Hutt DM, Herman D, Rodrigues AP, *et al.* Reduced histone deacetylase 7 activity restores function to misfolded CFTR in cystic fibrosis. *Nat Chem Biol* 2010; 6: 25–33.

49. Wilschanski M, Yahav Y, Yaacov Y, *et al.* Gentamicin-induced correction of CFTR function in patients with cystic fibrosis and CFTR stop mutations. *N Engl J Med* 2003; 349: 1433–1441.

50. Welch EM, Barton ER, Zhuo J, *et al.* PTC124 targets genetic disorders caused by nonsense mutations. *Nature* 2007; 447: 87–91.

51. Sermet-Gaudelus I, Boeck KD, Casimir GJ, *et al.* Ataluren (PTC124) induces cystic fibrosis transmembrane conductance regulator protein expression and activity in children with nonsense mutation cystic fibrosis. *Am J Respir Crit Care Med* 2010; 182: 1262–1272.

52. Wilschanski M, Miller LL, Shoseyov D, et al. Chronic ataluren (PTC124) treatment of nonsense mutation cystic fibrosis. Eur Respir J 2011; 38: 59–69.

53. Rowe SM, Sloane P, Tang LP, et al. Suppression of CFTR premature termination codons and rescue of CFTR protein and function by the synthetic aminoglycoside NB54. J Mol Med (Berl) 2011; 89: 1149–1161.

54. Linde L, Boelz S, Nissim-Rafinia M, et al. Nonsense-mediated mRNA decay affects nonsense transcript levels and governs response of cystic fibrosis patients to gentamicin. J Clin Invest 2007; 117: 683–692.

55. Matsui H, Grubb BR, Tarran R, et al. Evidence for periciliary liquid layer depletion, not abnormal ion composition, in the pathogenesis of cystic fibrosis airways disease. Cell 1998; 95: 1005–1015.

56. Garcia MA, Yang N, Quinton PM. Normal mouse intestinal mucus release requires cystic fibrosis transmembrane regulator-dependent bicarbonate secretion. J Clin Invest 2009; 119: 2613–2622.

57. Gustafsson JK, Ermund A, Ambort D, et al. Bicarbonate and functional CFTR channel are required for proper mucin secretion and link cystic fibrosis with its mucus phenotype. J Exp Med 2012; 209: 1263–1272.

58. Pezzulo AA, Tang XX, Hoegger MJ, et al. Reduced airway surface pH impairs bacterial killing in the porcine cystic fibrosis lung. Nature 2012; 487: 109–113.

59. Elkins MR, Robinson M, Rose BR, et al. A controlled trial of long-term inhaled hypertonic saline in patients with cystic fibrosis. N Engl J Med 2006; 354: 229–224.

60. Daviskas E, Anderson SD, Brannan JD, et al. Inhalation of dry-powder mannitol increases mucociliary clearance. Eur Respir J 1997; 10: 2449–2454.

61. Daviskas E, Anderson SD, Jaques A, et al. Inhaled mannitol improves the hydration and surface properties of sputum in patients with cystic fibrosis. Chest 2010; 137: 861–868.

62. Robinson M, Daviskas E, Eberl S, et al. The effect of inhaled mannitol on bronchial mucus clearance in cystic fibrosis patients: a pilot study. Eur Respir J 1999; 14: 678–685.

63. Bilton D, Daviskas E, Anderson SD, et al. Phase 3 randomized study of the efficacy and safety of inhaled dry powder mannitol for the symptomatic treatment of non-cystic fibrosis bronchiectasis. Chest 2013; 144: 215–225.

64. Mason SJ, Paradiso AM, Boucher RC. Regulation of transepithelial ion transport and intracellular calcium by extracellular ATP in human normal and cystic fibrosis airway epithelium. Br J Pharmacol 1991; 103: 1649–1656.

65. Accurso FJ, Moss RB, Wilmott RW, et al. Denufosol tetrasodium in patients with cystic fibrosis and normal to mildly impaired lung function. Am J Respir Crit Care Med 2011; 183: 627–634.

66. Ratjen F, Durham T, Navratil T, et al. Long term effects of denufosol tetrasodium in patients with cystic fibrosis. J Cyst Fibros 2012; 11: 539–549.

67. Yang YD, Cho H, Koo JY, et al. TMEM16A confers receptor-activated calcium-dependent chloride conductance. Nature 2008; 455: 1210–1215.

68. Schroeder BC, Cheng T, Jan YN, et al. Expression cloning of TMEM16A as a calcium-activated chloride channel subunit. Cell 2008; 134: 1019–1029.

69. Caputo A, Caci E, Ferrera L, et al. TMEM16A, a membrane protein associated with calcium-dependent chloride channel activity. Science 2008; 322: 590–594.

70. Huang F, Rock JR, Harfe BD, et al. Studies on expression and function of the TMEM16A calcium-activated chloride channel. Proc Natl Acad Sci USA 2009; 106: 21413–21418.

71. Fischer H, Illek B, Sachs L, et al. CFTR and calcium-activated chloride channels in primary cultures of human airway gland cells of serous or mucous phenotype. Am J Physiol 2010; 299: L585–L594.

72. Yu K, Duran C, Qu Z, et al. Explaining calcium-dependent gating of anoctamin-1 chloride channels requires a revised topology. Circ Res 2012; 110: 990–999.

73. Tian Y, Kongsuphol P, Hug M, et al. Calmodulin-dependent activation of the epithelial calcium-dependent chloride channel TMEM16A. FASEB J 2011; 25: 1058–1068.

74. Jung J, Nam JH, Park HW, et al. Dynamic modulation of ANO1/TMEM16A HCO_3^- permeability by Ca^{2+}/calmodulin. Proc Natl Acad Sci USA 2013; 110: 360–365.

75. Huang F, Zhang H, Wu M, et al. Calcium-activated chloride channel TMEM16A modulates mucin secretion and airway smooth muscle contraction. Proc Natl Acad Sci USA 2012; 109: 16354–16359.

76. Scudieri P, Caci E, Bruno S, et al. Association of TMEM16A chloride channel overexpression with airway goblet cell metaplasia. J Physiol 2012; 590: 6141–6155.

77. Namkung W, Yao Z, Finkbeiner WE, et al. Small-molecule activators of TMEM16A, a calcium-activated chloride channel, stimulate epithelial chloride secretion and intestinal contraction. FASEB J 2011; 25: 4048–4062.

78. Veit G, Bossard F, Goepp J, et al. Proinflammatory cytokine secretion is suppressed by TMEM16A or CFTR channel activity in human cystic fibrosis bronchial epithelia. Mol Biol Cell 2012; 23: 4188–4202.

79. Wong XM, Younger S, Peters CJ, et al. Subdued, a TMEM16 family Ca^{2+}-activated Cl^- channel in Drosophila melanogaster with an unexpected role in host defense. Elife 2013; 2: e00862.

80. Alper SL, Sharma AK. The SLC26 gene family of anion transporters and channels. Mol Aspects Med 2013; 34: 494–515.

81. Anagnostopoulou P, Riederer B, Duerr J, et al. SLC26A9-mediated chloride secretion prevents mucus obstruction in airway inflammation. J Clin Invest 2012; 122: 3629–3634.

82. Bertrand CA, Zhang R, Pilewski JM, *et al.* SLC26A9 is a constitutively active, CFTR-regulated anion conductance in human bronchial epithelia. *J Gen Physiol* 2009; 133: 421–438.

83. Avella M, Loriol C, Boulukos K, *et al.* SLC26A9 stimulates CFTR expression and function in human bronchial cell lines. *J Cell Physiol* 2011; 226: 212–223.

84. Bakouh N, Bienvenu T, Thomas A, *et al.* Characterization of SLC26A9 in patients with CF-like lung disease. *Hum Mutat* 2013; 34: 1404–1414.

Disclosures: None declared.

Chapter 10

Potentiating and correcting mutant CFTR in patients with cystic fibrosis

Isabelle Sermet-Gaudelus[1,2,3], Jacques de Blic[2,3], Muriel LeBourgeois[2,3], Iwona Pranke[1,3], Aleksander Edelman[1,3] and Bonnie W. Ramsey[4]

Recent data have established proof of concept that rescue of the underlying defects in the cellular processing and channel function of mutant cystic fibrosis transmembrane conductance regulator (CFTR) can result in clinical benefit. Modulators of the CFTR protein include: correctors, which are mainly targeted at rescuing the Phe508del-CFTR at the plasma membrane; and potentiators, which aim to restore activity of mutants that impair channel gating. The potentiator ivacaftor proved safe in patients carrying the Gly551Asp mutation and demonstrated a significant change in sweat chloride and an improvement in lung function; an effect that was maintained for up to 144 weeks. This clinical benefit has also been demonstrated in patients with other mutations that resulted in defective channel gating or conductance. Ivacaftor acts as a modest potentiator for the small amount of Phe508del-CFTR channels trafficked to the cell surface. However its combination with the corrector lumacaftor resulted in improvement in the forced expiratory volume in 1 s (FEV1) in Phe508del homozygote patients. Such treatments provide rationale for a personalised medicine strategy in the treatment of cystic fibrosis (CF).

Cystic Fibrosis (CF) is an autosomal recessive disease that is caused by mutations in the cystic fibrosis transmembrane conductance regulator (CFTR) gene, which encodes for the CFTR protein and is one of the main chloride (Cl^-) and bicarbonate channels at the plasma membrane [1]. CF affects approximately 80 000 patients worldwide. The *CFTR* gene and the deletion of phenylalanine at residue 508 (Phe508del), the most frequent mutation in the Caucasian population, were both identified in 1989 [2]. Recent data have established the proof of concept that rescuing the underlying defects in the cellular processing and Cl^- channel function of CF-causing mutant *CFTR* alleles can result in clinical benefit [3]. CFTR modulators include correctors that target Phe508del cellular misprocessing to rescue the mutant CFTR at the plasma membrane and potentiators, which aim to restore Cl^- channel activity of the CFTR mutants that are located at the cell surface and impair CFTR gating. In 2012, one of those potentiator compounds, ivacaftor (also known as VX-770, trade name Kalydeco; Vertex Pharmaceuticals Inc., Boston, MA, USA), was approved by the US Food and Drug Administration (FDA) and the European Medicines Agency (EMA) for patients carrying the Gly551Asp-CFTR mutation, thus becoming the first available treatment to

[1]INSERM 1151, Paris, France. [2]Centre de Ressources et de Compétence de Mucoviscidose, Unité de Pneumo-Allergologie Pédiatrique, Hôpital Necker, Paris, France. [3]Faculté de Medecine René Descartes, Université Paris V, Paris, France. [4]Seattle Children's Research Institute, Seattle, WA, USA.

Correspondence: Isabelle Sermet-Gaudelus, INSERM 1151 and Centre de Ressources et de Compétence de Mucoviscidose, Unité de Pneumo-Allergologie Pédiatrique, Hôpital Necker, 149 rue de Sévres, Paris 75015, France. E-mail: isabelle.sermet@nck.aphp.fr

Copyright ERS 2014. Print ISBN: 978-1-84984-050-7. Online ISBN: 978-1-84984-051-4. Print ISSN: 2312-508X. Online ISSN: 2312-5098.

directly address the basic defect of the disease. The considerable improvements in patients carrying the Gly551Asp mutation treated with ivacaftor have raised hope of impacting the entire pathophysiological cycle and changing the course of the disease. Although this drug benefits a small minority of the CF population, the developmental pathway established by ivacaftor paves the way for other CFTR modulators that may improve many more patients [4].

After a brief review on how recent basic, scientific findings have helped to decipher the complex biogenesis and function of the wild-type protein, this chapter will focus on connecting the current understanding of the CFTR-mutant defects to the discovery of correctors and potentiators and their subsequent rapid advancement through the current therapeutic pipeline.

Targets for CFTR drug discovery

Wild-type CFTR protein structure

The CFTR protein is a member of the ATP-binding cassette (ABC) transporter superfamily, and is mainly expressed in the apical membrane of epithelia [5]. This 1480 amino acid multidomain glycoprotein architecture involves a dimeric organisation of two membrane-spanning domains (MSDs) that form the channel pore (fig. 1). MSDs are tightly associated with two cytoplasmic nucleotide-binding domains (NBDs), NBD1 and NBD2 that gate the channel and the dimerisation of which upon ATP binding drives channel opening [6]. The MSDs interact with the NBDs *via* intracellular loops (ICLs; ICL1/2 from MSD1 and ICL3/4 from MSD2). NBD1 associates with MSD2 *via* the coupling helix of ICL4 and with MSD1 *via* ICL1 [7]. These interfaces are involved in folding and relaying ATP-dependent conformational changes of the NBDs to the MSDs, therefore allowing channel activation and gating [8]. The Phe508 amino acid has a critical position in NBD1 because it is partially exposed on its surface, lining a hydrophobic groove that forms interface with ICL4 and ICL1.

An additional domain called the regulatory (R) domain, inserted between NBD1 and MSD2, links the two transporter domains. It contains serine residues that are phosphorylated by protein kinase A and protein kinase C. This mechanism is mandatory for gating of the channel to the open state. Because of its high content in charged amino acids, the R domain is an unstructured peptide that interacts with different regions of the protein simultaneously, as well as with other proteins, and enhances ATP binding to the NBDs [9].

Wild-type CFTR biogenesis

CFTR biogenesis is a complex and multistep process that provides insight into the design of targets for the CFTR modulators.

As a first step, CFTR is co-translationally inserted into the endoplasmic reticulum (ER) membrane and concomitantly N-linked to glycosyl groups. CFTR undergoes a cooperative folding process where domains of the protein fold during translation and interact together like pieces of a puzzle to form multidomain folding intermediates, which are continuously submitted to the fast ER-associated degradation (ERAD) (fig. 2) [10, 11].

Wild-type CFTR conformational maturation is highly inefficient: at least 80% of wild-type CFTR is degraded because of abnormal folding and quality control. This results from prolonged interaction with molecular chaperone complexes that ultimately condemns the

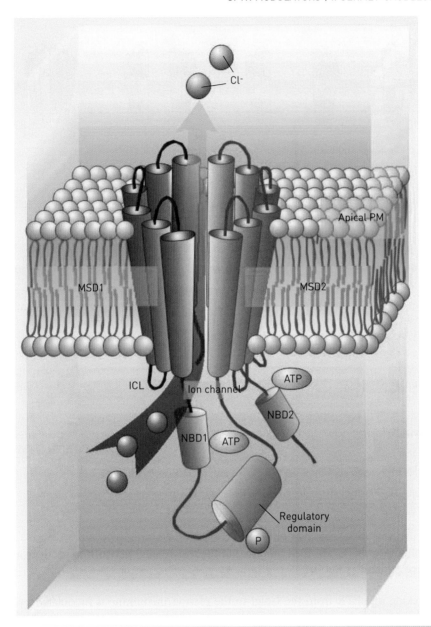

Figure 1. Protein structure. The cystic fibrosis transmembrane conductance regulator (CFTR) protein structure is composed of 12 helical domains belonging to two membrane-spanning domains (MSDs), intermediate extracellular loops, two cytoplasmic nucleotide-binding domains (NBDs) and four intracellular loops (ICL). NBD1 is connected to an intracellular domain called the regulatory (R) domain. The two NBDs form tightly interacting dimers in a head-to-tail configuration upon ATP binding at their interface, and dissociate upon ATP hydrolysis. The nonphosphorylated R domain interacts with the NBDs and inhibits channel activity by blocking heterodimerisation. Phosphorylation (P) shifts the equilibrium such that the R domain is excluded from the NBD dimer interface, facilitating ATP binding to the NBDs and gating of the channel. PM: plasma membrane.

permanently misfolded wild-type protein to final ubiquitination and proteasome degradation (fig. 3) [12–14]. CFTR is then transported to the Golgi complex *via* common cytosolic budding machinery, regulated by coat-protein II coated vesicles that form at the ER exit sites.

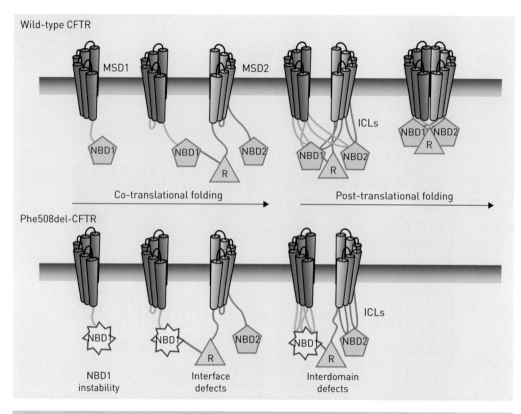

Figure 2. Model of the cooperative folding process [11]. Each cystic fibrosis transmembrane conductance regulator (CFTR) domain folds during translation with a relative energetic instability. Domain interactions facilitate intradomain folding and interdomain assembly. Attaining the stable CFTR native fold requires specific interdomain interactions that are critical to proper folding. The Phe508 residue and its surrounding area in nucleotide-binding domain (NBD)1 interfaces with the coupling helix of the cytoplasmic loops (CL)4 and CL1 in membrane spanning domain (MSD)2 and MSD1, respectively. This creates a hydrophobic patch. Destabilisation of this interface by Phe508 deletion impairs NBD1 energetics and interactions leading to the impairment of the four other domains and folding disruption. R: regulatory domain; ICL: intracellular loops.

The carbohydrate chains are then modified in the trans-Golgi network to produce a complex glycosylated protein [13, 14].

The trafficking of CFTR from the Golgi to the plasma membrane is modulated by dynamic interactions of its C-terminal amino acid sequence with PDZ-domain-containing proteins, such as Na^+/H^+ exchanger regulatory factor isoform (NHERF)1 and NHERF2 [15]. (PDZ (postsynaptic density Drosophila disc large tumour suppressor zona occludens) domains are modular protein interaction domains that play a role in protein targeting and protein complex assembly). NHERF1, ezrin and F-actin form a complex that is essential for stabilising CFTR by facilitating anterograde trafficking, anchoring the CFTR protein to the apical membrane and to the actin cytoskeleton [16]. This complex is also critical for the compartmentalisation of sufficient levels of cAMP, and its effector protein kinase A in the appropriate subcortical membrane compartment. All these mechanisms allow tight modulation of CFTR-plasma membrane levels and fine-tuning regulation of its channel function.

The mature CFTR is very stable and the proteins that are endocytosed (10% of the plasma membrane CFTR each minute) are recycled back to the cell surface. In contrast, misfolded

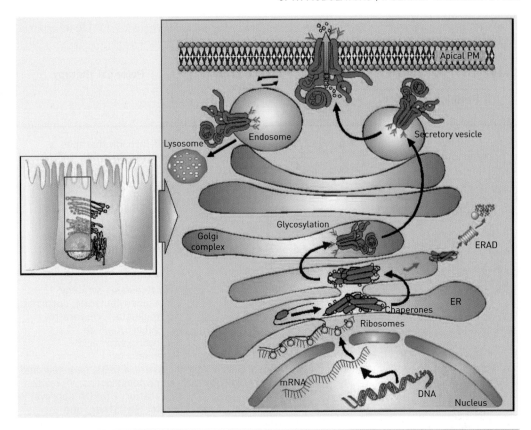

Figure 3. The cystic fibrosis transmembrane conductance regulator (CFTR) is inserted into the endoplasmic reticulum (ER) membrane during translation. The energetic instability of individual domains, the slow domain assembly contrasting with the fast ER-associated degradation (ERAD) kinetics of folding intermediates explains the inefficient folding yield of wild-type CFTR in the ER. CFTR is folded and core-glycosylated with assistance of chaperones in the ER. A large portion of misfolded proteins is degraded by ERAD after previous ubiquitination. Properly folded CFTR is subsequently transported to the Golgi complex for further maturation and glycosylation. Finally, a mature channel is trafficked in secretory vesicles to the apical plasma membrane (PM). Membrane protein is continuously endocytosed and recycled or degraded in lysosomes if misfolded.

CFTR that has escaped ERAD is rapidly eliminated from the plasma membrane by a peripheral ubiquitination-related protein quality-control system, which triggers lysosomal degradation and serves as a final check point [17, 18].

Classification of CFTR mutations

The most frequent mutation is the deletion of phenylalanine at residue 508, known as Phe508del, which accounts for 70% of CF alleles in Caucasian patients with CF. Among the remaining alleles, fewer than 20 mutations occur at a worldwide frequency of $\geqslant 0.1\%$ [19].

CF mutations cause loss of CFTR function by different mechanisms that include: defective protein production, impaired CFTR processing in the cell, and defective channel gating. Five mutation subclasses can be considered: defective protein production (class 2), defective protein processing (class 2), defective protein regulation (class 3), defective protein conductance (class 4), and reduced amounts of functional CFTR protein (class 5) (table 1 and fig. 4) [20]. These classes are not mutually exclusive and, therefore, a mutation can combine two defects, *i.e.* be classified as classes 2 and 3 like Phe508del. Classes 1, 2 and 5

Table 1. Classification of cystic fibrosis transmembrane conductance regulator (CFTR) mutations and corresponding CFTR modulators

Class	CFTR			Mutation protein name	Potential therapy
	Protein	Function	Apical expression		
1	Defective production	No	No	Gly542X, Trp1282X, Arg553X, Arg1162X, Glu822X, 1717-1G>A, 711+1G>T, 621+1G>T	Read-through therapy: gentamycin, ataluren[#], NMD inhibitors
2	Impaired processing	No	No	Phe508del, Asn1303Lys, Ile507del, Arg1066Cys, Ser549Arg, Gly85Glu	Correctors: *In vitro*: glycerol, Corr-4, VRT-325, glafenine, phenylhydrazone RDR1 Ongoing clinical development: lumacaftor, VX-661 Proteostasis strategy 4-phenylbutyrate, cucurmin, miglustat[¶], resveratrol, suberoylanilide hydroxamic acid
3	Defective regulation	No	Yes	Gly551Asp, Gly178Arg, Ser549Asn, Ser549Arg, Gly551Ser, Gly970Arg, Gly1244Glu, Ser1251Asn, Ser1255Pro, Gly1349Asp	Potentiators: *In vitro*: PG-01, genistein and phytoestrogens, VRT-532 Ivacaftor: US FDA approval for Gly551Asp, and ongoing clinical development for other gating mutations
4	Defective conductance	Reduced	Yes	Arg117His, Asp110His, Arg117Cys, Arg347His, Arg352Gln, Asp1152His,	Potentiators: Ongoing clinical development: ivacaftor
5	Reduced amount	Reduced	Reduced	3272-26A>G, 3849+10kbC>T, Ala455Glu, Asp565Gly, 5T	NMD inhibitors Splicing modulators

NMD: nonsense-mediated mRNA decay; US FDA: US Food and Drug Administration. [#]: formerly known as PTC124 (PTC Therapeutics, South Plainfield, NJ, USA); [¶]: Actelion, Allschwil, Switzerland.

decrease the quantity of CFTR (little or none for classes 1 and 2; residual expression for class V). Classes 3 and 4 mutated proteins do not have any conformational or trafficking defects but decrease function by impaired gating (class 3) or conductance (class 4). This classification based on structure function provides a rationale for mutation-targeted therapeutic strategy [21].

Mutations disturbing the gating of the Cl⁻ channel and potentiator therapies

Gly551Asp mutation and potentiator therapy

Class 3 mutations are frequently located in the ATP-binding domain of NBDs and, thus, are referred to as gating mutations (table 1 and fig. 4). The Gly551Asp mutation is the most

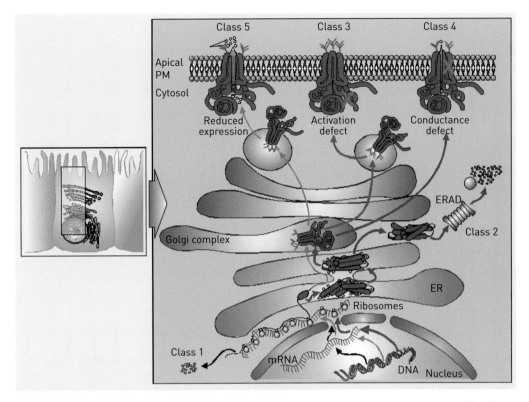

Figure 4. Cystic fibrosis transmembrane conductance regulator mutation classes. PM: plasma membrane; ER: endoplasmic reticulum; ERAD: ER-associated degradation.

prevalent and accounts for ~4% of mutations in CF patients. It is caused by the substitution of the amino acid glycine by aspartate at position 551 at a crucial point in the NBD1, the interface with NBD2 [22]. It abolishes ATP-dependent gating, resulting in an open probability that is ~100-fold lower than that of wild-type channels.

Among the compounds identified by high-throughput screening (table 1) [23], the most promising is ivacaftor, which increases the Gly551Asp channel opening probability [24] by possibly enhancing the ATP-independent opening probability [25].

Acute addition of ivacaftor increases CFTR-mediated Cl⁻ secretion in Gly551Asp/Phe508del human bronchial epithelium (HBE) cells from 0–5% to levels 35–50% of that measured in non-CF HBE and reduces Na^+ absorption [24]. This pharmacological effect is associated with an enhanced height in the apical airway surface liquid (ASL) sufficient to increase cilia beating to levels observed in non-CF airway epithelium.

Clinical trials with ivacaftor in Gly551Asp patients

Ivacaftor was first evaluated in a phase II clinical trial that used both a crossover component and a confirmatory parallel group design. 39 adults carrying at least one Gly551Asp-CFTR allele were randomised to receive placebo or oral ivacaftor every 12 h at a dose of 25, 75 or 150 mg for 14 days in part 1 of the study, and placebo or ivacaftor every 12 h at a dose of 150 or 250 mg for 28 days in part two of the study (table 2) [26]. Ivacaftor proved safe and well

Table 2. Main clinical trials of ivacaftor monotherapy in patients with cystic fibrosis

Trial name	Phase	Design	Genotype	Main inclusion criteria	Treatment duration	Patients n	Δ FEV1[#] %	Other selected outcomes[#]
VX06-770-101	1	Randomised, placebo-controlled, double-blind, multiple-dose study Part 1: crossover Part 2: parallel	Gly551Asp in at least 1 allele	Aged ≥18 years FEV1 ≥40%	Part 1: 28 days Part 2: 28 days	39	10.8% relative improvement at the maximally effective dose	Sweat chloride: -55 mEq·L⁻¹ at the maximally effective dose
STRIVE	III	Randomised, placebo-controlled, double-blind, parallel study Open-label, rollover study [PERSIST]	Gly551Asp in at least 1 allele	Aged ≥12 years FEV1 40–90%	48 weeks 96 weeks	161	10.6% absolute improvement, 16.7% relative improvement	Pulmonary exacerbation: -55% Sweat chloride: -48 mEq·L⁻¹ Weight: 2.7 kg
ENVISION	IV	Randomised, placebo-controlled, double-blind, parallel study Open-label, rollover study [PERSIST]	Gly551Asp in at least 1 allele	Aged 6–11 years FEV1 40–105%	48 weeks 96 weeks	52	10% adjusted absolute improvement	Sweat Cl⁻: -53 mEq·L⁻¹ Weight: 2.8 kg
KONDUCT	III	Randomised, placebo-controlled, double-blind, parallel study Open-label, rollover study [KONTINUE]	Arg117His in at least 1 allele	Aged ≥6–11 years and FEV1 40–105% ≥12 years and FEV1 40–90%	24 weeks 104 weeks	69	5% absolute improvement in all the patients, 9.1% absolute improvement in patients aged >18 years	
KONNECTION	III	Randomised, placebo-controlled, double-blind, crossover study Open-label 16-week treatment period Open-label, rollover study [KONTINUE]	Non-Gly551Asp gating mutation in at least 1 allele¶	Aged ≥6 years	8 weeks 16 weeks 96 weeks	39	10.7% absolute improvement	Sweat chloride: -53 mEq·L⁻¹ BMI 0.66
DISCOVER	II	Randomised, placebo-controlled, double-blind, parallel study Open-label study for suitable patients	Phe508del homozygous	Aged ≥12 years FEV1 ≥40%	16 weeks 96 weeks	140	1.3% absolute improvement	Sweat chloride: -2.9 mEq·L⁻¹

Table 2. Continued

Trial name	Phase	Design	Genotype	Main inclusion criteria	Treatment duration	Patients n	Δ FEV1 # %	Other selected outcomes #
VX10-770-106	II	Randomised, placebo-controlled, double-blind, crossover study	Gly551Asp in at least 1 allele FEV1 >90%, LCI upper limit of normal	Aged ⩾6 years FEV1 >90%	Two periods of 28 days	21	LCI improved (-2.1)	FEV1%: 7% (absolute improvement)
KIWI	III	Open-label study	1 gating mutation in at least 1 allele+	2–5 years	24 weeks	NA	FEV1 % pred	Sweat chloride, CFQ-R, BMI and time to first pulmonary exacerbation
VX12-770-113	II	Single-centre, randomised, double-blind, multiple within-subject (N-of-one) crossover study Open-label treatment period	Residual CFTR function§	Aged ⩾12 years FEV1 ⩾40% Phenotypic or molecular evidence of residual function§	Two periods of 2 weeks	NA	FEV1 % pred	LCI and weight
VX10-770-107	II	Placebo-controlled, single-blind study Open-label follow-up study	Gly551Asp in at least 1 allele	Aged ⩾12 years FEV1 ⩾40% pred	4 weeks 48 weeks	NA	^{3}He-MRI total ventilation defect	FEV1 % pred, sweat chloride and CFQ-R

ΔFEV1: change in forced expiratory volume in 1 s; BMI: body mass index; LCI: lung clearance index; CFQ-R: Cystic Fibrosis Questionnaire Revised; CFTR: cystic fibrosis transmembrane conductance regulator; NA: study not completed, the main end-points are listed; ^{3}He-MRI: helium-3 magnetic resonance imaging. #: mean difference between treatment and placebo group. ¶: one of the following: Gly178Arg, Gly551Ser, Ser549Arg, Ser549Asn, Gly970Arg, Gly1244Glu, Ser1251Asn, Ser1255Pro, Gly1349Asp. +: one of the following: Gly551Asp, Gly178Arg, Ser549Arg, Ser549Asn, Gly551Ser, Gly970Arg, Gly1244Glu, Ser1251Asn, Ser1255Pro, Gly1349Asp. §: one of the following: clinically documented exocrine pancreatic function and/or sweat chloride ⩽80 mM·L^{-1} and/or one of the following mutations with defective residual function or defective mRNA splicing: Arg117His, Glu56Lys, Pro67Leu, Asp110Glu, Asp110His, Arg117Cys, Arg110His, Arg347His, Arg352Gln, Ala455Glu, Asp579Gly, Ser945Leu, Leu206Trp, Arg1070Trp, Phe1074Leu, Asp1152His, Ser1235Arg, Asp1270Asn, 2789+5G>A, 3849+10kbC>T, 3272-26A>G, 711+5G>A, 3120G>A, 1811+1.6kbA>G, 711+3A>G, 1898+3A>G, 1898+1G>A, 1717-1G>A, 1717-8G>A, 1342-2A>C, 405+3A>C, 1716G/A 1811+1G>C, 1898+5G>T, 3850-3T>G, IVS14b+5G>A, 1898+1G>T, 4005+2T>C, 621+3A>G, 621+1G>T.

tolerated. Dose-dependent within-subject improvements were observed in channel function in both the nasal and the sweat gland epithelia, *i.e.* trend to normalisation in the sweat test and nasal potential difference (NPD). The median reduction in sweat chloride of 59 mEq at the maximally effective dose resulted in a mean sweat chloride of 55 mEq. Interestingly, measures of lung function also showed significant improvements. Dosage with 150 mg a day proved the best responsive and was then chosen for phase III clinical trials.

Two 48-week randomised, double-blind, placebo-controlled trials were conducted in adolescents/adults with a forced expiratory volume in 1 s (FEV1) of 40–90% of the predicted normal (STRIVE study) [3] and in children with an FEV1 40–105% of the predicted normal (ENVISION study) [27]. At the end of the 48-week study period, patients were offered the opportunity to rollover into an optional open-label study (PERSIST) designed to monitor the long-term impact of ivacaftor treatment over a period 96 weeks (tables 2 and 3).

In the STRIVE study, the primary end-point was achieved. At week 24, the FEV1 % pred showed a statistically significant treatment effect of 10.6% points (p<0.001). This ivacaftor-dependent improvement was noted as early as 15 days and was maintained throughout the study; with a treatment effect through to week 48 [3, 27]. Nearly 75% of adults treated with ivacaftor had a mean improvement of 5% points. Interestingly, improvements in patients with poor pulmonary function were similar to those in patients with only mild functional impairment (table 2).

Secondary end-points also showed significant improvement, including a reduction in the risk of pulmonary exacerbation by more than two-fold, a positive change in patient-reported quality-of-life index and a significant weight gain. Similar to the phase II trial, sweat chloride levels demonstrated a rapid and sustained response below the diagnostic threshold of CF in comparison to placebo (table 3). This effect was seen as early as day 15 and maintained through to week 48. However, no direct correlation was observed between sweat chloride concentration modifications and pulmonary improvement [28].

A similar pattern of data, with a similar magnitude as those seen in the adult study, was observed in the paediatric ENVISION study for FEV1, weight gain and sweat test. Interestingly, improvements in FEV1 were, despite baseline lung function, within the normal range suggesting a silent asymptomatic lung disease [27]. This was confirmed in a specific study in patients with mild disease at the age of ⩾6 years, who showed a significant improvement in FEV1 and forced expiratory flow at 25–75% of forced vital capacity (FEF25-75%) in association with a dramatic improvement in lung clearance index (LCI) [29].

The adults/adolescents who switched from placebo to ivacaftor in the long-term PERSIST study showed an improvement in FEV1, weight and exacerbation rate, which were similar to those observed in the patients treated with ivacaftor during the 48 weeks prior to the study, further supporting the beneficial effect of ivacaftor [30]. Response was sustained through to 96 weeks (and 144 weeks for those who received the treatment in the previous study) (table 2).

These remarkable results established the proof of concept that molecular transformation, *i.e.* increase in the channel open probability and epithelial CFTR function rescue, can translate into outstanding clinical improvements. This was obvious from the second week of treatment, even in patients who were asymptomatic. These successes led to US FDA/EMA approval of ivacaftor monotherapy to treat CF patients aged >6 years with the Gly551Asp mutation on at least one allele.

Table 3. Treatment effects in patients with cystic fibrosis carrying the Gly551Asp mutation, in at least one allele, enrolled in phase III clinical trials STRIVE or ENVISION and continued in the PERSIST trial

Treatment assigned	Patients n	Duration of ivacaftor weeks	FEV1 % predicted	BMI[#] kg·m^{-2}
STRIVE[¶] to PERSIST[+]				
Ivacaftor to ivacaftor	77	48	9.4±8.3	1.0±1.6
	74	96	9.1±10.8	1.0±2.1
	72	144	9.4±10.8	1.2±2.2
Placebo to ivacaftor	67	0	-1.2±7.8	-0.1±1.0
	63	48	9.4±8.5	1.2±1.3
	55	96	9.5±11.2	1.0±1.6
ENVISION[§] to PERSIST[+]				
Ivacaftor to ivacaftor	26	48	10.2±15.7	1.5±1.2
	25	96	9.0±15.2	2.0±1.6
	25	144	14.8±5.7	2.5±1.6
Placebo to ivacaftor	22	0	-0.6±10.1	0.1±0.8
	22	48	8.8±12.5	1.4±1.0
	21	96	10.5±11.5	2.0±1.2

Data are presented as mean absolute change from baseline ± SD, unless otherwise stated. FEV1: forced expiratory volume in 1 s; BMI: body mass index. [#]: at 48 weeks (end of the phase III trial), 96 weeks and 144 weeks (follow-up in the rollover study); [¶]: enrolled adolescents/adults aged >12 years with FEV1 40–90% of the predicted normal; [+]: extension study; [§]: enrolled children aged 6–11 years with FEV1 40–105% of the predicted normal.

A cohort of patients who had been newly prescribed ivacaftor were monitored for the initial 6 months in a phase IV observational cohort study. The 151 observed patients' data demonstrated an improvement in FEV1, body mass index (BMI) and sweat test with a magnitude similar to the phase III clinical trial [31]. The percentage of patients hospitalised decreased from 25% during the previous 6 months to 8%. Interestingly, the rate of *Pseudomonas aeruginosa* positive cultures dropped from 52% to 34%. This result, still under investigation, suggests that CFTR modulators might help clearance and elimination of *P. aeruginosa*, a crucial result that could be a decisive step in changing the course of the disease. A peripheral mucociliary clearance substudy showed impressive improvement at 1 and 3 months, which substantiates the mechanism of action of ivacaftor. Importantly the intestinal pH, which is more acidic in patients with CF, increased significantly in patients taking ivacaftor. This suggests that this potentiator may increase pancreatic extracts efficiency and, more generally, opens the question of whether absorptive capacity across intestinal epithelia can be changed by modulators. Ongoing studies in patients carrying the Gly551Asp mutation are described in table 2.

Other class 3 mutations and ivacaftor

Other class 3 *CFTR* gating mutations are potentiated by ivacaftor as assessed by the increased probability of channel opening and cAMP activated Cl⁻ transport after the addition of the compound [32].

Clinical benefits of ivacaftor were evaluated in 39 patients aged >6 years with other gating mutations (table 2). The KONNECTION study showed a significant improvement in FEV1, BMI and sweat test after 8 weeks of treatment in a similar range as for Gly551Asp. At least one patient was found to have improved for each mutation [33]. Ongoing studies in patients carrying gating mutations are described in table 2.

Phe508del and ivacaftor

Ivacaftor acts as a modest potentiator for the small amount of Phe508del-CFTR channels trafficked to the cell surface. It increases the CFTR channel open probability of the Phe508del channel by five-fold and CFTR-mediated Cl⁻ secretion in cultured HBE of some Phe508del-homozygous CF patients to levels >10% of that observed in non-CF HBE [24]. A phase II clinical trial (DISCOVER) in patients who were homozygous for the Phe508del-CFTR mutation did not show any significant improvements in FEV1 or other clinical end-points including Cystic Fibrosis Questionnaire Revised (CFQ-R) or rate of pulmonary exacerbations (table 2) [34]. Although a small reduction in sweat chloride concentration was noted in the first part of the study, this was not observed in the open-label extension.

Class 4: mutations altering the conduction of the Cl⁻ channel

Class 4 mutations, mostly located within membrane spanning domains, have defective conductance but display a residual function with normal regulation. Therefore, therapies aimed at increasing their activity might be effective. This was demonstrated in a panel of Fischer rat thyroid (FRT) cells that carried such a mutation [35]. However, the magnitude of the responses to ivacaftor, as assessed by Cl⁻ transport *via* Ussing chambers, varied widely according to residual activity and, very probably, to the association of a gating defect counteracted by ivacaftor. Arg117His was one of the most responsive mutations. CFTR Cl⁻ transport increased from 33% to 134% of the normal; this is most probably due to the mutation affecting both the conductance and the gating of the channel [36].

The efficacy of ivacaftor was tested in 69 patients, aged ⩾6 years, carrying the Arg117His mutation on at least one allele (KONDUKT study) (table 2). In the 50 patients aged ⩾18 years, the mean treatment difference in FEV1 was 9.1% (p=0.008) [37]. However, for the whole population the treatment effect was at the limit of significance. Ongoing studies in patients carrying other mutations with residual function are described in table 2.

Class 2: mutations altering the cellular processing of the protein and corrector therapies

Phe508del defect

Phe508del leads to abnormal intradomain interfaces resulting in energetic and kinetic instability of the NBD1 and ultimately impaired intrinsic NBD1 folding (table 1 and fig. 2) [38]. This impairs the assembly of the interface between NBD1 and ICL4/MSD2, and destabilises the NBD1-NBD2 dimerisation interface that is critical for both channel activation and gating [39, 40]. Almost 100% of the newly synthesised misfolded Phe508del-CFTR protein is retained in the ER and retro-translocated into the cytoplasm to be degraded by ERAD [41, 42] (fig. 4). This results from an increased associations with the heat shock protein (Hsp) 70/90 chaperone-ER quality control machinery [43] and SUMOylation (SUMO: small ubiquitin-like modifier) of Phe508del-CFTR [44]. Finally, misfolded Phe508del-CFTR fails to exit the ER because of exposure of the ER retention motifs [45]. Interestingly, the preferential association of cytokeratin-8 with Phe508del-CFTR plays a role in sending misfolded Phe508del-CFTR conformers for degradation as downregulation of this interaction contributes to the restoration of Phe508del-CFTR trafficking [46]. Phe508del-CFTR presents accelerated endocytic retrieval from the plasma membrane, because of defective surface anchoring, and is then prevented from re-routing back to the membrane by recycling to endosomes and lysosomal degradation [47, 48]. Finally, once at the membrane, Phe508del presents a gating defect [49] and disabled activation because of relocalisation of cAMP and protein kinase A in the cytosol due to disorganised cortical actin cytoskeleton [16].

Goal of correction

Obviously, identification and development of correctors of Phe508del-CFTR cellular misprocessing is far more challenging than that for potentiators because of the multistep misfolding and the involvement of multiple components of the cellular quality-control machinery, both in the cytoplasm and at the membrane [50, 51].

At least three major defects need to be repaired: 1) efficient rescue to the cell surface, which may involve improving the folding of the protein and/or escaping ER quality-control mechanisms by other means; 2) increase the compromised activity of the Phe508del-CFTR channels; and 3) increase the stability of the mutant protein on the cell surface.

Corrector efficiency of lumacaftor

High-throughput screening has identified pharmacological chaperones working at different points in the folding process (table 1) [52]. The most promising compound is lumacaftor (former name VX-809; Vertex Pharmaceuticals Inc.) and its pharmacokinetic optimised derivative VX-661 [53, 54]. These are the first corrector molecules to be tested in CF patients.

Lumacaftor does not restore the thermostability of Phe508del-NBD1 and, therefore, does not act by stabilising NBD1 [40, 55]. Instead it restores the interaction of the protein with ICL4 and thus stabilises the interaction between NBD1 and MSD. An interpretation supported by the additive effect of lumacaftor with revertant mutations located at the NBD1-MSD2 interface [40] and the correction by the compound of missense mutations primarily destabilising the NBD1-MSD1/2 interface [55]. Recently, it was suggested that lumacaftor could alter the conformation of MSD1 and suppress the folding defects in Phe508del-CFTR through allosteric interdomain communication [56].

The corrector potency of the compound was validated in primary HBE derived from Phe508del homozygotes patients [54]. Lumacaftor promoted conformational maturation of the protein and decreased ER-associated degradation. Residence time in the plasma membrane of Phe508del-CFTR was increased and Phe508del-CFTR gating was significantly improved. It restored up to 15% of CFTR-dependent Cl⁻ transport, a channel activity found in patients with mild disease. This result is further supported by the increase in ASL height. However, it must be pointed out that in comparison with the rescue of channel activity by ivacaftor in Gly551Asp HBE cells, this restoration level is modest [24, 55].

Monotherapy with lumacaftor was evaluated in a 28-day randomised, double-blind, placebo-controlled study in 89 adult patients homozygous for the Phe508del-CFTR mutation. *In vivo* bioactivity studies showed a small, dose-dependent improvement in CFTR function in sweat gland epithelium with a maximal reduction in sweat Cl⁻ by 8 mEq·L^{-1}, but no significant change was observed, in CFTR function either in the nasal epithelium or improvement in lung function [57].

Combination studies

The marginal clinical effects that have been observed argued for the use of a combination of therapies. Ivacaftor, aimed at normalising defective Phe508del-CFTR Cl⁻ channel gating, might potentiate the effect of the lumacaftor corrector, which rescues the traffic of the protein to the membrane. This rationale was based on *in vitro* studies showing that lumacaftor increased Cl⁻ transport in cultured Phe508del-HBE pretreated with lumacaftor by approximately 25% of that measured in non-CF HBE [54].

A complex phase II randomised, multiple-dose, placebo-controlled, double-blind study in Phe508del homozygotes was undertaken to test the ivacaftor/lumacaftor combination therapy (table 4). This resulted in a dose-dependent improvement in FEV1 during the combination therapy. The greatest effect was obtained when 400 mg or 600 mg of lumacaftor was taken once daily in combination with ivacaftor 250 mg every 12 h (increase in absolute percentage predicted by ~9% in comparison to the end of monotherapy), whereas lumacaftor alone had no effect. It was observed that 25% of the patients had improvements >10% and 55% of the patients had improvements >5%. However, when the change was referenced to baseline, FEV1 improvement decreased to around 6%. There was also a significant decrease in sweat chloride, which was maximal with the 400 mg dosage. However, it should be noted that is dosage was low (not more than 10 mmol·L^{-1}) [58].

These findings supported the initiation of two large ongoing confirmatory phase III studies with ivacaftor and lumacaftor in 1000 patients who were homozygous for Phe508del (TRAFFIC and TRANSPORT) to support registration for the combination in patients homozygous for the Ph508del mutation in the second half of 2014 (table 4).

These combination therapies might also be theoretically considered for compound heterozygotes. However, this deserves further investigation because the ivacaftor-lumacaftor therapy did not improve Ph508del heterozygotes [58].

VX-661

VX-661 is an optimised derivative of lumacaftor that is less sensitive to cytochrome P4503A, but provides similar improvements as lumacaftor. Indeed, fundamental studies show that VX-661 improves Cl⁻ transport in cells at 10% of the normal rate, an increase that is further enhanced to 27% by the addition of ivacaftor (Scott Donaldson, University of North Carolina Chapel Hill, NC, USA; personal communication).

A phase II multiple ascending-dose trial demonstrated an increase in FEV1, which was maximum at the combined therapy of 100 mg or 150 mg lumacaftor once daily in combination with ivacaftor 150 mg every 12 h (table 4) [59]. The decrease in the sweat test was found to be best with 100 mg monotherapy. Further development of VX-661 includes a study in combination with ivacaftor in patients carrying the Gly551Asp and Phe508del mutation.

Table 4. Clinical trials of ivacaftor in combination with cystic fibrosis transmembrane conductance regulator correctors in patients with cystic fibrosis

Trial name	Design	Genotype	Inclusion criteria	Treatment dosage/duration	Patients n	ΔFEV_1 % predicted	Secondary outcomes
VX09-809-102	Randomised, placebo-controlled, double-blind, multiple-ascending dose	Phe508del homozygous Phe508del heterozygote	Aged ⩾ 18 years FEV1 ⩾40%	Cohort 1: 200 mg lumacaftor once daily for 14 days followed by 200 mg lumacaftor once daily and 150 mg or 250 mg ivacaftor every 12 h for 7 days Cohort 2: 200 mg or 400 mg or 600 mg lumacaftor once daily for 28 days followed by 200 mg or 400 mg or 600 mg lumacaftor once daily and 250 mg ivacaftor every 12 h for 28 days Cohort 3: 400 mg lumacaftor every 12 h for 28 days followed by both 400 mg of lumacaftor and 250 mg ivacaftor every 12 h for 28 days	109	Cohort 2: Phe508del homozygotes end of combination therapy with the most effective combination, ivacaftor+lumacaftor 600 mg once daily mean absolute change from day 28 baseline was +6.1%[#] and mean relative change is 9.7%[#], mean absolute treatment effect versus placebo was +8.6 (p<0.001) Cohort 3: Phe508del homozygotes end of combination therapy mean absolute change from day 28 baseline 9%[#] Cohort 2: Phe508del heterozygotes 600 mg lumacaftor once daily followed by 600 mg lumacaftor once daily and 250 mg ivacaftor every 12 h the mean absolute change from day 1 was -1.3%[¶]	Maximum sweat chloride decrease was -8.4 mEq·L^{-1}[#] for cohort 2 600 mg lumacaftor once daily monotherapy
VX12-809 103 / TRAFFIC VX12-809-104/ TRANSPORT	Randomised, placebo-controlled, double-blind Open-label rollover study	Phe508del homozygous	Aged ⩾12years FEV1 40-90%	600 mg once daily or 400 mg lumacaftor every 12 h and 250 mg ivacaftor once daily for 24 weeks 600 mg once daily or 400 mg lumacaftor every 12 h and 250 mg ivacaftor once daily for 96 weeks	1000	A relative change from baseline in at 24 weeks of treatment	BMI CFQ-R Number of exacerbations Safety
VX13-809-011	Open-label, single group	Phe508del homozygous	Aged 6–12 years FEV1 70–105%	200 mg lumacaftor and 250 mg ivacaftor, both every12 h for 14 days	NA	Pharmacokinetics parameters	Protein kinase parameters Safety
VX11-661-101	Randomised, placebo-controlled, double-blind multiple escalating-dose, three-part study	Phe508del homozygous	Aged ⩾18 years FEV1 40–90%	10 mg, 30 mg, 100 mg and 150 mg VX-661 once daily with 150 mg ivacaftor every 12 h for 28 days 10 mg or 30 mg or 100 mg or 150 mg VX-661 once daily monotherapy for 28 days	128	End of combination therapy with the most effective combination 100 mg ivacaftor+100 mg VX-661 both once daily, mean relative change from day 28 baseline was +9%[+]	Maximum sweat chloride decrease was -15 mEq·l^{-1} for 100 mg lumacaftor once daily monotherapy

ΔFEV_1: change in forced expiratory volume in 1 s; NA: study not completed; BMI: body mass index; CFQ-R: Cystic Fibrosis Questionnaire Revised. [#]: p<0.05; [¶]: not significant; [+]: p=0.01.

Future prospects and new challenges

Novel correctors and co-therapy development

Future prospects are to develop correctors and potentiators that achieve near wild-type processing and function. One challenge for the discovery of therapies that target the Phe508del mutation is to design molecules based on 3-dimensional (3D) structural information, allowing design of *in silico* structure-targeted molecules to "complement" the defects due to Phe508del [60]. A recent study based on Phe508del-NBD1 interaction-sites mapping enabled the design of specific compounds, docking directly to NBD1, which efficiently corrected the CFTR trafficking defects and partially restored CFTR function [61].

Identifications of correctors that target complementary conformational defects could overcome their individually modest effects. Different pathways can give additive and even synergistic effects that overcome the modest "ceiling" of each individual component and achieve therapeutically useful levels [42, 62–64]. Such dual-corrector regimens may be combined with potentiators. This bifunctional corrector–potentiator strategy is based on *in vitro* data that showed how a combination of two correctors with ivacaftor increased Cl⁻ transport in Phe508del homozygous HBEs, compared with the use of a single corrector in combination with ivacaftor. Altogether, the ideal corrector therapy would be to develop a compound that: 1) rescues folding as much as possible, 2) promotes maximal surface stability of the rescued protein, and 3) maximises the regulated channel activity of that surface targeted protein.

A novel approach is the association of "molecular" correctors with proteostasis regulators that act as "pharmacological chaperones" to modulate the quality control machinery and alter Phe508del-CFTR recognition and processing [65]. As a monotherapy this might not be sufficient, as demonstrated by inconclusive clinical trials, with already clinically available molecules including: 4-phenylbutyrate, an inhibitor of Hsc70 [66]; cucurmin, a sarcoplasmic/ER calcium (SERCA) pump inhibitor [67]; and miglustat (Actelion, Allschwil, Switzerland), an α-glucosidase inhibitor already used in Gaucher lysosomal storage disease [68]. New targets for proteostasis regulation might be down-regulation of Aha1, an Hsp90 co-chaperone ATPase regulator [69], and the reduction of the histone deacetylation level [70]. Interestingly, many histone deacetylases (HDAC) inhibitors are drugs already used in numerous diseases such as resveratrol, valproic acid and suberoylanilide hydroxamic acid (SAHA), a compound already approved by the US FDA for lymphoma.

Novel biomarkers and new trials designs

Electrophysiological measurements on primary HBE cell cultures were helpful in directly linking drug efficacy with the CFTR genotypic background [24, 54].

However, data from the phase IIa clinical trial of monotherapy with lumacaftor suggest that the level of *in vitro* correction in HBEs is below that needed to achieve clinical efficacy. This demonstrates the necessity of novel preclinical surrogate biomarkers to predict clinical efficacy on a patient-specific basis and to help define study populations suitable for pivotal studies [58]. In this perspective, restoration of fluid secretion in patient tissues, such as rectal biopsies or organoids, might be useful as an *ex vivo* assay [71, 72]. There also remains a need to better understand the threshold of CFTR activation, which is required to produce sustained clinical benefit. Moreover, newer pig and ferret animal models have provided the opportunity to investigate at novel biomarkers, such as ASL pH and early bacterial killing, in the neonatal period.

There is also a need for meaningful end-points that are sensitive to compound exposure, since the sweat test is not reliable. LCI and magnetic resonance imaging (MRI) might provide sensitive *in vivo* markers of mucus plugging and volume, and perform as surrogate end-points for the restoration of efficient mucociliary clearance, the main cause of the initial phase of lung damage [73, 74].

Novel clinical trial approaches are needed to detect, as quickly as possible, the efficacy of CFTR modulators selected in preclinical settings. Previous studies with potentiators have demonstrated that results at 8 weeks are comparable with 24 weeks, therefore, enabling the use of shorter trials. Adaptive trial design with unbalanced randomisation and multiple ascending doses could constitute pivotal proof-of-concept studies. Crossover trials, ensuring on- and off-drug periods could address the issues of heterogeneity whilst decreasing the number of patients needed to enrol in a trial. For ultra-rare mutations with residual function, n-of-one design, (to test each person as his/her own control) is being considered since the availability of human derived airway cells for efficacy testing is limited and, therefore, the translation from preclinical models systems to patients is challenging.

Long-term challenges

Before considering prescription of such treatments in newborns with the aim that targeting the basic disease prevents organ damage, long-term efficacy and, above all, long-term tolerances need to be determined. This is clearly one of the most important challenges of mutation-targeted therapeutic strategies. Combined corrector–potentiator therapy could lead to the interaction with drugs binding to other nearby targets. Moreover, as these drugs impact on proteic properties and on cellular pathways necessary for proper folding of many other proteins, they may have nonspecific off-target effects that may only be revealed after long periods of time [75].

Last but not the least, an emerging and unsolved question is how to best administer these therapies. The progression of the disease, in which periodic exacerbations are experienced by patients, may require the administration of corrector and potentiator treatments separately, thereby alternating different correctors and wash-out periods for more efficient rescue. Fortunately, the CF community is in an ideal position for long-term phase IV clinical trial safety monitoring because of the robust worldwide registries permitting the vast majority of patients internationally to be followed closely for years.

Extend CFTR modulators to all the patients

The last challenge announced at the 2013 North American Cystic Fibrosis meeting was to bring CFTR modulators to all CF patients. Ivacaftor monotherapy benefits only 7% of the patients with gating mutations and responsive class 4 mutations. As 90% of the patients worldwide have at least one Phe508del copy, successful corrector and potentiator therapies could potentially cover over 90% of CF patients.

The remaining mutations to be addressed are class 1 and 5 mutations. The former include nonsense mutations generating premature termination codons and frame-shift mutations that lead to truncated and/or nonfunctional proteins [20, 76]. Some nonsense mutations (3%)

may be "suppressed" by drugs interrupting the normal proofreading function or inhibitors of the nonsense-mediated mRNA decay (NMD) pathway [77, 78]. Ataluren (formerly known as PTC124; PTC Therapeutics, South Plainfield, NJ, USA), an orally bioavailable drug with diminished toxicity when compared with gentamycin, seems to be effective in patients not receiving inhaled aminoglycosides [79–81]. However, the interpretation of the data requires caution as patients under placebo experienced a large fall in FEV1. Further studies will clarify its role in the management of class 1 mutations. Most of the class 5 mutations cause alternative splicing and can be improved by ivacaftor and can be targeted more specifically by an antisense oligonucleotide approach [82]. More than 20 years after the gene discovery we can dream of soon being able to offer therapies for the treatment of basic trafficking defects to most of the CF patients.

Conclusion

Amazing progress has been made in the past decade in the discovery of CFTR correctors and potentiators and their rapid advancement in clinical trials. We now know that improving CFTR function at the molecular level is decisive in changing the course of the disease. This new paradigm heralds a new era in CF care, where therapeutic choices will be driven by genetic information. Target-specific drug discovery research is expanding and drugs are moving rapidly into the therapeutic pipeline, providing rationale for a personalised medicine strategy specifically tailored for each CF patient in the very near future [4].

It is exciting that such drug development may also have wider implications for other areas of medicine and for the pharmaceutical industry, both because of contributions to new research and development of paradigms, but also because these advances may be applied to other disorders caused by trafficking-deficient surface proteins. CF is a rare disease, but a multitude of other diseases are caused by protein-folding defects and, therefore, novel therapies for CF hold promise for improved treatments of many other patients, the ultimate goal for medical research.

References

1. O'Sullivan BP, Freedman SD. Cystic fibrosis. *Lancet* 2009; 373: 1891–1904.
2. Riordan JR, Rommens JM, Kerem B, *et al.* Identification of the cystic fibrosis gene: cloning and characterization of complementary DNA. *Science* 1989; 245: 1066–1073.
3. Ramsey BW, Davies J, McElvaney NG, *et al.* A CFTR potentiator in patients with cystic fibrosis and the *G551D* mutation. *N Engl J Med* 2011; 365: 1663–1672.
4. Green DM. Cystic fibrosis: a model for personalized genetic medicine. *Nat Med J* 2013; 74: 486–487.
5. Gadsby DC, Vergani P, Csanády L. The ABC protein turned chloride channel whose failure causes cystic fibrosis. *Nature* 2006; 440: 477–483.
6. Mornon JP, Lehn P, Callebaut I. Molecular models of the open and closed states of the whole human CFTR protein. *Cell Mol Life Sci* 2009; 66: 3469–3486.
7. Billet A, Mornon JP, Jollivet M, *et al.* CFTR: effect of ICL2 and ICL4 amino acids in close spatial proximity on the current properties of the channel. *J Cyst Fibros* 2013; 12: 737–745.
8. Vergani P, Nairn AC, Gadsby DC. On the mechanism of MgATP-dependent gating of CFTR Cl⁻ channels. *J Gen Physiol* 2003; 121: 17–36.
9. Ostedgaard LS, Baldursson O, Vermeer DW, *et al.* A functional R domain from cystic fibrosis transmembrane conductance regulator is predominantly unstructured in solution. *Proc Natl Acad Sci USA* 2000; 97: 5657–5662.
10. Cui L, Aleksandrov L, Chang XB, *et al.* Domain interdependence in the biosynthetic assembly of CFTR. *J Mol Biol* 2007; 365: 981–994.
11. Okiyoneda T, Lukacs G. Fixing cystic fibrosis by correcting CFTR domain assembly. *J Cell Biol* 2012; 199: 199–204.
12. Ward CL, Omura S, Kopito RR. Degradation of CFTR by the ubiquitin-proteasome pathway. *Cell* 1995; 83: 121–127.
13. Farinha C, Matos P, Amaral M. Control of cystic fibrosis transmembrane conductance regulator membrane trafficking: not just from the endoplasmic reticulum to the Golgi. *FEBS J* 2013; 280: 4396–4406.

14. Chong A, Kota P, Dokholyan N, *et al.* Dynamics intrinsic to cystic fibrosis transmembrane conductance regulator function and stability. *Cold Spring Harb Perspect Med* 2013; 3: a009522.

15. Raghuram V, Mak DO, Foskett JK. Regulation of cystic fibrosis transmembrane conductance regulator single-channel gating by bivalent PDZ-domain-mediated interaction. *Proc Natl Acad Sci USA* 2001; 98: 1300–1305.

16. Monterisi S, Favia M, Guerra L, *et al.* CFTR regulation in human airway epithelial cells requires integrity of the actin cytoskeleton and compartmentalized cAMP and PKA activity. *J Cell Sci* 2012; 125: 1106–1117.

17. Okiyoneda T, Barrière H, Bagdány M, *et al.* Peripheral protein quality control removes unfolded CFTR from the plasma membrane. *Science* 2010; 329: 805–810.

18. Okiyoneda T, Lukacs GL. Cell surface dynamics of CFTR: the ins and outs. *Biochim Biophys Acta* 2007; 1773: 476–479.

19. Castellani C, Cuppens H, Macek M Jr, *et al.* Consensus on the use and interpretation of cystic fibrosis mutation analysis in clinical practice. *J Cyst Fibros* 2008; 7: 179–196.

20. Welsh MJ, Smith AE. Molecular mechanisms of CFTR chloride channel dysfunction in cystic fibrosis. *Cell* 1993; 73: 1251–1254.

21. Riordan JR. CFTR function and prospects for therapy. *Annu Rev Biochem* 2008; 77: 701–726.

22. Bompadre SG, Sohma Y, Li M, *et al.* G551D and G1349D, two CF-associated mutations in the signature sequences of CFTR, exhibit distinct gating defects. *J Gen Physiol* 2007; 129: 285–298.

23. Pedemonte N, Sonawane ND, Taddei A, *et al.* Phenylglycine and sulfonamide correctors of defective ΔF508 and G551D cystic fibrosis transmembrane conductance regulator chloride-channel gatings. *Mol Pharmacol* 2005; 67: 1797–1807.

24. Van Goor F, Hadida S, Grootenhuis PD, *et al.* Rescue of CF airway epithelial cell function *in vitro* by a CFTR potentiator, VX-770. *Proc Natl Acad Sci USA* 2009; 106: 18825–18830.

25. Lin W, Jih K, Hwang T. Unraveling the mechanism of VX-770 on WT- and G551D-CFTR. *Pediatr Pulmonol* 2013; 48: Suppl. 36, 210.

26. Accurso FJ, Rowe SM, Clancy JP, *et al.* Effect of VX-770 in persons with cystic fibrosis and the *G551D-CFTR* mutation. *N Engl J Med* 2010; 363: 1991–2003.

27. Davies JC, Wainwright CE, Canny GJ, *et al.* Efficacy and safety of ivacaftor in patients aged 6 to 11 years with cystic fibrosis with a *G551D* mutation. *Am J Respir Crit Care Med* 2013; 187: 1219–1225.

28. Durmowicz AG, Witzmann KA, Rosebraugh CJ, *et al.* Change in sweat chloride as a clinical end point in cystic fibrosis clinical trials: the ivacaftor experience. *Chest* 2013; 143: 14–18.

29. Davies JC, Sheridan H, Lee PJ, *et al.* Lung clearance index to evaluate the effect of ivacaftor on lung function in subjects with CF who have the *G551D-CFTR* mutation and mild lung disease. *Pediatr Pulmonol* 2012; 47: Suppl. 35, 311.

30. McKone EF, Borowitz D, Drevinek P, *et al.* Long-term safety and efficacy of ivacaftor in patients with cystic fibrosis who have the G551D-CFTR mutation: response through 144 weeks of treatment (96 weeks of persist). *Pediatr Pulmonol* 2013; 48: Suppl. 36, 287.

31. Rowe SM, Heltshe SL, Gonska T, *et al.* Results of the G551D observational study: the effect of ivacaftor in G551D patients following FDA approval. *Pediatr Pulmonol* 2013; 48: Suppl. 36, 278.

32. Yu H, Burton B, Huang CH, *et al.* Ivacaftor potentiation of multiple CFTR channels with gating mutations. *J Cyst Fibros* 2012; 1: 237–245.

33. De Boeck K, Paskavitz J, Chen X, *et al.* Ivacaftor, a CFTR potentiator, in cystic fibrosis patients who have a non-*G551D-CFTR* gating mutation: phase 3, part 1 results. *Pediatr Pulmonol* 2013; 48: Suppl. 36, 292.

34. Flume PA, Liou TG, Borowitz DS, *et al.* Ivacaftor in subjects with cystic fibrosis who are homozygous for the F508del-CFTR mutation. *Chest* 2012; 142: 718–724.

35. Van Goor F, Yu H, Burton B, *et al.* Effect of ivacaftor on CFTR forms with missense mutations associated with defects in protein processing or function. *J Cyst Fibros* 2014; 13: 29–36.

36. Sheppard DN, Rich DP, Ostedgaard LS, *et al.* Mutations in CFTR associated with mild-disease-form Cl- channels with altered pore properties. *Nature* 1993; 362: 160–164.

37. Cystic Fibrosis Foundation. Vertex announces results from phase 3 study of ivacaftor in people with the R117H mutation of CF. www.cff.org/aboutCFFfoundation/NewsEvents/12-19-Vertex-Anounces-Results-from-Study-R117H. cfm Date last updated: December 19, 2013. Date last accessed: January 5, 2014.

38. Protasevich I, Yang Z, Wang C, *et al.* Thermal unfolding studies show the disease causing F508del mutation in CFTR thermodynamically destabilizes nucleotide-binding domain 1. *Protein Sci* 2010; 19: 1917–1931.

39. Thibodeau PH, Richardson JM, Wang W, *et al.* The cystic fibrosis-causing mutation ΔF508 affects multiple steps in cystic fibrosis transmembrane conductance regulator biogenesis. *J Biol Chem* 2010; 285: 35825–35835.

40. He L, Aleksandrov LA, Cui L, *et al.* Restoration of domain folding and interdomain assembly by second-site suppressors of the ΔF508 mutation in CFTR. *FASEB J* 2010; 24: 3103–3112.

41. Younger JM, Chen L, Ren HY, *et al.* Sequential quality-control checkpoints triage misfolded cystic fibrosis transmembrane conductance regulator. *Cell* 2006; 126: 571–578.

42. Farinha CM, King-Underwood J, Sousa M, *et al.* Revertants, low temperature, and correctors reveal the mechanism of F508del-CFTR rescue by VX-809 and suggest multiple agents for full correction. *Chem Biol* 2013; 20: 943–955.

43. El Khouri E, Le Pavec G, Toledano MB, *et al.* RNF185 is a novel E3 ligase of endoplasmic reticulum-associated degradation (ERAD) that targets cystic fibrosis transmembrane conductance regulator (CFTR). *J Biol Chem* 2013; 288: 31177–31191.

44. Ahner A, Gong X, Schmidt BZ, *et al.* Small heat shock proteins target mutant cystic fibrosis transmembrane conductance regulator for degradation *via* a small ubiquitin-like modifier-dependent pathway. *Mol Biol Cell* 2013; 24: 74–84.

45. Kim Chiaw P, Huan LJ, Gagnon S, *et al.* Functional rescue of DeltaF508-CFTR by peptides designed to mimic sorting motifs. *Chem Biol* 2009; 16: 520–530.

46. Colas J, Faure G, Saussereau E, *et al.* Disruption of cytokeratin-8 interaction with F508del-CFTR corrects its functional defect. *Hum Mol Genet* 2012; 21: 623–634.

47. Sharma M, Pampinella F, Nemes C, *et al.* Misfolding diverts CFTR from recycling to degradation: quality control at early endosomes. *J Cell Biol* 2004; 164: 923–933.

48. Moniz S, Sousa M, Moraes BJ, *et al.* HGF stimulation of Rac1 signaling enhances pharmacological correction of the most prevalent cystic fibrosis mutant F508del-CFTR. *ACS Chem Biol* 2013; 8: 432–442.

49. Dalemans W, Barbry P, Champigny G, *et al.* Altered chloride ion channel kinetics associated with the ΔF508 cystic fibrosis mutation. *Nature* 1991; 354: 526–528.

50. Lukacs GL, Verkman AS. CFTR: folding, misfolding and correcting the ΔF508 conformational defect. *Trends Mol Med* 2012; 18: 81–91.

51. Molinski S, Eckford PD, Pasyk S, *et al.* Functional rescue of F508del-CFTR using small molecule correctors. *Front Pharmacol* 2012; 3: 160.

52. Pedemonte N, Lukacs GL, Du K, *et al.* Small-molecule correctors of defective ΔF508-CFTR cellular processing identified by high-throughput screening. *J Clin Invest* 2005; 115: 2564–2571.

53. Van Goor F, Straley KS, Cao D, *et al.* Rescue of ΔF508-CFTR trafficking and gating in human cystic fibrosis airway primary cultures by small molecules. *Am J Physiol Lung Cell Mol Physiol* 2006; 290: L1117–L1130.

54. Van Goor F, Hadida S, Grootenhuis PD, *et al.* Correction of the F508del-CFTR protein processing defect *in vitro* by the investigational drug VX-809. *Proc Natl Acad Sci USA* 2011; 108: 18843–18848.

55. He L, Kota P, Aleksandrov AA, *et al.* Correctors of ΔF508 CFTR restore global conformational maturation without thermally stabilizing the mutant protein. *FASEB J* 2013; 27: 536–545.

56. Ren HY, Grove DE, De La Rosa O, *et al.* VX-809 corrects folding defects in cystic fibrosis transmembrane conductance regulator protein through action on membrane-spanning domain 1. *Mol Biol Cell* 2013; 24: 3016–3024.

57. Clancy JP, Rowe SM, Accurso FJ, *et al.* Results of a phase IIa study of VX-809, an investigational CFTR corrector compound, in subjects with cystic fibrosis homozygous for the F508del-CFTR mutation. *Thorax* 2012; 67: 12–18.

58. Boyle MP, Bell SC, Konstan MW, *et al.* The investigational CFTR corrector, VX-809 (lumacaftor) co-administered with the oral potentiator ivacaftor improved CFTR and lung function in *F508del* homozygous patients: phase II study results. *Pediatr Pulmonol* 2012; 47: Suppl. 35, 315.

59. Clancy JP. Bridging novel CFTR therapies to CF patients. *Pediatr Pulmonol* 2013; 48: Suppl. 36, 175.

60. Kalid O, Mense M, Fischman S, *et al.* Small molecule correctors of F508del-CFTR discovered by structure-based virtual screening. *J Comput Aided Mol Des* 2010; 24: 971–991.

61. Odolczyk N, Fritsch J, Norez C, *et al.* Discovery of novel potent ΔF508-CFTR correctors that target the nucleotide binding domain. *EMBO Mol Med* 2013; 5: 1484–1501.

62. Rabeh WM, Bossard F, Xu H, *et al.* Correction of both NBD1 energetics and domain interface is required to restore ΔF508 CFTR folding and function. *Cell* 2012; 148: 150–163.

63. Mendoza JL, Schmidt A, Li Q, *et al.* Requirements for efficient correction of ΔF508 CFTR revealed by analyses of evolved sequences. *Cell* 2012; 148: 164–174.

64. Lin S, Sui J, Cotard S, *et al.* Identification of synergistic combinations of F508del cystic fibrosis transmembrane conductance regulator (CFTR) modulators. *Assay Drug Dev Technol* 2010; 8: 669–684.

65. Balch WE, Roth DM, Hutt DM. Emergent properties of proteostasis in managing cystic fibrosis. *Cold Spring Harb Perspect Biol* 2011; 3: a004499.

66. Rubenstein RC, Egan ME, Zeitlin PL. *In vitro* pharmacologic restoration of CFTR-mediated chloride transport with sodium 4-phenylbutyrate in cystic fibrosis epithelial cells containing delta F508-CFTR. *J Clin Invest* 1997; 100: 2457–2465.

67. Egan ME, Pearson M, Weiner SA, *et al.* Curcumin, a major constituent of turmeric, corrects cystic fibrosis defects. *Science* 2004; 304: 600–602.

68. Leonard A, Lebecque P, Dingemanse J, *et al.* A randomized placebo-controlled trial of miglustat in cystic fibrosis based on nasal potential difference. *J Cyst Fibros* 2012; 11: 231–236.

69. Wang X, Venable J, LaPointe P, *et al.* Hsp90 cochaperone Aha1 downregulation rescues misfolding of CFTR in cystic fibrosis. *Cell* 2006; 127: 803–815.

70. Hutt DM, Herman D, Rodrigues AP, *et al.* Reduced histone deacetylase 7 activity restores function to misfolded CFTR in cystic fibrosis. *Nat Chem Biol* 2010; 6: 25–33.

71. Dekkers JF, Wiegerinck CL, de Jonge HR, *et al.* A functional CFTR assay using primary cystic fibrosis intestinal organoids. *Nat Med* 2013; 19: 939–945.

72. Clancy JP, Szczesniak RD, Ashlock MA, *et al.* Multicenter intestinal current measurements in rectal biopsies from CF and non-CF subjects to monitor CFTR function. *PLoS One* 2013; 8: e73905.

73. Dasenbrook EC, Lu L, Donnola S, *et al.* Normalized T1 magnetic resonance imaging for assessment of regional lung function in adult cystic fibrosis patients – a cross-sectional study. *PLoS One* 2013; 8: e73286.

74. Kent L, Reix P, Innes JA, *et al.* Lung clearance index: evidence for use in clinical trials in cystic fibrosis. *J Cyst Fibros* 2014; 13: 123–138.

75. Loo TW, Bartlett MC, Clarke DM. Correctors enhance maturation of ΔF508 CFTR by promoting interactions between the two halves of the molecule. *Biochemistry* 2009; 48: 9882–9890.

76. Linde L, Boelz S, Nissim-Rafinia M, *et al.* Nonsense-mediated mRNA decay affects nonsense transcript levels and governs response of cystic fibrosis patients to gentamicin. *J Clin Invest* 2007; 117: 683–692.

77. Wilschanski M, Yahav Y, Blau H, *et al.* Gentamicin-induced correction of CFTR function in patients with cystic fibrosis and CFTR stop mutations. *N Engl J Med* 2003; 349: 1433–1441.

78. Sermet-Gaudelus I, Renouil M, Fajac A, *et al. In vitro* prediction of stop-codon suppression by intravenous gentamicin in patients with cystic fibrosis: a pilot study. *BMC Med* 2007; 5: 5.

79. Kerem E, Hirawat S, Armoni S, *et al.* Effectiveness of PTC124 treatment of cystic fibrosis caused by nonsense mutations: a prospective phase II trial. *Lancet* 2008; 372: 719–727.

80. Sermet-Gaudelus I, Boeck KD, Casimir GJ, *et al.* Ataluren (PTC124) induces cystic fibrosis transmembrane conductance regulator protein expression and activity in children with nonsense mutation cystic fibrosis. *Am J Respir Crit Care Med* 2010; 182: 1262–1272.

81. Rowe SM, Sermet-Gaudelus I, Konstan MW, *et al.* Results of the phase 3 study of Ataluren in nonsense mutation cystic fibrosis (NMCF). *Pediatr Pulmonol* 2012; 47: Suppl. 35, 290.

82. Irony TS, Wilton S, Kerem B. Restoration of the CFTR function by antisense oligonucleotide splicing modulation. *Pediatr Pulmonol* 2013; 48: Suppl. 36, 265–265.

Acknowledgements: We would like to acknowledge and thank Jean Pierre Laigneau (INSERM, IFR94, Université Paris V, Paris, France) for the illustrations. We would also like to thank Charlotte Sumida for checking the manuscript.

Disclosures: B.W. Ramsey reports outside of the submitted work that the Seattle Children's Hospital (Seattle, WA, USA) has contracts with the following companies: 12th Man Technologies, Achaogen, Apartia, Bayer HealthCare AG, Bristol-Myers Squibb, Celtaxsys, Cornerstone Therapeutics, CSL Behring LLC, Eli Lilly, Genentech, Gilead Sciences Inc., GlaxoSmithKline, Hall Bioscience, Insmed Inc., KaloBios, Rempex Pharmaceuticals Inc., N30 Pharmaceuticals LLC, Nikan Pharmaceuticals, Nordmark, Novartis Pharmaceuticals Corp, Pharmagenesis, Pulmatrix, Pulmoflow, Savara Pharmaceuticals, Talecris, Vectura Ltd, Vertex Pharmaceuticals Inc., B.W. Ramsey also reports outside of the submitted work receiving grants from the Cystic Fibrosis Foundation and the National Institutes of Health.

Chapter 11

New horizons for cystic fibrosis gene and cell therapy

Uta Griesenbach, Rosanna F. Featherstone and Eric W.F.W. Alton

In this chapter, we will review key studies that have contributed to our current know-how on the feasibility of gene therapy in cystic fibrosis (CF). We have learnt that the lung is a more difficult target organ than originally anticipated and have gathered significant information on the strengths and weaknesses of the different gene transfer vectors in pre-clinical and clinical research. The important question of whether nonviral gene transfer can improve CF lung disease has not yet been answered, but a large multidose clinical trial is currently ongoing to address this question. Cell therapy, defined as the administration of stem/progenitor cells to correct cystic fibrosis transmembrane conductance regulator (CFTR) dysfunction in the lung, is a comparatively new concept and may be an alternative or an addition to gene therapy. Key studies related to cell therapy and bioengineering will also be discussed.

The first gene therapy-based drug, an adeno-associated virus (AAV) carrying the lipoprotein lipase gene, also known as Glybera, obtained European marketing authorisation for the treatment of patients with severe lipoprotein lipase deficiency in 2012. Through advances in recombinant DNA technology, gene therapy is being developed for a large number of inherited and acquired diseases. Although cystic fibrosis (CF) gene therapy has been at the forefront of gene therapy research since cloning of the cystic fibrosis transmembrane conductance regulator (*CFTR*) gene in 1989 (see table 1 for key publications), other disease targets, including immune deficiencies, degenerative eye disorders and haemophilia [8], have made advances with respect to demonstrating some degree of clinical efficacy [9]. This is in part due to the lung being a more difficult-to-treat target organ than originally anticipated and due to conclusive phase IIB clinical trials being expensive and difficult to perform because of the large surface area to be treated. This realisation has, over the last 10 years, led to a waning enthusiasm for CF gene therapy, which is currently only being performed by a small number of committed mainly academic groups.

In contrast to many other strategies that aim to treat the downstream consequences of mutated CFTR, such as rehydration of the airways and treatment of infection and inflammation, gene replacement has the potential to tackle the disease at its origin and, if successful, may allow for amelioration of existing disease or, if given early enough, prevent

Dept of Gene Therapy, National Heart and Lung Institute, Imperial College London, London, UK, and the UK Cystic Fibrosis Gene Therapy Consortium.

Correspondence: Uta Griesenbach, Dept of Gene Therapy, Imperial College London, Manresa Road, London, SW3 6LR, UK. E-mail: u.griesenbach@imperial.ac.uk

Copyright ERS 2014. Print ISBN: 978-1-84984-050-7. Online ISBN: 978-1-84984-051-4. Print ISSN: 2312-508X. Online ISSN: 2312-5098.

Table 1. Key milestone studies since cloning of the cystic fibrosis transmembrane conductance regulator (*CFTR*) in 1989

Time after cloning years	First author [ref.]	Summary
1	DRUMM [1]	Established proof-of-principle that retrovirus-mediated gene transfer of *CFTR* can correct cAMP-mediated chloride conductance *in vitro*
3	ROSENFELD [2]	Provided evidence of successful *CFTR* mRNA and protein expression after adenovirus-mediated *CFTR* cDNA transfer into cotton rats
4	HYDE [3]	Showed that nonviral *CFTR* cDNA transfer was able to partially correct the chloride transport in tracheal epithelium of CF knockout mice
4	ZABNER [4]	First, albeit small and not placebo-controlled, CF gene therapy trial in three patients: a first-generation adenoviral vector carrying the *CFTR* cDNA was administered to the nasal epithelium and shown to partially restore cAMP-mediated chloride transport
5	CRYSTAL [5]	First phase I dose-escalation CF gene therapy study: first and foremost a safety study and showed transient inflammatory responses at the highest dose (5×10^9 plaque-forming units/patient)
6	CAPLEN [6]	Provided first evidence that a nonviral gene transfer agent (DC-Chol:DOPE) complexed with *CFTR* cDNA could partially correct cAMP-mediated chloride transport in nasal epithelium of CF patients
10	ALTON [7]	Demonstrated that a nonviral gene transfer agent (GL67A) complexed with *CFTR* cDNA could partially correct cAMP-mediated chloride transport in the lungs of CF patients; this study remains the only study assessing CFTR function after gene transfer into lower airways

CF: cystic fibrosis.

the development of lung disease. In addition, gene therapy may help to reduce the overall treatment burden and improve compliance, particularly if infrequent treatments will suffice. Proof-of-concept for targeting the genetic defect has recently been established. Ivacaftor (under the brand name Kalydeco; manufactured by Vertex Pharmaceuticals Inc., Boston, MA, USA) is a CFTR potentiator and improves lung function in patients with certain types of CFTR mutations (*i.e.* class 3 mutations such as Gly551Asp) [10]. However, these mutations are only found in approximately 4% of CF patients. CFTR "corrector" molecules (such as lumacaftor, formerly known as VX-809, manufactured by Vertex Pharmaceuticals Inc., Boston, MA, USA), which aim to refold the common class 2 CFTR mutations, have been unable to demonstrate clinical efficacy to date, confirming the broad consensus that efficiently promoting correct folding through small molecules is intrinsically more challenging than correcting class 3 mutations [11]. Importantly, gene therapy is independent of CFTR mutational class and is thus likely to be applicable for treating lung disease in all CF individuals, regardless of the mutation class.

Although a comparatively large number of clinical trials have been performed over the last 20 years to establish proof-of-concept for gene transfer into airway epithelium, these were generally not designed to answer the question of whether gene therapy can help CF patients by improving lung disease severity, and the results of an ongoing trial designed to assess clinical efficacy (described in this chapter) are eagerly awaited.

The repopulation of airway epithelium following administration of gene-corrected stem/ progenitor cells may be an alternative to classical gene therapy or may be used in combination with gene therapy. Systemic and topical cell administration routes have been assessed, albeit currently with limited success. Most recently, significant advances in lung and airway *ex vivo* bioengineering have been made, which may in the future benefit CF patients.

The lung is a challenging target organ

The lung has evolved to fight invasion of foreign particles, and gene transfer agents (GTAs) have to overcome a number of extra- and intracellular barriers to achieve their

Table 2. Extra- and intracellular barriers to airway gene transfer agents (GTAs)

Barrier	Explanation	[Ref.]
Extracellular		
Mucin secretions	• Component of natural host defence, but further enhanced by infection and inflammation (cystic fibrosis sputum) • Mucus and sputum prevent migration of GTAs to the cell surface • Does not affect all GTAs to the same degree	[12, 13]
Cilia	• Component of natural host defence but mucociliary clearance has an impact on GTAs	[14, 15]
Immune surveillance	• Pre-existing neutralising antibodies may affect GTAs • Induced adaptive immune responses are a particular problem for viral GTAs and can prevent efficacy on repeat administration	[16–18]
Cell entry	• Airway epithelial cells have comparatively low endocytosis rates at the apical membrane • Viral vectors generally require receptors, which are not always present on the apical membrane of airway epithelial cells • Receptor availability is a key determinant for efficient gene expression	[13, 19, 20]
Intracellular		
Cytoplasmic migration	• Generally more efficient for viral than for nonviral GTAs • In contrast to nonviral GTAs, viral vectors have evolved specific mechanisms for efficient cytoplasmic transport • Different viruses have evolved different strategies	[21–24]
Nuclear entry	• Generally more efficient for viral than for nonviral GTAs • Different viruses have evolved different strategies • Some viruses remain in the cytoplasm	[21–24]

objective (table 2) [25]. In general, viral vectors are more efficient than nonviral GTAs, which is in part related to their relative strengths and weaknesses in overcoming these barriers. However, sputum obstruction, particularly in patients with more advanced disease, will impair both viral and nonviral GTAs and gene therapy will, therefore, be most efficient in young CF patients before disease has established (preventative therapy). However, this patient group is not suitable for early-phase clinical trials and careful selection of patient populations to establish proof-of-principle is a critical aspect of the trial design.

Although it is difficult to identify the most important extra- or intracellular barrier, it has become clear that induction of adaptive immune responses after administration of most viral vectors prevents efficient repeated administration and therefore renders these vectors ineffective for CF gene therapy. However, induction of immune responses is vector specific and will be discussed in the relevant sections of this chapter. Importantly, nonviral vectors are less likely to induce immune responses and consistent efficacy after repeat administration has been demonstrated in pre-clinical [17] and clinical studies [18].

To date, we do not know if the levels of lung gene transfer that can be achieved are sufficient for generating clinical benefit (i.e. improvement in lung function). However, a body of evidence suggests that even modest amounts of CFTR expression may suffice to improve lung disease. First, CF individuals with certain "mild" mutations that retain as little as 10% of normal CFTR expression per cell do not generally suffer from lung disease, although other organs such as the vas deferens may be affected [26]. Secondly, in vitro cell mixing experiments suggest that 6–10% of non-CF cells intermixed with CF cells restore CFTR-mediated chloride secretion to non-CF levels [27, 28]. However, it is important to note that CFTR has to be expressed in at least 25% of cells grown in monolayer in vitro to restore mucus transport [29] and that correction of sodium hyperabsorption requires substantially higher numbers (close to 100%) of non-CF cells [28, 30]. Thirdly, adenovirus-mediated CFTR gene transfer into 20–30% of sinus epithelial cells extracted from CF knockout pigs corrects chloride transport to 50% of non-CF levels. Even low levels of gene transfer (~7%) produced detectable levels of correction (~6% of non-CF) [31, 32].

These considerations led us to conclude that there may be a nonlinear relationship between the level of CFTR function and disease severity and to infer that low-level CFTR expression may be sufficient to significantly improve lung disease severity [33]. This also argues that clinical trials using nonviral GTAs (which are generally less efficient than viral vectors) are well worth pursuing considering the potential advantages of these formulations, including the reduced risk of inducing immune responses, easier scale-up of manufacturing and potentially better safely profiles.

In addition, it is also important to consider several additional questions. 1) Which cells have to express functional CFTR? CFTR is expressed in various lung regions and cell types [34–38]. In our view, airway epithelial cells are currently the most likely target cell for gene replacement. 2) Is a low level ($\leqslant$10%) of CFTR required in all cells (as in CF subjects with milder mutations), or are normal levels (100%) of CFTR expression required in ~10% of cells (maybe the more likely scenario after gene therapy)? 3) Does the correction of chloride transport translate into correction of fluid transport, as well as improvements in mucus obstruction, inflammation and bronchiectasis? 4) Does the "low volume" hypothesis underpin disease aetiology or are intrinsic defects, for example in the immune system [39, 40] or airway pH [41], also important factors? 5) Is delivery to a sufficient area of the bronchial/ bronchiolar tree feasible, considering that most patients suffer from air trapping from an early age?

Gene therapy

Viral vectors

Adenoviral vectors

Adenoviral vectors were the first viral vectors to be assessed for CF gene therapy. Various viral genes have been deleted over the years, culminating in the generation of "gut-less" viruses that are completely devoid of viral genome [42]. Adenoviral vectors do not integrate into the host genome, but remain episomal. Due to a natural tropism for the target organ, adenoviral vectors were an obvious first choice for CF gene therapy and the first ever CF gene therapy trial was carried out with an adenoviral vector just a couple of years after cloning the *CFTR* gene in 1989. ZABNER *et al.* [4] administered adenovirus-CFTR to the nasal epithelium of three CF patients. The nasal epithelium was initially chosen as a target organ, because the cell composition is similar to the lower airways and efficacy end-points were easier to assess [43]. Due to the low number of subjects (n=3) treated by ZABNER *et al.* [4], conclusions about efficacy were difficult to draw, but the study opened the door for the additional nine adenovirus CF gene therapy trials that were carried out in the nose and lungs of CF patients between 1993 and 2001 [44].

Taken together, these trials showed the following: 1) low-level gene transfer can be achieved in some subjects, based on detection of vector-specific *CFTR* mRNA and protein; 2) partial correction of the CF ion transport defect, specifically the chloride transport, can be achieved in the nasal epithelium of some patients; 3) adenovirus administration can cause side-effects (lung inflammation), but this effect is dose-dependent; 4) efficacy in general was lower than originally predicted by the pre-clinical models, due to the absence of the relevant receptor (coxsackie adenovirus receptor (CAR)) on the apical surface of human airway epithelial cells; 5) administration of adenoviral vectors induced humoral and cellular immune responses; and 6) these immune responses affect efficacy after re-administration of the virus.

In parallel to these clinical adenovirus studies, a large body of pre-clinical work has been conducted, in an attempt to overcome the shortcomings of the vector for CF gene therapy [45]. However, in our view, to date there is no strong evidence that adenoviral vectors will be useful for CF gene therapy, although the vector has been very useful for pre-clinical proof-of-concept studies. For example, POTASH *et al.* [31] have recently shown that *ex vivo* adenovirus-mediated CFTR transfer can partially correct the chloride transport defect in the sinus epithelium of CF pigs. In addition, CAO *et al.* [46] have shown that helper-dependent adenoviral vectors efficiently transduce pig airway epithelium and submucosal glands, which express high levels of CFTR and may, therefore, be useful to address basic pathophysiology questions in the CF pig model.

Adeno-associated viral vectors

Adenoviral vectors were superceded by AAV vectors, which are depleted of viral genes and remain largely episomal once inside the nucleus [47–49]. A large number of serotypes have now been identified [50], and capsids from serotypes 1, 5, 6, 8 and 9 appear to be most efficient in transducing airway epithelial cells [51]. What is now termed AAV serotype 2 (AAV2) was the first serotype, and this is currently the most extensively studied. Between 1999 and 2007, six clinical studies were carried out, mainly led by Targeted Genetics, Corp. (Seattle, WA, USA), in which the vector was administered to the nose, sinuses and lungs of CF patients [52]. Initial single-dose phase I trials demonstrated that virus administration to the CF airways was safe, but provided little opportunity to assess efficiency of vector-specific CFTR expression. A large repeat-administration study (100 subjects), sufficiently powered to detect significant changes in lung function, did not meet its primary efficacy end-point (improvement in lung function) [53].

There may be several reasons for these disappointing results: 1) AAV2 is too inefficient in transducing airway epithelial cells *via* the apical membrane; 2) the LTR (long terminal repeat) promoter, which was used to drive expression of the 4.7-kb *CFTR* cDNA due to the limited packaging capacity (about 5 kb) of the virus, is too weak; and/or 3) repeat administration of AAV2 to the lung is not possible due to the development of an anti-viral immune response. No additional AAV lung trials have been performed since 2005, but research aimed at addressing and improving these potential limitations of AAV has been actively pursued (extensively reviewed in [45]) and some progress, particularly related to improving transduction efficiency, has been made.

However, on balance we would argue that AAV vectors may face problems with repeat administrations similar to adenovirus vectors, but a clinical trial assessing repeat administration of an AAV vector, proven to transduce the human airway epithelium efficiently, is the only way to address this question reliably. Interestingly, LIU *et al.* [54] have shown that AAV vectors may be able to transduce progenitor cells in the mouse lung, which, if efficient, may help to overcome the repeat administration problem. Recently, FAUST *et al.* [55] have shown that depletion of CpG dinucleotides from the AAV vector (a strategy that reduced inflammation and prolonged gene expression of nonviral vectors) reduced adaptive immune responses and inflammation after intramuscular injection of AAV vectors. It remains to be seen if CpG-depleted AAV vectors offer any advantages for lung applications. Despite the assumption that most AAV vectors remain episomal upon nuclear entry, KAEPPEL *et al.* [56] assessed the integration site profile in patients treated intramuscularly with Glybera (an AAV vector carrying lipoprotein lipase) and showed that integration occurred but was random and, in contrast to gamma-oncoretroviral vectors, which have been associated with cases of insertional mutagenesis, not associated with preferential integration close to transcription start sites. KAEPPEL *et al.* [56] also noticed significant integration into mitochondrial genomes, which was surprising and raises further questions related to AAV biology.

Other viral vectors for CF gene therapy
In addition to adenovirus and AAV, various cytoplasmic RNA viruses have been validated for airway gene transfer. The murine parainfluenza virus type 1 (or Sendai virus (SeV)), the human respiratory syncytial virus (RSV) and the human parainfluenza virus (PIV) have all been shown to transfect airway epithelial cells efficiently *via* the apical membrane [20, 57] using sialic acid and cholesterol, which are abundantly expressed on the apical surface of airway epithelial cells. These viruses have a negative strand RNA genome and, in contrast to other viral vectors, replicate in the cytoplasm. Only SeV has been assessed in animal models *in vivo*, and is arguably the most efficient vector for transducing airway epithelial cells, but repeated administration was not feasible (extensively reviewed in [45]); therefore, the vector did not progress further.

Promising lentiviral vectors

Recently, lentiviral vectors, which integrate into the host genome, have gained interest and in our view, for reasons described hereafter, hold promise for CF gene therapy. Recombinant human immunodeficiency virus (HIV) is most commonly used, but in the context of lung gene transfer, simian (SIV) [58, 59], feline (FIV) [60] and equine (EIAV) [61] immunodeficiency viruses have also been studied. Lentiviral vectors are commonly pseudotyped with an envelope glycoprotein from the vesicular stomatitis virus G (VSV-G), allowing for a broad tissue tropism. However, VSV-G-pseudotyped vectors only poorly transduce airway epithelial cells and require the addition of tight junction openers such as lysophosphatidylcholine (LPC) to allow virus entry into airway cells [62, 63]. Several groups have replaced VSV-G with other envelope proteins to improve airway transduction [59–61, 64, 65]. We, for example, used the Sendai virus-derived F (fusion) and HN (haemagglutinin-neuraminidase) envelope proteins (fig. 1) and achieved efficient and persistent gene expression in mice (life-long expression after a single dose) and relevant human airway models [59] (fig. 2). STOCKER et al. [67] have demonstrated that lentivirus-mediated CFTR expression in the nasal epithelium of CF knockout mice allows partial correction of the chloride transport to persist for at least 12 months. In preparation for experiments in CF knockout pigs, SINN et al. [68] have recently shown that FIV pseudotyped with the baculovirus GP64 envelope protein can transduce porcine airways. In a small pilot study, FARROW et al. [69] showed that VSV-G-pseudotyped lentivirus transduced airway and alveolar epithelium in a nonhuman primate model (marmoset), although this required pre-treatment with the tight junction opener LPC. In contrast to SeV, adenovirus and AAV vectors, we and others have shown that lentiviral vectors can be repeatedly administered to murine airways [59, 60], which is a major requirement for the treatment of chronic diseases such as CF, although it remains to be assessed if repeat administration is feasible in humans.

Before progression into clinical trials, several major points have to be addressed. The first is the safety of genomic intergration of lentiviral vectors in the lung. Encouragingly, we have not observed any side-effects in a 2-year mouse study [70]. The second is the scale-up of vector production, because comparatively high virus titres will be required to treat the lung, due to its large surface area. Finally, the risk/benefit ratio needs to be carefully discussed and agreed, before regulatory approval for progression into clinical trials can be obtained.

Nonviral vectors

Nonviral gene transfer formulations have two components: 1) the nucleic acid, *i.e.* the therapeutic cDNA and appropriate regulatory elements; and 2) a carrier molecule that binds to the DNA.

A large number of carrier molecules have been developed that broadly fall into either cationic lipids or cationic polymers. Both classes of molecules bind to negatively charged plasmid DNA through charge interaction and either encapsulate or condense the DNA to generate lipoplexes and polyplexes. The mechanism of nonviral gene transfer is poorly understood, but it is thought that lipoplexes and polyplexes bind to the cell membrane, are endocytosed and subsequently escape from endosomes by inducing rupture of the endosomal membrane [71]. Nonviral vectors are generally less efficient than viral GTAs. This is due to a lack of specific components that would help with cell entry, endosomal escape, movement through the cytoplasm and nuclear uptake, all stages for which viruses have evolved efficient strategies

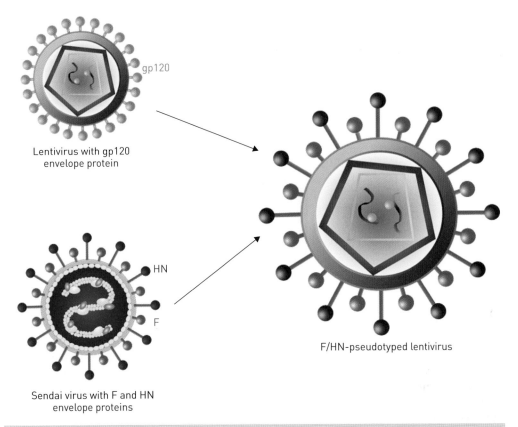

Figure 1. Generation of F/HN-pseudotyped lentiviral vector. Sophisticated molecular techniques enable the replacement of the gp120 envelope glycoprotein, which supports lentivirus entry into T-cells but is not suitable for entry into airway epithelial cells, with the F (fusion) and HN (haemagglutinin-neuraminidase) proteins from the Sendai virus, which support efficient entry into airway epithelial cells. This process is called pseudotyping and leads to the generation of a chimeric pseudotyped F/HN lentiviral vector. Figure courtesy of A.C. Boyd, UK CF Gene Therapy Consortium.

and specific proteins [72]. The simpler composition of nonviral vectors, however, may be an advantage. If free of "nonhuman" protein components, successful re-administration may be easier to achieve than with viral vectors (although a case-by-case assessment will be necessary to determine efficacy on repeat administration). Importantly, proof-of-principle for repeat administration of liposome-based gene transfer in human airways has been established in clinical studies [18]. A flurry of activity in the 1990s led to the development of a myriad of nonviral GTAs [73]. However, it is our impression that progress in developing novel formulations for airway gene therapy over the last 5–10 years has been modest (see [72] for a more comprehensive review).

In addition to the nonviral carrier, the nucleic acid component is a key factor in nonviral gene transfer. Most pre-clinical and clinical studies have relied on the use of viral promoters such as the cytomegalovirus (CMV) promoter/enhancer to regulate gene expression. These generally lead to comparatively high-level gene expression at early time-points (1–2 days), but expression is very transient [7, 74]. Loss of transgene expression cannot simply be explained through plasmid degradation [75]. PRINGLE et al. [75] assessed whether plasmid silencing may be due to methylation of the DNA, which can cause silencing of integrating

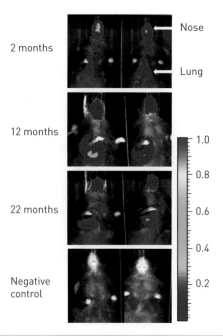

Figure 2. F/HN-SIV transduction leads to persistent gene expression in mouse airways. Mice were transduced with F/HN-SIV-Lux (simian immunodeficiency virus pseudotyped with F (fusion) and HN (haemagglutinin-neuraminidase) proteins from the Sendai virus, and carrying the bacterial luciferase (lux) reporter system) (5×10^8 transduction units per mouse) by nasal sniffing, or received PBS (negative controls). Luciferase expression was visualised using bioluminescence *in vivo* imaging, 2–22 months after transduction. Colour scale indicates photon emission in $\times 10^6$ photons·s^{-1}·cm^{-2}. Reproduced and modified from [66] with permission from the publisher.

viral vectors [76], but did not find any evidence for *de novo* methylation after nonviral gene transfer. It has been shown, however, that vector-induced secretion of inflammatory cytokines silences the CMV promoter/enhancer [77]. Importantly, problems related to transient lung expression after nonviral gene transfer have been overcome by the use of endogenous mammalian promoters [78, 79] or, more recently, through the use of viral and mammalian hybrid regulatory elements [74]. This study led to selection of a hybrid promoter consisting of a human CMV enhancer and the human elongation factor 1α promoter (the resulting promoter/enhancer being termed hCEFI). This chimeric promoter/enhancer supports prolonged gene expression in mice (lasting for months) [74] and was selected for our ongoing clinical trial programme (described later in this chapter). Unmethylated nucleotides (CpG motifs) in the plasmid can activate the innate immune system *via* Toll-like receptor (TLR)9 and lead to production of pro-inflammatory cytokines. CpG-free plasmids not only reduce inflammation, but also lead to longer lasting gene expression when administered to the mouse lung [74].

It is undisputed that gene transfer into dividing cells is significantly more efficient than into fully differentiated, nondividing cells. It has, therefore, been postulated that the nuclear membrane is a significant barrier to nonviral gene transfer. A more detailed understanding of how plasmid DNA moves from the cytoplasm into the nucleus of nondividing cells may help to improve gene transfer into differentiated airway epithelium. It has been hypothesised that DNA-binding proteins, destined to move into the nucleus, bind to plasmid DNA in the cytoplasm and support nuclear uptake of the DNA using the nuclear import machinery [80, 81].

However, these experiments were carried out in *in vitro* models and it is currently unclear if and how these findings translate into airways *in vivo*.

Nine clinical trials have evaluated nonviral gene transfer to nasal or lung epithelium [44]. These studies were largely single-dose phase I safety studies, but in most cases included some molecular or bioelectrical efficacy end-points: detection of vector-specific *CFTR* mRNA or potential difference measurements to assess correction of the ion transport defect. However, detection of vector-specific mRNA proved difficult in most studies. This may be due to patchy gene transfer combined with comparatively small numbers of cells from a limited region being collected, although in some studies technical difficulties prevented extraction of mRNA. Interestingly, the majority of the studies have shown partial correction of the chloride transport defect in nasal epithelium. In addition, we were able to demonstrate approximately 25% correction of the chloride transport defect in the lung [7]. These findings provide proof-of-principle for nonviral *CFTR* gene transfer to the airways of CF patients and may argue that potential difference measurements may be more sensitive than RT-PCR.

More recently, several publications have highlighted the potential for using chemically modified mRNA as a therapeutic agent. KORMANN *et al.* [82] provided proof-of-concept that intratracheal administration of surfactant protein (SP)-B mRNA twice weekly restored expression of wild-type SP-B protein and survival in a SP-B knockout mouse. In addition, MAYS *et al.* [83] showed that administration of Foxp3 mRNA, which encodes a regulatory T-cell transcription factor, ameliorated asthma symptoms in mouse models. Interestingly, the treatment was effective when administered either before or after the allergen challenge, implying that this strategy may have preventative, as well as therapeutic benefit. It is conceivable that transfer of *CFTR* mRNA may also lead to production of CFTR protein. However, the size of the coding region (~4.7 kb), as well as protein/mRNA stability, may be limiting factors. Despite these promising results it is currently unknown whether nonviral GTAs will be able to improve CF lung disease, because none of the trials were designed to assess clinical efficacy of gene therapy.

Ongoing clinical trials

A critical observer may question whether the field has benefited from the large number of nonviral phase I proof-of-principle studies and may suggest a more co-ordinated and joined-up strategy. In an attempt to join up CF gene therapy across the UK, we formed the UK CF Gene Therapy Consortium and are currently conducting the only active CF gene therapy clinical trial.

From the outset, we assumed that one-time administration of a GTA (single dose) to the lung will be unlikely to lead to significant improvements in CF lung disease severity and, therefore, planned our clinical trial programme to culminate in a multidose clinical trial sufficiently powered to support a clinically relevant primary end-point.

In an extensive pre-clinical research programme, we determined that the cationic lipid formulation GL67A (Genzyme Corp., Cambridge, MA, USA), a comparatively old lipid that we had already used 15 years ago in a CF clinical trial [7], was still the most efficient nonviral vector currently available. We also showed that repeat aerosolisation of GL67A/pDNA complexes was feasible without loss of efficacy [84]. In regulatory-compliant multidose murine and ovine toxicology studies, we showed that administration of 12 doses (over 6 months) and nine doses (over 9 months) of GL67A/pDNA to mice and sheep, respectively, was safe [84, 85].

In addition, we further optimised the DNA component. Key modifications included: 1) incorporation of the hybrid promoter/enhancer hCEFI; and 2) CpG motif depletion to limit inflammatory responses in humans [74]. The final completely CpG-depleted plasmid carrying the *CFTR* cDNA under control of the hCEFI promoter is called pGM169.

We have completed a single-dose phase I/IIa safety pilot trial (n=36 subjects) and have succeeded in identifying a safe dose suitable for progression into a multidose trial (manuscript in preparation). The phase IIb multidose trial is a double-blinded placebo-controlled study [86]. Recruitment of more than 120 trial participants has recently been completed and trial recruitment is now closed. Trial participants are receiving 12 monthly doses of GL67A/pGM169 or placebo over a 1-year period. The primary end-point is a change from baseline in forced expiratory volume in 1 s (FEV1) % predicted. Secondary end-points include lung clearance index (LCI), computed tomography (CT) and quality-of-life (QoL) questionnaires. By December 2013, approximately 50% of patients had completed all 12 doses and no safety problems were observed. The trial will be completed in June 2014, with final results expected to be available in October 2014.

While conducting what is the largest CF gene therapy trial, we have learnt important lessons. First, although the UK CF community was eager to participate, the required long-term commitment to this trial (at least 16 hospital visits over the 12-month trial period) was one of a number of factors which made recruitment challenging. Secondly, education of nursing staff, who were not familiar with the concept of gene therapy and had not handled gene therapy products, was required to ensure that those with first-hand patient contact were able to confidently discuss the treatment with patients and families. If the trial is successful, an early education programme of relevant healthcare professionals will assist with a smooth introduction of CF gene therapy into the clinical setting. Longer term, CF gene therapy may lead to reduced treatment burden, improved patient compliance and fewer hospital admissions, which may change the work of CF healthcare professionals. Thirdly, infrastructure to handle gene therapy products in hospital pharmacies is not readily available. Pharmacists and associated staff have to be trained and infrastructure put into place to allow transition of CF gene therapy into mainstream clinical care.

Cell therapy

Various cell types, including bone marrow stem cells (BMSCs), embryonic stem (ES) cells and induced pluripotent stem (iPS) cells, are being studied in the context of cell therapy for CF and other lung diseases. To date, these various cell types have been administered to wild-type mice (sometimes after induction of lung injury) using intravenous or topical delivery methods.

Intravenous cell therapy

The finding that, under certain circumstances, BMSCs or umbilical cord blood-derived stem cells may have the capacity to transdifferentiate and repopulate various organs has triggered research into the development of stem cell-based therapies for a large number of diseases, including CF. It has been shown that these cells may have the capacity to induce expression of lung epithelial cell-specific markers when cultured appropriately (reviewed in [87]).

In addition, WONG et al. [88] identified a population of cells positive for the club cell-specific marker, club cell secretory protein (CCSP), in human and murine bone marrow. The number of circulating CCSP-positive bone marrow cells increased after cell injury, and these cells may be an interesting choice for cell therapy of lung disease. WANG et al. [89] have shown that mesenchymal stem cells of CF patients can, after ex vivo gene correction and co-culture with primary CF airway epithelial cells in air–liquid interface cultures, generate CFTR-mediated chloride channel activity.

Several groups have attempted to assess whether BMSCs can transdifferentiate into airway epithelium after intravenous administration, but results have been conflicting, in part due to methodological artefacts [87, 90]. BRUSCIA et al. [91] have reported that systemic administration of CFTR-positive BMSCs into irradiated CF knockout mice may lead to very modest correction of the CF chloride transport defect in intestinal epithelium; however, to the best of our knowledge, these studies have not been reproduced in other laboratories. The same group also assessed whether BMSC transplantation into newborn mice increased engraftment into various organs, including lung, liver and intestine, but showed that detection of bone marrow-derived epithelial cells remained a very rare event even in myeloablated newborn mice [91]. Along similar lines, LOI et al. [92] showed that bone marrow cells isolated from non-CF donor mice restored very low levels of CFTR expression in CF-knockout mice recipients. Combined data generated over the last few years illustrate that systemic administration of BMSCs currently does not hold great promise for CF therapy.

Topical cell therapy

Interestingly, systemic administration of stem cells has been superseded by studies assessing topical administration of various types of stem cell, which may be a more efficient route to deliver cell therapy to the airways. This was supported in studies by WONG et al. [88] and REJMAN et al. [93]. However, even after topical administration, the detection of transplanted cells in the recipient lung remained a rare event. DUCHESNEAU et al. [94] extended these studies and showed that destruction of endogenous club cells with naphthalene 2 days prior to transplantation, in combination with busulfan-induced myeloablation 1 day prior to transplantation, achieved maximal retention in the lung. However, the retention frequency of transplanted cells remained low and the differentiation status largely unresolved. In addition, it is unclear if and how these aggressive protocols can be translated into clinical applications. It has recently been reported that retention of bone marrow-derived progenitor cells is increased in the presence of Pseudomonas aeruginosa-induced lung infection [93], which may be particularly relevant for CF. However, despite more efficient retention after topical administration, the convincing detection and characterisation of cells retained in the lung remains a problem. Although sensitive PCR-based methods can detect low levels of transplanted cells, these methods provide little information about engraftment and differentiation status of these cells. In contrast, microscopy-based methods, even when coupled with sophisticated immunohistochemistry-based cell visualisation and characterisation, suffer from low sensitivity and problems associated with reliable interpretation of images.

Differentiation of ES cells into airway cells

In addition to the adult stem cells described above, ES cells have been studied. RIPPON et al. [95] published preliminary work following the fate of intravenously injected mouse ES cells and showed that a small number of transplanted, but not further characterised, cells were detectable in the distal lung for a few days. Similarly, LEBLOND *et al.* [96] assessed intratracheal administration of murine ES cells and mesenchymal stem cells in uninjured and injured (treated with 2% polidocanol) murine lungs, and showed some retention of transplanted cells (not further characterised) in injured but not uninjured murine lungs. Several studies have shown that, under certain circumstances, ES cells can be induced to express lung-specific proteins such as SP-B and -C as well as club cell protein 10 [97, 98]. WANG *et al.* [99] have shown that intratracheal administration of human ES cell-derived alveolar type II cells improved survival and reduced inflammation and fibrosis in a bleomycin-induced murine lung injury model. Although it is currently unclear whether the protective effect is due to cell engraftment and differentiation or an undefined paracrine effect, this study is, to the best of our knowledge, the first to demonstrate amelioration of lung injury using ES cells.

Maybe more relevant in the context of CF is a recent study by WONG *et al.* [100], who showed that after careful optimisation of culture conditions, human ES cells can generate conducting airway epithelium expressing functional CFTR. Combined with studies that have generated a human ES cell line from a CF embryo [101] and iPS cells from dermal fibroblasts of a CF subject [102], this technology may become powerful for disease modelling and drug screening. This is further supported in a recent study by MOU *et al.* [103], who established proof-of-concept for generation of human lung progenitors from CF iPS cells. The key to success was the careful recapitulation of endogenous signalling events, which were based on knowledge derived from murine studies. Importantly, the disease-specific human lung progenitor cells generated respiratory epithelium when subcutaneously engrafted into immunodeficient mice. In the short term, these cells will be more applicable to model disease and generate *ex vivo* models for drug testing than for *in vivo* transplantation strategies.

Ex vivo bioengineering of airways

Ex vivo bioengineered lungs are a dream for the future. However, early steps towards lung tissue engineering have been taken. A variety of synthetic scaffold materials have been developed [104]. However, the use of decellularised lung scaffolds currently appears to be most promising for recapitulating and re-generating the complex lung structure. Protocols for the decellularisation of rodent and nonhuman primate lungs have been developed [105, 106], and early proof-of-concept for regeneration of a bioartificial lung has recently been demonstrated in two high-profile publications [107, 108]. In both studies, decellularised rodent lungs were re-seeded with epithelial and endothelial cells *via* trachea and vasculature, respectively. After a few days in a bioreactor, re-seeding of the scaffolds was observed and gas exchange measurable. Following orthotopic transplantation, the bioengineered lung supported *in vivo* gas exchange for a few hours.

Importantly, MACCHIARINI *et al.* [109] have reported the successful transplantation of an *ex vivo*-engineered airway into a stenosed main bronchus of a female recipient. In this study, a donor trachea was de-cellularised and subsequently incubated with airway epithelial cells and bone marrow-derived chondrocytes from the recipient, which led to reconstitution of normal cell architecture on the tracheal scaffold. Recently, the results after 5 years' follow-up were reported [110]. GONFIOTTI *et al.* [110] reported that, although stenosis requiring repeated endoluminal stenting in the native trachea occurred close to the site of anastomosis, the tissue-engineered trachea remained open, well vascularised and had normal ciliary function and mucus clearance. Importantly, there was no evidence of teratoma or anti-donor antibody formation. The same group also used a synthetic polymer scaffold re-seeded with autologous bone marrow mononuclear cells to treat a patient with inoperable tracheal carcinoma [111]. Although information about graft integrity could not be provided, the 4-month follow-up report stated that the patient was free of obstructive symptoms and had resumed daily activities.

It is obviously far too early to speculate about the use of tissue-engineered lung in the context of CF therapy, but the reports are encouraging and the less ambitious airway engineering strategies outlined above may pave the way.

Cell therapy for CF comorbidities

Due to the constant development of better treatments, the survival of CF patients over the last 50 years has significantly increased. However, as survival increases, comorbidities such as CF-related diabetes mellitus (CFRD) and progressive liver disease become more prevalent [112, 113]. CF patients may therefore benefit from pancreatic islet transplantation. Proof-of-principle for this approach has recently been demonstrated. KESSLER et al. [114] reported that four end-stage CF patients with severe CFRD received a lung and pancreatic islet transplant from the same donor. Three out of four patients showed improved glucose control and reduced need for insulin several years after transplant. In addition, transplantation of autologous liver stem cells is advancing [115]. Although cell therapy may be far from being suitable for treating CF lung disease, it may, more immediately, be more appropriate for treating CF-related comorbidities such as CFRD and liver disease.

Bone marrow transplantation

It is easy to forget that bone marrow transplantation also falls under the definition of cell therapy and may have a role in treating CF. Although published studies are currently conflicting, it has been suggested that macrophages and neutrophils express CFTR and may have defective phagolysosomal function and phagosome acidification, leading to impaired host defence [38, 39, 116]. It is therefore conceivable that correction of CFTR function in bone marrow-derived haematopoietic stem cells through *ex vivo* transduction of autologous bone marrow with a lentivirus expressing CFTR may correct this host defence defect.

Conclusion

Over the last 20 years, the field has spent a significant amount of time evaluating, characterising and understanding the strengths and weaknesses of various viral and nonviral GTAs for CF gene therapy. We have learnt to appreciate that the lung has powerful defence mechanisms that make efficient gene transfer more difficult than originally predicted. The outcome of the multidose clinical trial performed by the UK CF Gene Therapy Consortium will determine whether nonviral GTAs are suitable for CF gene therapy. Results from this trial will significantly contribute to directing the field into a large phase III trial or into more phase II studies targeting "responders" or into focusing on lentiviral vectors. The latter are, in our view, currently the only viral vectors that warrant assessment in CF gene therapy trials, providing that the risk/benefit ratio, which will be assessed in pre-clinical studies, is favourable.

Cell therapy or the generation of bioengineered lungs are some way from translating into CF clinical trials, but early proof-of-concept studies for the generation of bioengineered tracheal segments look encouraging. Developed technologies, including the differentiation of ES and iPS cells into lung cells will, in the first instance, be more applicable for generation of *ex vivo* human lung models and, thereafter, for the treatment of CF-related comorbidities in organs other than the lung.

References

1. Drumm ML, Pope HA, Cliff WH, *et al*. Correction of the cystic fibrosis defect *in vitro* by retrovirus-mediated gene transfer. *Cell* 1990; 62: 1227–1233.
2. Rosenfeld MA, Yoshimura K, Trapnell BC, *et al*. *In vivo* transfer of the human cystic fibrosis transmembrane conductance regulator gene to the airway epithelium. *Cell* 1992; 68: 143–155.
3. Hyde SC, Gill DR, Higgins CF, *et al*. Correction of the ion transport defect in cystic fibrosis transgenic mice by gene therapy. *Nature* 1993; 362: 250–255.
4. Zabner J, Couture LA, Gregory RJ, *et al*. Adenovirus-mediated gene transfer transiently corrects the chloride transport defect in nasal epithelia of patients with cystic fibrosis. *Cell* 1993; 75: 207–216.
5. Crystal RG, McElvaney NG, Rosenfeld MA, *et al*. Administration of an adenovirus containing the human CFTR cDNA to the respiratory tract of individuals with cystic fibrosis. *Nat Genet* 1994; 8: 42–51.
6. Caplen NJ, Alton EW, Middleton PG, *et al*. Liposome-mediated CFTR gene transfer to the nasal epithelium of patients with cystic fibrosis. *Nat Med* 1995; 1: 39–46.
7. Alton EW, Stern M, Farley R, *et al*. Cationic lipid-mediated CFTR gene transfer to the lungs and nose of patients with cystic fibrosis: a double-blind placebo-controlled trial. *Lancet* 1999; 353: 947–954.
8. Nathwani AC, Tuddenham EG, Rangarajan S, *et al*. Adenovirus-associated virus vector-mediated gene transfer in hemophilia B. *N Engl J Med* 2011; 365: 2357–2365.
9. Seymour LW, Thrasher AJ. Gene therapy matures in the clinic. *Nat Biotechnol* 2012; 30: 588–593.
10. Accurso FJ, Rowe SM, Clancy JP, *et al*. Effect of VX-770 in persons with cystic fibrosis and the G551D-CFTR mutation. *N Engl J Med* 2010; 363: 1991–2003.
11. Clancy JP, Rowe SM, Accurso FJ, *et al*. Results of a phase IIa study of VX-809, an investigational CFTR corrector compound, in subjects with cystic fibrosis homozygous for the F508del-CFTR mutation. *Thorax* 2012; 67: 12–18.
12. Stern M, Ulrich K, Geddes DM, *et al*. Poly (D, L-lactide-co-glycolide)/DNA microspheres to facilitate prolonged transgene expression in airway epithelium *in vitro, ex vivo* and *in vivo*. *Gene Ther* 2003; 10: 1282–1288.
13. Yonemitsu Y, Kitson C, Ferrari S, *et al*. Efficient gene transfer to airway epithelium using recombinant Sendai virus. *Nat Biotechnol* 2000; 18: 970–973.
14. Sinn PL, Shah AJ, Donovan MD, *et al*. Viscoelastic gel formulations enhance airway epithelial gene transfer with viral vectors. *Am J Respir Cell Mol Biol* 2005; 32: 404–410.
15. Griesenbach U, Meng C, Farley R, *et al*. The use of carboxymethylcellulose gel to increase non-viral gene transfer in mouse airways. *Biomaterials* 2010; 31: 2665–2672.
16. Chirmule N, Propert K, Magosin S, *et al*. Immune responses to adenovirus and adeno-associated virus in humans. *Gene Ther* 1999; 6: 1574–1583.
17. Davies LA, Hyde SC, Nunez-Alonso G, *et al*. The use of CpG-free plasmids to mediate persistent gene expression following repeated aerosol delivery of pDNA/PEI complexes. *Biomaterials* 2012; 33: 5618–5627.
18. Hyde SC, Southern KW, Gileadi U, *et al*. Repeat administration of DNA/liposomes to the nasal epithelium of patients with cystic fibrosis. *Gene Ther* 2000; 7: 1156–1165.
19. Pickles RJ, McCarty D, Matsui H, *et al*. Limited entry of adenovirus vectors into well-differentiated airway epithelium is responsible for inefficient gene transfer. *J Virol* 1998; 72: 6014–6023.
20. Ferrari S, Griesenbach U, Shiraki-Iida T, *et al*. A defective nontransmissible recombinant Sendai virus mediates efficient gene transfer to airway epithelium *in vivo*. *Gene Ther* 2004; 11: 1659–1664.
21. Mudhakir D, Harashima H. Learning from the viral journey: how to enter cells and how to overcome intracellular barriers to reach the nucleus. *AAPS J* 2009; 11: 65–77.
22. Lam AP, Dean DA. Progress and prospects: nuclear import of nonviral vectors. *Gene Ther* 2010; 17: 439–447.
23. Ding W, Zhang L, Yan Z, *et al*. Intracellular trafficking of adeno-associated viral vectors. *Gene Ther* 2005; 12: 873–880.
24. Lee K, Ambrose Z, Martin TD, *et al*. Flexible use of nuclear import pathways by HIV-1. *Cell Host Microbe* 2010; 7: 221–233.
25. Sanders N, Rudolph C, Braeckmans K, *et al*. Extracellular barriers in respiratory gene therapy. *Adv Drug Deliv Rev* 2009; 61: 115–127.
26. Chu CS, Trapnell BC, Curristin S, *et al*. Genetic basis of variable exon 9 skipping in cystic fibrosis transmembrane conductance regulator mRNA. *Nat Genet* 1993; 3: 151–156.

27. Johnson LG, Olsen JC, Sarkadi B, *et al.* Efficiency of gene transfer for restoration of normal airway epithelial function in cystic fibrosis. *Nat Genet* 1992; 2: 21–25.

28. Farmen SL, Karp PH, Ng P, *et al.* Gene transfer of CFTR to airway epithelia: low levels of expression are sufficient to correct Cl- transport and overexpression can generate basolateral CFTR. *Am J Physiol Lung Cell Mol Physiol* 2005; 289: L1123–L1130.

29. Zhang L, Button B, Gabriel SE, *et al.* CFTR delivery to 25% of surface epithelial cells restores normal rates of mucus transport to human cystic fibrosis airway epithelium. *PLoS Biol* 2009; 7: e1000155.

30. Johnson LG, Boyles SE, Wilson J, *et al.* Normalization of raised sodium absorption and raised calcium-mediated chloride secretion by adenovirus-mediated expression of cystic fibrosis transmembrane conductance regulator in primary human cystic fibrosis airway epithelial cells. *J Clin Invest* 1995; 95: 1377–1382.

31. Potash AE, Wallen TJ, Karp PH, *et al.* Adenoviral gene transfer corrects the ion transport defect in the sinus epithelia of a porcine CF model. *Mol Ther* 2013; 21: 947–953.

32. Bombieri C, Claustres M, De Boeck K, *et al.* Recommendations for the classification of diseases as CFTR-related disorders. *J Cyst Fibros* 2011; 10: Suppl. 2, S86–S102.

33. Griesenbach U, Alton EWFW. Gene and stem cell therapy in cystic fibrosis. *In*: Bush A, Bilton D, Hodson M, eds. Cystic Fibrosis. 4th Edn. Boca Raton, Taylor and Francis Group, 2014 (In press).

34. Engelhardt JF, Yankaskas JR, Ernst SA, *et al.* Submucosal glands are the predominant site of CFTR expression in the human bronchus. *Nat Genet* 1992; 2: 240–248.

35. Kreda SM, Mall M, Mengos A, *et al.* Characterization of wild-type and ΔF508 cystic fibrosis transmembrane regulator in human respiratory epithelia. *Mol Biol Cell* 2005; 16: 2154–2167.

36. Penque D, Mendes F, Beck S, *et al.* Cystic fibrosis F508del patients have apically localized CFTR in a reduced number of airway cells. *Lab Invest* 2000; 80: 857–868.

37. Deriy LV, Gomez EA, Zhang G, *et al.* Disease-causing mutations in the cystic fibrosis transmembrane conductance regulator determine the functional responses of alveolar macrophages. *J Biol Chem* 2009; 284: 35926–35938.

38. Painter RG, Valentine VG, Lanson NA Jr, *et al.* CFTR expression in human neutrophils and the phagolysosomal chlorination defect in cystic fibrosis. *Biochemistry* 2006; 45: 10260–10269.

39. Di A, Brown ME, Deriy LV, *et al.* CFTR regulates phagosome acidification in macrophages and alters bactericidal activity. *Nat Cell Biol* 2006; 8: 933–944.

40. Hartl D, Latzin P, Hordijk P, *et al.* Cleavage of CXCR1 on neutrophils disables bacterial killing in cystic fibrosis lung disease. *Nat Med* 2007; 13: 1423–1430.

41. Pezzulo AA, Tang XX, Hoegger MJ, *et al.* Reduced airway surface pH impairs bacterial killing in the porcine cystic fibrosis lung. *Nature* 2012; 487: 109–113.

42. Brunetti-Pierri N, Ng P. Progress and prospects: gene therapy for genetic diseases with helper-dependent adenoviral vectors. *Gene Ther* 2008; 15: 553–560.

43. Weiss L, ed. Cell and Tissue Biology. A Text Book of Histology. 6th Edn. Baltimore, Urban and Schwarzenberg Inc., 1988.

44. Griesenbach U, Alton EW. Gene transfer to the lung: lessons learned from more than 2 decades of CF gene therapy. *Adv Drug Deliv Rev* 2009; 61: 128–139.

45. Griesenbach U, Alton EW. Progress in gene and cell therapy for cystic fibrosis lung disease. *Curr Pharm Des* 2012; 18: 642–662.

46. Cao H, Machuca TN, Yeung JC, *et al.* Efficient gene delivery to pig airway epithelia and submucosal glands using helper-dependent adenoviral vectors. *Mol Ther Nucleic Acids* 2013; 2: e127.

47. Duan D, Sharma P, Yang J, *et al.* Circular intermediates of recombinant adeno-associated virus have defined structural characteristics responsible for long-term episomal persistence in muscle tissue. *J Virol* 1998; 72: 8568–8577.

48. Flotte TR. Recent developments in recombinant AAV-mediated gene therapy for lung diseases. *Curr Gene Ther* 2005; 5: 361–366.

49. McCarty DM, Young SM Jr, Samulski RJ. Integration of adeno-associated virus (AAV) and recombinant AAV vectors. *Annu Rev Genet* 2004; 38: 819–845.

50. Gao G, Vandenberghe LH, Wilson JM. New recombinant serotypes of AAV vectors. *Curr Gene Ther* 2005; 5: 285–297.

51. Limberis MP, Vandenberghe LH, Zhang L, *et al.* Transduction efficiencies of novel AAV vectors in mouse airway epithelium *in vivo* and human ciliated airway epithelium *in vitro*. *Mol Ther* 2009; 17: 294–301.

52. Moss RB, Rodman D, Spencer LT, *et al.* Repeated adeno-associated virus serotype 2 aerosol-mediated cystic fibrosis transmembrane regulator gene transfer to the lungs of patients with cystic fibrosis: a multicenter, double-blind, placebo-controlled trial. *Chest* 2004; 125: 509–521.

53. Moss RB, Milla C, Colombo J, *et al.* Repeated aerosolized AAV-CFTR for treatment of cystic fibrosis: a randomized placebo-controlled phase 2B trial. *Hum Gene Ther* 2007; 18: 726–732.

54. Liu X, Luo M, Guo C, *et al.* Analysis of adeno-associated virus progenitor cell transduction in mouse lung. *Mol Ther* 2009; 17: 285–293.

55. Faust SM, Bell P, Cutler BJ, *et al.* CpG-depleted adeno-associated virus vectors evade immune detection. *J Clin Invest* 2013; 123: 2994–3001.

56. Kaeppel C, Beattie SG, Fronza R, *et al.* A largely random AAV integration profile after LPLD gene therapy. *Nat Med* 2013; 19: 889–891.

57. Zhang L, Bukreyev A, Thompson CI, *et al.* Infection of ciliated cells by human parainfluenza virus type 3 in an *in vitro* model of human airway epithelium. *J Virol* 2005; 79: 1113–1124.

58. Kobayashi M, Iida A, Ueda Y, *et al.* Pseudotyped lentivirus vectors derived from simian immunodeficiency virus SIVagm with envelope glycoproteins from paramyxovirus. *J Virol* 2003; 77: 2607–2614.

59. Mitomo K, Griesenbach U, Inoue M, *et al.* Toward gene therapy for cystic fibrosis using a lentivirus pseudotyped with Sendai virus envelopes. *Mol Ther* 2010; 18: 1173–1182.

60. Sinn PL, Arias AC, Brogden KA, *et al.* Lentivirus vector can be readministered to nasal epithelia without blocking immune responses. *J Virol* 2008; 82: 10684–10692.

61. McKay T, Patel M, Pickles RJ, *et al.* Influenza M2 envelope protein augments avian influenza hemagglutinin pseudotyping of lentiviral vectors. *Gene Ther* 2006; 13: 715–724.

62. Limberis M, Anson DS, Fuller M, *et al.* Recovery of airway cystic fibrosis transmembrane conductance regulator function in mice with cystic fibrosis after single-dose lentivirus-mediated gene transfer. *Hum Gene Ther* 2002; 13: 1961–1970.

63. Cmielewski P, Anson DS, Parsons DW. Lysophosphatidylcholine as an adjuvant for lentiviral vector mediated gene transfer to airway epithelium: effect of acyl chain length. *Respir Res* 2010; 11: 84.

64. Medina MF, Kobinger GP, Rux J, *et al.* Lentiviral vectors pseudotyped with minimal filovirus envelopes increased gene transfer in murine lung. *Mol Ther* 2003; 8: 777–789.

65. Patel M, Giddings AM, Sechelski J, *et al.* High efficiency gene transfer to airways of mice using influenza hemagglutinin pseudotyped lentiviral vectors. *J Gene Med* 2013; 15: 51–62.

66. Griesenbach U, Alton EW. Moving forward: cystic fibrosis gene therapy. *Hum Mol Genet* 2013; 22: R52–R58.

67. Stocker AG, Kremer KL, Koldej R, *et al.* Single-dose lentiviral gene transfer for lifetime airway gene expression. *J Gene Med* 2009; 11: 861–867.

68. Sinn PL, Cooney AL, Oakland M, *et al.* Lentiviral vector gene transfer to porcine airways. *Mol Ther Nucleic Acids* 2012; 1: e56.

69. Farrow N, Miller D, Cmielewski P, *et al.* Airway gene transfer in a non-human primate: lentiviral gene expression in marmoset lungs. *Sci Rep* 2013; 3: 1287.

70. Griesenbach U, Inoue M, Meng C, *et al.* Assessment of F/HN-pseudotyped lentivirus as a clinically relevant vector for lung gene therapy. *Am J Respir Crit Care Med* 2012; 186: 846–856.

71. Pichon C, Billiet L, Midoux P. Chemical vectors for gene delivery: uptake and intracellular trafficking. *Curr Opin Biotechnol* 2010; 21: 640–645.

72. Griesenbach U, Alton EW. Expert opinion in biological therapy: update on developments in lung gene transfer. *Expert Opin Biol Ther* 2013; 13: 345–360.

73. Jin L, Zeng X, Liu M, *et al.* Current progress in gene delivery technology based on chemical methods and nano-carriers. *Theranostics* 2014; 4: 240–255.

74. Hyde SC, Pringle IA, Abdullah S, *et al.* CpG-free plasmids confer reduced inflammation and sustained pulmonary gene expression. *Nat Biotechnol* 2008; 26: 549–551.

75. Pringle IA, Raman S, Sharp WW, *et al.* Detection of plasmid DNA vectors following gene transfer to the murine airways. *Gene Ther* 2005; 12: 1206–1214.

76. Stein S, Ott MG, Schultze-Strasser S, *et al.* Genomic instability and myelodysplasia with monosomy 7 consequent to EVI1 activation after gene therapy for chronic granulomatous disease. *Nat Med* 2010; 16: 198–204.

77. Qin L, Ding Y, Pahud DR, *et al.* Promoter attenuation in gene therapy: interferon-γ and tumor necrosis factor-α inhibit transgene expression. *Hum Gene Ther* 1997; 8: 2019–2029.

78. Gill DR, Smyth SE, Goddard CA, *et al.* Increased persistence of lung gene expression using plasmids containing the ubiquitin C or elongation factor 1α promoter. *Gene Ther* 2001; 8: 1539–1546.

79. Yew NS, Przybylska M, Ziegler RJ, *et al.* High and sustained transgene expression *in vivo* from plasmid vectors containing a hybrid ubiquitin promoter. *Mol Ther* 2001; 4: 75–82.

80. Munkonge FM, Amin V, Hyde SC, *et al.* Identification and functional characterization of cytoplasmic determinants of plasmid DNA nuclear import. *J Biol Chem* 2009; 284: 26978–26987.

81. Badding MA, Lapek JD, Friedman AE, *et al.* Proteomic and functional analyses of protein-DNA complexes during gene transfer. *Mol Ther* 2013; 21: 775–785.

82. Kormann MS, Hasenpusch G, Aneja MK, *et al.* Expression of therapeutic proteins after delivery of chemically modified mRNA in mice. *Nat Biotechnol* 2011; 29: 154–157.

83. Mays LE, Ammon-Treiber S, Mothes B, *et al.* Modified Foxp3 mRNA protects against asthma through an IL-10-dependent mechanism. *J Clin Invest* 2013; 123: 1216–1228.

84. Alton EW, Boyd AC, Cheng SH, *et al.* Toxicology study assessing efficacy and safety of repeated administration of lipid/DNA complexes to mouse lung. *Gene Ther* 2014; 21: 89–95.

85. Alton EW, Baker A, Baker E, *et al.* The safety profile of a cationic lipid-mediated cystic fibrosis gene transfer agent following repeated monthly aerosol administration to sheep. *Biomaterials* 2013; 34: 10267–10277.

86. Alton EW, Boyd AC, Cheng SH, *et al.* A randomised, double-blind, placebo-controlled phase IIB clinical trial of repeated application of gene therapy in patients with cystic fibrosis. *Thorax* 2013; 68: 1075–1077.

87. Weiss DJ. Stem cells and cell therapies for cystic fibrosis and other lung diseases. *Pulm Pharmacol Ther* 2008; 21: 588–594.

88. Wong AP, Keating A, Lu WY, *et al.* Identification of a bone marrow-derived epithelial-like population capable of repopulating injured mouse airway epithelium. *J Clin Invest* 2009; 119: 336–348.

89. Wang G, Bunnell BA, Painter RG, *et al.* Adult stem cells from bone marrow stroma differentiate into airway epithelial cells: potential therapy for cystic fibrosis. *Proc Natl Acad Sci USA* 2005; 102: 186–191.

90. Kotton DN, Fine A. Lung stem cells. *Cell Tissue Res* 2008; 331: 145–156.

91. Bruscia EM, Price JE, Cheng EC, *et al.* Assessment of cystic fibrosis transmembrane conductance regulator (CFTR) activity in CFTR-null mice after bone marrow transplantation. *Proc Natl Acad Sci USA* 2006; 103: 2965–2970.

92. Loi R, Beckett T, Goncz KK, *et al.* Limited restoration of cystic fibrosis lung epithelium *in vivo* with adult bone marrow-derived cells. *Am J Respir Crit Care Med* 2006; 173: 171–179.

93. Rejman J, Colombo C, Conese M. Engraftment of bone marrow-derived stem cells to the lung in a model of acute respiratory infection by *Pseudomonas aeruginosa*. *Mol Ther* 2009; 17: 1257–1265.

94. Duchesneau P, Wong AP, Waddell TK. Optimization of targeted cell replacement therapy: a new approach for lung disease. *Mol Ther* 2010; 18: 1830–1836.

95. Rippon HJ, Lane S, Qin M, *et al.* Embryonic stem cells as a source of pulmonary epithelium *in vitro* and *in vivo*. *Proc Am Thorac Soc* 2008; 5: 717–722.

96. Leblond AL, Naud P, Forest V, *et al.* Developing cell therapy techniques for respiratory disease: intratracheal delivery of genetically engineered stem cells in a murine model of airway injury. *Hum Gene Ther* 2009; 20: 1329–1343.

97. Lin YM, Zhang A, Bismarck A, *et al.* Effects of fibroblast growth factors on the differentiation of the pulmonary progenitors from murine embryonic stem cells. *Exp Lung Res* 2010; 36: 307–320.

98. Samadikuchaksaraei A, Cohen S, Isaac K, *et al.* Derivation of distal airway epithelium from human embryonic stem cells. *Tissue Eng* 2006; 12: 867–875.

99. Wang D, Morales JE, Calame DG, *et al.* Transplantation of human embryonic stem cell-derived alveolar epithelial type II cells abrogates acute lung injury in mice. *Mol Ther* 2010; 18: 625–634.

100. Wong AP, Bear CE, Chin S, *et al.* Directed differentiation of human pluripotent stem cells into mature airway epithelia expressing functional CFTR protein. *Nat Biotechnol* 2012; 30: 876–882.

101. Pickering SJ, Minger SL, Patel M, *et al.* Generation of a human embryonic stem cell line encoding the cystic fibrosis mutation deltaF508, using preimplantation genetic diagnosis. *Reprod Biomed Online* 2005; 10: 390–397.

102. Somers A, Jean JC, Sommer CA, *et al.* Generation of transgene-free lung disease-specific human induced pluripotent stem cells using a single excisable lentiviral stem cell cassette. *Stem Cells* 2010; 28: 1728–1740.

103. Mou H, Zhao R, Sherwood R, *et al.* Generation of multipotent lung and airway progenitors from mouse ESCs and patient-specific cystic fibrosis iPSCs. *Cell Stem Cell* 2012; 10: 385–397.

104. Song JJ, Ott HC. Bioartificial lung engineering. *Am J Transplant* 2012; 12: 283–288.

105. Song JJ, Ott HC. Organ engineering based on decellularized matrix scaffolds. *Trends Mol Med* 2011; 17: 424–432.

106. Bonvillain RW, Danchuk S, Sullivan DE, *et al.* A nonhuman primate model of lung regeneration: detergent-mediated decellularization and initial *in vitro* recellularization with mesenchymal stem cells. *Tissue Eng Part A* 2012; 18: 2437–2452.

107. Ott HC, Clippinger B, Conrad C, *et al.* Regeneration and orthotopic transplantation of a bioartificial lung. *Nat Med* 2010; 16: 927–933.

108. Petersen TH, Calle EA, Zhao L, *et al.* Tissue-engineered lungs for *in vivo* implantation. *Science* 2010; 329: 538–541.

109. Macchiarini P, Jungebluth P, Go T, *et al.* Clinical transplantation of a tissue-engineered airway. *Lancet* 2008; 372: 2023–2030.

110. Gonfiotti A, Jaus MO, Barale D, *et al.* The first tissue-engineered airway transplantation: 5-year follow-up results. *Lancet* 2014; 383: 238–244.

111. Jungebluth P, Alici E, Baiguera S, *et al.* Tracheobronchial transplantation with a stem-cell-seeded bioartificial nanocomposite: a proof-of-concept study. *Lancet* 2011; 378: 1997–2004.

112. Moran A, Dunitz J, Nathan B, *et al.* Cystic fibrosis-related diabetes: current trends in prevalence, incidence, and mortality. *Diabetes Care* 2009; 32: 1626–1631.

113. Parisi GF, Di Dio G, Franzonello C, *et al.* Liver disease in cystic fibrosis: an update. *Hepat Mon* 2013; 13: e11215.

114. Kessler L, Bakopoulou S, Kessler R, *et al.* Combined pancreatic islet-lung transplantation: a novel approach to the treatment of end-stage cystic fibrosis. *Am J Transplant* 2010; 10: 1707–1712.

115. Moore JK, Stutchfield BM, Forbes SJ. Systematic review: the effects of autologous stem cell therapy for patients with liver disease. *Aliment Pharmacol Ther* 2014; 39: 673–685.

116. Haggie PM, Verkman AS. Cystic fibrosis transmembrane conductance regulator-independent phagosomal acidification in macrophages. *J Biol Chem* 2007; 282: 31422–31428.

Acknowledgements: We thank Samia Soussi (Dept of Gene Therapy, Imperial College London, London, UK) for help with preparing this manuscript. The views expressed in this chapter are those of the authors and not necessarily those of the National Health Service, the NIHR or the Dept of Health.

Support statement: U. Griesenbach, R.F. Featherstone and E.W.F.W. Alton have received grants from the Cystic Fibrosis Trust, the Medical Research Council's Developmental Pathway Funding Scheme (MRC-DPFS) and the National Institute for Health Research Efficacy and Mechanism Evaluation Programme (NIHR-EME). This project was supported by the National Institute for Health Research (NIHR) Respiratory Disease Biomedical Research Unit at the Royal Brompton and Harefield NHS Foundation Trust and Imperial College London, London, UK.

Disclosures: U. Griesenbach and E.W.F.W. Alton have been issued patents for cystic fibrosis treatment, for gene transfer into airway epithelial stem cells using a lentiviral vector pseudotyped with RNA virus or DNA virus spike protein, and for minus strand RNA viral vectors carrying a gene with altered hypermutable region. R.F. Featherstone reports receiving grants from the Cystic Fibrosis Trust, grants from MRC-DPFS and grants from NIHR-EME during the conduct of the study.

Chapter 12

Improving airway clearance in cystic fibrosis lung disease

Judy M. Bradley[1], Katherine O'Neill[2], Ruth Dentice[3] and Mark Elkins[4,5,6]

In cystic fibrosis (CF) the mucociliary clearance mechanism is impaired and airway clearance techniques aim to compensate for this by promoting secretion clearance. A substantial body of research has been unable to provide clear evidence for one technique over another. This is in part due to limitations in the study designs used to assess the effects of the techniques. There is great variability in the airway clearance techniques used at patient, centre and country level. Adherence to airway clearance techniques is consistently low and there is an urgent need to focus research on interventions to overcome key barriers to non-adherence. Airway clearance techniques also need to be coordinated with mucoactive medications to ensure the overall effect is optimised. Recent trials have identified the challenges related to using forced expiratory volume in 1 s (FEV_1) as a primary outcome measure for airway clearance trials. New testing methods, for example multiple-breath washout and radio-imaging studies, may improve our understanding of the mechanisms underlying airway clearance as well as offering potential alternate clinical end-points.

The key aims of airway clearance techniques are to compensate for impaired mucociliary clearance by promoting secretion clearance. In cystic fibrosis (CF), facilitating secretion clearance is intended to reduce bacterial load, thereby decreasing inflammation and airway damage, in order to delay progression of the disease process [1]. There has been much research conducted in airway clearance in CF, yet many techniques still do not have a strong evidence base. This chapter focuses on current themes in practice related to airway clearance and explores the challenges of research in this area, with a view to highlighting considerations relating to research design, outcome measures and funding needed to conduct research that will answer important clinical questions and make a real impact on practice. This chapter will also review the evidence related to coordinating airway clearance techniques with mucoactive medications, so that interactions between the two interventions can be used to increase the benefit obtained by the patient.

[1]Centre for Health and Rehabilitation Technologies, Institute Nursing and Health Research, University of Ulster and Dept of Respiratory Medicine, Belfast Health and Social Care Trust, Newtownabbey, UK. [2]Centre for Infection and Immunity, School of Medicine, Dentistry and Biomedical Sciences, Queen's University Belfast, Belfast, UK. [3]Dept of Physiotherapy, Royal Prince Alfred Hospital, Sydney Local Health Network, Camperdown, Sydney, Australia. [4]Royal Prince Alfred Hospital, Camperdown, Sydney, Australia. [5]Sydney Medical School, University of Sydney, Sydney, Australia. [6]Centre for Evidence-Based Physiotherapy, George Institute of Global Health, Sydney, Australia.

Correspondence: Judy M. Bradley, 1F117 University of Ulster, Shore Road, Newtownabbey, BT37 0QB, UK. E-mail: jm.bradley@ulster.ac.uk

Mucociliary clearance

The mucociliary system is responsible for transport of mucus along the airways and so has an essential role for bronchial hygiene. Healthy individuals produce 10–100 mL of airway secretions daily, which are cleared by the action of the mucociliary escalator [2]. A functioning mucociliary clearance system requires hydration of the airway surface liquid (ASL) layer, normal functioning of the cilia and adequate rheology of the sputum for clearance. This should be supplemented by an effective cough as a back-up mechanism for when the secretion load is too great for the mucociliary system alone. In CF, the usual mucociliary defence mechanisms are impaired. The causes of impaired mucociliary clearance in CF are multifactorial and are likely to link to abnormalities of the ASL layer (which includes periciliary liquid (PCL) layer and mucus layer). In healthy individuals, the PCL layer is slightly thinner than the length of the cilia (5–7 µm) and the mucus layer is 2–3 µm. In CF, cystic fibrosis transmembrane conductance regulator (CFTR) abnormalities in sodium and chloride transport lead to dehydration of the ASL layer, which disrupts the normal interaction between the cilia and mucus, subsequently impairing mucociliary transport (fig. 1) [4]. Mucus that is not cleared from the airways continues to trap inhaled bacteria, becoming a nidus for chronic infection. Acidic ASL pH resulting from defective or absent CFTR function may also impair bacterial killing in the airway [5]. This results in a pro-inflammatory environment within the lung, which leads to progressive lung damage. In addition, dysregulation of the host inflammatory response may be a direct consequence of CFTR dysfunction, leading to inflammation independent of infection [6, 7]. Although the initiating event is debated, the resulting large amounts of DNA and inflammatory substances alter sputum rheology, increasing viscosity, spinability and adhesivity, which makes the sputum more difficult to clear. Cough, which is dependent on expiratory flow rates, can often be rendered less effective because of reduced expiratory flow rates and altered sputum rheology. Furthermore, large volumes of neutrophilic inflammatory products overwhelm the antiprotease activity of the lung, resulting in airway wall destruction and bronchiectasis, which provide an environment that is favourable to bacterial colonisation and hence the infection becomes chronic in nature [8].

Theory underlying airway clearance techniques

There are a variety of airway clearance techniques used in CF. These include independent techniques (*e.g.* active cycle of breathing techniques and autogenic drainage), device-dependent techniques (*e.g.* positive expiratory pressure (PEP) and oscillating PEP) and assistive components that can be used in conjunction with other techniques (*e.g.* chest percussion/clapping and vibrations). Airway clearance techniques use physical and/or mechanical means to dislodge adhered secretions and to manipulate airflow, in order to mobilise secretions towards more proximal airways to facilitate evacuation by expiratory manoeuvres such as coughing. A number of theoretical concepts are hypothesised to provide a rationale for mechanisms underlying airway clearance techniques. These concepts include interdependence (*i.e.* during inspiration, expanding alveoli exert a force on adjacent alveoli, which may assist in the re-expansion of collapsed ventilatory units), collateral ventilation (*i.e.* the ventilation of alveolar structures through passages or channels that bypass the normal airways, which may increase air behind impacted secretions making them more amenable to dislodgement) and positioning (*i.e.* additional gravitational forces affect secretions in vertically positioned bronchi, which may enhance impaired mucociliary transport) [9].

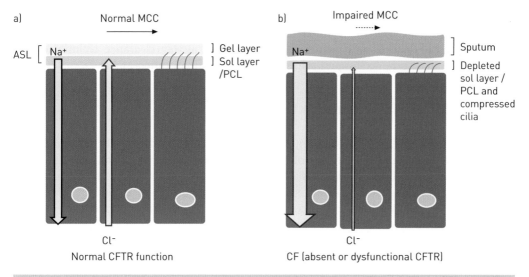

Figure 1. Depletion of the airway surface liquid (ASL) [3]. a) Healthy epithelium, b) Cystic fibrosis (CF) epithelium. MCC: mucociliary clearance; PCL: periciliary liquid; CFTR: cystic fibrosis transmembrane conductance regulator.

Airway clearance techniques also incorporate strategies to increase expiratory flow rate. Huffing, first introduced in the 1970s and defined as a forced expiration with an open glottis, is a component of many airway clearance techniques. It uses the concept of the equal pressure point to compress airways, increasing airflow velocity and turbulence through peripheral airways and moving secretions proximally [10]. Many airway clearance techniques invariably incorporate oscillation (manually or *via* mechanisms built into the device) and there is increasing evidence from laboratory and animal models that oscillation can improve mucociliary clearance. TARRAN *et al.* [11] conducted an *in vitro* study demonstrating that manoeuvres generating motion and shear forces facilitated regulation of the PCL in CF. There is also evidence that oscillations alter the rheology of sputum and increase ciliary beat through stimulation of ciliated epithelial cells [12, 13]. McCARREN and ALISON [14] also suggest that the oscillations produced by commonly used devices are within the range of frequencies that optimally impact on mucociliary clearance (table 1).

Table 1. The frequency of oscillation of the physiotherapy interventions as determined by frequency spectral analysis

Intervention	Frequency Hz
Vibration	8.4 ± 0.4 (7.3–10.0)
Percussion	7.3 ± 0.3 (6.5–8.0)
Flutter	11.3 ± 1.5 (7.5–13.7)
Acapella	13.5 ± 1.7 (10.0–18.3)

Data are presented as mean ± SD (range) of means of each subject. Reproduced and modified from [14] with permission from the publisher.

Higher ratios of peak expiratory flow rate (PEFR) to peak inspiratory flow rate (PIFR) promote mucociliary clearance compared to lower ratios. MCCARREN and ALISON [14] have explored the PEFR/PIFR ratio achieved by a range of airway clearance techniques and demonstrated that some techniques achieve higher ratios than others (table 2).

Evidence for airway clearance techniques

In the last three decades there has been a plethora of randomised clinical trials conducted that focus on examining the efficacy of different methods of airway clearance. The trials have been summarised in a series of six Cochrane reviews [15–20]. The characteristics of the included trials of airway clearance techniques are summarised in table 3. This table shows that this pool of evidence is directed mostly towards establishing "proof of concept" of the airway clearance techniques, with few of the trials able to assess the clinical efficacy of the techniques. For example, most of the trials use a crossover design, which is reasonable for single-treatment studies to assess whether a technique increases secretion clearance from the airways in the short term but would be confounded by carryover effects and the inherently unstable clinical course of CF if used to assess long-term effects. Regardless of the study design used, most of the intervention periods are of too short a duration (median 11 days) to assess long-term effects. Most trials are underpowered, with the median sample size being only 18 participants, and have marked heterogeneity in age range and disease severity. The outcomes measured in these trials, which are discussed in more detail below, also tend to reflect immediate secretion clearance effects rather than important clinical end-points.

One of the reviews summarised in table 3 focuses on the efficacy of "chest physiotherapy" compared to "no chest physiotherapy" and presents evidence to support the short-term beneficial effects of chest physiotherapy on mucus transport in CF. However, it highlights that there is currently no robust evidence regarding the long-term effects of chest physiotherapy [17].

Table 2. Effects of physiotherapy interventions on peak flow rate respiratory volumes and stimulation of cough

Intervention	Subjects n	PEFR $L \cdot s^{-1}$	PIFR $L \cdot s^{-1}$	PEFR/ PIFR	Inspired volume L	Expired volume L	Coughs stimulated
Vibration	17	1.58 ± 0.73	1.06 ± 0.27	1.51	1.78 ± 0.87	2.44 ± 1.06	0.7 ± 1.0
Percussion	18	$0.83 \pm 0.14^{***}$	0.84 ± 0.10	0.99	$0.91 \pm 0.37^{***}$	1.03 ± 0.50	0.5 ± 0.9
PEP	18	$0.44 \pm 0.15^{***}$	0.96 ± 0.20	0.47	1.64 ± 0.40	1.96 ± 0.57	0.5 ± 0.6
Flutter	17	$1.13 \pm 0.30^{\#}$	1.05 ± 0.27	1.15	1.62 ± 0.52	1.81 ± 0.57	0.4 ± 0.7
Acapella	18	$0.59 \pm 0.08^{***}$	0.98 ± 0.27	0.64	1.55 ± 0.46	1.68 ± 0.50	0.8 ± 1.0
TLCrelax	15	0.66 ± 0.16	1.01 ± 0.40	0.73	1.79 ± 0.66	2.24 ± 0.79	0

Data are presented as mean ± SD of means of each subject, unless otherwise stated. PEFR: peak expiratory flow rate; PIFR: peak inspiratory flow rate; PEP: positive expiratory pressure; TLCrelax: inspiration to total lung capacity followed by passive expiration (acts as a control manoeuvre to account for the effects of lung recoil on expiratory flow). p-values are significantly different from vibration. ***: $p < 0.001$; #: $p = 0.002$. Reproduced and modified from [14] with permission from the publisher.

Table 3. Characteristics of clinical trials of airway clearance techniques

Study characteristic	Studies n (%)	Mean ± SD	Median (range)	Studies not reporting n
Design				
Parallel	21 (30)			0
Crossover	49 (70)			
Sample size		25 ± 23	18 (5–166)	0
Participant age years		19 ± 7	20 (0.2–30)	20
Participant age group				12
Infant	1 (4)			
Paediatric	0 (0)			
Paediatric and adolescent	9 (5)			
Adolescent	0 (0)			
Adolescent and adult	25 (43)			
Adult	3 (5)			
Paediatric, adolescent and adult	20 (34)			
Participant age span# years		19 ± 10	17 (6–46)	13
FEV1 % pred		57 ± 18	53 (25–88)	13
FEV1 span# % pred		65 ± 23	68 (12–99)	54
Clinical status				0
Stable	53 (67)			
Exacerbation	17 (24)			
Intervention period days		96 ± 190	11 (0.5–876)	0
Intervention arms				0
2	47 (67)			
3	13 (19)			
4	6 (9)			
5	4 (6)			
Control intervention				0¶
Spontaneous cough	8 (80)			
Matched cough	2 (20)			

FEV1: forced expiratory volume in 1 s. #: calculated as highest minus lowest age or FEV1 reported; if only SD was reported, this was converted to an age or FEV1 span by multiplying by 4. ¶: note that this was only relevant to 10 studies because the remainder of studies compared two or more groups receiving active interventions but no control group. The cohort of trials (n=70) were those included in six Cochrane systematic reviews of airway clearance techniques for people with cystic fibrosis [15–20].

The other reviews summarised in table 3 focus on the efficacy of one technique *versus* other techniques. The consistent conclusions of these reviews are that there is no clear evidence of greater benefit of one technique over another. RAND et al. [1] describe how this has led to clinicians adopting a more dynamic and individualised approach to airway clearance, often involving the combination of more than one technique and alteration in a patient's airway clearance regimen during onset of new symptoms or during acute exacerbations. While this use of clinical reasoning to individualise the airway clearance regimen for each patient is appropriate because of variation in how treatments are performed, tolerated and adhered to, clinicians should remember that it is based on the absence of evidence to dictate whether one intervention is better, not on the assumption that all treatment approaches are equally effective. This assumption has not been necessarily borne out when clinical trials of adequate size and rigour have been conducted.

As an example, a 1-year 12-site Canadian randomised controlled study was designed to determine the long-term efficacy of using high-frequency chest wall oscillation (HFCWO) as compared to PEP mask therapy in the treatment of CF [21]. In terms of research design, this study scores highly in terms of quality, with a Physiotherapy Evidence Database (PEDro) score of 7/10 [22]. Although participants were not blinded as to the arm of the study to which they were randomised (which is not possible in many physiotherapy trials), physicians and respiratory therapists performing the outcome measure were blinded to treatment allocation. The study adopted a computer-generated, blocked randomisation within each centre to control for treatment difference between centres. The intervention had good fidelity with delivery of a protocol-defined intervention, using study-trained principal investigators and research co-ordinators. 107 patients were randomised to two groups, PEP (n=51) and HFCWO (n=56). Although there were some dropouts in this 1-year trial (nine from the PEP group and 10 from the HFCWO group), follow-up of patients and key results relating to primary and secondary outcome measures were comprehensively reported in this study. There was a significant difference between groups in the primary outcome measure, which was the number of exacerbations requiring antibiotics (p<0.007). There was no significant difference in secondary outcomes, including change in pulmonary function or health-related quality of life (HRQoL), between the two groups during the 1-year treatment period. This study does not support the use of HFCWO as a primary means of airway clearance in CF and perfectly highlights the importance of examining the efficacy of new interventions within the context of well-designed and powered clinical trials, with a scientific rigour equivalent to that applied to pharmaceutical studies.

The trial by SONTAG et al. [23] is an example of a well-designed trial that has not been fortunate in obtaining a clear answer to the question posed. In a recent review, MAIN [24] provides a comprehensive overview of the reasons for this. This paper makes excellent reading for those considering embarking on or funding a future airway clearance clinical trial. The review highlights that despite rigorous designs, recent trials have faced several challenges, including dropouts, use of lung function to determine sample size and/or as a key outcome measure, and the influence of patient preference. These challenges have all affected the outcomes of recent airway clearance clinical trials [23, 25]. The review highlights the fundamental need of future studies to consider alternate trial designs, such as the design of RÜCKER [26], which will address these issues and help delineate more clearly the comparative benefits of different treatments.

Current usage of airway clearance techniques

As discussed above, the current pool of evidence does not contain many clear recommendations for the use of one technique over another. Consequently, choice of airway clearance treatments is influenced by a range of factors, including local availability and cost of devices, availability of therapists and therapist training. Origin of the device and strength of marketing in the country may also be more influential than evidence of efficacy [24].

These factors rationalise, at least in part, the different approaches to airway clearance between centres and more dramatic differences between countries. The "primary" airway clearance therapy recorded for patients in the UK CF registry has recently been explored (J.M. Bradley, unpublished data). Few people with CF used postural drainage and a clear preference was shown towards some devices that allow independent treatment (PEP and oscillating PEP). Few used HFCWO. Patients reported using forced expiratory techniques as their primary airway clearance technique; however, it is notable that forced expiratory techniques are incorporated into the majority of other airway clearance techniques. It is notable that a proportion of the population used exercise as their primary airway clearance technique or reported doing no airway clearance (J.M. Bradley, unpublished data). In other countries, other techniques are more popular, *e.g.* in Canada, McILWAINE *et al.* [27] showed that people had a preference for the use of PEP therapy and only a small proportion was using HFCWO. This contrasts to available data from the USA, which shows that over 40% of patients use HFCWO for airway clearance [28].

Adherence to airway clearance therapies

Existing research, which has relied on self-reporting, has demonstrated that adherence to airway clearance is poor across childhood, adolescence and adulthood for patients with CF. School-age children demonstrate adherence to airway clearance techniques of 51–74%, adolescents 50% and adults 30–32%, with increasing age associated with worse adherence [29–31]. Few studies have identified longitudinal patterns of adherence [32]. There is strong evidence that self-reporting overestimates adherence, so technological advances to improve the ability to objectively measure adherence to airway clearance are a crucial first step towards improving adherence to airway clearance. SAWICKI and TIDDENS [33] have provided a tabular overview of the key barriers to optimal treatment in CF and have themed these according to whether they are patient-, clinician- or treatment-related barriers (table 4). Many of these barriers affect adherence, so targeted interventions to overcome particular barriers could help improve adherence and optimise treatments. There is emerging evidence that independent treatments can facilitate adherence, *e.g.* recommendations and self-reported patient adherence were in best agreement when PEP and flutter devices were used [34]. Supporting adherence is complex and investment is needed into the development of effective adherence interventions.

What outcome measures should be used in trials of airway clearance techniques?

Studies aiming to assess the effectiveness of airway clearance techniques are challenging due to the lack of consensus on the appropriate outcome measure to use, resulting in studies using a large number of measures, as presented in figure 2. Furthermore, many of the available measures lack the appropriate clinimetric properties (*i.e.* demonstrated validity, reliability, sensitivity and responsiveness) to be able to accurately reflect the changes resulting from airway clearance techniques [35].

A review by MARQUES *et al.* [36] examined the clinical utility of a range of outcome measures for airway clearance techniques, and concluded that no one measure currently available met the requirements of a robust outcome measure for use in trials of airway clearance techniques. A number of other important reviews in CF to date have highlighted the need for consensus on which outcome measures are best to use and emphasised the need for further evidence to assess the physiological effects of airway clearance techniques [37, 38]. Since these summaries, the clinimetric properties of a number of available measures have been further studied and a number of new tools have emerged, which could offer further data to inform the choice of outcome measures for future airway clearance technique trials.

Table 4. Overview of barriers to optimal treatment in cystic fibrosis

Patient-related	Clinician-related	Treatment-related
• Unacceptable treatment burden • Symptoms (*e.g.* depression) • Lack of adequate training, particularly during transition from paediatric to adult care • Poor understanding of concept behind treatment • Social embarrassment • Difficulty maintaining correct inhalation technique during nebulisation • Adolescent behaviour, *e.g.* denial, risk taking, difficulty communicating • Restricted peer support due to infection avoidance	• Lack of time and resources to support patients • Lack of therapies targeting the cause of CF • Lack of accurate/sensitive end-points to effectively compare treatments • Difficulty extrapolating data from clinical trials to individual patients • Lack of biomarkers to tailor treatments to individual patients	• Complex treatment regimens • Time-consuming administration • Inconvenient delivery systems, *e.g.* due to lack of portability • Drug interactions • Adverse events, toxicity • Unpleasant taste

Reproduced and modified from [33] with permission from the publisher.

Pulmonary function tests

Forced expiratory volume in 1 s (FEV1) is an important surrogate marker of disease severity, due to its link with mortality [39]. It remains the only accepted surrogate outcome measure of lung function for trials in CF by the European Medicines Agency (EMA) and the US Food and Drug Administration (FDA). FEV1 has been used as a primary outcome for many trials of airway clearance techniques in CF; however, its relevance to physiotherapy respiratory

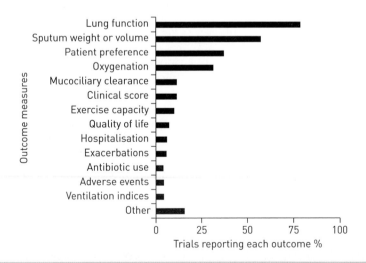

Figure 2. The proportion of randomised trials of airway clearance techniques that report specific outcome measures. The cohort of trials (n=70) were those included in six Cochrane systematic reviews of airway clearance techniques for people with cystic fibrosis [15–20].

interventions has been questioned [37]. Results from four recent trials of airway clearance techniques have highlighted the unsuitability of FEV1 as an assessment tool in this context [21, 23, 25, 40]. In many patients, the rate of FEV1 decline has slowed with improved standards of care, meaning that measuring a change becomes more difficult and greater numbers of patients are required to power a study. Furthermore, it is established that FEV1 is insufficiently sensitive to detect changes in the peripheral airways, as the smaller airways contribute little to the overall resistance to flow, highlighting that some effects of airway clearance techniques could go undetected by FEV1. For these reasons, there is consensus that FEV1 is not a suitable primary outcome measure for use in airway clearance technique trials [37].

Forced expiratory flows during the middle half of the forced vital capacity (FVC) manoeuvre (FEF25-75%) are largely effort independent [41] and provide a reflection of small airways function; however, the level of variability observed with this parameter can be unacceptably high, with reported intra-visit coefficients of variation of up to 10% and poor repeatability in children and adolescents with CF [42]. FEF25-75% is measured at a different lung volume if there are changes in FVC, so it is only valid to compare FEF25-75% measures at two time-points if FVC does not change over the same period. It also has no established clinically worthwhile threshold for change.

Exacerbations

It is frequently noted in Cochrane reviews of clinical trials in CF that a clear definition of an exacerbation is lacking as an important outcome measure. Exacerbations are irregular, acute increases in pulmonary symptoms that are probably related to a complex relationship between host defence and airway microbiology that impacts on sputum production and airflow obstruction [43]. Importantly, the frequency of acute exacerbations is predictive of survival: each acute pulmonary exacerbation within a year has a negative impact on 5-year survival equal to a 12% reduction in FEV1 [44]. Defining when an increase in pulmonary symptoms should be considered to be an exacerbation is challenging and difficult to standardise. Clinical trials are increasingly using multiple signs, symptoms and test results to provide an exacerbation score. An example is the score described by FUCHS et al. [45] in 1994, which requires at least four out of 12 items to define an exacerbation. Researchers performing trials in airway clearance techniques should use an established exacerbation definition to facilitate both comparison and meta-analysis of data across trials.

Ventilation distribution indices

Inert gas washout tests
In respiratory disease, changes in the peripheral airways result in inhomogeneous ventilation of parallel airways. Subsequent inhomogeneous emptying of these lung units on expiration causes ventilation inhomogeneity [46, 47]. This inhomogeneity of ventilation distribution is reflected as a delayed clearance of a tracer gas in a multiple-breath washout (MBW) test (fig. 3). Although a number of indices can be measured, the lung clearance index (LCI) is the most widely studied and robust index of ventilation inhomogeneity.

Lung clearance index
Research to date has demonstrated the LCI to be a reliable measure in CF. It has a narrow normal range [48–50] and greater sensitivity to abnormalities in lung function across the age ranges compared with spirometry [46, 49, 51, 52], and is feasible to carry out, requiring only relaxed tidal breathing.

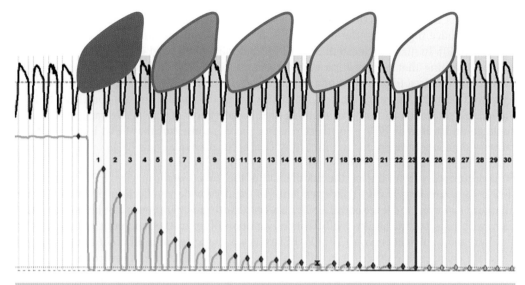

Figure 3. Clearance of a tracer gas from the lungs during a multiple-breath washout test to measure lung clearance index. Image reproduced from Simple Washout software (Nick Bell, Bristol Royal Infirmary, University Hospitals, Bristol, UK; personal communication).

LCI has been used as a primary outcome measure in clinical trials of inhaled therapies (hypertonic saline and dornase alfa) and small molecule therapies (ivacaftor) in CF, measuring significant improvements more demonstrable than those of FEV1 % predicted, with effect sizes ranging from 0.5 to 2.2 lung volume turnovers [53–56].

A small number of studies have been carried out to investigate the short-term effect of airway clearance interventions on LCI, showing no change or a variable change (increase and decrease) in LCI [57–60], highlighting that airway clearance techniques cause alterations in gas mixing that are greater than in those who do not undergo airway clearance. Airway clearance may open up previously "blocked off" areas caused by mucus plugging, or relieve areas of atelectasis, opening up poorly ventilated areas, thereby causing a rise (worsening) in LCI (fig. 4).

This evidence highlights a potential limitation of LCI as an outcome measure for airway clearance techniques, as there is potential for a bidirectional response to therapy. However, the studies to date have assessed short-term effects only and were not powered to detect effect of therapy. Further studies of the medium- to long-term effect of airway clearances techniques on LCI would be beneficial in informing physiotherapists whether there is a place for LCI as an outcome measure in airway clearance technique trials.

Guidance on equipment, procedure and protocols on inert gas washout testing has been comprehensively outlined in the recent European Respiratory Society (ERS)/American Thoracic Society (ATS) consensus document, facilitating the implementation of these tests into centres [62]. Furthermore, the literature on the clinimetric properties of LCI as an outcome measure has been summarised, demonstrating the usefulness of incorporating this measure into clinical trials in CF [63].

Single-breath washout

The single-breath washout (SBW) test requires only a single vital capacity manoeuvre and is an attractive alternative to MBW. The phase III slope of the expired inert gas during the

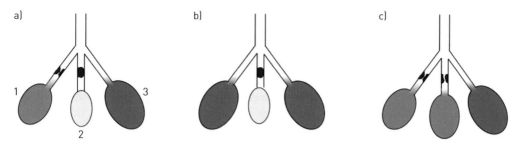

Figure 4. Possible effects of airway clearance on ventilation inhomogeneity (lung clearance index (LCI)) and functional residual capacity (FRC). a) Three lung units pre-treatment: 1) partially obstructed and poorly ventilated; 2) completely obstructed and unventilated; 3) unobstructed. b) One possible outcome of treatment of the same three lung units: the partially obstructed unit has been cleared and is now normally ventilated. This should reduce ventilation inhomogeneity (and hence LCI) and increase FRC. c) Another possible outcome of treatment: the unventilated unit has now been partially opened up and is poorly ventilated. This will therefore increase FRC, but will also increase ventilation inhomogeneity, leading to an increase in LCI. Reproduced and modified from [61] with permission.

single breath is analysed. SBW has reported utility in patients during clinical stability and acute exacerbation [64, 65]. ABBAS et al. [64] assessed the effect of routine airway clearance techniques on the phase III slope of a double tracer gas mixture of helium and sulfur hexafluoride, as obtained from a novel tidal volume SBW manoeuvre in 25 clinically stable children with CF. They demonstrated a significant decrease (improvement) in phase III double tracer gas z-scores with treatment, suggesting that airway clearance techniques improve gas mixing immediately after treatment. Therefore, SBW provides indices that show some promise as a potential outcome measure for airway clearance trials but more research on their clinimetric properties is required.

Patient-reported outcomes: symptoms and HRQoL

A patient-reported outcome (PRO) is any measure of a patient's health status obtained directly from the patient. It assesses how they feel or function with respect to their health condition, and is an important measure of the clinical efficacy of airway clearance techniques as it directly assesses benefit to the patient. Chronic cough, expectoration of sputum and breathlessness can affect how an individual functions and socialises. As airway clearance techniques aim to facilitate the clearance of sputum and reduce associated symptoms and potential impact on daily living, this effect can be evaluated. The Cystic Fibrosis Questionnaire Revised (CFQ-R) is the most widely available, validated instrument, encompassing a wide age range (patients aged $\geqslant 6$ years) and including parental perspectives [66].

Measures of expectorated sputum

Expectorated sputum can help to indicate how an airway clearance technique might work. If expectorated sputum has better rheological properties for mucociliary clearance, then presumably this is due to the applied technique, as discussed above in relation to airway clearance techniques with an oscillating component. Bacterial load can also be assessed, although if the mucus load is reduced by an effective airway clearance therapy, it may become difficult to assess bacterial load adequately. One of the most commonly used measures of expectorated sputum is its amount, measured either by volume or wet weight, which are confounded by unintentional expectoration of saliva with the sample, or dry weight, which avoids this confounding because the dry weight of saliva is negligible. Regardless of which measure of sputum amount is chosen, however, two problems remain. One is that sputum can easily be swallowed unintentionally or subconsciously, introducing error. The other is that the measure is only interpretable over a very short intervention period. If a trial involves regular use of an airway clearance therapy over months and the amount of sputum expectorated increases over time, is that a sign that the treatment is effective, or a sign that the treatment is ineffective because the underlying infection in the lung is increasing? Conversely, if the amount of sputum expectorated decreases over time, is that a sign that the treatment is becoming less effective, or a sign that the underlying infection is clearing up so the sputum load is decreasing? There is no way to know from expectorated sputum measures. The bacterial density in sputum can also be measured but it is confounded by sampling issues. If a particular airway clearance treatment works by dislodging long-impacted sputum, which is known to become a nidus for infection, the intervention may be associated with an increase in bacterial density, even if it decreases the overall bacterial load in the lungs.

To solve the confounding caused by expectorated saliva and swallowed secretions, some investigators have developed methods of radioactively labelling airway secretions so that their movement can be scanned with a gamma camera. There are complex issues involved in administering and interpreting this measure, so very few centres in the world use it. Despite this key advantage, there are several important limitations of the technique. These cannot be covered adequately in this chapter, but an excellent summary of them has been published [67].

Technegas

In addition to reducing the overall bacterial load in the lungs, the benefits of dislodging impacted or adhered airway secretions and clearing them from the airways is that airflow resistance decreases and a greater proportion of the lung can participate in gas exchange. To some extent, the indices of ventilation discussed above could capture this. However, they only provide data for the lungs as a whole; regional improvements are more difficult to localise. Another method might be able to illustrate that a region of the bronchial tree has been returned to participation in ventilation after dislodgement of secretions by an airway clearance technique. In this method, participants inhale a controlled dose of tiny (100-nm) radioactively labelled carbon particles with a maximal inhalation from functional residual capacity (FRC). These particles label all parts of the bronchial tree that are reached by the inhaled breath. Therefore, the regions of the lungs participating in gas exchange can be quantified and localised with scanning. This technique has only been used to measure regions of lung that stop participating in ventilation by inducing an asthmatic response in volunteers [68], but it would work equally well to identify re-recruitment of previously obstructed lung regions by dislodgement of secretions.

Magnetic resonance imaging of pulmonary perfusion

Although most physiotherapy interventions for airway clearance are not intended to influence pulmonary perfusion directly, measures of regional pulmonary perfusion caused by hypoxic vasoconstriction can be used as an indirect marker of impaired regional ventilation and may thus serve as a sensitive outcome measure for airway mucus plugging [69]. Automated assessment can provide percentage-based estimates of the severity of regional perfusion defects, particularly for early and subtle functional impairment [69]. This form of assessment has been incorporated into an automated magnetic resonance scoring system that is reproducible and applicable for semi-quantitative evaluation of a large spectrum of CF lung disease severity.

Mucoactive medications

Dornase alfa

The enzyme recombinant human DNase (dornase alfa), has been shown to reduce the viscosity of sputum taken from people with CF by digesting the DNA released from neutrophils [70]. Although radio-aerosol studies have not shown a significant increase in mucociliary clearance from dornase alfa, regular use over a 1-, 6- or 12-month period is associated with an improvement in lung function in CF [71]. Long-term use is also associated with a significant reduction in pulmonary exacerbations and an improvement in HRQoL [71]. Dornase alfa is expensive, requires refrigeration during storage, and requires nebulised delivery.

Hypertonic saline

In CF, hypertonic saline of a concentration of 3% or higher is generally used. When inhaled as an aerosol, hypertonic saline increases the osmotic pressure of the ASL above isotonicity, creating an osmotic gradient that draws water into the airway, restoring the ASL and re-establishing the ciliary clearance action [4]. However, hypertonic saline has several other mechanisms of action: reducing *Pseudomonas aeruginosa* motility [72] and viability [73]; improving bactericidal efficiency of some peptides [74]; and disrupting established bacterial biofilms and inhibiting formation of new ones [75]. Hypertonic saline accelerates mucociliary clearance immediately [76] and for at least 8 h after dosing with regular use [77]. Premedication with bronchodilators is recommended, as hypertonic saline can induce transient airway narrowing in some patients. Regular use of hypertonic saline improves lung function within 2 weeks [78] and a significant benefit is maintained while the nebulisations are continued [79]. Hypertonic saline also markedly reduces exacerbations, lessens the severity of CF-related symptoms and significantly improves HRQoL [79]. Hypertonic saline is available at a low cost, does not require refrigeration, and is delivered by nebuliser.

Mannitol

Mannitol is a naturally occurring non-ionic sugar alcohol that is available in 40-mg capsules. It is inhaled with a close to full inspiration, with an inspiratory flow above normal (45–60 L·min^{-1} or more), followed by a breath hold of 5 s. The standard dose of 400 mg therefore requires 10 capsules to be inhaled sequentially. Mannitol is a powerful trigger of asthma so a bronchodilator should be inhaled before the series of 10 capsules is commenced. Mannitol shares the osmotic action of hypertonic saline and has been shown to improve mucociliary clearance [80]. Regular use of mannitol improves lung function substantially, but despite this, mannitol did not improve the HRQoL of people with CF [81, 82]. The pooled effect on exacerbations is disappointing, with no significant effect on exacerbation frequency. The confidence interval around the reduction in exacerbation risk ranged from clinically worthwhile to clinically trivial [83], so it is unclear whether any worthwhile effect on exacerbations exists. However, mannitol does not need a nebuliser or fridge and uses a weekly disposable device, which potentially reduces cross-infection issues, so some patients may consider the reduced range of benefits outweighed by the greater convenience. Cost to the healthcare system and eligibility should also be considerations. For example, mannitol dry powder for inhalation is recommended by the UK National Institute for Health and Care Excellence (NICE) for those who cannot use dornase alfa because of ineligibility, intolerance or inadequate response to dornase alfa, whose lung function is rapidly declining (FEV1 decline greater than 2% annually) and for whom other osmotic agents are not considered appropriate [84].

Interactions between mucoactive medications and airway clearance techniques

Timing of hypertonic saline and airway clearance techniques

A recent Cochrane review described several theoretical rationales as to why alternatives to the traditional order of hypertonic saline inhalation before airway clearance techniques could influence the clinical effect [85]. Inhalation of the hypertonic saline during airway clearance could save time and may make the most of the immediate peak in the ASL volume caused by the osmotic effect. Inhalation after airway clearance techniques may take advantage of the reduction in airway obstruction by mucus and therefore allow delivery of the saline to a larger surface area in the lung. One randomised trial involving 50 adult CF patients assessed the change in lung function (FEV1 % predicted) and perceived effectiveness and satisfaction of three treatment regimens (hypertonic saline before, during and after airway clearance techniques) at the end of a hospital admission [86]. In the study for inhalation of hypertonic saline during airway clearance techniques, patients alternated between the nebuliser and the airway clearance technique (which was PEP). The study found that effects on lung function were nonsignificant. Satisfaction was rated significantly worse when hypertonic saline was inhaled after airway clearance techniques compared to before or during airway clearance techniques. Perceived effectiveness of treatment showed similar effects. The authors concluded that patients could be encouraged to inhale hypertonic saline before or during airway clearance techniques to maximise perceived satisfaction and efficacy.

Timing of dornase alfa and airway clearance techniques

Four trials of dornase alfa administration before *versus* after physiotherapy techniques for airway clearance have been performed in people with CF [87]. The duration of the studies varied from 2 to 8 weeks. Inhalation after instead of before airway clearance did not significantly change FEV1, FVC, FEF25-75%, HRQoL or most other secondary outcomes. Another small airways measure, forced expiratory flow at 25% of FVC (FEF25%), was significantly worse with dornase alfa inhalation after airway clearance. However, this was based on data from two small studies and the effect was only identified in children with well-preserved lung function [87]. In addition, FEF25% has high variability, the studies had variable follow-up, and the effect was not reflected in the FEF25-75% measure of small airway function. Therefore, most people with CF could take dornase alfa before or after airway clearance techniques. In one additional trial, morning *versus* evening inhalation had no impact on lung function or symptoms [88].

For most people with CF, the majority of evidence indicates that the effectiveness of dornase alfa is not influenced by when it is administered with respect to airway clearance or time of day. Therefore, the timing of dornase alfa inhalation can be largely based on pragmatic reasons (such as fitting around other medications in the airway clearance regimen) or individual preference. However, for children with well-preserved lung function, who are unlikely to be on other medications, inhalation before airway clearance could be recommended as it may be more beneficial for small airway function.

Timing of other medications

Although based on clinical reasoning alone, it is widely agreed that bronchodilators should precede other medications so that the deposition of other medications might be maximised and as protection against any airway narrowing induced by other medications. Inhaled steroids and antibiotics are generally given last, so that their deposition is maximised and so that they are not cleared by the airway clearance techniques.

Adherence to inhaled medications

The median number of daily treatments prescribed for patients with CF is seven [1]. Studies have consistently shown that ≤50% of patients are taking <40% of prescribed inhaled medications, leading to hospitalisation for rescue treatment. A CF consensus report in 2012 identified adherence as the number one research priority; however, development of strategies to assess and improve adherence is challenging [35]. Traditionally, most reports of adherence to inhaled medications have been based on self-reporting, which is known to overestimate actual adherence. New nebuliser technologies, such as adaptive aerosol delivery devices, allow clinicians and patients to get feedback on the treatment time, duration and dose completion, which can be used to provide accurate and detailed longitudinal adherence data. Using this technology, DANIELS et al. [89] have shown a wide discrepancy between median self-reported adherence of 80% (interquartile range (IQR) 60–95%) and actual downloaded adherence of 36% (IQR 5–84.5%). Technology is also being developed to chip other nebuliser devices such as eFlow (PARI Medical Ltd, West Byfleet, UK) and inhalers. These technologies make the time and date of each treatment visible, allowing accurate assessment of adherence and facilitating feedback to the patient. In the future they will facilitate the assessment of the efficacy of adherence interventions and they could also be used to provide patients with electronic feedback on their adherence.

Conclusion

Airway clearance incorporating mucoactive medications is an important but burdensome aspect of CF treatment and adherence is poor. Research has been unable to provide clear evidence of efficacy of one airway clearance technique over another. This is in part due to limitations in the study designs used to assess the effects of the techniques. Future research needs to ensure the appropriate choice of outcome measures. Short-term studies aiming to assess physiological effect may be better using ventilation indices, mucociliary clearance indices or expiratory flows. Outcomes of HRQoL, lung volumes and pulmonary exacerbation rates may be more appropriate for longer term trials.

References

1. Rand S, Hill L, Prasad SA. Physiotherapy in cystic fibrosis: optimising techniques to improve outcomes. *Paediatr Respir Rev* 2013; 14: 263–269.

2. Strickland SL, Rubin BK, Drescher GS, *et al.* AARC clinical practice guideline: effectiveness of nonpharmacologic airway clearance therapies in hospitalized patients. *Respir Care* 2013; 58: 2187–2193.

3. Treacy K, Tunney M, Elborn JS, *et al.* Mucociliary clearance in cystic fibrosis: physiology and pharmacological treatments. *Paediatr Child Health* 2011; 21: 425–430.

4. Button B, Cai LH, Ehre C, *et al.* A periciliary brush promotes the lung health by separating the mucus layer from airway epithelia. *Science* 2012; 337: 937–941.

5. Pezzulo AA, Tang XX, Hoegger MJ, *et al.* Reduced airway surface pH impairs bacterial killing in the porcine cystic fibrosis lung. *Nature* 2012; 487: 109–113.

6. Elizur A, Cannon CL, Ferkol TW. Airway inflammation in cystic fibrosis. *Chest* 2008; 133: 489–495.

7. Cohen-Cymberknoh M, Kerem E, Ferkol T, *et al.* Airway inflammation in cystic fibrosis: molecular mechanisms and clinical implications. *Thorax* 2013; 68: 1157–1162.

8. Hilliard TN, Regamey N, Shute JK, *et al.* Airway remodelling in children with cystic fibrosis. *Thorax* 2007; 62: 1074–1080.

9. Rogers D, Doull IJM. Physiological principles of airway clearance techniques used in the physiotherapy management of cystic fibrosis. *Curr Paediatr* 2005; 15: 233–238.

10. Pryor JA, Webber BA, Hodson ME, *et al.* Evaluation of the forced expiration technique as an adjunct to postural drainage in treatment of cystic fibrosis. *Br Med J* 1979; 2: 417–418.

11. Tarran R, Button B, Picher M, *et al.* Normal and cystic fibrosis airway surface liquid homeostasis. The effects of phasic shear stress and viral infections. *J Biol Chem* 2005; 280: 35751–35759.

12. Sanderson MJ, Chow I, Dirksen ER. Intercellular communication between ciliated cells in culture. *Am J Physiol* 1988; 254: C63–C74.

13. Sanderson MJ, Charles AC, Dirksen ER. Mechanical stimulation and intercellular communication increases intracellular Ca^{2+} in epithelial cells. *Cell Regul* 1990; 1: 585–596.

14. McCarren B, Alison JA. Physiological effects of vibration in subjects with cystic fibrosis. *Eur Respir J* 2006; 27: 1204–1209.

15. Morrison L, Agnew J. Oscillating devices for airway clearance in people with cystic fibrosis. *Cochrane Database Syst Rev* 2009; 1: CD006842.

16. McKoy NA, Saldanha IJ, Odelola OA, *et al.* Active cycle of breathing technique for cystic fibrosis. *Cochrane Database Syst Rev* 2012; 12: CD007862.

17. Warnock L, Gates A, van der Schans CP. Chest physiotherapy compared to no chest physiotherapy for cystic fibrosis. *Cochrane Database Syst Rev* 2013; 9: CD001401.

18. Elkins MR, Jones A, van der Schans CP. Positive expiratory pressure physiotherapy for airway clearance in people with cystic fibrosis. *Cochrane Database Syst Rev* 2006; 2: CD003147.

19. Main E, Prasad A, van der Schans CP. Conventional chest physiotherapy compared to other airway clearance techniques for cystic fibrosis. *Cochrane Database Syst Rev* 2005; 1: CD002011.

20. Moran F, Bradley JM, Piper AJ. Non-invasive ventilation for cystic fibrosis. *Cochrane Database Syst Rev* 2013; 4: CD002769.

21. McIlwaine MP, Alarie N, Davidson GF, *et al.* Long-term multicentre randomised controlled study of high frequency chest wall oscillation *versus* positive expiratory pressure mask in cystic fibrosis. *Thorax* 2013; 68: 746–751.

22. Moseley AM, Herbert RD, Maher CG, *et al.* Reported quality of randomized controlled trials of physiotherapy interventions has improved over time. *J Clin Epidemiol* 2011; 64: 594–601.

23. Sontag MK, Quittner AL, Modi AC, *et al.* Lessons learned from a randomized trial of airway secretion clearance techniques in cystic fibrosis. *Pediatr Pulmonol* 2010; 45: 291–300.

24. Main E. What is the best airway clearance technique in cystic fibrosis? *Paediatr Respir Rev* 2013; 14: Suppl. 1, 10–12.

25. Pryor JA, Tannenbaum E, Scott SF, *et al.* Beyond postural drainage and percussion: airway clearance in people with cystic fibrosis. *J Cyst Fibros* 2010; 9: 187–192.

26. Rücker G. A two-stage trial design for testing treatment, self-selection and treatment preference effects. *Stat Med* 1989; 8: 477–485.

27. McIlwaine MP, Agnew JL, Black C. Use of airway clearance techniques in cystic fibrosis clinics in Canada. *Pediatr Pulmonol* 2008; 43: Suppl. S31, 392–393.

28. Sawicki GS, Sellers DE, Robinson WM. High treatment burden in adults with cystic fibrosis: challenges to disease self-management. *J Cyst Fibros* 2009; 8: 91–96.

29. Modi AC, Quittner AL. Barriers to treatment adherence for children with cystic fibrosis and asthma: what gets in the way? *J Pediatr Psychol* 2006; 31: 846–858.

30. White T, Miller J, Smith GL, *et al.* Adherence and psychopathology in children and adolescents with cystic fibrosis. *Eur Child Adolesc Psychiatry* 2009; 18: 96–104.

31. Myers LB, Horn SA. Adherence to chest physiotherapy in adults with cystic fibrosis. *J Health Psychol* 2006; 11: 915–926.

32. Modi AC, Cassedy AE, Quittner AL, *et al.* Trajectories of adherence to airway clearance therapy for patients with cystic fibrosis. *J Pediatr Psychol* 2010; 35: 1028–1037.

33. Sawicki GS, Tiddens H. Managing treatment complexity in cystic fibrosis: challenges and opportunities. *Pediatr Pulmonol* 2012; 47: 523–533.

34. Flores JS, Teixeira FA, Rovedder PM, *et al.* Adherence to airway clearance therapies by adult cystic fibrosis patients. *Respir Care* 2013; 58: 279–285.

35. Bradley JM, Madge S, Morton AM, *et al.* Cystic fibrosis research in allied health and nursing professions. *J Cyst Fibros* 2012; 11: 387–392.

36. Marques A, Bruton A, Barney A. Clinically useful outcome measures for physiotherapy airway clearance techniques: a review. *Phys Ther Rev* 2006; 11: 299–307.

37. Main E. Airway clearance research in CF: the "perfect storm" of strong preference and effortful participation in long-term, non-blinded studies. *Thorax* 2013; 68: 701–702.

38. McIlwaine M. Chest physical therapy, breathing techniques and exercise in children with CF. *Paediatr Respir Rev* 2007; 8: 8–16.

39. Kerem E, Reisman J, Corey M, *et al.* Prediction of mortality in patients with cystic fibrosis. *N Engl J Med* 1992; 326: 1187–1191.

40. McIlwaine M, Wong LT, Chilvers M, *et al.* Long-term comparative trial of two different physiotherapy techniques; postural drainage with percussion and autogenic drainage, in the treatment of cystic fibrosis. *Pediatr Pulmonol* 2010; 45: 1064–1069.

41. Bakker EM, Borsboom GJ, van der Wiel-Kooij EC, *et al.* Small airway involvement in cystic fibrosis lung disease: routine spirometry as an early and sensitive marker. *Pediatr Pulmonol* 2013; 48: 1081–1088.

42. Sanders DB, Rosenfeld M, Mayer-Hamblett N, *et al.* Reproducibility of spirometry during cystic fibrosis pulmonary exacerbations. *Pediatr Pulmonol* 2008; 43: 1142–1146.

43. Flume PA, Mogayzel PJ Jr, Robinson KA, *et al.* Cystic fibrosis pulmonary guidelines: treatment of pulmonary exacerbations. *Am J Respir Crit Care Med* 2009; 180: 802–808.

44. Liou TG, Adler FR, FitzSimmons SC, *et al.* Predictive 5-year survivorship model of cystic fibrosis. *Am J Epidemiol* 2001; 153: 345–352.

45. Fuchs HJ, Borowitz DS, Christiansen DH, *et al.* Effect of aerosolized recombinant human DNase on exacerbations of respiratory symptoms and on pulmonary function in patients with cystic fibrosis. The Pulmozyme Study Group. *N Engl J Med* 1994; 331: 637–642.

46. Gustafsson PM, Aurora P, Lindblad A. Evaluation of ventilation maldistribution as an early indicator of lung disease in children with cystic fibrosis. *Eur Respir J* 2003; 22: 972–979.

47. Robinson PD, Goldman MD, Gustafsson PM. Inert gas washout: theoretical background and clinical utility in respiratory disease. *Respiration* 2009; 78: 339–355.

48. Aurora P, Gustafsson P, Bush A, *et al.* Multiple breath inert gas washout as a measure of ventilation distribution in children with cystic fibrosis. *Thorax* 2004; 59: 1068–1073.

49. Horsley AR, Gustafsson PM, Macleod KA, *et al.* Lung clearance index is a sensitive, repeatable and practical measure of airways disease in adults with cystic fibrosis. *Thorax* 2008; 63: 135–140.

50. Fuchs SI, Eder J, Ellemunter H, *et al.* Lung clearance index: normal values, repeatability, and reproducibility in healthy children and adolescents. *Pediatr Pulmonol* 2009; 44: 1180–1185.

51. Aurora P, Bush A, Gustafsson P, *et al.* Multiple-breath washout as a marker of lung disease in preschool children with cystic fibrosis. *Am J Respir Crit Care Med* 2005; 171: 249–256.

52. Lum S, Gustafsson P, Ljungberg H, *et al.* Early detection of cystic fibrosis lung disease: multiple-breath washout *versus* raised volume tests. *Thorax* 2007; 62: 341–347.

53. Amin R, Subbarao P, Jabar A, *et al.* Hypertonic saline improves the LCI in paediatric patients with CF with normal lung function. *Thorax* 2010; 65: 379–383.

54. Subbarao P, Stanojevic S, Brown M, *et al.* Lung clearance index as an outcome measure for clinical trials in young children with cystic fibrosis. A pilot study using inhaled hypertonic saline. *Am J Respir Crit Care Med* 2013; 188: 456–460.

55. Amin R, Subbarao P, Lou W, *et al.* The effect of dornase alfa on ventilation inhomogeneity in patients with cystic fibrosis. *Eur Respir J* 2011; 37: 806–812.

56. Davies J, Sheridan H, Bell N, *et al.* Assessment of clinical response to ivacaftor with lung clearance index in cystic fibrosis patients with a G551D-CFTR mutation and preserved spirometry: a randomised controlled trial. *Lancet Respir Med* 2013; 1: 630–638.

57. Mentore K, Froh DK, de Lange EE, *et al.* Hyperpolarized HHe 3 MRI of the lung in cystic fibrosis: assessment at baseline and after bronchodilator and airway clearance treatment. *Acad Radiol* 2005; 12: 1423–1429.

58. Main E, Tannenbaum E, Aurora P, *et al.* Evaluation of lung clearance index as an outcome measure for airway clearance intervention studies. *J Cyst Fibros* 2004; 3: Suppl. 1, A334.

59. Main E, Tannenbaum E, Stanojevic S, *et al.* The effects of positive expiratory pressure or oscillatory positive pressure on FEV1 and lung clearance index over a twelve month period in children with cystic fibrosis. *Paediatr Pulmonol* 2006; 41: Suppl. S29, 351.

60. Fuchs SI, Toussaint S, Edlhaimb B, *et al.* Short-term effect of physiotherapy on variability of the lung clearance index in children with cystic fibrosis. *Pediatr Pulmonol* 2010; 45: 301–306.

61. Horsley A. Non-invasive assessment of ventilation maldistribution in lung disease using multiple breath inert gas washouts. PhD thesis. Edinburgh University, 2009.

62. Robinson PD, Latzin P, Verbanck S, *et al.* Consensus statement for inert gas washout measurement using multiple- and single-breath tests. *Eur Respir J* 2013; 41: 507–522.

63. Kent L, Reix P, Innes JA, *et al.* Lung clearance index: evidence for use in clinical trials in cystic fibrosis. *J Cyst Fibros* 2014; 13: 123–138.

64. Abbas C, Singer F, Yammine S, *et al.* Treatment response of airway clearance assessed by single-breath washout in children with cystic fibrosis. *J Cyst Fibros* 2013; 12: 567–574.

65. Gozal D, Bailey SL, Keens TG. Evolution of pulmonary function during an acute exacerbation in hospitalized patients with cystic fibrosis. *Pediatr Pulmonol* 1993; 16: 347–353.

66. Quittner AL, Buu A, Messer MA, *et al.* Development and validation of The Cystic Fibrosis Questionnaire in the United States: a health-related quality-of-life measure for cystic fibrosis. *Chest* 2005; 128: 2347–2354.

67. Robinson M, Bye PT. Mucociliary clearance in cystic fibrosis. *Pediatr Pulmonol* 2002; 33: 293–306.

68. Farrow CE, Salome CM, Harris BE, *et al.* Airway closure on imaging relates to airway hyperresponsiveness and peripheral airway disease in asthma. *J Appl Physiol* 2012; 113: 958–966.

69. Bauman G, Puderbach M, Heimann T, *et al.* Validation of Fourier decomposition MRI with dynamic contrast-enhanced MRI using visual and automated scoring of pulmonary perfusion in young cystic fibrosis patients. *Eur J Radiol* 2013; 82: 2371–2377.

70. Lieberman J. Dornase aerosol effect on sputum viscosity in cases of cystic fibrosis. *JAMA* 1968; 205: 312–313.

71. Jones AP, Wallis C. Dornase alfa for cystic fibrosis. *Cochrane Database Syst Rev* 2010; 3: CD001127.

72. Havasi V, Hurst CO, Briles TC, *et al.* Inhibitory effects of hypertonic saline on *P. aeruginosa* motility. *J Cyst Fibros* 2008; 7: 267–269.

73. Behrends V, Ryall B, Wang X, *et al.* Metabolic profiling of *Pseudomonas aeruginosa* demonstrates that the anti-sigma factor MucA modulates osmotic stress tolerance. *Mol Biosyst* 2010; 6: 562–569.

74. Bergsson G, Reeves EP, McNally P, *et al.* LL-37 complexation with glycosaminoglycans in cystic fibrosis lungs inhibits antimicrobial activity, which can be restored by hypertonic saline. *J Immunol* 2009; 183: 543–551.

75. Anderson GG, O'Toole GA. Innate and induced resistance mechanisms of bacterial biofilms. *Curr Top Microbiol Immunol* 2008; 322: 85–105.

76. Robinson M, Hemming AL, Regnis JA, *et al.* Effect of increasing doses of hypertonic saline on mucociliary clearance in patients with cystic fibrosis. *Thorax* 1997; 52: 900–903.

77. Donaldson SH, Bennett WD, Zeman KL, *et al.* Mucus clearance and lung function in cystic fibrosis with hypertonic saline. *N Engl J Med* 2006; 354: 241–250.

78. Eng PA, Morton J, Douglass JA, *et al.* Short-term efficacy of ultrasonically nebulized hypertonic saline in cystic fibrosis. *Pediatr Pulmonol* 1996; 21: 77–83.

79. Elkins MR, Robinson M, Rose BR, *et al.* A controlled trial of long-term inhaled hypertonic saline in patients with cystic fibrosis. *N Engl J Med* 2006; 354: 229–240.

80. Robinson M, Daviskas E, Eberl S, *et al.* The effect of inhaled mannitol on bronchial mucus clearance in cystic fibrosis patients: a pilot study. *Eur Respir J* 1999; 14: 678–685.

81. Aitken ML, Bellon G, De Boeck K, *et al.* Long-term inhaled dry powder mannitol in cystic fibrosis: an international randomized study. *Am J Respir Crit Care Med* 2012; 185: 645–652.

82. Bilton D, Robinson P, Cooper P, *et al.* Inhaled dry powder mannitol in cystic fibrosis: an efficacy and safety study. *Eur Respir J* 2011; 38: 1071–1080.

83. Bilton D, Bellon G, Charlton B, *et al.* Pooled analysis of two large randomised phase III inhaled mannitol studies in cystic fibrosis. *J Cyst Fibros* 2013; 12: 367–376.

84. Mannitol dry powder for inhalation for cystic fibrosis. Manchester, National Institute for Health and Clinical Excellence, 2012.

85. Elkins M, Dentice R. Timing of hypertonic saline inhalation for cystic fibrosis. *Cochrane Database Syst Rev* 2012; 2: CD008816.

86. Dentice RL, Elkins MR, Bye PT. Adults with cystic fibrosis prefer hypertonic saline before or during airway clearance techniques: a randomised crossover trial. *J Physiother* 2012; 58: 33–40.

87. Dentice R, Elkins M. Timing of dornase alfa inhalation for cystic fibrosis. *Cochrane Database Syst Rev* 2011; 5: CD007923.

88. van der Giessen LJ, Gosselink R, Hop WC, *et al.* Recombinant human DNase nebulisation in children with cystic fibrosis: before bedtime or after waking up? *Eur Respir J* 2007; 30: 763–768.

89. Daniels T, Goodacre L, Sutton C, *et al.* Accurate assessment of adherence: self-report and clinician report *vs* electronic monitoring of nebulizers. *Chest* 2011; 140: 425–432.

Disclosures: None declared.

Chapter 13

Antibiotic treatment of cystic fibrosis lung disease

Christopher Orchard and Diana Bilton

Cystic fibrosis (CF) is a complex multisystem genetic disorder, with the major burden of morbidity and mortality resulting from destructive pulmonary disease associated with chronic airway infections. Successful treatment of pulmonary infections is one of the major reasons for improved life expectancy. In the past decades, we have embraced the principles of early treatment of infection and successful eradication regimens aimed at reducing the number of patients with chronic *Pseudomonas aeruginosa* infection.

In this chapter, we discuss current strategies and possible future developments for management of airway infection, focusing mainly on *P. aeruginosa* as the most prevalent pathogen. The principles of antibiotic therapy derived from treating *P. aeruginosa* infection are discussed with regard to other pathogens.

Most people with cystic fibrosis (CF) die from respiratory failure, which is a consequence of progressive lung damage resulting from chronic airway infection and inflammation. The airways of people with CF are susceptible to initial infection by organisms that are acquired from the environment and not adequately cleared. The range of microorganisms causing infection is quite distinct in CF, with *Staphylococcus aureus* being a common childhood infection and *Pseudomonas aeruginosa* becoming the dominant pathogen as patients move into adulthood (fig. 1) [1].

Currently, antibiotic therapy is focussed on treating the bacteria that are present in standard microbiological cultures. In the future, different strategies may be adopted as we begin to understand the role of the multiple bacterial species now recognised on molecular testing (discussed elsewhere in this *Monograph* [2]) (not shown in fig. 1), most particularly anaerobes such as *Prevotella* spp. Further studies examining the benefits of treating bacteria revealed by molecular tests alone are urgently required. In this chapter, we examine the evidence regarding treatment of bacteria in the CF patient. Where there are no randomised studies, we comment on consensus documents and clinical expertise. Treating CF lung infections can represent a complex challenge for a physician used to treating acute pneumonia, for example, or a single-organism blood infection. It is important to remember that infections in the airway can be in a biofilm growth and that there may be more than one organism present on culture, and we do not have, as yet, a good way of measuring in a patient whether one bacterial species may be suppressing or facilitating growth of another species.

Dept of Adult CF, Royal Brompton Hospital, London, UK.

Correspondence: Diana Bilton, Dept of Adult CF, Royal Brompton Hospital, Sydney Street, London, SW3 6NP, UK.
E-mail: d.bilton@rbht.nhs.uk

Copyright ERS 2014. Print ISBN: 978-1-84984-050-7. Online ISBN: 978-1-84984-051-4. Print ISSN: 2312-508X. Online ISSN: 2312-5098.

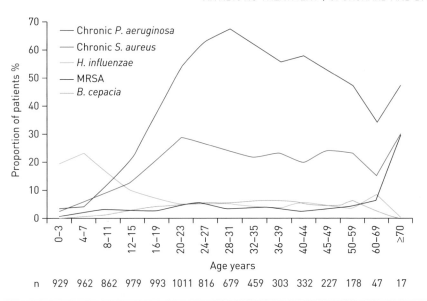

Figure 1. UK Cystic Fibrosis Registry 2012 data for chronic *Pseudomonas aeruginosa* (n=3041, 35.5%), chronic *Staphylococcus aureus* (n=1454, 17.1%), *Haemophilus influenzae* (n=899, 10.2%), methicillin-resistant *S. aureus* (MRSA) (n=286, 3.3%) and *Burkholderia cepacia* (n=306, 3.5%). Reproduced and modified from [1] with permission from the publisher.

Although we have evidence for some of what is recommended and trials to guide broad approaches, there remains much work to do in developing the optimum treatment approach for each patient. Thus, at times, CF physicians have to choose antibiotics knowing that a sputum culture and susceptibility result, which has been the holy grail of infectious disease training, will not predict a clinical response to treatment. In antibiotic trials in chronic airway infection in CF, the end-points that determine success or failure of a particular antibiotic regimen, namely lung function and time to next exacerbation, are not directly correlated to a change in bacterial numbers.

The study by AARON *et al.* [3], where patients were randomised to receive therapy based on synergy tests *versus* physician clinical choice with no difference in outcome, ably demonstrates the problem of CF airway infections remaining a conundrum for the microbiology laboratories in terms of determining best antibiotic choice. The complexities of multiple species growing in a biofilm, antibiotic effects on virulence factors (*i.e.* non-killing effects) and the possibilities of one species suppressing or facilitating another all explain the absence of correlation between laboratory predictions and clinical response. Thus, clinicians need to continue to practice an art of treating infections in CF while scientists continue to unravel these complexities.

In each of the following sections, we will provide information on what is known about treating a specific bacterial species in CF but highlight some of the discussions around the approaches recommended. In addition, it is important to recognise that patients may harbour mixtures of these species on standard culture, so the different approaches recommended may need to be adapted and rationalised.

Antibiotic strategies for *S. aureus*

S. aureus was one of the first bacteria to be detected in infants and children with CF and is a common cause of early airway infection [1]. The impact of *S. aureus* in the CF airway continues to be debated. It is recognised that there may be an increase in symptoms but less evidence of decline in lung function despite an inflammatory response to the infection. The presence of S. aureus in airway secretions from children with CF has prompted clinicians to consider the use of prophylactic antibiotics to prevent and control staphylococcal infection [4, 5]. Though the evidence in support of clinical improvements is weak, one randomised study in infants demonstrated that continuous flucloxacillin reduced the number of hospital admissions and additional courses of antibiotics [4]. The practice has remained controversial as a clinical trial of cephalexin, a more broad-spectrum antibiotic, which did not demonstrate any clinical efficacy, demonstrated an increase in the frequency of new infections with P. aeruginosa [6]. In addition, a German registry study confirmed that while continuous antistaphylococcal therapy may reduce the number of positive S. aureus cultures, there was an associated increase in P. aeruginosa cultures [7].

A Cochrane review of S. aureus prophylaxis concluded that antistaphylococcal prophylaxis with a narrow-spectrum antibiotic such as flucloxacillin is effective at reducing infection with S. aureus [5]. With this narrow-spectrum regimen, there has been no definitive evidence that there is an increase in the incidence of P. aeruginosa, but further studies are recommended. Registry data will play a part in examining the evidence and determining the best approach. This debate highlights the potential for complications of antibiotic therapy in CF. Successful treatment of one pathogen may facilitate emergence of another organism, which may require further therapy.

P. aeruginosa eradication

Registry data demonstrate that more than 60% of people with CF become chronically infected with P. aeruginosa by the third decade in life (fig. 1) [1, 8]. There is international consensus and compelling rationale that P. aeruginosa infection should be treated aggressively, as this infection is associated with more rapid decline in lung function, worsening quality of life (QoL) and decreased survival [9]. Thus, interventions to prevent chronic infection by treating and eradicating first or early isolates are worthwhile. The Copenhagen group first introduced the practice of treatment on first isolation, and reported success of eradication of P. aeruginosa using a combination of inhaled colistimethate sodium and oral ciprofloxacin [10]. Subsequently, the approach of regular surveillance of respiratory samples facilitating strict segregation to prevent cross-infection, combined with antibiotic treatment from the first isolate of P. aeruginosa, has been associated with reduction of the prevalence of chronic P. aeruginosa infection. Recent registry data from the UK demonstrate this changing prevalence in young adults with CF (fig. 2).

A variety of regimens have been studied and found to be effective in eradicating P. aeruginosa, and these are discussed in the following sections. Eradication therapy is now a recommended part of most guidelines for the treatment of new or repeated infection with P. aeruginosa, but it is clearly acknowledged that no particular regimen has superiority over another [9].

Oral ciprofloxacin and nebulised colistimethate sodium

This combination of antibiotics has been used in Europe for many years. VALERIUS et al. [10] documented the efficacy of twice-daily oral ciprofloxacin and nebulised colistimethate sodium for 3 weeks. Further experience showed more effective eradication of P. aeruginosa when the duration of treatment was increased to 3 months and the frequency of nebulised colomycin dosage to three times daily. After 3.5 years, only 16% of treated patients had developed chronic P. aeruginosa infection in comparison to 72% of untreated historical controls [11].

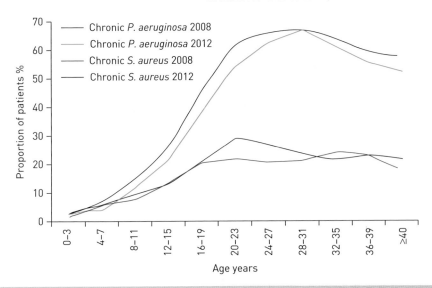

Figure 2. UK Cystic Fibrosis Registry 2012 data comparing chronic *Pseudomonas aeruginosa* and chronic *Staphylococcus aureus* infections between 2008 with 2012 among young adults, aged 16–19 years and 20–23 years. This demonstrates a statistically significant reduction in the proportion of patients chronically infected with *P. aeruginosa* between 2008 and 2012 for young adults aged 16–19 years (p=0.004) and 20–23 years (p=0.014). Reproduced and modified from [1] with permission from the publisher.

Nebulised tobramycin

Eradication of *P. aeruginosa* with tobramycin was first suggested in 2001 [12] and a subsequent randomised study showed effective eradication of early infection with tobramycin solution for inhalation of 300 mg twice daily for 28 days [13]. The ELITE (Early Inhaled Tobramycin for Eradication) trial compared the efficacy of a 28-day regime of tobramycin for inhalation *versus* a 56-day regime and found no difference between the regimes [14]. Two recent studies [15, 16] have shown no difference between nebulised colistimethate sodium and tobramycin for eradication purposes.

Intravenous eradication

Intravenous eradication of *P. aeruginosa,* most often with a combination of ceftazidime and tobramycin, is a relatively commonly used approach, particularly if the patient is unwell, with symptoms at the time of the first isolate. There are no trials, however, demonstrating that this is more effective than nebulised therapies. There is currently an on-going multicentre randomised trial (TORPEDO-CF, ISRCTN02734162) comparing 14 days of ceftazidime/tobramycin with 3 months of oral ciprofloxacin; both groups receive nebulised colistimethate sodium.

Chronic suppressive antibiotic therapy for *P. aeruginosa*

Inhaled therapy

Inhaled antibiotics are recommended in guidelines for use in chronic *P. aeruginosa* infection because large randomised trials have demonstrated a positive effect on bacterial load, lung function, QoL and frequency of pulmonary exacerbations [9].

Tobramycin

Tobramycin for inhaled use was first licenced in the form Tobi (Novartis, Basel, Switzerland) in 1998 for use in patients chronically infected with *P. aeruginosa*. Large randomised controlled trials (RCTs) demonstrated improvement in forced expiratory volume in 1 s (FEV1), decrease in *P. aeruginosa* colony-forming units and decrease in hospitalisations [17]. Tobi was well tolerated with limited side-effects. Despite high peak sputum levels of tobramycin, almost all 10 times greater than the minimum inhibitory concentration (MIC) of the organisms present, there was minimal systemic absorption.

Tobi is nebulised twice daily by jet nebuliser. This takes between 15 and 20 min per treatment, and the equipment then needs to be cleaned and sterilised. A newer formulation, Bramitob (Chiesi, Parma, Italy), was introduced in 2003, which is a 75-mg·mL^{-1}, 300-mg formulation. This was shown to be well tolerated and reduced treatment time *via* the LC Plus nebuliser (Pari, Starnberg, Germany) to around 12 min. Subsequently, patient demand has required clinicians to move to use both agents through nebulisers with vibrating mesh technology, which only take 5 min or less to administer the required dose.

More recently, tobramycin inhalation powder (TOBI Podhaler) has been developed by Novartis, and removes the need for nebulisation with an aim to reduce the time required for treatment and, therefore, increase adherence. The dry-powder inhaler is more efficiently delivered to the lung, allowing the equivalent dosage to be given in a four-capsule (112 mg) dose in roughly 5 min without the need for nebulisation or cleaning of the delivery device.

Two phase III trials of the TOBI Podhaler have been carried out. The first, the EVOLVE trial, showed significant improvement in FEV1, sputum *P. aeruginosa* density, respiratory-related hospitalisation and antipseudomonal antibiotic use [18]. The second, EAGER, comparing tobramycin solution for nebulisation *versus* the dry-powder inhaler showed comparable efficacy, but higher rates of patient satisfaction with the dry-powder inhaler [19].

Colistimethate sodium

Colistimethate sodium is a polymyxin antibiotic. It has been used for many years, throughout Europe as a treatment for chronic *P. aeruginosa* infection. However, there have been limited RCTs to confirm efficacy. The only placebo-controlled study was a small one that showed significant improvement in forced vital capacity (FVC) and a symptom score but only provided maintenance of FEV1 following *i.v.* therapy in the active group [20]. A comparative study of Tobi *versus* colistimethate sodium demonstrated that both caused a reduction in *P. aeruginosa* density but only the tobramycin demonstrated improvement in lung function [21]. A major limitation to this trial was that the patients were naïve to Tobi but had been taking colistimethate sodium prior to enrolment. A head-to-head comparison of naïve patients has not been performed and is unlikely to be possible.

Aztreonam lysine

Aztreonam is a monobactam antibiotic that has been used parenterally for decades to treat *P. aeruginosa*. It has recently been reformulated as a lysine salt for inhalation and labelled Cayston (Gilead, Foster City, CA, USA).

In a phase I, double-blind, placebo-controlled trial, Gibson *et al.* [22] reported that Cayston was well tolerated and that sputum concentrations exceeded the MIC for *P. aeruginosa*. A phase II, placebo-controlled, dose-ranging study identified the optimal dose as 75 mg three times daily. Two randomised, double-blind, placebo-controlled trials with 246 patients [23] and 164 patients [24], each with a 75-mg dose three times daily, showed improvement in FEV1, patient symptom score and *P. aeruginosa* density. A further 18-month, open-label trial showed that long-term use was well tolerated and again, at the end of each treatment cycle, there was improvement in FEV1, symptom scores and *P. aeruginosa* density [25]. Importantly, there was no increase in MIC of *P. aeruginosa* throughout the course of these studies. Cayston is approved for use in CF patients with *P. aeruginosa* over the age of 6 years.

Choice of regimen for chronic suppressive therapy

It should be noted that many of the nebulised antibiotics, including Tobi and Cayston, were studied as month-on/month-off regimens as opposed to continuous or alternating regimens. Colistimethate sodium is frequently used on a continuous basis and many centres alternate between two different types of nebulised antibiotics, *i.e.* nebulised colistimethate sodium for one month and nebulised tobramycin solution for the next. There are no trials to determine if this is the most appropriate way to use these antimicrobials. The principle of chronic suppressive therapy suggests it would be best to have continued, every-day administration of an antibiotic active against *P. aeruginosa*, but concerns about development of resistance resulting from long-term use drove a belief that the month-on/month-off regimen would be the best compromise to ensure long-term clinical effectiveness with minimal resistance. However, many patients describe increased symptoms and reduced lung function during the month off tobramycin, and require rescue therapy. Thus, the development of alternating regimens has been clinically driven without randomised trials. The optimal regimen for combining and sequencing inhaled antibiotic therapy as long-term suppressive therapy has yet to be determined. Direct comparisons between a range of regimens will be difficult but there is a current industry-sponsored study comparing an alternating regimen of Cayston and Tobi on alternate months with a month-on/month-off Tobi regimen (www.clinicaltrials. gov identifier number NCT01641822). Registry data could be used to provide some insights as regards the clinical outcomes of different regimens.

Patients are keen to reduce treatment burden and the licensing of a preparation of colistimethate sodium in a dry-powder inhaler (Colobreathe; Forest, London, UK) in Europe following a noninferiority study against nebulised Tobi [26], means that patients may be treated with a choice of dry-powder inhalers, either tobramycin or colistimethate sodium.

Future inhaled antibiotic therapies

Liposomal amikacin

Liposomal amikacin (Arikace; Insmed, Monmouth Junction, NJ, USA) is a sustained-release liposomal formulation of amikacin for inhalation for the treatment of *P. aeruginosa* that is currently being evaluated. It is administered once daily through a fast nebuliser using vibrating mesh technology. Liposomal forms of antibiotics have the advantage of greater penetration into the biofilm, thereby increasing the deliverable dose of antibiotic. Meers *et al.* [27] found superior *in vivo* efficacy of liposomal amikacin *versus* the free drug. Further advantages include sustained release, which reduces the frequency of dosing, and the site-specific release of drug from the liposomes by bacterial rhamnolipids. A phase II, placebo-controlled trial of 66 patients was carried out with two concentrations being tested (280 mg and 560 mg) over a 28-day period [28]. Those patients on Arikace demonstrated increased FEV1, reduced *P. aeruginosa* density, decreased exacerbations and a prolonged time to rescue antibiotics. The increase in FEV1 was sustained at day 56 in the higher dose group. An open-label extension study confirmed that Arikace was well tolerated and showed significant improvement in FEV1 of 11.7% at the end of six cycles. A phase III trial has recently completed in which Arikace was compared with Tobi on a month-on/month-off basis (NCT01315678).

Inhaled fluoroquinolones

Levofloxacin is a fluoroquinolone with potent activity against *P. aeruginosa*. In addition, it is not deactivated by CF sputum, biofilms or anaerobic conditions, conferring on it a possible advantage over other agents [29]. A novel formulation of levofloxacin, MP-376 (Aeroquin; Mpex Pharmaceuticals, Inc., San Diego, CA, USA), has been developed that contains high concentrations of levofloxacin alongside magnesium chloride, enabling rapid administration. A recent, multicentre, randomised, dose-ranging study of MP-376 in 151 patients found the optimum dose was 240 mg twice daily and this led to an 8.7% increase in FEV1 compared with placebo. Significant reductions in the need for other antipseudomonal antibiotics were observed in all treatment groups, and it was well tolerated [29]. Two phase III trials of inhaled levofloxacin have been completed (NCT01180634 and NCT01270347).

Ciprofloxacin is currently being evaluated for inhalation therapy in two formulations in non-CF bronchiectasis rather than CF. One is a dry-powder formulation using similar techniques to tobramycin inhalation power. The second is a liposomal formulation for nebulisation.

Fosfomycin/tobramycin

Fosfomycin is a phosphonic acid antibiotic, which works by inhibiting bactericidal cell wall synthesis; it is active against Gram-negative, Gram-positive and anaerobic bacteria, including methicillin-resistant *S. aureus* (MRSA). Fosfomycin in combination with tobramycin for inhalation (FTI), in a 4:1 ratio, has been developed for use in patients chronically infected with *P. aeruginosa*. In a recent placebo-controlled, multicentre study, following a 4-week run-in period on Cayston, 119 patients were randomised to FTI twice daily (160/40 mg, n=41; 80/20 mg, n=38) or placebo (n=40). There was significant improvement with Cayston but this was only maintained in the FTI groups, with the biggest improvement being in the 80/20-mg group (with a 7.5% improvement in FEV1; p<0.001). *P. aeruginosa* density also decreased significantly in the FTI 80/20-mg group (p=0.02). There were fewer side-effects in the 80/20-mg group than the 160/40-mg group and this may have been the reason for the greater apparent efficacy. In addition to the effect on *P. aeruginosa*, the FTI had significant impact on both MRSA and methicillin-sensitive *S. aureus* [30].

The development of these new agents through to a license requires large randomised trials showing at least noninferiority against the accepted gold-standard licenced agent. Thus, for the last few agents discussed, the regulatory authorities have required comparison with alternating-month Tobi therapy. The clinical community then has the challenge of attempting to find the best regimen for individual patients from the options available. In making that choice, patient preferences regarding nebuliser use *versus* inhaled use, clinical response and side-effects will be taken into account.

Chronic oral therapy in P. aeruginosa *infection*

Azithromycin has been used in patients chronically colonised with *P. aeruginosa* as an immunomodulatory agent. It has shown to be efficacious in reducing rates of pulmonary exacerbations, and improving in FEV1 and body weight [31]. Although *P. aeruginosa* is not conventionally considered to be sensitive to this agent, data demonstrate that organisms growing as a biofilm may be [32]. Furthermore, it is possible that some of the beneficial effects relate to an antibiotic effect on other, non-*Pseudomonas* bacteria present in the CF airway. Chronic azithromycin therapy is recommended in guidelines for maintaining lung function and preventing exacerbations in CF, with the strongest evidence being in patients with chronic *P. aeruginosa* infection [33]. Long-term treatment with oral ciprofloxacin is not recommended because of rapid loss of both microbiological susceptibility and clinical response.

Antibiotic treatment of exacerbations in *P. aeruginosa* infection

Optimising antibiotic selection for treatment of exacerbations is currently a difficult task for clinicians. We know that susceptibility testing may be unhelpful, and that around 25% of pulmonary exacerbations result in a failure to return to baseline lung function and/or rapid relapse [34–36]. There is a large unmet need in terms of laboratory tests that will reliably predict clinical response in exacerbation therapy.

Oral therapy for mild exacerbations of *P. aeruginosa* infection

There are few RCTs comparing the efficacy of oral antibiotics to alternative treatments. However, data from trials performed in the 1980s and 1990s [37] suggested equivalence of oral ciprofloxacin to a variety of parenteral antibiotics in the treatment of pulmonary exacerbations. We recognise that the usefulness of oral ciprofloxacin diminishes with repeated frequent use. Other oral antibiotics that are used in the management of pulmonary exacerbations in patients chronically infected with *P. aeruginosa* include co-trimoxazole and chloramphenicol. However, there are very few data to support their use and both these drugs are more commonly prescribed on a pragmatic basis.

Intravenous therapy for exacerbations of *P. aeruginosa* infection

Intravenous antibiotics have played an important role for decades in the management of acute exacerbations in CF patients chronically infected with *P. aeruginosa*. Clinical experience and expertise indicate that patients with pulmonary exacerbations benefit from the use of *i.v.* antibiotics. Intravenous antibiotics are usually delivered as a combination of a β-lactam (*i.e.* ceftazidime) or a carbapenem (*i.e.* meropenem) combined with an aminoglycoside. There are no RCTs determining the optimal length of antibiotic treatment but, conventionally, this therapy has been given for 14 days. In a recent registry-based study, it seemed that 10 days may be a sufficient period of time for many patients [38], at least in terms of lung function improvement. Time to next exacerbation may also be an important end-point for future studies in determining the optimal length of therapy. Some patients with more severe exacerbations may require longer courses. Intravenous antibiotics may be administered either at home or in hospital, as evidence suggests that both are effective [39–41].

The role of susceptibility testing when using oral and intravenous antibiotics for *P. aeruginosa*

The role of antimicrobial antibiotic susceptibility testing to help choose antibiotics is controversial. It has been demonstrated that for the majority of patients suffering an infective exacerbation, the infecting agent is the same as that chronically infecting the lung. Therefore, one would expect a similar antibiotic susceptibility profile between samples if no new antibiotics have been given. However, a seminal study demonstrated significant variability in antibiotic susceptibility profiles of *P. aeruginosa* taken from a single sputum sample [42]. In addition, the only robust study to correlate antibiotic resistance to clinical response showed that lung function improved in spite of treatment with antibiotics to which their *P. aeruginosa* were resistant *in vitro* [43]. Although antibiotic susceptibility does not appear to assist with antibiotic choice, both multidrug-resistant and pan-drug-resistant *P. aeruginosa* were associated with a worse outcome in pulmonary exacerbations [34]. In addition, there is no evidence that synergy testing of antibiotics is helpful [3] and the current US Cystic Fibrosis Foundation (CFF) guidelines on treating exacerbations do not recommend this [44]. The choice of antibiotics to treat a pulmonary exacerbation, or change in antibiotics if a patient is not responding, is determined by knowledge of previous combinations of antibiotics that resulted in a good response to treatment, and limitations due to antibiotic allergy and toxicity rather than *in vitro* antimicrobial sensitivity.

Furthermore, this lack of influence of antibiotic susceptibility patterns on treatment outcome may help explain why some oral antibiotics appear to be effective despite apparent *P. aeruginosa* resistance.

MRSA

Infection with MRSA is becoming an increasing problem, with the prevalence in the USA now estimated at 25% although in the UK and Europe numbers are much lower, around 2.6% (fig. 1). There is clear evidence that infection with MRSA is associated with lower and more rapidly declining lung function, higher rates of hospitalisation, and greater use of antibiotics in all forms [45, 46]. In addition, known MRSA infection is one of the factors associated with failure to recover after an exacerbation [35, 46] and a study published in 2010 concluded that MRSA infection was associated with an increased mortality [47].

MRSA eradication

There are no published RCTs of MRSA eradication to guide us as to the best regimen. There are, however, two eradication studies ongoing in the USA. One study is comparing an eradication protocol *versus* observation in early MRSA infection while the other is examining the effect of inhaled vancomycin *versus* placebo in addition to a combination of oral antibiotics (NCT01349192 and NCT01594827).

One group of centres published their experience of MRSA eradication [48], showing successful eradication in 81% of patients, even among those who had had MRSA infection for some time. Approximately 19% of patients required more than one treatment course to achieve this. There was no standardised regimen but all used a combination of two oral antibiotics, with the first line being fusidic acid 500 mg three times daily, and rifampicin 300 mg twice daily or trimethoprim 200 mg twice daily. Nebulised vancomycin was also used.

In addition, there is also a phase II, placebo-controlled safety and efficacy study of AeroVanc (Savara Pharmaceuticals, Austin, TX, USA), a novel vancomycin inhalation powder, in CF patients with persistent MRSA being performed in the USA (NCT01746095).

MRSA exacerbations

There are no trials confirming superiority of one treatment regime for MRSA over others but the antibiotics available for the treatment of acute infection include the glycol peptides vancomycin and teicoplanin, and the oxazolidinone linezolid. There are concerns about further antibiotic resistance in MRSA strains. There have been two studies describing decreased susceptibility of CF patients with respiratory tract MRSA to glycopeptides [49, 50] and two studies documenting linezolid-resistant MRSA strains. In one, in as many as 11 out of 77 patients treated with linezolid, resistance developed [51, 52]. The monitoring of use of such agents to try and prevent the development of these resistant strains is vital. The reasons proposed for development of resistance by authors of these papers are a combination of prolonged use and subtherapeutic doses.

Burkholderia cepacia complex

Burkholderia cepacia complex (BCC) is a relatively uncommon but very important group of bacteria causing airway infection in CF. The CFF registry reports the current rate of infection is around 2.5% in the USA with similar levels in the UK and Europe. Taxonomic studies revealed genotypic differences between several *B. cepacia* species leading to the identification of at least 17 different species [53] referred to as the BCC. The most frequently occurring are *Burkholderia cenocepacia* (~50%), *Burkholderia multivorans* (~38%) and *Burkholderia vietnamienesis* (~5%). Treatment of BCC is difficult as the species are intrinsically resistant, therefore prevention is preferable and most CF clinics now employ strict infection control procedures.

BCC eradication

Once a new growth of BCC has been identified in our centre, we recommend an attempt at eradication but there are no trials evaluating this approach. There are anecdotal reports of successful eradication with a regimen of three *i.v.* antibiotics [54].

BCC exacerbations

Again, there are no trials confirming the optimal regimen for treatment of exacerbations. The UK Cystic Fibrosis Trust recommends that antimicrobial therapy be directed by *in vitro* testing. The antibiotics to which BCC species may be susceptible include the carbapenems, quinolones, piperacillin, ceftazidime, trimethoprim-sulfamethoxazole and minocycline [55–57]. Although some strains show resistance to these antibiotics, combinations may be effective.

Chronic suppressive therapy for BCC

A recent trial of Cayston for management of chronic infection has been completed and the results were disappointing, demonstrating no significant benefit overall [58]. Reasons for the lack of efficacy may have related to the wide variety of subspecies included in the study, and the wide variety of concomitant nebulised and oral antibiotics already in use in many patients. Anecdotally, a number of nebulised regimens seem beneficial, including ceftazidime and temocillin, and oral minocycline may have benefits. We are therefore left with an evidence gap and clinicians having to make empirical choices.

Achromobacter xylosoxidans

Achromobacter xylosoxidans has been recognised for many years a causative agent of pulmonary infections in CF. Its prevalence is around 6.2% in US centres, rising to 10% in some other areas, but it appears to be on the increase [59].

The clinical significance of *A. xylosoxidans* is unclear. A review by TAN *et al.* [60] found no evidence to suggest an increased rate of decline in lung function, although another report found a subgroup in a case–control study that did experience a more rapid decline [59].

Eradication of *A. xylosoxidans*

Due to concerns about possible decline in lung function, many clinicians will attempt eradication, usually with *i.v.* antibiotics, in the absence of evidence from controlled trials. However, *A. xylosoxidans* is a multiresistant organism and there are few data to suggest optimum therapy. *In vitro* testing suggests the most appropriate antibiotics may be *i.v.* meropenem, piperacillin-tazobactam, colomycin, oral chloramphenicol and minocycline. The Copenhagen group have very recently reported successful eradication therapy with inhaled ceftazidime or colistimethate sodium or tobramycin [61].

Stenotrophomonas maltophilia

Stenotrophomonas maltophilia is an important nosocomial pathogen, affecting immuno-compromised patients and those on ventilator support. It has intrinsic resistance to broad-spectrum antibiotic agents including the carbapenems. The increase of *S. maltophilia* in CF has been linked to the use of antipseudomonal drugs and in particular meropenem [62].

No evidence has been found to suggest either an increase in mortality or a faster rate of decline in lung function with chronic *S. maltophilia* infection [63, 64]. In individual cases, treatment may be warranted, but this is usually a matter of individual clinical judgment. Co-trimoxazole is a very useful agent for treatment.

Nontuberculous mycobacteria

The nontuberculous mycobacteria, in particular *Mycobacterium avium-intracellulare* and *Mycobacterium abscessus* complex, have emerged as troublesome pathogens in the last few years. Treatment decisions are complex, as are the antibiotic regimens, and beyond the scope of this chapter.

Challenges of antibiotic therapy

Antibiotic toxicity is an increasing challenge in CF and particularly relates to the use of *i.v.* aminoglycosides.

Toxicity is a much greater challenge with *i.v.* antibiotics and a number of studies have highlighted the risk of chronic renal disease in patients with CF, particularly those with high lifetime doses of aminoglycosides [65]. All aminoglycosides can cause renal tubular damage, although recent studies suggest the strongest factor in development of chronic renal disease in CF is diabetes [66]. Gentamicin should not be used for *i.v.* therapy as a case–control study has suggested that acute renal failure is mainly associated with gentamicin [67]; therefore, tobramycin is used in preference. Once-daily use of tobramycin for treatment of exacerbations reduces the risk of renal damage [68]. Hearing impairment is also commonly found in individuals with CF who receive aminoglycosides, and annual screening with a pure-tone audiogram can be performed in those receiving frequent *i.v.* antibiotic courses that include aminoglycosides. Care should also be taken to ensure that other nephrotoxic drugs are not co-prescribed, and that estimated glomerular filtration rate and plasma magnesium are monitored.

Antibiotic allergy

Allergic reactions to antibiotics are thought to be more common in CF patients than in the general population, though the increased prevalence of allergic reactions may be due to more frequent exposure to antibiotics. Certainly, antibiotic choice can become limited by allergies as CF patients with chronic *P. aeruginosa* infection get older and require frequent *i.v.* courses. Allergic reactions can occur to most of the antibiotics used in CF but are particularly frequent with the β-lactam piperacillin. Antibiotic allergies should be clearly documented in patients' notes. Allergic reactions can be investigated with serum and skin-prick testing [69]. Importantly, desensitisation, although time consuming, is possible [70].

Conclusion

Treating respiratory infection in CF is an important and ongoing concern. While there is excitement over the potential of novel disease-modifying treatments, it is vital that we continue to work on developing new antibiotics and strategies to manage respiratory infection. It is clear that for those bacteria we know are harmful, early and aggressive eradication should be attempted. But, for many infections, their significance and optimal management are still unknown and, even for those bacteria that have been extensively investigated, there are still many unanswered questions. More research is required to attempt to ensure we have identified optimal regimens to treat specific bacteria.

References

1. UK Cystic Fibrosis Registry. Annual data report 2012. https://cysticfibrosis.org.uk/media/316760/scientific%20Registry%20Review%202012.pdf Date last updated: January 2013.
2. Zhao J, Elborn JS, LiPuma JJ. Airway infection and the microbiome. *In:* Mall MA, Elborn JS, eds. Cystic Fibrosis. *ERS Monogr* 2014; 64: 32–46.
3. Aaron SD, Vandemheen KL, Ferris W, *et al.* Combination antibiotic susceptibility testing to treat exacerbations of cystic fibrosis associated with multiresistant bacteria: a randomised, double-blind, controlled clinical trial. *Lancet* 2006; 366: 463–471.
4. Weaver T, Green MR, Nicholson K, *et al.* Prognosis in cystic fibrosis treated with continuous flucloxacillin from the neonatal period. *Arch Dis Child* 1994; 70: 84–89.
5. Smyth AR, Walters S. Prophylactic anti-staphylococcal antibiotics for cystic fibrosis. *Cochrane Database Syst Rev* 2012; 12: CD001912.
6. Stutman HR, Lieberman JM, Nussbaum E, *et al.* Antibiotic prophylaxis in infants and young children with cystic fibrosis: a randomized controlled trial. *J Pediatr* 2002; 140: 299–305.
7. Ratjen F, Comes G, Paul K, *et al.* Effect of continuous antistaphylococcal therapy on the rate of *P. aeruginosa* acquisition in patients with cystic fibrosis. *Pediatr Pulmonol* 2001; 31: 13–16.
8. Cystic Fibrosis Foundation. Patient registry 2011 annual data report. Bethesda, CFF, 2012.
9. Döring G, Flume P, Heijerman H, *et al.* Treatment of lung infection in patients with cystic fibrosis: current and future strategies. *J Cyst Fibros* 2012; 11: 461–479.

10. Valerius NH, Koch C, Høiby N. Prevention of chronic *Pseudomonas aeruginosa* colonisation in cystic fibrosis by early treatment. *Lancet* 1991; 338: 725–726.

11. Frederiksen B, Koch C, Høiby N. Antibiotic treatment of initial colonization with *Pseudomonas aeruginosa* postpones chronic infection and prevents deterioration of pulmonary function in cystic fibrosis. *Pediatr Pulmonol* 1997; 23: 330–335.

12. Ratjen F, Döring G, Nikolaizik WH. Effect of inhaled tobramycin on early *Pseudomonas aeruginosa* colonisation in patients with cystic fibrosis. *Lancet* 2001; 358: 983–984.

13. Gibson RL, Emerson J, McNamara S, et al. Significant microbiological effect of inhaled tobramycin in young children with cystic fibrosis. *Am J Respir Crit Care Med* 2003; 167: 841–849.

14. Ratjen F, Munck A, Kho P, et al. Treatment of early *Pseudomonas aeruginosa* infection in patients with cystic fibrosis: the ELITE trial. *Thorax* 2010; 65: 286–291.

15. Proesmans M. Comparison of two treatment regimens for eradication of *Pseudomonas aeruginosa* infection in children with cystic fibrosis. *J Cyst Fibros* 2013; 12: 29–34.

16. Taccetti G, Bianchini E, Cariani L, et al. Early antibiotic treatment for *Pseudomonas aeruginosa* eradication in patients with cystic fibrosis: a randomised multicentre study comparing two different protocols. *Thorax* 2012; 67: 853–859.

17. Ramsey BW, Pepe MS, Quan JM, et al. Intermittent administration of inhaled tobramycin in patients with cystic fibrosis. *N Engl J Med* 1999; 340: 23–30.

18. Konstan MW, Geller DE, Mini P, et al. Tobramycin inhalation powder for *P. aeruginosa* infection in cystic fibrosis: the EVOLVE trial. *Pediatr Pulmonol* 2011; 46: 230–238.

19. Konstan MW, Flume PA, Kappler M, et al. Safety, efficacy and convenience of tobramycin inhalation powder in cystic fibrosis patients: the EAGER trial. *J Cyst Fibros* 2011; 10: 54–61.

20. Jensen T, Pedersen SS, Garne S, et al. Colistin inhalation therapy in cystic fibrosis patients with chronic *Pseudomonas aeruginosa* lung infection. *J Antimicrob Chem* 1987; 19: 831–838.

21. Hodson ME, Gallagher CG, Govan JRW. A randomised clinical trial of nebulised tobramycin or colistin in cystic fibrosis. *Eur Respir J* 2002; 20: 658–664.

22. Gibson RL, Retsch-Bogart GZ, Oermann C, et al. Microbiology, safety, and pharmacokinetics of aztreonam lysinate for inhalation in patients with cystic fibrosis. *Pediatr Pulmonol* 2006; 41: 656–665.

23. McCoy KS, Quittner AL, Oermann CM, et al. Inhaled aztreonam lysine for chronic airway *Pseudomonas aeruginosa* in cystic fibrosis. *Am J Respir Crit Care Med* 2008; 178: 921–928.

24. Retsch-Bogart GZ, Quittner AL, Gibson RL, et al. Efficacy and safety of inhaled aztreonam lysine for airway *Pseudomonas* in cystic fibrosis. *Chest* 2009; 135: 1223–1232.

25. Oermann CM, Retsch-Bogart GZ, Quittner AL, et al. An 18-month study of the safety and efficacy of repeated courses of inhaled aztreonam lysine in cystic fibrosis. *Pediatr Pulmonol* 2010; 45: 1121–1134.

26. Schuster A, Haliburn C, Döring G, et al. Safety, efficacy and convenience of colistimethate sodium dry powder for inhalation (Colobreathe DPI) in patients with cystic fibrosis: a randomised study. *Thorax* 2013; 68: 344–350.

27. Meers P, Neville M, Malinin V, et al. Biofilm penetration, triggered release and *in vivo* activity of inhaled liposomal amikacin in chronic *Pseudomonas aeruginosa* lung infections. *J Antimicrob Chem* 2008; 61: 859–868.

28. Clancy JP, Dupont L, Konstan MW, et al. Phase II studies of nebulised Arikace in CF patients with *Pseudomonas aeruginosa* infection. *Thorax* 2013; 68: 818–825.

29. Geller DE, Flume PA, Staab D, et al. Levofloxacin inhalation solution (MP-376) in patients with cystic fibrosis with *Pseudomonas aeruginosa*. *Am J Respir Crit Care Med* 2011; 183: 1510–1516.

30. Trapnell BC, McColley SA, Kissner DG, et al. Fosfomycin/tobramycin for inhalation in patients with cystic fibrosis with *Pseudomonas* airway infection. *Am J Respir Crit Care Med* 2012; 185: 171–178.

31. Saiman L. Azithromycin in patients with cystic fibrosis chronically infected with *Pseudomonas aeruginosa*: a randomized controlled trial. *JAMA* 2003; 290: 1749–1756.

32. Nalca Y, Jänsch L, Bredenbruch F, et al. Quorum-sensing antagonistic activities of azithromycin in *Pseudomonas aeruginosa* PAO1: a global approach. *Antimicrob Agents Chemother* 2006; 50: 1680–1688.

33. Mogayzel PJ, Edward T, Naureckas ET, et al. Cystic fibrosis pulmonary guidelines. Chronic medications for maintenance of lung health. *Am J Respir Crit Care Med* 2013; 187: 680–689.

34. Parkins MD, Rendall JC, Elborn JS. Incidence and risk factors for pulmonary exacerbation treatment failures in patients with cystic fibrosis chronically infected with *Pseudomonas aeruginosa*. *Chest* 2012; 141: 485–493.

35. Sanders DB, Bittner RC, Rosenfeld M, et al. Failure to recover to baseline pulmonary function after cystic fibrosis pulmonary exacerbation. *Am J Respir Crit Care Med* 2010; 182: 627–632.

36. Sanders DB, Hoffman LR, Emerson J, et al. Return of FEV_1 after pulmonary exacerbation in children with cystic fibrosis. *Pediatr Pulmonol* 2010; 45: 127–134.

37. Hodson M, Butland RJA, Roberts CM, et al. Oral ciprofloxacillin compared with conventional intravenous treatment for *Pseudomonas aeruginosa* infection in adults with cystic fibrosis. *Lancet* 1987; 329: 235–237.

38. VanDevanter DR, O'Riordan MA, Blumer JL, et al. Assessing time to pulmonary function benefit following antibiotic treatment of acute cystic fibrosis exacerbations. *Respir Res* 2010; 11: 137.

39. Collaco JM, Green DM, Cutting GR, *et al.* Location and duration of treatment of cystic fibrosis respiratory exacerbations do not affect outcomes. *Am J Respir Crit Care Med* 2010; 182: 1137–1143.

40. Riethmueller J, Busch A, Damm V, *et al.* Home and hospital antibiotic treatment prove similarly effective in cystic fibrosis. *Infect* 2002; 30: 387–391.

41. Wolter JM, Bowler SD, Nolan PJ, *et al.* Home intravenous therapy in cystic fibrosis: a prospective randomized trial examining clinical, quality of life and cost aspects. *Eur Respir J* 1997; 10: 896–900.

42. Foweraker JE, Laughton CR, Brown DFJ, *et al.* Phenotypic variability of *Pseudomonas aeruginosa* in sputa from patients with acute infective exacerbation of cystic fibrosis and its impact on the validity of antimicrobial susceptibility testing. *J Antimicrob Chem* 2005; 55: 921–927.

43. Smith AL, Fiel SB, Mayer-Hamblett N, *et al.* Susceptibility testing of *Pseudomonas aeruginosa* isolates and clinical response to parenteral antibiotic administration. *Chest* 2003; 123: 1495–1502.

44. Flume PA, Mogayzel PJ, Robinson KA, *et al.* Cystic fibrosis pulmonary guidelines. *Am J Respir Crit Care Med* 2009; 180: 802–808.

45. Ren CL, Morgan WJ, Konstan MW, *et al.* Presence of methicillin resistant *Staphylococcus aureus* in respiratory cultures from cystic fibrosis patients is associated with lower lung function. *Pediatr Pulmonol* 2007; 42: 513–518.

46. Dasenbrook EC, Merlo CA, Diener-West M, *et al.* Persistent methicillin-resistant *Staphylococcus aureus* and rate of FEV1 decline in cystic fibrosis. *Am J Respir Crit Care Med* 2008; 178: 814–821.

47. Dasenbrook EC, Checkley W, Merlo CA, *et al.* Association between respiratory tract methicillin-resistant *Staphylococcus aureus* and survival in cystic fibrosis. *JAMA* 2010; 303: 2386–2392.

48. Doe SJ, McSorley A, Isalska B, *et al.* Patient segregation and aggressive antibiotic eradication therapy can control methicillin-resistant *Staphylococcus aureus* at large cystic fibrosis centres. *J Cyst Fibros* 2010; 9: 104–109.

49. Cafiso V, Bertuccio T, Spina D, *et al.* Methicillin resistance and vancomycin heteroresistance in *Staphylococcus aureus* in cystic fibrosis patients. *Eur J Clin Microbiol Infect Dis* 2010; 29: 1277–1285.

50. Filleron A, Chiron Rl, Reverdy ME., et al. *Staphylococcus aureus* with decreased susceptibility to glycopeptides in cystic fibrosis patients. *J Cyst Fibros* 2011; 10: 377–382.

51. Endimiani A, Blackford M, Dasenbrook EC, *et al.* Emergence of linezolid-resistant *Staphylococcus aureus* after prolonged treatment of cystic fibrosis patients in Cleveland, Ohio. *Antimicrob Agents Chemother* 2011; 55: 1684–1692.

52. Hill RLR, Kearns AM, Nash J, *et al.* Linezolid-resistant ST36 methicillin-resistant *Staphylococcus aureus* associated with prolonged linezolid treatment in two paediatric cystic fibrosis patients. *J Antimicrob Chemother* 2010; 65: 442–445.

53. Vandammea P, Dawyndtb P. Classification and identification of the *Burkholderia cepacia* complex: past, present and future. *Syst Appl Microbiol* 2011; 34: 87–95.

54. Etherington C, Peckham DG, Conway SP, *et al.* *Burkholderia cepacia* complex infection in adult patients with cystic fibrosis – is early eradication possible? *J Cyst Fibros* 2003; 2: 220–221.

55. Vermis K, Vandamme PAR, Nelis HJ. *Burkholderia cepacia* complex genomovars: utilization of carbon sources, susceptibility to antimicrobial agents and growth on selective media. *J Appl Microbiol* 2003; 95: 1191–1199.

56. Lewin C, Doherty C, Govan J. *In vitro* activities of meropenem, PD 127391, PD 131628, ceftazidime, chloramphenicol, co-trimoxazole, and ciprofloxacin against *Pseudomonas cepacia*. *Antimicrob Agents Chemother* 1993; 37: 123–125.

57. Pitt TL, Kaufmann ME, Patel PS, *et al.* Type characterisation and antibiotic susceptibility of *Burkholderia* (*Pseudomonas*) *cepacia* isolates from patients with cystic fibrosis in the United Kingdom and the Republic of Ireland. *J Med Microbiol* 1996; 44: 203–210.

58. Tullis DE, Burns JL, Retsch-Bogart GZ, *et al.* Inhaled aztreonam for chronic *Burkholderia* infection in cystic fibrosis: a placebo-controlled trial. *J Cyst Fibros* 2014; 13: 296–305.

59. De Baets F, Schelstraete P, Van Daele S, *et al.* *Achromobacter xylosoxidans* in cystic fibrosis: prevalence and clinical relevance. *J Cyst Fibros* 2007; 6: 75–78.

60. Tan K, Conway SP, Brownlee KG, *et al.* *Alcaligenes* infection in cystic fibrosis. *Pediatr Pulmonol* 2002; 34: 101–104.

61. Wang M, Ridderberg W, Hansen CR, *et al.* Early treatment with inhaled antibiotics postpones next occurrence of *Achromobacter* in cystic fibrosis. *J Cyst Fibros* 2013; 12: 638–643.

62. Denton M, Todd NJ, Littlewood JM. Role of anti-pseudomonal antibiotics in the emergence of *Stenotrophomonas maltophilia* in cystic fibrosis patients. *Eur J Clin Microbiol Infect Dis* 1996; 15: 402–405.

63. Goss CH, Otto K, Aitken ML, *et al.* Detecting *Stenotrophomonas maltophilia* does not reduce survival of patients with cystic fibrosis. *Am J Respir Crit Care Med* 2002; 166: 356–361.

64. Goss CH, Mayer-Hamblett N, Aitken ML, *et al.* Association between *Stenotrophomonas maltophilia* and lung function in cystic fibrosis. *Thorax* 2004; 59: 955–959.

65. Al-Aloul M, Miller H, Alapati S, *et al.* Renal impairment in cystic fibrosis patients due to repeated intravenous aminoglycoside use. *Pediatr Pulmonol* 2005; 39: 15–20.

66. Quon BS, Mayer-Hamblett N, Aitken ML, *et al.* Risk factors for chronic kidney disease in adults with cystic fibrosis. *Am J Respir Crit Care Med* 2011; 184: 1147–1152.

67. Smyth A, Lewis S, Bertenshaw C, *et al.* A case control study of acute renal failure in cystic fibrosis patients in the United Kingdom. *Thorax* 2008; 63: 532–535.

68. Smyth A, Tan KH, Hyman-Taylor P, *et al.* Once *versus* three-times daily regimens of tobramycin treatment for pulmonary exacerbations of cystic fibrosis – the TOPIC study: a randomized controlled trial. *Lancet* 2005; 365: 573–578.

69. Parmar JS, Nasser S. Antibiotic allergy in cystic fibrosis. *Thorax* 2005; 60: 517–520.

70. Whitaker P, Naisbitt D, Peckham D. Nonimmediate β-lactam reactions in patients with cystic fibrosis. *Curr Opin Allergy Clin Immunol* 2012; 12: 369–375.

Disclosures: D. Bilton reports receiving advisory board fees from: Gilead regarding the use of nebulised antibiotics in the UK; Novartis regarding the design of trials in non-CF bronchiectasis; and Pharmaxis regarding CF and complications of inhaled therapy. The authors' institution received a grant from Insmed to conduct a clinical trial.

Exercise in cystic fibrosis

Helge Hebestreit

Physical activity and exercise have become part of standard treatment in many centres caring for people with cystic fibrosis (CF). Observed benefits include positive effects on exercise capacity, pulmonary disease and health-related quality of life (HRQoL). Furthermore, some data also suggest improvements in bone mineral density and psychological well-being. However, exercise may carry some risks in CF. Most of the adverse events associated with exercise are more common in individuals with advanced disease. In addition to knowing a patient's medical history and actual health status, standardised cardiopulmonary exercise testing can identify patients at risk for many of the potential complications, as well as the reasons for a reduced exercise capacity. The Godfrey protocol for cycle ergometry is employed by many international experts. A proper individual risk assessment, as well as patient education and counselling, will foster an active and healthy lifestyle.

The importance of habitual physical activity and a good physical fitness for health and longevity has been well established for the general population. In fact, regular exercise can reduce the risk of conditions such as cardiovascular disease, obesity, diabetes mellitus, osteoporosis and some types of cancer, and reduces overall mortality. In cystic fibrosis (CF), accumulating evidence has also led to a general understanding that high levels of physical activity and a good physical fitness are beneficial for patients [1, 2].

Habitual physical activity

In healthy European children and adolescents, activity levels decline during adolescence, and boys are more physically active than girls at all ages [3]. In healthy adults, physical activity is even lower than in adolescents [4]. For prepubescent children with CF and older individuals with mild lung disease (*i.e.* forced expiratory volume in 1 s (FEV_1) $\geqslant 70\%$ predicted), physical activity levels seem to be similar to or even higher than those of healthy controls [5]. In pubescent or post-pubescent patients with more advanced disease, physical activity appears to be reduced [5]. As in the healthy population, lower levels of physical activity have been reported for females compared with males with CF [6]. The sex difference may be less relevant for prepubescent children but appears to be larger in adolescents [5].

High levels of physical activity in people with CF have been linked to a slower rate of decline in FEV_1 in a long-term longitudinal study [7]. Furthermore, cross-sectional data suggest that

Paediatrics, University of Würzburg, Würzburg, Germany.

Correspondence: Helge Hebestreit, Paediatrics, University of Würzburg, Josef-Schneider-Str. 2, 97080 Würzburg, Germany.
E-mail: hebestreit@uni-wuerzburg.de

Copyright ERS 2014. Print ISBN: 978-1-84984-050-7. Online ISBN: 978-1-84984-051-4. Print ISSN: 2312-508X. Online ISSN: 2312-5098.

physical activity is positively related to bone mineral density, as assessed by dual-energy X-ray absorptiometry, in CF [8, 9]. However, conclusive evidence for a role of physical activity in fracture prevention in CF is still lacking.

Fitness

Some, but not all, people with CF have reduced aerobic [10, 11] and/or anaerobic fitness [10, 12] compared with their healthy counterparts. In fact, some individuals with CF can even perform competitively at a high level or complete extremely demanding tasks, like running a marathon.

Aerobic fitness, usually assessed by measuring peak oxygen uptake ($V'O_2$peak), may be limited in CF by respiratory disease (*e.g.* CF lung disease), cardiovascular disease (*e.g.* ventricular dysfunction and cardiac arrhythmia), poor muscle performance (*e.g.* muscle wasting) and lack of training [13]. However, respiratory limitations and deconditioning appear to be much more common than cardiovascular limitations in CF.

In a way, $V'O_2$peak can be viewed as an integrated measure reflecting disease severity and activity behaviour in an individual patient. It is therefore not surprising that aerobic fitness has been associated with survival in the general CF population [14, 15] and also in people pre-transplant [16]. However, it remains unclear whether $V'O_2$peak can be of prognostic value, in addition to established predictors such as FEV1, body mass index (BMI) and *Pseudomonas aeruginosa* status, to model survival in CF. Nevertheless, a high $V'O_2$peak is linked to a lower risk for hospitalisation in children with CF, even in a multivariate analysis [17]. Furthermore, $V'O_2$peak correlated better with changes on thin-section computed tomography (CT) images than other clinical measures including FEV1 and BMI [18].

Factors limiting performance

As outlined above, exercise capacity may be limited for several reasons in people with CF.

Limitation of ventilation and gas exchange
Several studies have established an association between physical fitness and measures of pulmonary function such as FEV1 in CF [11, 13, 19–21]. This association is explained in several ways.

With advancing lung disease in CF, peak minute ventilation ($V'E$) is limited due to high airway resistance and hyperinflation/reduced vital capacity. Dynamic hyperinflation may further reduce tidal volume (VT) during exertion [22]. In many patients with advanced lung disease, $V'E$ approaches or even exceeds maximal voluntary ventilation (MVV) at peak exercise. Due to the relatively higher dead space with decreasing VT, ventilation becomes less efficient during exercise in people with advanced lung disease. This is reflected in increased ventilatory equivalents for oxygen and carbon dioxide [10, 23]. Last but not least, the oxygen cost attributable to ventilation during exercise in people with lung disease can be more than double that in healthy individuals [24]. Since total oxygen uptake is often reduced in such conditions, up to 40% of total oxygen uptake ($V'O_2$) may be utilised by the respiratory muscles in the presence of lung disease, compared to 10–15% in healthy people. This fact may partly explain the higher $V'O_2$ over work rate ratio in CF patients compared with controls [10].

Cardiovascular dysfunction

Several studies indicate that stroke volume may be lower in people with CF compared with healthy controls for any given $V'O_2$ [25–27], while cardiac output relative to $V'O_2$ does not seem to be impaired [27, 28]. Even though malnutrition might explain some of the stroke volume impairment [27], there may also be some additional CF-related factors. KOELLING et al. [29] have demonstrated impaired left ventricular distensibility in people with advanced CF using radionuclide ventriculography, possibly indicating myocardial fibrosis. There are some data to suggest that left ventricular dysfunction may start early in CF and could progress with advancing disease in some patients.

In addition to cardiac abnormalities, pulmonary vascular disease may contribute to exercise limitations in CF. Pulmonary arterial pressure may increase from rest to exercise in people with severe lung disease [30]. The increase in pulmonary arterial pressure has shown a negative correlation with measures of exercise capacity [31].

Muscular limitations

Nutritional status and, as a result, muscle mass have a strong impact on exercise capacity [12, 20, 32]. However, there might also be a direct functional impairment of CF muscle [33]. Using magnetic resonance imaging (MRI) spectroscopy, deficiencies in CF muscle metabolism have been described in the absence of malnutrition [34]. Furthermore, cystic fibrosis transmembrane conductance regulator (CFTR) channels have been identified in human sarcoplasmic reticulum, which may play a role in Ca^{2+} release [35, 36]. Interestingly, muscle from CFTR-deficient mice infected with *P. aeruginosa* showed a significant decrease in force generation compared with muscle from infected control mice [35], while there was no impairment in force generation in the absence of infection in CFTR-deficient mice. In the infected CFTR-deficient mice, a hyperinflammatory phenotype of CFTR-deficient muscle was observed, possibly leading to muscle wasting and an alteration of contractile properties [35]. In line with this finding, VAN DE WEERT-VAN LEEUWEN et al. [37] showed that chronic *P. aeruginosa* infection and IgG levels, a marker of inflammation, were both negatively associated with $V'O_{2peak}$ in a longitudinal study on patients with CF.

Lack of physical activity/regular exercise

Physical activity is associated with aerobic exercise capacity in CF [13, 38] and randomised controlled trials have shown that an increase in regular exercise can improve exercise capacity [39–43]. It is likely that nearly every individual with CF can improve their fitness with the use of an appropriate exercise programme, irrespective of disease stage.

Exercise-associated risks

Table 1 summarises the potential exercise-related risks in CF.

Sprains, strains and fractures

In theory, people with CF carry the same risk of suffering sprains and strains with exercise and sports as healthy individuals. Conversely, osteoporosis and osteopenia are common in CF [44], thus, an increased risk for exercise-related fractures might be assumed. However, a survey on exercise-related injuries, including fractures, reported a surprisingly low incidence of 0.4% per 1000 patient-years and a lifetime incidence of 6.3% [45]. These incidences are

Table 1. Exercise-related risks in cystic fibrosis

- Sprains, strains and fractures
- Worsening of arthritis
- Exercise-induced hypoxaemia and cardiac arrhythmia
- Exercise-induced bronchoconstriction
- Pneumothorax and haemoptysis
- Fluid and electrolyte losses
- Weight loss
- Hypoglycaemia
- Injury to spleen and oesophageal haemorrhage

lower than expected from epidemiological studies on healthy people. Possible explanations for the low incidences of reported injuries in CF might include problems with recall, less participation in injury prone activities, and less engagement in vigorous activities in general [45]. Furthermore, coordination skills preventing injuries might be better in people with CF compared with their healthy peers, at least in preschool children [46]. Finally, the low bone mineral density observed in CF is probably different from post-menopausal osteoporosis, and may confer a lower fracture risk.

Worsening of arthritis

Arthritis in CF is a comorbidity that may severely affect physical activity. There are only very sparse data on the effects of exercise on CF-related arthritis. Based on a survey with 256 respondents, RUF et al. [45] reported an incidence rate for arthritis manifesting or worsening with exercise of 0.14% per 1000 patient-years.

Exercise-induced hypoxaemia and cardiac arrhythmia

Hypoxaemia during exercise, defined as a decrease in oxygen saturation by $>4\%$ and/or to below 90%, is relatively common in CF, affecting about 20–25% of patients [47, 48]. Although conclusive data are lacking, it has been suggested that prolonged periods with an oxygen saturation $<90\%$ during exercise may pose a risk and should be avoided [49]. In fact, cardiac arrhythmias have been associated with exercise-related desaturations [48].

A drop in oxygen saturation below 90% with exercise mainly manifests in patients with severely impaired lung function, but patients showing hypoxaemia with exercise can have an FEV1 of $\geqslant 60\%$ predicted. Furthermore, these patients cannot be identified from resting spirometry alone, standardised exercise testing is required [48].

Exercise-induced bronchoconstriction

Some studies [50, 51], but not all [52, 53], report a relatively high incidence of exercise-induced bronchoconstriction in CF. Whether these responses are related to atopy and/or sensitisation to *Aspergillus* antigens and whether inhaled steroids or pretreatment with β_2-agonists may be beneficial in CF has not been formally assessed. Some data suggest that exercise-induced bronchoconstriction in CF may be different from that in bronchial asthma, at least in some cases [51, 53], so an individual evaluation will be necessary before treatment decisions can be made.

Pneumothorax and haemoptysis

Approximately 3–4% of people with CF may suffer from a pneumothorax and also 3–4% may suffer from massive haemoptysis sometime during their life [45, 54]. Although these conditions may occur during exercise, additional predisposing factors such as recent exacerbation and cough may be involved [45]. There are also anecdotal reports of pneumothoraces associated with the "wrong" breathing technique (a pressing breath-hold) during weight training.

After mild or moderate haemoptysis or pneumothorax, some consensus exists to withhold exercise [55]. In case of massive haemoptysis, most experts would stop exercise. However, no guidance is available on when to start exercise again. Naturally, all decisions on restarting exercise are based on the decisions of the treating physician(s) based on the individual's situation. However, in my experience, starting light aerobic type exercises 3–7 days after a mild or moderate haemoptysis will usually not induce a recurrence. After about 2 days, exercise intensity can be gradually increased if no adverse reactions occur. In massive haemoptysis, time to restart of exercise will usually have to be longer, often around 2 weeks or even more, depending on the underlying condition and the measures taken (conservative treatment, embolisation, *etc.*). In pneumothorax, once a chest drain has been removed and the pneumothorax has resolved light leg exercises may be started under close supervision for leaks. Exercise intensity can then be gradually increased and upper body exercises may be introduced. We would also ask our patients to refrain from lifting weights for 2–4 weeks after a pneumothorax and start weight lifting or upper body resistance exercise under the supervision of an experienced physiotherapist.

Fluid and electrolyte losses

People with CF tend to dehydrate more than healthy individuals, especially when exercising in a warm climate [56]. It has been shown that the excessive loss of electrolytes with sweating in CF results in less increase in serum osmolality during exercise-induced dehydration compared with healthy controls [57] or, if drinking is allowed, even in a decrease in serum osmolality [58]. Fluid intake during [56] and after [57] exercise is diminished in CF, which might reflect mechanisms targeting preservation of salt balance over volume restoration [57]. Adding salt to drinks might increase fluid intake in CF [58], thus, it has been suggested to provide exercising CF patients with drinks that contain NaCl (preferably $\geqslant 50$ mmol·L^{-1}) to prevent dehydration.

Weight loss

Exercising increases energy expenditure so that weight loss is a common concern when an exercise programme is suggested. However, many studies show that a reasonable increase in exercise time per week (*e.g.* 2–3 hours per week) will not induce weight loss [39, 59]. Resistance training with optimal nutrition may even increase muscle mass [42]. However, it is possibly that excessive vigorous physical activity can induce weight loss so nutritional counselling is warranted in highly active people, especially if they are losing weight.

Hypoglycaemia

An over-proportional decrease in blood glucose with exercise is a common finding in people treated for diabetes mellitus. Symptomatic exercise-induced hypoglycaemia does occur in CF

[45], even though no reliable information on incidence is available. Thus, counselling of CF patients with diabetes should include the management of exercise sessions and prolonged episodes of activities.

Injury to spleen and oesophageal haemorrhage

With hepatic cirrhosis and portal hypertension, oesophageal and gastric varices develop and the spleen enlarges. In such cases, rupture of the spleen or haemorrhage from varices is a concern in contact sports or when intra-abdominal pressure changes rapidly. Conceivably, impaired blood clotting associated with advanced liver disease and thrombocytopaenia from hypersplenism could further increase the risk of haemorrhage. However, no systematic assessments are available to better understand the exercise-related risks from hepatic cirrhosis.

Activity assessment

Most experts concerned with physical activity and exercise in CF would agree that determining the level of physical activity (and inactivity) is valuable for understanding the consequences of disease on daily life and for individual counselling. However, assessment of physical activity is difficult and no gold standard is available. Most studies on physical activity in CF have relied on questionnaires or objective instruments, such as accelerometers or systems integrating several signals.

Activity questionnaires

Many different questionnaires have been employed to determine activity behaviour in CF. At least three questionnaires have been assessed for their validity in this population. The Habitual Activity Estimation Scale (HAES) and the Seven Day Physical Activity Recall questionnaire were both found to provide some valid information on activity when compared with objective measurements [60, 61], but the associations were only moderate. However, habitual activity determined by the HAES has also been linked to lung function decline in a longitudinal observational study [7]. Thus, it has been suggested that activity questionnaires might be useful for epidemiological research but not for assessment of physical activity in individuals [61]. In addition, activity questionnaires may have their place in initiating a discussion with the patient about activity during clinic visits.

Objective methods to assess physical activity, *i.e.* pedometers, accelerometers and more complex systems, were all used to assess physical activity in CF [13, 39, 61–64]. Available data show that these systems may be used for research and might also have some value in individual patient care. The most informed choices are the SenseWear armband (BodyMedia Inc., Pittsburgh, PA, USA) and the actigraph accelerometers (ActiGraph, Pensacola, FL, USA) [13, 39, 61–63]. However, more research and standardisation of procedures is necessary to identify the best system and approach.

Exercise testing

As exercise capacity is affected by pulmonary function, nutritional state, physical activity and infection/inflammation (see earlier), determining exercise capacity in a standardised fashion can provide an integral measure of a patient's health. Furthermore, exercise testing can identify patients with a low fitness level as well as those with adverse reactions to exertion, such as exercise-induced hypoxaemia [48]. Finally, exercise testing can motivate patients to become more active and give positive feedback during an exercise programme. Thus, exercise testing is a key component in exercise counselling. It is, therefore, not surprising that several national expert groups have recommended annual exercise testing in CF [65–67].

Cardiopulmonary exercise testing

The gold standard for exercise testing is a full cardiopulmonary exercise test (CPET). Both the European Respiratory Society and the American Thoracic Society have issued documents on CPET that address indications, contraindications, methodology and interpretation of results in detail [68, 69]. These documents can also guide testing in CF, especially with respect to indications and contraindications, as well as laboratory set-up and safety measures. Some issues relevant for CF are addressed below.

Selection of protocol

Both the cycle ergometer and the treadmill are used for CPET in CF. However, most published CPET data relate to cycle ergometry using the Godfrey protocol [70] or a modification thereof (table 2) [13, 14, 39, 40, 71]. Many centres use this protocol to test people with CF.

In the absence of CPET equipment, a cycle ergometer test employing the Godfrey protocol without gas exchange measures might be an alternative and would be preferred over field testing by many experts.

Test interpretation

V'_{O_2peak}, the commonly reported measure of exercise capacity determined during a CPET, and peak work rate (W_{peak}) are usually expressed as per cent predicted [70, 72]. It is usually assumed that a V'_{O_2peak} <82% predicted and a W_{peak} <93% predicted indicate reduced exercise capacity [14].

V'_{O_2peak} is linked to physical activity [13], pulmonary function and structural lung damage [13, 18], the risk of future hospitalisations [17] and survival [14, 15]. Thus, a low V'_{O_2peak} in a patient should trigger some additional thoughts and possibly an intervention.

In order to understand the factors limiting exercise capacity, it is important to first ascertain that the test was maximal. For lung diseases, a V'_E approaching or exceeding the predicted MVV during exercise is used as a criterion, in addition to a heart rate reaching the predicted maximal heart rate or a respiratory exchange ratio exceeding 1.03 or 1.05 in children and adults, respectively [69, 73, 74]. In addition, a high rating of perceived exertion may be used as a criterion [69, 74].

If the test was stopped due to an adverse reaction to exercise before the patient was exercising maximally this reaction indicates a limitation to exercise (e.g. hypoxaemia, haemoptysis, cardiac arrhythmia and joint pain). In all patients who have a reduced exercise capacity but fulfil the criteria of a maximal effort, the reason for the exercise limitation can be identified from the CPET data (table 3). Figure 1 is an example of a patient with moderately impaired pulmonary function and deconditioning.

Table 2. The modified Godfrey protocol for cycle ergometry

	Increment per minute
FEV1 >30% predicted	
Stature <120 cm	10 W
Stature 120–150 cm	15 W
Stature >150 cm	20 W
FEV1 ⩽30% predicted	
All	10 W

Pre-exercise resting measurements are taken over 3 min. The exercise test starts with 3 min of unloaded pedalling. Thereafter, work rate is increased minute by minute depending on lung function and stature. FEV1: forced expiratory volume in 1 s.

Field tests

In addition to standardised laboratory-based exercise tests, field tests such as walk tests, shuttle tests and step tests are also used to assess exercise capacity in CF. These tests are performed with minimal equipment and at relatively low costs. They have their value in pre-transplant evaluation [75] and functional assessments and may also help in exercise counselling. However, none of these tests are able to identify causes of a reduced exercise capacity and many are not suitable for all patients, *e.g.* very young patients or those who are very fit or very sick.

Physical activity interventions and physical training programmes

Physical activity and exercise have been increasingly recognised as part of CF treatment over the past years [1, 2]. Many centres counsel their patients to include more physical activity in daily life and start some formal training. In Germany, the national patient organisation Mukoviszidose e.V. has not only produced a booklet [65] and a DVD on physical activity and sports in CF to educate patients, their families and care team members but also started an exercise counselling service *via* telephone to all patients. Unfortunately, none of these efforts have been evaluated scientifically.

In contrast, several studies have looked at the effects of formal exercise recommendations and supervised training interventions. To administer physical training programmes different

Table 3. Interpretation of cardiopulmonary exercise test data in patients with reduced exercise capacity

	Respiratory limitation	Cardiovascular limitation	Peripheral (muscular) limitation	Deconditioned
Peak HR	May be reduced	May be reduced	Reduced	Normal
S_pO_2 at peak exercise	May be reduced	Normal	Normal	Normal
$\Delta V'O_2/\Delta WR$ slope	Normal	Often reduced	Often normal	Normal
$\Delta V'E/\Delta V'CO_2$ slope	Often increased	May be increased	Increased	Normal
$V'E$ % MVV	>85%	<85%	<85%	<85%

HR: heart rate; S_pO_2: arterial oxygen saturation measured by pulse oximetry; $V'O_2$: oxygen uptake; WR: work rate; $V'E$: minute ventilation; $V'CO_2$: carbon dioxide production; MVV: maximal voluntary ventilation.

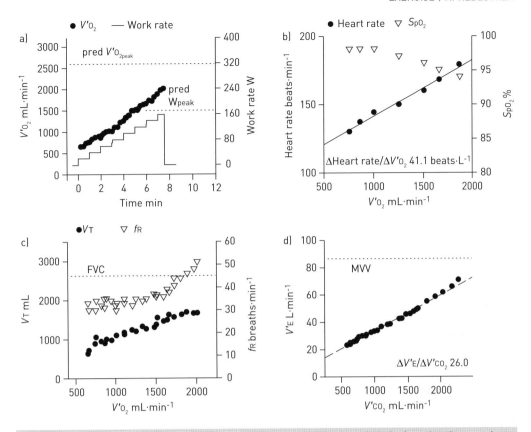

Figure 1. Results of an exercise test in a 16-year-old patient with cystic fibrosis and a forced expiratory volume in 1 s of 57% predicted. Forced vital capacity (FVC) was 65% predicted. The test was maximal since respiratory exchange ratio at peak exercise was 1.12 and rating of perceived exertion was 10 on a Borg CR10 scale. The data indicate deconditioning. a) Peak oxygen uptake (V'_{O_2peak}) (76% predicted) and peak work rate (W_{peak}) (88% predicted) were slightly reduced. b) The Δheart rate/Δoxygen uptake (V'_{O_2}) slope was below the predicted maximal slope of 51.5 beats·L^{-1} and peak heart rate (179 beats·min^{-1}) was in the normal range (92% predicted) indicating normal cardiac function. Arterial oxygen saturation measured by pulse oximetry (S_{pO_2}) decreased from 98% at rest to 94% at peak exercise, which still reflects a normal response (maximum normal drop in S_{pO_2} is 4%). c) There was a normal response in tidal volume (V_T) and respiratory frequency (f_R) with exercise. d) The Δminute ventilation (V'_E)/Δcarbon dioxide production (V'_{CO_2}) slope was within the normal range (it should be <28.6) and V'_E reached 82% of the predicted maximal voluntary ventilation (MVV). Based on this test, the patient started individualised exercise intervention adding 2 h of vigorous activities per week to his routine. Within 7 months, V'_{O_2peak} had increased to 91% predicted without significant changes in lung function. At the re-test, however, there were some signs of respiratory limitation (drop in S_{pO_2} of 5% and V'_E exceeding estimated MVV).

settings have been used, such as inpatient stays for intravenous antibiotic therapy [42] or pulmonary rehabilitation [43, 76], a fully supervised programme in an outpatient setting [40, 77] or a fitness centre [71], and partially supervised programmes at home [39, 78, 79]. Exercise modes predominantly included aerobic training, strength training and anaerobic training, or a combination of these [41, 59, 71, 78, 79]. Training interventions have included children and adults with mild to quite severe lung disease.

Randomised controlled trials showed that programmes were usually effective in improving aerobic fitness [39–42, 71, 77], strength [42] and anaerobic performance [41]. Many programmes also improved pulmonary function, with forced vital capacity (FVC) being improved more often [42, 59, 71, 78] than FEV1 [42, 71]. In contrast to common beliefs that regular exercise leads to weight loss, body weight or BMI did not change and even improved in the patients engaging in an exercise programme compared with the control group [39, 42, 59]. Furthermore, several studies indicate that health-related quality of life (HRQoL) improves with conditioning [39, 41, 42].

All these benefits may last for some time beyond the intervention period [39]. Figure 2 summarises the effects of a 6-month partially supervised, individualised, mainly aerobic exercise intervention on anthropometry, lung function and exercise capacity 12–18 months after the end of the programme.

Possible mechanisms involved in the effects of regular exercise on pulmonary disease

Several effects of exercise have been observed that might explain, at least in part, the benefits of physical activity and exercise in CF on lung function.

Exercise for airway clearance

Some evidence indicates that sputum expectoration might be augmented by an exercise bout compared with rest [80, 81]. It has been speculated that these effects might be the consequence of whole body vibrations and an increase in ventilation with exercise.

Exercise inhibits epithelial sodium channels

The most common hypothesis explaining CF airway pathophysiology assumes a depleted periciliary liquid (PCL) volume due to a failure to secrete chloride and a hyperabsorption of sodium. Using measurements of nasal potential difference (NPD) at rest and during exercise, an inhibition of amiloride-sensitive epithelial sodium channels during exercise has been observed in healthy people and those with CF [82, 83]. It is possible that the exercise-induced increase in ventilation results in increased phasic shear stress to the epithelial cells. This has been shown to reduce the amiloride-sensitive sodium transport in CF epithelial cells, possibly *via* shear stress induced ATP-release interacting with P2 receptors [84].

Modulation of immune function

It has been suggested that exercise exerts anti-inflammatory effects [85], which may also be relevant in people with CF participating in regular exercise [86]. However, much more research is needed.

Exercise counselling and prescription

Some "unscheduled" exercise counselling often occurs during clinic visits. The patient is asked for his or her activities and symptoms related to exercise. Based on this information, the clinical findings and diagnostic results, some exercise-related recommendations are given to the patient. In many centres, more structured assessments and counselling occur once or twice a year.

In my opinion, four groups of patients may warrant more intense work-up with respect to exercise counselling: 1) those with very low activity/low fitness levels; 2) those with extremely high exercise levels including competitive athletes; 3) those reporting adverse reactions to exercise or with newly diagnosed risk factors; and 4) those with severe disease.

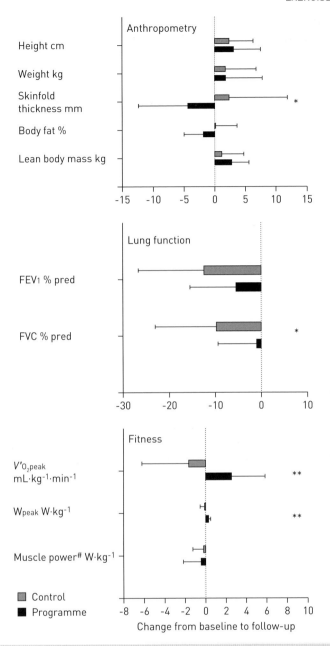

Figure 2. Effects of a 6-month partially supervised conditioning programme, compared with control, on several outcomes determined 12–18 months after the programme had finished. FEV1: forced expiratory volume in 1 s; FVC: forced vital capacity; $V'O_2peak$: peak oxygen uptake; W_{peak}: peak work rate. Data are presented as mean±SD. #: mean power during a 30-s Wingate test. *: p<0.05; **: p<0.01. Data from [39].

Patients with low activity/fitness levels

These individuals may be identified based on interviews during the clinic visit, activity questionnaires, objective activity assessments, or exercise testing. The approach many centres currently take during exercise counselling in this group is to perform a motivational interview to identify activities that are enjoyable and feasible for the individual, and which could easily be incorporated into weekly routines. Obviously, activities with a perceived risk should not be encouraged. Selecting activities that can be done with friends and that do not depend on specific weather conditions are likely to yield more success than those carried out alone outdoors. Especially in adolescents and young adults, these activities might also include weight/resistance training to bulk-up muscles and exercises employing active video games [87, 88]. An inpatient stay for routine antibiotic therapy or other reasons can be used to introduce these activities to patients and to train them in the correct performance of the exercises to reduce risks. It is important to stress during the session that some activity is better than none, and that the patient is not required to engage in a specific sport for x hours per week since many of the patients in this group have negative feelings about "sports". It is also important to set realistic goals and, in some individuals, motivational tools like step counters or smartphone apps may help to boost adherence. It is likely that only a few patients in this group will benefit from a formal exercise prescription.

Since some CF centres do not have the expertise or time to counsel patients on physical activity, the German CF organisation Mukoviszidose e.V. has established a central office which can help patients to become more active.

Patients with extremely high activity levels including competitive athletes

These patients need to be especially aware of their individual risks and possible means of precaution. In other words, they need very specific guidance on what to do during exercise, such as how to adjust fluid/salt intake during a long distance run in hot weather or how to modify insulin dosage during a day of hiking. Furthermore, proper counselling on training regimes is necessary to ensure that individual goals can be reached without doing (risking) too much. It has been shown that injuries due to overtraining and overuse may occur in highly motivated individuals [89].

Patients reporting adverse reactions to exercise or with newly diagnosed risk factors

Patients reporting adverse reactions to exercise may require additional diagnostic procedures, including exercise testing, depending on the symptoms reported. Based on the understanding of individual factors underlying the reported symptom (see earlier), counselling addresses the possible measures to prevent problems and treat symptoms.

It is important to realise that some exercise-associated problems reported may not be reproduced in the clinical setting and require true field observations (*e.g.* a video clip recorded on the smartphone). However, some reports of adverse events are anxiety driven. In these cases, proving that there is no danger during exercise may help the patient, their family and/or teachers and staff to allow more activities to be undertaken.

Patients with severe lung disease

Although there is limited scientific evidence, some studies suggest that patients with severe lung disease may benefit from structured exercise programmes [43, 90]. In this population, additional oxygen or even noninvasive ventilation may be required during exercise. Individuals may also use strength training involving only small muscle groups, such as training only elbow flexors of one arm at a time or interval training to reduce dyspnoea. Interval training with 10 sets of 20–30 s of relatively intense cycling or treadmill walking followed by 60 s of active recovery has also been found to be feasible and effective in improving fitness in this group [43].

Conclusions

Physical activity and exercise are beneficial for people with CF and, thus, important for CF care. There may be several reasons for a reduced exercise capacity, including: respiratory limitations, cardiovascular limitations, peripheral (muscular) limitations and infection/inflammation, as well as deconditioning. CPET may help to distinguish among these. Furthermore, CPET can reveal adverse reactions to exercise such as exercise-induced hypoxaemia and can motivate patients to become more active. Additional risks associated with exertion may be identified from a patient's clinical condition and their preferred activities. Exercise counselling should motivate towards exercise, identify barriers and facilitators to becoming active, set realistic goals, and find an achievable and enjoyable way to lead an active life for each individual.

References

1. Barker M, Hebestreit A, Gruber W, *et al.* Exercise testing and training in German CF centres. *Pediatr Pulmonol* 2004; 37: 351–355.
2. Stevens D, Oades PJ, Armstrong N, *et al.* A survey of exercise testing and training in UK cystic fibrosis clinics. *J Cyst Fibros* 2010; 9: 302–306.
3. Armstrong N, Welsman JR. The physical activity patterns of European youth with reference to methods of assessment. *Sports Med* 2006; 36: 1067–1086.
4. Spittaels H, van Cauwenberghe E, Verbestel V, *et al.* Objectively measured sedentary time and physical activity time across the lifespan: a cross-sectional study in four age groups. *Int J Behav Nutr Phys Act* 2012; 9: 149.
5. Selvadurai HC, Blimkie CJ, Cooper PJ, *et al.* Gender differences in habitual activity in children with cystic fibrosis. *Arch Dis Child* 2004; 89: 928–933.
6. Schneiderman-Walker J, Wilkes DL, Strug L, *et al.* Sex differences in habitual physical activity and lung function decline in children with cystic fibrosis. *J Pediatr* 2005; 147: 321–326.
7. Schneiderman JE, Wilkes DL, Atenafu DE, *et al.* Longitudinal relationship between physical activity and lung health in patients with cystic fibrosis. *Eur Respir J* 2014; 43: 817–823.
8. Buntain HM, Greer RM, Schluter PJ, *et al.* Bone mineral density in Australian children, adolescents and adults with cystic fibrosis: a controlled cross-sectional study. *Thorax* 2004; 59: 149–155.
9. García ST, Giráldez Sánchez MA, Cejudo P, *et al.* Bone health, daily physical activity, and exercise tolerance in patients with cystic fibrosis. *Chest* 2011; 140: 475–481.
10. de Meer K, Gulmans VA, van der Laag J. Peripheral muscle weakness and exercise capacity in children with cystic fibrosis. *Am J Respir Crit Care Med* 1999; 159: 748–754.
11. Freeman W, Stableforth DE, Cayton RM, *et al.* Endurance exercise capacity in adults with cystic fibrosis. *Respir Med* 1993; 87: 541–549.
12. Cabrera ME, Lough MD, Doershuk CF, *et al.* Anaerobic performance assessed by the Wingate Test in patients with cystic fibrosis. *Pediatr Exerc Sci* 1993; 5: 78–87.
13. Hebestreit H, Kieser S, Rüdiger S, *et al.* Physical activity is independently related to aerobic capacity in cystic fibrosis. *Eur Respir J* 2006; 28: 734–739.
14. Nixon PA, Orenstein DM, Kelsey SF, *et al.* The prognostic value of exercise testing in patients with cystic fibrosis. *N Engl J Med* 1992; 327: 1785–1788.
15. Moorcroft AJ, Dodd ME, Webb AK. Exercise testing and prognosis in adult cystic fibrosis. *Thorax* 1997; 52: 291–293.
16. Rüter K, Staab D, Magdorf K, *et al.* The 12-min walk test as an assessment criterion for lung transplantation in subjects with cystic fibrosis. *J Cyst Fibros* 2003; 2: 8–13.
17. Pérez M, Groeneveld IF, Santana Sosa E, *et al.* Aerobic fitness is associated with lower risk of hospitalization in children with cystic fibrosis. *Pediatr Pulmonol* 2013 [In press DOI: 10.1002/ppul.22878].
18. Dodd JD, Barry SC, Barry RB, *et al.* Thin-section CT in patients with cystic fibrosis: correlation with peak exercise capacity and body mass index. *Radiology* 2006; 240: 236–245.
19. Lands LC, Heigenhauser GJF, Jones NL. Analysis of factors limiting maximal exercise performance in cystic fibrosis. *Clin Sci* 1992; 83: 391–397.

20. Shah AR, Gozal D, Keens TG. Determinants of aerobic and anaerobic exercise performance in cystic fibrosis. *Am J Respir Crit Care Med* 1998; 157: 1145–1150.

21. Pianosi P, LeBlanc J, Almudevar A. Relationship between FEV1 and peak oxygen uptake in children with cystic fibrosis. *Pediatr Pulmonol* 2005; 40: 324–329.

22. Alison JA, Regnis JA, Donnelly PM, *et al.* End-expiratory lung volume during arm and leg exercise in normal subjects and patients with cystic fibrosis. *Am J Respir Crit Care Med* 1998; 158: 1450–1458.

23. Bradley S, Solin P, Wilson J, *et al.* Hypoxemia and hypercapnia during exercise and sleep in patients with cystic fibrosis. *Chest* 1999; 116: 647–654.

24. Levison H, Cherniack RM. Ventilatory cost of exercise in chronic obstructive pulmonary disease. *J Appl Physiol* 1968; 25: 21–27.

25. Hortop J, Desmond KJ, Coates AL. The mechanical effects of expiratory airflow limitation on cardiac performance in cystic fibrosis. *Am Rev Respir Dis* 1988; 137: 132–137.

26. Marcotte JE, Canny GJ, Grisdale R, *et al.* Effects of nutritional status on exercise performance in advanced cystic fibrosis. *Chest* 1986; 90: 375–379.

27. Pianosi P, Pelech A. Stroke volume during exercise in cystic fibrosis. *Am J Respir Crit Care Med* 1996; 153: 1105–1109.

28. Lands LC, Heigenhauser GJF, Jones NL. Cardiac output determination during progressive exercise in cystic fibrosis. *Chest* 1992; 102: 1118–1123.

29. Koelling TM, Dec GW, Ginns LC, *et al.* Left ventricular diastolic function in patients with advanced cystic fibrosis. *Chest* 2003; 123: 1488–1494.

30. Hayes D Jr, Daniels CJ, Mansour HM, *et al.* Right heart catheterization measuring central hemodynamics in cystic fibrosis during exercise. *Respir Med* 2013; 107: 1365–1369.

31. Manika K, Pitsiou GG, Boutou AK, *et al.* The impact of pulmonary arterial pressure on exercise capacity in mild-to-moderate cystic fibrosis: a case control study. *Pulm Med* 2012; 2012: 252345.

32. Boas SR, Joswiak ML, Nixon PA, *et al.* Factors limiting anaerobic performance in adolescent males with cystic fibrosis. *Med Sci Sports Exerc* 1996; 28: 291–298.

33. Moser C, Tirakitsoontorn P, Nussbaum E, *et al.* Muscle size and cardiorespiratory response to exercise in cystic fibrosis. *Am J Respir Crit Care Med* 2000; 162: 1823–1827.

34. Selvadurai HC, Sachinwalla T, Macauley J, *et al.* Muscle function and resting energy expenditure in female athletes with cystic fibrosis. *Am J Respir Crit Care Med* 2003; 168: 1476–1480.

35. Divangashi M, Balghi H, Danialou G, *et al.* Lack of CFTR in skeletal muscle predisposes to muscle wasting and diaphragm muscle pump failure in cystic fibrosis mice. *PLoS Genet* 2009; 5: e1000586.

36. Lamhonwah AM, Bear CE, Huan LJ, *et al.* Cystic fibrosis transmembrane conductance regulator in human muscle: dysfunction causes abnormal metabolic recovery in exercise. *Ann Neurol* 2010; 67: 802–808.

37. van de Weert-van Leeuwen PB, Slieker MG, Hulzebos HJ, *et al.* Chronic infection and inflammation affect exercise capacity in cystic fibrosis. *Eur Respir J* 2012; 39: 893–898.

38. Fournier C, Bosquet L, Leroy S, *et al.* Évaluation de l'activité physique quotidienne de patients adultes atteints de mucoviscidose [Measurement of daily physical activity in patients with cystic fibrosis]. *Rev Mal Respir* 2005; 22: 63–69.

39. Hebestreit H, Kieser S, Junge S, *et al.* Long-term effects of a partially supervised conditioning programme in cystic fibrosis. *Eur Respir J* 2010; 35: 578–583.

40. Orenstein DM, Franklin BA, Doerchuk CF, *et al.* Exercise conditioning and cardiopulmonary fitness in cystic fibrosis. The effects of a three-month supervised running program. *Chest* 1981; 80: 392–398.

41. Klijn PH, Oushoorn A, van der Ent CK, *et al.* Effects of anaerobic training in children with cystic fibrosis: a randomized controlled study. *Chest* 2004; 125: 1299–1305.

42. Selvadurai HC, Blimkie CJ, Meyers N, *et al.* Randomized controlled study of in-hospital exercise training programs in children with cystic fibrosis. *Pediatr Pulmonol* 2002; 33: 194–200.

43. Gruber W, Orenstein D, Braumann KM, *et al.* Interval exercise training in cystic fibrosis – effects on exercise capacity in severely affected adults. *J Cyst Fibros* 2014; 13: 86–91.

44. Conway SP, Morton AM, Oldroyd B, *et al.* Osteoporosis and osteopenia in adults and adolescents with cystic fibrosis: prevalence and associated factors. *Thorax* 2000; 55: 798–804.

45. Ruf K, Winkler B, Hebestreit A, *et al.* Risks associated with exercise testing and sports participation in cystic fibrosis. *J Cyst Fibros* 2010; 9: 339–345.

46. Gruber W, Orenstein DM, Paul K, *et al.* Motor performance is better than normal in preschool children with cystic fibrosis. *Pediatr Pulmonol* 2010; 45: 527–535.

47. Lebecque P, Lapierre JG, Lamarre A, *et al.* Diffusion capacity and oxygen desaturation effects on exercise in patients with cystic fibrosis. *Chest* 1987; 91: 693–697.

48. Ruf K, Hebestreit H. Exercise-induced hypoxemia and cardiac arhythmia in cystic fibrosis. *J Cyst Fibros* 2009; 8: 83–90.

49. Boas SR. Exercise recommendations for individuals with cystic fibrosis. *Sports Med* 1997; 24: 17–37.

50. Silverman M, Hobbs FDR, Gordon IRS, *et al.* Cystic fibrosis, atopy, and airway lability. *Arch Dis Child* 1978; 53: 873–877.

51. Kaplan TA, Moccia G, McKey RM. Unique pattern of pulmonary function after exercise in patients with cystic fibrosis. *Pediatr Exerc Sci* 1994; 6: 275–286.

52. Price JF, Weller PH, Harper SA, *et al.* Response to bronchial provocation and exercise in children with cystic fibrosis. *Clin Allergy* 1979; 9: 563–570.

53. MacFarlane PI, Heaf D. Changes in airflow obstruction and oxygen saturation in response to exercise and bronchodilators in cystic fibrosis. *Pediatr Pulmonol* 1990; 8: 4–11.

54. Flume PA, Strange C, Ye X, *et al.* Pneumothorax in cystic fibrosis. *Chest* 2005; 128: 720–728.

55. Flume PA, Mogayzel PJ Jr, Robinson KA, *et al.* Cystic fibrosis pulmonary guidelines: pulmonary complications: hemoptysis and pneumothorax. *Am J Respir Crit Care Med* 2010; 182: 298–306.

56. Bar-Or O, Blimkie CJ, Hay JA, *et al.* Voluntary dehydration and heat intolerance in cystic fibrosis. *Lancet* 1992; 339: 696–699.

57. Brown MR, McCarty NA, Millard-Stafford M. High-sweat Na^+ in cystic fibrosis and healthy individuals does not diminish thirst during exercise in the heat. *Am J Physiol Regul Integr Comp Physiol* 2011; 301: R1177–R1185.

58. Kriemler S, Wilk B, Schurer W, *et al.* Preventing dehydration in children with cystic fibrosis who exercise in the heat. *Med Sci Sports Exerc* 1999; 31: 774–779.

59. Moorcroft AJ, Dodd ME, Morris J, *et al.* Individualized unsupervised exercise training in adults with cystic fibrosis: a 1 year randomized controlled trial. *Thorax* 2004; 59: 1074–1080.

60. Wells GD, Wilkes DL, Schneiderman-Walker J, *et al.* Reliability and validity of the habitual activity estimation scale (HAES) in patients with cystic fibrosis. *Pediatr Pulmonol* 2008; 43: 345–353.

61. Ruf KC, Fehn S, Bachmann M, *et al.* Validation of activity questionnaires in patients with cystic fibrosis by accelerometry and cycle ergometry. *BMC Med Res Methodol* 2012; 12: 43.

62. Dwyer TJ, Alison JA, McKeough ZJ, *et al.* Evaluation of the SenseWear activity monitor during exercise in cystic fibrosis and in health. *Respir Med* 2009; 103: 1511–1517.

63. Savi D, Quattrucci S, Internullo M, *et al.* Measuring habitual physical activity in adults with cystic fibrosis. *Respir Med* 2013; 107: 1888–1894.

64. Quon BS, Patrick DL, Edwards TC, *et al.* Feasibility of using pedometers to measure daily step counts in cystic fibrosis and an assessment of its responsiveness to changes in health state. *J Cyst Fibros* 2012; 11: 216–222.

65. Gruber W, Hebestreit A, Hebestreit H, *et al.* Leitfaden Sport bei Mukoviszidose. Bonn, Muko e.V., 2004.

66. Karila C, Gautthier R, Denjean A. Épreuve d'effort et mucoviscidose [Exercise testing in patients with cystic fibrosis]. *Rev Pneumol Clin* 2008; 64: 195–201.

67. Agent P, Morrison L, Prasad A, eds. Standards of Care and Good Clinical Practice for the Physiotherapy Management of Cystic Fibrosis. 2nd Edn. London, Cystic Fibrosis Trust, 2011.

68. Clinical exercise testing with reference to lung diseases: indications, standardization and interpretation strategies. ERS Task Force on Standardization of Clinical Exercise Testing. European Respiratory Society. *Eur Respir J* 1997; 10: 2662–2289.

69. American Thoracic Society, American College of Chest Physicians. ATS/ACCP statement on cardiopulmonary exercise testing. *Am J Respir Crit Care Med* 2003; 167: 211–277.

70. Godfrey S, Davies CT, Wozniak E, *et al.* Cardio-respiratory response to exercise in normal children. *Clin Sci* 1971; 40: 419–431.

71. Kriemler S, Kieser S, Junge S, *et al.* Effect of supervised training on FEV1 in cystic fibrosis: a randomised controlled trial. *J Cyst Fibros* 2013; 12: 714–720.

72. Orenstein DM. Assessment of exercise pulmonary function. *In*: Rowland TW, ed. Pediatric Laboratory Exercise Testing. Clinical Guidelines. Champaign, Human Kinetics Publishers, 1993; pp. 141–163.

73. Rowland TW, ed. Developmental Exercise Physiology. Champaign, Human Kinetics Publishers, 1996.

74. Nes BM, Janszky I, Wisloff U, *et al.* Age-predicted maximal heart rate in healthy subjects: the HUNT Fitness Study. *Scand J Med Sci Sports* 2013; 23: 697–704.

75. Radtke T, Faro A, Wong J, *et al.* Exercise testing in pediatric lung transplant candidates with cystic fibrosis. *Pediatr Transplant* 2011; 15: 294–299.

76. Gruber W, Orenstein DM, Braumann KM, *et al.* Health-related fitness and trainability in children with cystic fibrosis. *Pediatr Pulmonol* 2008; 43: 953–964.

77. Santana Sosa E, Groenefeld IF, Gonzales-Saiz L, *et al.* Intrahospital weight and aerobic training in children with cystic fibrosis: a randomized controlled trial. *Med Sci Sports Exerc* 2012; 44: 2–11.

78. Schneiderman-Walker J, Pollock SL, Corey M, *et al.* A randomized controlled trial of a three year home exercise program in cystic fibrosis. *J Pediatr* 2000; 136: 304–310.

79. Orenstein DM, Hovell MF, Mulvihill M, *et al.* Strength *vs* aerobic training in children with cystic fibrosis. A randomized controlled trial. *Chest* 2004; 126: 1204–1214.

80. Baldwin DR, Hill AL, Peckham DG, *et al.* Effect of addition of exercise to chest physiotherapy on sputum expectoration and lung function in adults with cystic fibrosis. *Respir Med* 1994; 88: 49–53.

81. Zach M, Purrer B, Oberwalder B. Effect of swimming on forced expiration and sputum clearance in cystic fibrosis. *Lancet* 1981; 2: 1201–1203.

82. Hebestreit A, Kersting U, Basler B, *et al.* Exercise inhibits epithelial sodium channels in patients with cystic fibrosis. *Am J Respir Crit Care Med* 2001; 164: 443–446.

83. Schmitt L, Wiebel M, Frese F, *et al.* Exercise reduces airway sodium ion absorption in cystic fibrosis but not in exercise asthma. *Eur Respir J* 2011; 37: 342–348.

84. Tarran R, Button B, Picher M, *et al.* Normal and cystic fibrosis airway surface liquid homeostasis. The effects of phasic shear stress and viral infections. *J Biol Chem* 2005; 280: 35751–35759.

85. Walsh NP, Gleeson M, Shephard RJ, *et al.* Position stand: Part one: Immune function and exercise. *Exerc Immunol Rev* 2011; 17: 6–63.

86. van de Weert-van Leeuwen PB, Arets HG, van der Ent CK, *et al.* Infection, inflammation and exercise in cystic fibrosis. *Respir Res* 2013; 14: 32.

87. Holmes H, Wood J, Jenkins S, *et al.* Xbox Kinect™ represents high intensity exercise for adults with cystic fibrosis. *J Cyst Fibros* 2013; 12: 604–608.

88. O'Donovan C, Greally P, Canny G, *et al.* Active video games as an exercise tool for children with cystic fibrosis. *J Cyst Fibros* 2014; 13: 341–346.

89. Neubauer H, Wirth C, Ruf K, *et al.* Acute muscle trauma due to overexercise in an otherwise healthy patient with cystic fibrosis. *Case Rep Pediatr* 2012; 2012: 527989.

90. Mathur S, Hornblower E, Levy RD. Exercise training before and after lung transplantation. *Phys Sportsmed* 2009; 37: 78–87.

Disclosures: H. Hebestreit reports personal fees and presentation and advisory board fees from Vertex Pharmaceuticals (€4000) and Pharmaxis Ltd (€3000). He has been a principal investigator in studies, with financial compensation of study activities paid to his employer. H. Hebestreit is a principal investigator of the IgY study; compensation for study activities were paid to his employer by Mukoviszidose e.V. Outside the submitted work he is a coordinator of the European Cystic Fibrosis Society Exercise Working Group and a member of the Working Group on Exercise of the German patient organisation Mukoviszidose e.V.

Chapter 15

Extrapulmonary manifestations of cystic fibrosis

Barry J. Plant[1] and Michael D. Parkins[2]

This chapter details the key manifestations of extrapulmonary cystic fibrosis (CF), which include the following. 1) Nasal polyposis: an increasing prevalence from 18% in patients aged <6 years to 45% in adolescents/adults. 2) Focal biliary fibrosis: progresses to multilobular biliary cirrhosis in 5–10% of affected individuals. 3) Pancreatic insufficiency: occurs in 80–85% of infants and leads to malabsorption. 4) CF-related diabetes mellitus: an increasing prevalence from 2–3% in patients aged 6–10 years to 13.5–17.5% in patients aged 18–24 years. 5) Acute kidney injury: common with an estimated incidence of 4.6–10.1 cases in 10 000 children per year; chronic kidney disease is concentrated in adults. 6) Gastro-oesophageal reflux disease: observed in up to 80% of CF patients. 7) Obstructive azoospermia: results in infertility in ~98% of males with CF. Stress urinary incontinence remains an under-reported issue in female CF patients. 8) Osteoporosis: suggested to have a pooled prevalence of 23.5% in adult CF patients. 9) Gastro-intestinal cancer: risk was found to be significantly increased in CF patient cohorts. 10) Macrovascular complications: emerging issue for CF patients. 11) Anxiety and depression: rates range from 10% to 30%.

Although cystic fibrosis (CF) is most recognisable for its pulmonary manifestations, the first symptoms that are apparent and its very namesake derive from extrapulmonary pathology. Aberrant chloride transport across epithelial surfaces owing to cystic fibrosis transmembrane conductance regulator (CFTR) mutations in various organ systems results in a wide range of phenotypes. The spectrum of extrapulmonary diseases in CF patients varies both in prevalence and presentation (fig. 1). With the observed improved survival of patients in recent decades, the impact of chronic inflammation, chronic CFTR dysfunction and nutritional compromises on other organ systems over a lifetime are increasingly apparent and important. The long-term complications associated with lung transplantation are covered in another chapter in this *Monograph* [1]. Many of the extrapulmonary manifestations of CF may be further accentuated under cytotoxic immunosuppressive treatments that are required. In this chapter we summarise the most salient points regarding each of the classic extrapulmonary manifestations of CF and how their prevalence changes with age (fig. 2), focusing on a pre-transplant CF population. Extrapulmonary manifestations are detailed in a cranial–caudal progression.

[1]Adult Cystic Fibrosis Centre, Dept of Medicine, Cork University Hospital, University College Cork, Cork, Ireland. [2]Dept of Medicine, The University of Calgary, Calgary, AB, Canada.

Correspondence: Barry J. Plant, Adult Cystic Fibrosis Centre, Dept of Medicine, Cork University Hospital, University College Cork, Cork, Ireland. E-mail: b.plant@ucc.ie

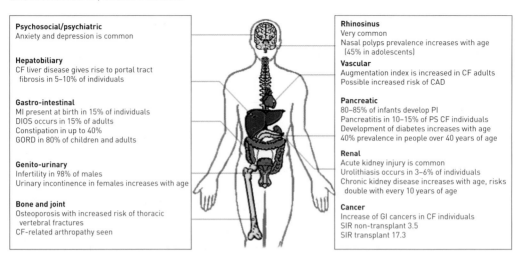

Psychosocial/psychiatric
Anxiety and depression is common

Hepatobiliary
CF liver disease gives rise to portal tract
  fibrosis in 5–10% of individuals

Gastro-intestinal
MI present at birth in 15% of individuals
DIOS occurs in 15% of adults
Constipation in up to 40%
GORD in 80% of children and adults

Genito-urinary
Infertility in 98% of males
Urinary incontinence in females increases with age

Bone and joint
Osteoporosis with increased risk of thoracic
  vertebral fractures
CF-related arthropathy seen

Rhinosinus
Very common
Nasal polyps prevalence increases with age
  (45% in adolescents)

Vascular
Augmentation index is increased in CF adults
Possible increased risk of CAD

Pancreatic
80–85% of infants develop PI
Pancreatitis in 10–15% of PS CF individuals
Development of diabetes increases with age
40% prevalence in people over 40 years of age

Renal
Acute kidney injury is common
Urolithiasis occurs in 3–6% of individuals
Chronic kidney disease increases with age, risks
  double with every 10 years of age

Cancer
Increase of GI cancers in CF individuals
SIR non-transplant 3.5
SIR transplant 17.3

Figure 1. Key nonpulmonary manifestations of cystic fibrosis (CF). MI: meconium ileus; DIOS: distal intestinal obstruction syndrome; GORD: gastro-oesophageal reflux disease; CAD: coronary artery disease; PI: pancreatic insufficiency; PS: pancreatic sufficiency; GI: gastro-intestinal; SIR: standardised incidence ratios. Figure courtesy of James Finn (University College Cork, Cork, Ireland).

Rhinosinus manifestations

Sinus involvement in CF is very common at all ages [3], presenting symptoms including nasal obstruction and snoring, rhinorrhoea, headache and anosmia. Symptomatic disease is rarely self-reported, suggesting adaptation to chronic circumstances [4].

CF rhinosinus has distinguishing characteristics, including medial displacement of the lateral nasal wall, demineralisation of the uncinate, hypoplasia of the frontal and sphenoid sinuses, and the formation of mucoceles. The majority of patients benefit from chronic sinus irrigation with saline/hypertonic saline, and/or corticosteroids [5]. Recalcitrant cases may require antipseudomonal antibiotics and DNase used as irrigants. Aerosolised therapies, in

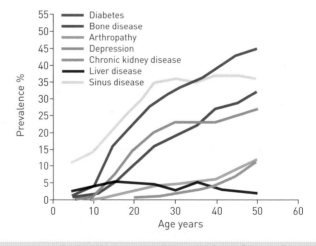

Figure 2. Extrapulmonary complications by age according to the Cystic Fibrosis Foundation Patient Registry. Reproduced and modified from [2] with permission from the publisher.

the absence of ostial surgical widening, are not typically delivered to the sinuses [6]. Although, new pulsating nebulisers designed for sinus administration hold promise for conservative management, many patients require surgery when conservative measures fail to settle symptoms.

Increasing evidence supports the argument that sinuses may be the initial portal for pathogen entry and development of chronic sinopulmonary colonisation. Extensive functional endoscopic sinus surgery (FESS) increases access to the sinuses for the administration of intranasal topical antibiotics, mucolytics and airway rehydrants, and aggressive treatment may reduce chronic infection development [7–9].

Nasal polyposis (NP) is a common feature in CF patients and may result in a CF diagnosis in those individuals presenting outside of infancy with NP, as NP is relatively obscure in the general population. The prevalence increases with age in CF patients, from 18% in those aged <6 years to 45% in adolescents and adults [10]. Unlike asthma, CF NP consists of neutrophilic as opposed to eosinophilic infiltrates and leads to an increase in epithelial mucus [11]. Risk factors include severe CF genotype, and both *Pseudomonas aeruginosa* colonisation and duration of colonisation [12]. The presence of NP does not portend a poorer prognosis [13]. Treatment includes saline irrigations and the topical application of inhaled corticosteroids, with surgical resection reserved for those cases failing conservative management as they frequently recur [5].

Hepatobiliary manifestations

Liver involvement is reported in up to a third of the CF population [14, 15]. Hepatobiliary diseases in CF patients may include: hepatic steatosis, sclerosing cholangitis, cholelithiasis, biliary tract or ductal stones or stenosis, micro-gallbladder and complications of drugs [16]. However, focal biliary cirrhosis leading to portal hypertension is the pathognomonic and most significant complication of cystic fibrosis liver disease (CFLD). The lack of consensus definitions in the literature make exact reporting difficult as some studies include patients with any evidence of liver biochemistry abnormalities or use of ursodeoxycholic acid (URSO), whereas others use strict definitions involving ultrasonographic features such as hepatosplenomegaly.

The pathophysiology of CFLD is thought to be related to impaired cholangiocyte chloride transport with sluggish bile flow resulting in peribiliary fibrosis [17]. Focal biliary fibrosis may progress to multilobular biliary cirrhosis and in 5–10% of individuals this can culminate in portal tract fibrosis with preserved hepatic architecture [14]. Accordingly, advanced CFLD is typified by complications of portal hypertension, whereas hepatocellular synthetic dysfunction is observed to a much lesser degree. The diagnosis is made through a combination of biochemical enzyme surveillance, routine ultrasonography and transient elastography (fibroscan; Echosens, Paris, France) [18, 19]. Current recommendations for screening include annual clinical exam and liver biochemical testing with ultrasounds in those with suspicion of existing or evolving disease [19].

Proposed diagnostic criteria [19], include two or more of: clinical evidence of hepatosplenomegaly, ultrasonographic evidence of CF hepatic parenchymal nodularity or an irregular edge, a liver biopsy showing classic histopathological findings, and/or three consecutive apparent elevations in biochemical testing performed over 1 year.

It is reported that ~30% of children with a diagnosis of CFLD will develop complications of portal hypertension and 10–20% of these children may die from complications of CFLD [20, 21]. Risk factors for development and progression of CFLD in children are not clear but include severe CFTR mutation class, CF modifier genes, such as the Z-allele of *Serpina1*, and environmental factors, and may also include others such as meconium ileus and male sex [14, 22, 23]. Considerable data exist suggesting that *de novo* CFLD does not develop in adults without prior evident disease [24]. Outcomes of CFLD vary somewhat in the literature, which can be attributed to varying definitions used. However, increasing evidence suggests that CFLD is associated with increased risk of mortality [21, 25, 26], and may be associated with more advanced respiratory disease. CFLD with portal hypertension should not be viewed as an absolute contraindication to lung transplantation as outcomes for these individuals may be similar [27].

Management of CFLD should focus on oesophageal and gastric varices. Although the role of URSO is unclear, it continues to be a recommended therapy [19]. Whilst shown to be effective in diminishing and reversing biochemical abnormalities, long-term studies demonstrating the impact on progression of CFLD are lacking [28]. Liver transplantation is a viable strategy for end-stage CFLD. Survival 5 years post-transplantation is approaching 75%, although individuals with advancing lung disease generally do worse. Critically, CF lung disease does not appear to progress disproportionally in liver transplant recipients [29].

Pancreatic and nutritional manifestations

In CF, pancreatic ductal secretions containing enzymes and bicarbonate are blocked by inspissated mucins due to defective CFTR function, thereby resulting in pancreatic autodigestion. This process may even begin *in utero*, and is the basis of many newborn screening assays. Accordingly, 80–85% of infants are born with or quickly develop pancreatic insufficiency (PI) leading to malabsorption, particularly of fats and fat soluble vitamins [30]. PI has the strongest genotype–phenotype correlation observed in CF patients [31]. Symptoms include foul greasy stools, abdominal pain, diarrhoea, weight loss and failure to thrive. PI can be diagnosed with multiple modalities including faecal elastase, fat balance/coefficient of fat absorption and 72-h faecal-fat tests.

Treatment of PI includes pancreatic enzyme replacement therapy (PERT), a high calorie diet that is rich in protein and fat, and optimisation of fat soluble vitamins. PERT consists of porcine-derived formulations of lipase, amylase and proteases, required for the efficient digestion of macromolecules into absorbable elemental components. Enteric-coated preparations of PERT and acid-suppressing agents have improved potency. Standard therapy ($<$10 000 lipase IU·kg^{-1} per day) is highly effective and safe. A rare complication involving the proximal colon termed fibrosing colonopathy was observed in the early 1990s in centres using very high-dose therapy [32]. Monitoring and supplementation of the fat soluble vitamins (vitamins A, D, E and K) is also necessary. In addition, the use of oral nutritional supplements is common. Nocturnal enteral supplementation *via* percutaneous endoscopic gastrostomy (PEG) tubes is used in up to 8% of children who fail to thrive or adults with advancing lung disease to optimise and/or maintain nutrition [33]. Multiple datasets support the importance of nutrition in both pulmonary and overall health outcomes including survival [34–36]. Other factors contributing to nutritional deficiencies in CF are summarised in table 1.

Table 1. Factors contributing to malabsorption in cystic fibrosis

Factor	Aetiology	Result	Management considerations
Pancreatic insufficiency	Physical destruction of acinar tissue replaced with adipose/connective tissue	Loss of endogenous lipase/amylase/protease	PERT Acid-suppressing agents: H2 blockers and PPI
Increased duodenal acidity	Altered bicarbonate transport	Reduced efficacy of enzymes	Acid-suppressing agents: H2 blockers and PPI
Bile salt abnormalities	Increased bile salt loss, secondary to intestinal mucosal anomalies	Reduced solubilisation ability of bile potentiating steatorrhoea	Unknown Taurine supplementation?
Impaired bowel transit	Insufficient digestion in proximal small bowel, owing to pancreatic insufficiency and bicarbonate deficiencies	Impaired transit particularly through distal small intestine	PERT Promotility agents
Small bowel bacterial overgrowth	Synthesis of bacterial-derived enterotoxins and unabsorbable metabolites	Results in intestinal mucosal damage and impedance of digestion and absorption	Lifestyle and dietary changes Judicious use of antibacterials

PERT: pancreatic enzyme replacement therapy; PPI: proton pump inhibitors.

Pancreatitis is a recognisable complication in 10–15% of pancreatic sufficient (PS) CF individuals [34, 37, 38]. They may have milder CFTR mutations (class 4 and 5) with partially active pancreatic enzymatic secretions, which are semi-viscous, resulting in PS that is potentially punctuated by episodes of intermittent ductal obstruction and acute pancreatitis [39]. To develop pancreatitis, CF patients must possess at least 5% of residual pancreatic acinar tissue [40]. Over time these individuals may progress to PI, as repeated pancreatitis results in destruction of residual acinar tissue [37]. Treatment is primarily supportive.

Diabetic manifestations

Cystic fibrosis-related diabetes mellitus (CFRD) represents a unique entity, with some features of both type 1 and type 2 diabetes mellitus [41–43]. Progressive fibrotic disruption and fatty infiltration of the pancreas result in a loss of islet cells, as well as an increasing relative insulin deficiency [41]. Residual insulin production prevents the occurrence of diabetic ketoacidosis. CFRD exists as a spectrum that may evolve from impaired glucose intolerance (IGT) to CFRD with or without fasting hyperglycaemia.

Age is one of the most important factors associated with the development of CFRD and, therefore, CFRD prevalence varies considerably in different cohorts [44, 45]. Cystic Fibrosis Foundation Patient Registry data show that the prevalence increases from 2% to 3% in patients aged 6–10 years, from 5% to 10% in patients aged 11–17 years, and from 13.5% to 17.5% in patients aged 18–24 years. In CF adults aged >40 years this prevalence range is 27–52% [46, 47]. Incidences plateau in the fourth decade of life [48]. Other risk factors for CFRD include advancing lung disease, PI, severe CFTR mutations as well as modifier genes with linkages to diabetes mellitus type II, female sex, CFLD and receipt of systemic steroids [48, 49].

Importantly CFRD has been associated with increased rates of pulmonary function decline, pulmonary exacerbations and the inability to recover lung function after an exacerbation [50–52]. Critically, CFRD is an independent predictor of mortality with a relative risk of up to six-fold greater than non-CFRD [50, 53, 54]. Diagnosis and correction of dysglycaemia can partially reverse the pulmonary function decline in CF, suggesting that CFRD independently contributes to disease progression of lung disease and is not just a marker for advanced disease [55]. Its timely diagnosis has become increasingly stressed in the longitudinal management of CF patients; current recommendations and diagnostic criteria for CFRD are listed in table 2.

Microvascular complications attributable to CFRD are seen generally in those with CFRD of ⩾5–10 years' duration, and not usually before there is evidence of fasting hyperglycaemia. Neuropathy occurs in ~50%, retinopathy and nephropathy in ~15% of those with CFRD for >10 years [56]. Hypertension is relatively uncommon in patients with CF [57]. When present, it is more frequently encountered in patients with CFRD and those post-lung transplant [44]. In patients with CFRD and hypertension, the guidelines suggest treatment modalities similar to other patients with diabetes, with the exception that dietary salt restriction is not as necessary and is potentially harmful [44]. Macrovascular complications have, as yet, been infrequently reported; however, with improvements in survival these may become an important issue in the future, *i.e.* long-term vascular manifestations in CF patients; this is discussed in more detail later in the chapter.

Management goals in CFRD include control of dysglycaemia, avoidance of microvascular complication and maintenance of pulmonary and nutritional status. Importantly, diabetic regimens for CF patients must adjust to compensate for the calorie-dense CF diet as opposed to instituting a restricted diet. Insulin-based regimens are the standard of care recommended in treatment guidelines [44, 58, 59].

Table 2. Diagnostic criteria and recommended screening frequency for cystic fibrosis (CF)-related diabetes mellitus (CFRD)/impaired glucose intolerance (IGT) in a population without CFRD

Modality	When to screen	CF-related pathology diagnosis	
		IGT	CFRD
OGTT (2 h, 75 g)	Annually, when well Prior to transplant referral During pregnancy trimesters and *post partum*	7.8–11 mmol·L^{-1}	>11.1 mmol·L^{-1}
Postprandial (2 h) glucose monitoring	During significant therapeutic changes[#] During enteral feeds	7.8–11 mmol·L^{-1}	>11.1 mmol·L^{-1}
Fasting glucose	Annually, as part of OGTT	>6 mmol·L^{-1}	>7 mmol·L^{-1}
Random glucose	Between routine testing Symptoms of polyuria and/or polydipsia During enteral feeds	7.8–11 mmol·L^{-1}	>11.1 mmol·L^{-1}
HbA1c	Not routinely recommended, but insensitive	Not established	⩾6.5% (values <6.5% do not rule out)

OGTT: oral glucose tolerance test, HbA1c: haemoglobin A1c. [#]: significant therapeutic changes denote hospital admissions for pulmonary exacerbations, changes in systemic steroid therapy and changes in nocturnal enteral feeding. Data from [42, 44].

Renal manifestations

Although CFTR is extensively expressed in the kidney [60] and some functional consequences of its dysfunction can be demonstrated [59] there is no clear CF renal phenotype that obviously manifests with a particular clinical problem. Evidence suggests that CFTR malfunction leads to a defect in the proximal tubular handling of low-molecular weight proteins, leading to low-molecular weight proteinuria [61]. Traditionally, renal problems have not been viewed as being of particular importance in CF patients. However, with improved survival rates, multiple renal-disease syndromes are now being observed [62, 63].

Acute kidney injury (AKI) is common in CF patients, with an estimated incidence of 4.6–10.1 cases per 10 000 in children with CF per year [62], ~100-fold times greater than found in the general population [63]. This cohort is much more likely to have risk factors for AKI, including recent exposure to intravenous aminoglycosides, pre-existing renal disease, dehydration or the use of other nephrotoxic drugs (e.g. nonsteroidal anti-inflammatory drugs (NSAIDs)) [63], and to have sustained a pulmonary exacerbation. AKI should be treated in the standard fashion, including hydration monitoring with correction (or withdrawal) of other risk factors.

Electrolyte abnormalities with chloride depletion and associated metabolic alkalosis are prominent, especially with extremes of heat or exercise. Hyponatraemia, hypokalaemia and profound depletion of extracellular fluid volume can occur through an exaggerated loss in sweat [64] and may be a presenting feature in CF patients that is diagnosed late [65]. Hydration and electrolyte supplementation may prevent the precipitation of these events.

Urolithiasis occurs in 3–6% of individuals with CF each year, a rate three times that in the age-matched controls [66]. Urolithiasis is considered to be multifactorial in origin including decreased urine output, hypocitraturia and absorptive hyperoxaluria with antibiotic-induced loss of oxalate-degrading intestinal microflora [67]. A high fluid intake combined with a low-oxalate and high-calcium diet is an appropriate dietary modification for individuals with a history of calcium oxalate stones.

Permanent micro-albuminuria occurs in 6–14% of patients with CF, the majority of which either have had CFRD for $\geqslant 10$ years or an organ transplant [56, 68]. Proteinuria is very uncommon and almost always reflects established underlying kidney disease. A renal biopsy should be considered as a diagnostic tool. It has revealed a very wide range of pathologies in CF patients, including diabetic nephropathy [69], diffuse and nodular glomerulosclerosis, NSAID toxicity, amyloidosis, nephrocalcinosis, immunoglobulin (Ig)A nephropathy, fibrillary glomerulopathy and, after lung transplantation, IgA nephropathy, pigmented tubulopathy and calcineurin-phosphatase inhibitor toxicity [69, 70]. The presence of nodular glomerulosclerosis has been postulated to be a CF-specific nephropathy occurring in older patients with CF who do not have CFRD as a response to chronic inflammatory stimuli and oxidative stresses [71, 72].

Chronic kidney disease (CKD) increases with age and is concentrated in adults [73, 74]. The largest study of ~12 000 CF adults reported an overall prevalence of CKD stage 3 (estimated glomerular filtration rate (eGFR) <60 mL·min^{-1}·1.73 m^{-2}) of 2.3%. Risks doubled with every additional 10 years of age, particularly in those with CFRD, organ transplantation or in those with a previous diagnosis of AKI. Patients with CKD are more likely to be female and typically have poorer pulmonary function [75]. Interestingly, cumulative exposure to aminoglycosides over 4 years did not lead to a higher frequency of CKD [75]. This has been debated [76, 77], but it has been suggested that a longer-term reduction in the GFR may reflect the consequences of recurrent episodes of AKI rather than the cumulative antibiotic exposure [76]. Once CKD stage 3 is established it is typically progressive, with 53% of cases progressing to CKD stage 4 (eGFR<30 mL·min^{-1}·1.73 m^{-2}) and 44% to stage 5 (eGFR<15 mL·min^{-1}·1.73 m^{-2}) [75]. However, the prevalence of advanced CKD (stages 4 and 5) remains low at 0.7% and 0.6%, respectively.

Gastro-intestinal manifestations

Meconium ileus, distal intestinal obstruction syndrome (DIOS) and constipation in CF patients are all consequences of CFTR dysfunction, resulting in increased viscosity of intestinal mucous and prolonged bowel transit time [78]. Meconium ileus is characterised by complete intestinal obstruction occurring in neonates owing to accumulation of inspissated meconium; it presents at birth in 15% of individuals with CF [79, 80]. Meconium ileus is strongly associated with CFTR class but can also be partially explained by disease-modifying genes [78]; however, its presence in the past was associated with very low survival rates beyond 1 year, studies today show no difference in survival outcomes [81]. Traditional management focused on surgical intervention, but nonsurgical approaches are increasingly effective [82–84].

DIOS is the complete or incomplete obstruction of the terminal ileum/cecum and proximal colon with viscid faeces (table 3). DIOS presents with acute onset of abdominal pain, generally concentrated in the right lower quadrant, with a palpable mass of stool and vomiting. DIOS occurs in <10% of children and ~15% of adults, with an incidence of ~6–23 episodes per 1000 patient-years [86, 87]. Repeated episodes are common. Risk factors include PI, steatorrhoea and/or PERT noncompliance, meconium ileus history and dehydration [88]. Genetic determinants may also play a small role [80, 89]. Up to 20% of individuals experience DIOS in the peri-transplant period related to the culmination of dehydration, immobility and narcotic-induced slowing of intestinal transit [90]. Treatment approaches vary considerably but may include oral/nasogastric or enema-based therapies, such as laxatives including polyethylene glycol, or hyperosmotic water-soluble contrast, such as sodium meglumine diatrizoate (gastrografin; Bayer, Schering, Germany) or N-acetylcysteine (NAC) [89].

Constipation is a common problem in CF patients and can be found in up to 40% of individuals [88]. Differentiating it from DIOS can be difficult. DIOS is acute, whereas constipation starts as a gradual faecal impaction of the entire colon and generally presents with milder and longer standing symptoms. Constipation management focuses on chronic dietary changes emphasising fibre, fluid intake and the use of chronic laxatives.

Gastro-oesophageal reflux disease (GORD) is observed in up to 80% of children and adults with CF [91, 92]. Postulated mechanisms of GORD in CF include a reduced lower oesophageal sphincter pressure as well as reduced frequency of the lower oesophageal sphincter relaxation and delayed gastric emptying [91, 93]. A strong correlation between GORD and meconium ileus has been reported, which may support the notion that oesophageal motility abnormalities are the underlying mechanism [94]. CF patients have a high risk of microaspiration and the presence of bile acid in sputum is associated with increased airway inflammation and colonisation, with P. aeruginosa, of the lower airways [95, 96]. Furthermore, the presence of bile acid seems to be associated with increased cough frequency and worsening pulmonary function [91, 95].

Table 3. Requirement for the formal diagnosis of distal intestinal obstruction syndrome (DIOS) as defined by the ESPGHAN cystic fibrosis working group

	Complete intestinal obstruction with bilious vomiting and/or evident air fluid levels on AXR	Faecal mass in the ileocecum	Abdominal pain and/or distension
Incomplete DIOS	No	Yes	Yes
Complete DIOS	Yes	Yes	Yes

ESPGHAN: European Society for Paediatric Gastroenterology, Hepatology and Nutrition; AXR: abdominal chest radiograph. Data from [85].

Genito-urinary manifestations

Infertility in males with CF is an important issue. Whilst testicular histology is preserved and active spermatogenesis occurs, obstructive azoospermia due to the absence of the vas deferens results in infertility in 98% of males [97]. However, there are rare CFTR mutations associated with preserved fertility [98]. Recent studies suggest that >90% of males are aware of their infertility [97, 99, 100]; however, two-thirds of patients were unsure of its aetiology [101, 102]. Furthermore, 43% of males surveyed never discussed this topic with their healthcare team [100]. Issues surround who should inform the male patient and when males with CF should first be informed of potential infertility [103, 104]. Semen analysis is required to definitively establish infertility. However, studies suggest that only 27–53% have been tested [104, 105]. Semen analysis was more likely when the patient is married and/or was older (p<0.001). Assisted fertility techniques, including intracytoplasmic sperm injection, can support couples in achieving pregnancy [106, 107].

An under-reported but important issue in females with CF is stress urinary incontinence. Prevalence estimates vary 30–74% in different cohorts [108–110] but increase with age [109, 110] and decreasing forced expiratory volume in 1 s (FEV1) [109]. In a single-centre UK study, prevalence was 80–100% in CF females aged >35 years [111]. This involuntary leakage of urine is exacerbated with cough, pulmonary exacerbations or physiotherapy and may impede effective chest physiotherapy [112]. Proper identification of patients can enable teaching of pelvic floor muscle exercises, which can reduce symptoms and improve quality of life (QoL).

Bone and joint manifestations

The aetiology of CF-related metabolic bone diseases are multifactorial including exocrine PI, vitamin D, vitamin K and calcium insufficiency, inadequate accrual of peak bone mass in adolescence/young adulthood [113], recurrent infection with cytokine-stimulated osteoclast-mediated bone resorption, physical inactivity, steroid use, and CFRD [114–116]. There may also be a CFTR-mediated component [117, 118]. In a recent meta-analysis, pooled prevalence of osteoporosis was 23.5% and osteopenia was 38.0% in adults with CF. Interestingly, prevalence appears to be decreasing over time [119]. This is further supported by a recent large single-centre study showing a significant reduction in the prevalence of osteoporosis over 10 years from 18.8% to 5.8%, and of osteopenia from 48% to 34.5% [120, 121]. It is important to screen for and treat osteoporosis due to an increase in the incidence of fractures in this cohort, with thoracic vertebral being the most common (pooled prevalence 14%). However, fracture risk decreases in patients aged >30 years suggesting a survivor effect

[119]. Rib fractures and kyphosis are also important as any or all of these impact chest physiotherapy routines and may herald pulmonary exacerbations [122].

A combination of preventative strategies is critical for bone health in CF patients. These include: vitamin D, vitamin K and calcium supplementation; optimisation of nutritional status; tight glycaemic control (in patients with CFRD); aggressive treatment of pulmonary exacerbations; and exercise, which includes weight-bearing. Sex hormones and antiresorptive therapies should be considered, particularly in adults with a T/Z score $\leqslant$-2, or $\leqslant$-1 if a fragility fracture has occurred in patients awaiting transplant, and those with accelerated bone mass density (BMD) loss >3–5% per year where appropriate [114, 122].

Arthritis remains a relatively infrequent complication of CF but increases with age; however, it is a cause of significant morbidity when it does occur. Two distinct types of arthritis are classically described in CF patients: CF-related arthropathy (CFA) is more common than hypertrophic osteoarthropathy (HOA) (9% versus 7%, respectively) with an earlier age of onset (15 versus 20 years, respectively) [123]. CFA is a painful, typically relapsing and remitting asymmetric mono- or polyarthritis involving the large joints, which develops over 12–24 h and typically lasts up to 1 week [124]. Associated findings may rarely include fever and a skin rash similar to erythema nodosum. Radiographs are usually normal without evidence of joint destruction. The aetiology is unclear with proposed mechanisms including immune complex-mediated inflammation, induction of autoantibodies, or a reactive arthritis. Treatment with analgesics and anti-inflammatory agents may be needed. Glucocorticoids and disease-modifying antirheumatic drugs may be considered in refractory cases.

HOA is more common with severe lung disease and during acute pulmonary exacerbations [123], and usually involves large joints with insidious dull bony pain at the distal end of long bones in the extremities as the presenting feature [125]. Unlike CFA, a rash is not a feature with HOA and diagnostic imaging is useful with plain radiography or nuclear bone scanning demonstrating periosteal thickening and elevation. Treatment is similar to CFA. Interestingly, a recent single-centre German study, which included 70 patients with CF, demonstrated that the prevalence of rheumatic symptoms increased with age and CF severity, and that there was an association with P. aeruginosa and Aspergillus fumigatus infections. However, no association with CF and definite inflammatory joint or connective tissue diseases was observed, and no CF-specific pattern of musculoskeletal symptoms were seen [126].

Cancer manifestations

In healthy populations, the risk of malignancy with increasing age has been well established [127]. In CF patients these concerns have been documented, with early studies highlighting an increase in gastro-intestinal (GI) malignancies [128–130]. As a measure of relative risk, studies have employed the use of standardised incidence ratios (SIRs), the ratio of observed compared with expected cancers in a cohort, extrapolated from general population data. In a large USA Patient Registry study between 1990 and 1999 [131], there was a significantly increased number of cancers arising in the GI tract in non-transplant CF patients. This has recently been followed up with a further 10 years of registry data from the same population which, when pooled with original data, demonstrates a significant increase in GI cancers (n=45, 0 observed versus 12.8 expected; SIR 3.5, 95% CI 2.6–4.7) [132]. The increased risk was associated with cancers detected in the small intestine (SIR 11.5), biliary tract (SIR 11.4), colon (SIR 6.2) and oesophagus/stomach (SIR 3.1). Risk factors associated with the development of bowel cancer included previous DIOS and homozygosity for Phe508del mutation. Other prior GI conditions that include GORD, liver disease or CFRD, were not associated with a higher risk of GI malignancy [132]. However, the original 10-year data from this cohort suggested an increased risk of digestive cancers with increasing age. Pooling of the expanded data set over a 20-year period suggested that the SIR did not vary substantially with age; however, it was higher in males *versus* females (8.4 *versus* 4.6). Similar findings were seen in the post-transplant CF cohort (digestive tract cancer SIR 17.3) and this is further supported by a single-transplant centre study that reported an incidence in colon cancer in CF patients of 5.7% compared with 0.3% in post-lung transplant patients who did not have CF [133]. Screening by colonoscopy identified polyps in 35% of CF post-transplant patients, supporting the role of screening in this cohort.

One of the problems facing the CF clinician in diagnosing digestive tract malignancies relates to the frequency of bowel complications in CF patients. Anaemia is common in CF patients, and increases with age and may be associated with iron deficiency [134, 135]. Its assessment is complex due to the underlying inflammatory nature of CF, complicating the interpretation of iron status. Abdominal pain and constipation are common features of CF. The decision of when and how to investigate possible bowel pathology is a complex clinical dilemma [136]. Some centres advocate routine colonoscopy at 40 years of age as well as symptom-based investigations for noncolon complaints.

Currently, there are conflicting data on whether CF confers an increased risk of non-GI cancers [130, 131, 137]; however, recent studies have suggested an increased risk of testicular (SIR 1.7–2.6) and thyroid (SIR 9.6) cancers, and lymphoid leukaemia (SIR 2.0) [132, 137]. Given the location of these malignancies, the potential role of iatrogenic radiation has been raised as a contributor [138, 139]. A recent study from Ireland demonstrated that the mean annual cumulative effective dose (CED) per patient significantly and consecutively increased from 0.39 mSv·year^{-1} to 0.47 mSv·year^{-1} and to 1.67 mSv·year^{-1} over three equal tertiles from 1992 to 2009 [140]. In parallel, there was a 5.9-fold increase in the use of computed tomography (CT) scanning per patient during this period. With increased survival, the burden of radiograph investigations will need to be considered including adopting the use of low radiation-dose CT imaging where possible [141, 142].

Long-term vascular manifestations

Macrovascular complications (both arterial and venous) are emerging issues in CF patients.

With ongoing improvements in survival, coronary artery disease may become increasingly more recognised over the coming decades. A recent report highlighted the potential for dyslipidaemia in CF patients, in particular with increasing age, body mass index (BMI) and PS status [143]. In other inflammatory lung diseases [144], increased cardiovascular risk and premature vascular ageing are being observed. Augmentation index is a measure of vascular stiffness and in adults with CF it was increased when compared with control subjects. It further increased with age and/or in the presence of CFRD [57]. It is also important to highlight that right ventricular failure and pulmonary hypertension may occur in patients with end-stage lung disease, which is discussed further in another chapter in this *Monograph* [145].

Totally implantable venous access devices (TIVADs) offer long-term reliable central venous access. TIVAD-associated venous thrombosis rates between 0% and 13.6% have been reported. Whilst superior vena cava obstruction as a consequence has been considered to be rare, it may be catastrophic [146]. Careful attention to TIVAD maintenance and monitoring remains important.

Psychological and/or psychiatric manifestations

Anxiety and depression are common in CF patients, where reported rates range from 10% to 30% [147, 148]. These individuals are more likely to suffer increased perceived burden of illness, and have higher rates of noncompliance and healthcare utilisation [149]. Key to maintaining both mental and physical well-being is the early identification and the use of management strategies, as anxiety and depression have been shown to correlate with pulmonary function and pulmonary exacerbation frequency [147, 148].

Disordered eating may further compound the difficulties of nutritional management in CF patients, and this is particularly common amongst adolescents [150]. It may involve combinations of restricting, excess compensatory physical activity and medication manipulation (*i.e.* PERT).

Conclusions

Given the frequency and magnitude of the impact on CF outcomes, monitoring for and managing the extrapulmonary manifestations of CF is key to successful clinical outcomes. While progressive respiratory disease is responsible for the most significant attributable morbidity and mortality observed in CF patients, the extrapulmonary manifestations are increasingly recognised as modifiable contributors. Strategies such as routine annual reviews to prospectively evaluate and monitor for the emergence of extrapulmonary complications in CF are critical to the continued successes in clinical outcomes.

References

1. Gottlieb J, Greer M. Lung transplantation for cystic fibrosis. *In:* Mall MA, Elborn JS, eds. Cystic Fibrosis. *ERS Monogr* 2014; 64: 236–245.
2. Quon BS, Aitken ML. Cystic fibrosis: what to expect now in the early adult years. *Paediatr Respir Rev* 2012; 4: 206–214.
3. Eggesbø HB, Søvik S, Dølvik S, *et al.* CT characterization of developmental variations of the paranasal sinuses in cystic fibrosis. *Acta Radiol* 2001; 42: 482–493.
4. King VV. Upper respiratory disease, sinusitis, and polyposis. *Clin Rev Allergy* 1991; 9: 143–157.
5. Mainz JG, Koitschev A. Pathogenesis and management of nasal polyposis in cystic fibrosis. *Curr Allergy Asthma Rep* 2012; 12: 163–174.
6. Mainz JG, Schiller I, Ritschel C, *et al.* Sinonasal inhalation of dornase alfa in CF: a double-blind placebo-controlled cross-over pilot trial. *Auris Nasus Larynx* 2011; 38: 220–227.
7. Hansen SK, Rau MH, Johansen HK, *et al.* Evolution and diversification of *Pseudomonas aeruginosa* in the paranasal sinuses of cystic fibrosis children have implications for chronic lung infection. *ISME J* 2012; 6: 31–45.
8. Aanaes K. Bacterial sinusitis can be a focus for initial lung colonisation and chronic lung infection in patients with cystic fibrosis. *J Cyst Fibros* 2013; 12: Suppl. 2, S1–S20.
9. Aanaes K, Johansen HK, Skov M, *et al.* Clinical effects of sinus surgery and adjuvant therapy in cystic fibrosis patients – can chronic lung infections be postponed? *Rhinology* 2013; 51: 222–230.
10. Koitschev A, Wolff A, Koitschev C, *et al.* Standardisierte HNO-untersuchung bei patienten mit mukoviszidose [Routine otorhinolaryngological examination in patients with cystic fibrosis]. *HNO* 2006; 54: 361–368.
11. Beju D, Meek WD, Kramer JC. The ultrastructure of the nasal polyps in patients with and without cystic fibrosis. *J Submicrosc Cytol Pathol* 2004; 36: 155–165.
12. Henriksson G, Westrin KM, Karpati F, *et al.* Nasal polyps in cystic fibrosis: clinical endoscopic study with nasal lavage fluid analysis. *Chest* 2002; 121: 40–47.

13. Cimmino M, Cavaliere M, Nardone M, *et al.* Clinical characteristics and genotype analysis of patients with cystic fibrosis and nasal polyposis. *Clin Otolaryngol Allied Sci* 2003; 28: 125–132.

14. Colombo C, Battezzati PM, Crosignani A, *et al.* Liver disease in cystic fibrosis: a prospective study on incidence, risk factors, and outcome. *Hepatology* 2002; 36: 1374–1382.

15. Lindblad A, Glaumann H, Strandvik B. Natural history of liver disease in cystic fibrosis. *Hepatology* 1999; 30: 1151–1158.

16. Flass T, Narkewicz MR. Cirrhosis and other liver disease in cystic fibrosis. *J Cyst Fibros* 2013; 12: 116–124.

17. Lindblad A, Hultcrantz R, Strandvik B. Bile-duct destruction and collagen deposition: a prominent ultrastructural feature of the liver in cystic fibrosis. *Hepatology* 1992; 16: 372–381.

18. Malbrunot-Wagner AC, Bridoux L, Nousbaum JB, *et al.* Transient elastography and portal hypertension in pediatric patients with cystic fibrosis transient elastography and cystic fibrosis. *J Cyst Fibros* 2011; 10: 338–342.

19. Debray D, Kelly D, Houwen R, *et al.* Best practice guidance for the diagnosis and management of cystic fibrosis-associated liver disease. *J Cyst Fibros* 2011; 10: Suppl. 2, S29–S36.

20. Feigelson J, Anagnostopoulos C, Poquet M, *et al.* Liver cirrhosis in cystic fibrosis – therapeutic implications and long term follow up. *Arch Dis Child* 1993; 68: 653–657.

21. Chryssostalis A, Hubert D, Coste J, *et al.* Liver disease in adult patients with cystic fibrosis: a frequent and independent prognostic factor associated with death or lung transplantation. *J Hepatol* 2011; 55: 1377–1382.

22. Bartlett JR, Friedman KJ, Ling SC, *et al.* Genetic modifiers of liver disease in cystic fibrosis. *JAMA* 2009; 302: 1076–1083.

23. Corbett K, Kelleher S, Rowland M, *et al.* Cystic fibrosis-associated liver disease: a population-based study. *J Pediatr* 2004; 145: 327–332.

24. Wilschanski M, Durie PR. Patterns of GI disease in adulthood associated with mutations in the CFTR gene. *Gut* 2007; 56: 1153–1163.

25. Chamnan P, Shine BS, Haworth CS, *et al.* Diabetes as a determinant of mortality in cystic fibrosis. *Diabetes Care* 2010; 33: 311–316.

26. Rowland M, Gallagher CG, O'Laoide R, *et al.* Outcome in cystic fibrosis liver disease. *Am J Gastroenterol* 2011; 106: 104–109.

27. Nash EF, Volling C, Gutierrez CA, *et al.* Outcomes of patients with cystic fibrosis undergoing lung transplantation with and without cystic fibrosis-associated liver cirrhosis. *Clin Transplant* 2012; 26: 34–41.

28. Cheng K, Ashby D, Smyth RL. Ursodeoxycholic acid for cystic fibrosis-related liver disease. *Cochrane Database Syst Rev* 2012; 10: CD000222.

29. Miller MR, Sokol RJ, Narkewicz MR, *et al.* Pulmonary function in individuals who underwent liver transplantation: from the US cystic fibrosis foundation registry. *Liver Transpl* 2012; 18: 585–593.

30. Kraisinger M, Hochhaus G, Stecenko A, *et al.* Clinical pharmacology of pancreatic enzymes in patients with cystic fibrosis and *in vitro* performance of microencapsulated formulations. *J Clin Pharmacol* 1994; 34: 158–166.

31. Correlation between genotype and phenotype in patients with cystic fibrosis. The Cystic Fibrosis Genotype-Phenotype Consortium. *N Engl J Med* 1993; 329: 1308–1313.

32. FitzSimmons SC, Burkhart GA, Borowitz D, *et al.* High-dose pancreatic-enzyme supplements and fibrosing colonopathy in children with cystic fibrosis. *N Engl J Med* 1997; 336: 1283–1289.

33. White H, Morton AM, Conway SP, *et al.* Enteral tube feeding in adults with cystic fibrosis; patient choice and impact on long term outcomes. *J Cyst Fibros* 2013; 12: 616–622.

34. Gaskin K, Gurwitz D, Durie P, *et al.* Improved respiratory prognosis in patients with cystic fibrosis with normal fat absorption. *J Pediatr* 1982; 100: 857–862.

35. Corey M, McLaughlin FJ, Williams M, *et al.* A comparison of survival, growth, and pulmonary function in patients with cystic fibrosis in Boston and Toronto. *J Clin Epidemiol* 1988; 41: 583–591.

36. Konstan MW, Butler SM, Wohl ME, *et al.* Growth and nutritional indexes in early life predict pulmonary function in cystic fibrosis. *J Pediatr* 2003; 142: 624–630.

37. Durno C, Corey M, Zielenski J, *et al.* Genotype and phenotype correlations in patients with cystic fibrosis and pancreatitis. *Gastroenterology* 2002; 123: 1857–1864.

38. Dray X, Marteau P, Bienvenu T, *et al.* Discussion on genotype and phenotype correlations in patients with cystic fibrosis and pancreatitis. *Gastroenterology* 2003; 125: 1286.

39. Walkowiak J, Lisowska A, Blaszczynski M. The changing face of the exocrine pancreas in cystic fibrosis: pancreatic sufficiency, pancreatitis and genotype. *Eur J Gastroenterol Hepatol* 2008; 20: 157–160.

40. Augarten A, Ben Tov A, Madgar I, *et al.* The changing face of the exocrine pancreas in cystic fibrosis: the correlation between pancreatic status, pancreatitis and cystic fibrosis genotype. *Eur J Gastroenterol Hepatol* 2008; 20: 164–168.

41. Mohan K, Miller H, Dyce P, *et al.* Mechanisms of glucose intolerance in cystic fibrosis. *Diabet Med* 2009; 26: 582–588.

42. Kelly A, Moran A. Update on cystic fibrosis-related diabetes. *J Cyst Fibros* 2013; 12: 318–331.

43. Sterescu AE, Rhodes B, Jackson R, *et al.* Natural history of glucose intolerance in patients with cystic fibrosis: ten-year prospective observation program. *J Pediatr* 2010; 156: 613–617.

44. Moran A, Brunzell C, Cohen RC, *et al*. Clinical care guidelines for cystic fibrosis-related diabetes: a position statement of the American Diabetes Association and a clinical practice guideline of the Cystic Fibrosis Foundation, endorsed by the Pediatric Endocrine Society. *Diabetes Care* 2010; 33: 2697–2708.

45. Moran A, Becker D, Casella SJ, *et al*. Epidemiology, pathophysiology, and prognostic implications of cystic fibrosis-related diabetes: a technical review. *Diabetes Care* 2010; 33: 2677–2683.

46. Hodson ME, Simmonds NJ, Warwick WJ, *et al*. An international/multicentre report on patients with cystic fibrosis (CF) over the age of 40 years. *J Cyst Fibros* 2008; 7: 537–542.

47. Simmonds NJ, Cullinan P, Hodson ME. Growing old with cystic fibrosis - the characteristics of long-term survivors of cystic fibrosis. *Respir Med* 2009; 103: 629–635.

48. Adler AI, Shine BS, Chamnan P, *et al*. Genetic determinants and epidemiology of cystic fibrosis-related diabetes: results from a British cohort of children and adults. *Diabetes Care* 2008; 31: 1789–1794.

49. Blackman SM, Commander CW, Watson C, *et al*. Genetic modifiers of cystic fibrosis-related diabetes. *Diabetes* 2013; 62: 3627–3635.

50. Koch C, Rainisio M, Madessani U, *et al*. Presence of cystic fibrosis-related diabetes mellitus is tightly linked to poor lung function in patients with cystic fibrosis: data from the European Epidemiologic Registry of Cystic Fibrosis. *Pediatr Pulmonol* 2001; 32: 343–350.

51. Parkins MD, Rendall JC, Elborn JS. Incidence and risk factors for pulmonary exacerbation treatment failures in patients with cystic fibrosis chronically infected with *Pseudomonas aeruginosa*. *Chest* 2012; 141: 485–493.

52. Milla CE, Warwick WJ, Moran A. Trends in pulmonary function in patients with cystic fibrosis correlate with the degree of glucose intolerance at baseline. *Am J Respir Crit Care Med* 2000; 162: 891–895.

53. Rosenecker J, Höfler R, Steinkamp G, *et al*. Diabetes mellitus in patients with cystic fibrosis: the impact of diabetes mellitus on pulmonary function and clinical outcome. *Eur J Med Res* 2001; 6: 345–350.

54. Marshall BC, Butler SM, Stoddard M, *et al*. Epidemiology of cystic fibrosis-related diabetes. *J Pediatr* 2005; 146: 681–687.

55. Lanng S, Thorsteinsson B, Nerup J, *et al*. Diabetes mellitus in cystic fibrosis: effect of insulin therapy on lung function and infections. *Acta Paediatr* 1994; 83: 849–853.

56. Schwarzenberg SJ, Thomas W, Olsen TW, *et al*. Microvascular complications in cystic fibrosis-related diabetes. *Diabetes Care* 2007; 30: 1056–1061.

57. Hull JH, Garrod R, Ho TB, *et al*. Increased augmentation index in patients with cystic fibrosis. *Eur Respir J* 2009; 34: 1322–1328.

58. Laguna TA, Nathan BM, Moran A. Managing diabetes in cystic fibrosis. *Diabetes Obes Metab* 2010; 12: 858–864.

59. Onady GM, Stolfi A. Insulin and oral agents for managing cystic fibrosis-related diabetes. *Cochrane Database Syst Rev* 2013; 7: CD004730.

60. Morales MM, Falkenstein D, Lopes AG. The cystic fibrosis transmembrane regulator (CFTR) in the kidney. *An Acad Bras Cienc* 2000; 72: 399–406.

61. Jouret F, Devuyst O. CFTR and defective endocytosis: new insights in the renal phenotype of cystic fibrosis. *Pflugers Arch* 2009; 457: 1227–1236.

62. Bertenshaw C, Watson AR, Lewis S, *et al*. Survey of acute renal failure in patients with cystic fibrosis in the UK. *Thorax* 2007; 62: 541–545.

63. Smyth A, Lewis S, Bertenshaw C, *et al*. Case-control study of acute renal failure in patients with cystic fibrosis in the UK. *Thorax* 2008; 63: 532–535.

64. Quinton PM. Defective epithelial ion transport in cystic fibrosis. *Clin Chem* 1989; 35: 726–730.

65. Priou-Guesdon M, Malinge MC, Augusto JF, *et al*. Hypochloremia and hyponatremia as the initial presentation of cystic fibrosis in three adults. *Ann Endocrinol (Paris)* 2010; 71: 46–50.

66. Perez-Brayfield MR, Caplan D, Gatti JM, *et al*. Metabolic risk factors for stone formation in patients with cystic fibrosis. *J Urol* 2002; 167: 480–484.

67. Sidhu H, Hoppe B, Hesse A, *et al*. Absence of *Oxalobacter formigenes* in cystic fibrosis patients: a risk factor for hyperoxaluria. *Lancet* 1998; 352: 1026–1029.

68. Lind-Ayres M, Thomas W, Holme B, *et al*. Microalbuminuria in patients with cystic fibrosis. *Diabetes Care* 2011; 34: 1526–1528.

69. Stephens SE, Rigden SP. Cystic fibrosis and renal disease. *Paediatr Respir Rev* 2002; 3: 135–138.

70. Lefaucheur C, Nochy D, Amrein C, *et al*. Renal histopathological lesions after lung transplantation in patients with cystic fibrosis. *Am J Transplant* 2008; 8: 1901–1910.

71. Westall GP, Binder J, Kotsimbos T, *et al*. Nodular glomerulosclerosis in cystic fibrosis mimics diabetic nephropathy. *Nephron Clin Pract* 2004; 96: c70–c75.

72. O'Connell O, Magee CN, Fitzgerald B, *et al*. CF patient with progressive proteinuric renal disease: a CF-specific nodular glomerulosclerosis? *NDT Plus* 2010; 3: 354–356.

73. Andrieux A, Harambat J, Bui S, *et al*. Renal impairment in children with cystic fibrosis. *J Cyst Fibros* 2010; 9: 263–268.

74. O'Connell OJ, Harrison MJ, Murphy DM, *et al.* Peri-lung transplant renal issues in patients with cystic fibrosis. *Chest* 2013; 143: 271.

75. Quon BS, Mayer-Hamblett N, Aitken ML, *et al.* Risk factors for chronic kidney disease in adults with cystic fibrosis. *Am J Respir Crit Care Med* 2011; 184: 1147–1152.

76. Florescu MC, Lyden E, Murphy PJ, *et al.* Long-term effect of chronic intravenous and inhaled nephrotoxic antibiotic treatment on the renal function of patients with cystic fibrosis. *Hemodial Int* 2012; 16: 414–419.

77. Etherington C, Bosomworth M, Clifton I, *et al.* Measurement of urinary N-acetyl-b-D-glucosaminidase in adult patients with cystic fibrosis: before, during and after treatment with intravenous antibiotics. *J Cyst Fibros* 2007; 6: 67–73.

78. van der Doef HP, Kokke FT, van der Ent CK, *et al.* Intestinal obstruction syndromes in cystic fibrosis: meconium ileus, distal intestinal obstruction syndrome, and constipation. *Curr Gastroenterol Rep* 2011; 13: 265–270.

79. Kerem E, Corey M, Kerem B, *et al.* Clinical and genetic comparisons of patients with cystic fibrosis, with or without meconium ileus. *J Pediatr* 1989; 114: 767–773.

80. Blackman SM, Deering-Brose R, McWilliams R, *et al.* Relative contribution of genetic and nongenetic modifiers to intestinal obstruction in cystic fibrosis. *Gastroenterology* 2006; 131: 1030–1039.

81. Efrati O, Nir J, Fraser D, *et al.* Meconium ileus in patients with cystic fibrosis is not a risk factor for clinical deterioration and survival: the Israeli Multicenter Study. *J Pediatr Gastroenterol Nutr* 2010; 50: 173–178.

82. Karimi A, Gorter RR, Sleeboom C, *et al.* Issues in the management of simple and complex meconium ileus. *Pediatr Surg Int* 2011; 27: 963–968.

83. Carlyle BE, Borowitz DS, Glick PL. A review of pathophysiology and management of fetuses and neonates with meconium ileus for the pediatric surgeon. *J Pediatr Surg* 2012; 47: 772–781.

84. Burke MS, Ragi JM, Karamanoukian HL, *et al.* New strategies in nonoperative management of meconium ileus. *J Pediatr Surg* 2002; 37: 760–764.

85. van der Doef HP, Slieker MG, Staab D, *et al.* Association of the CLCA1 p.S357N variant with meconium ileus in European patients with cystic fibrosis. *J Pediatr Gastroenterol Nutr* 2010; 50: 347–349.

86. Houwen RH, van der Doef HP, Sermet I, *et al.* Defining DIOS and constipation in cystic fibrosis with a multicentre study on the incidence, characteristics, and treatment of DIOS. *J Pediatr Gastroenterol Nutr* 2010; 50: 38–42.

87. Dray X, Bienvenu T, Desmazes-Dufeu N, *et al.* Distal intestinal obstruction syndrome in adults with cystic fibrosis. *Clin Gastroenterol Hepatol* 2004; 2: 498–503.

88. Rubinstein S, Moss R, Lewiston N. Constipation and meconium ileus equivalent in patients with cystic fibrosis. *Pediatrics* 1986; 78: 473–479.

89. Colombo C, Ellemunter H, Houwen R, *et al.* Guidelines for the diagnosis and management of distal intestinal obstruction syndrome in cystic fibrosis patients. *J Cyst Fibros* 2011; 10: Suppl. 2, S24–S28.

90. Gilljam M, Chaparro C, Tullis E, *et al.* GI complications after lung transplantation in patients with cystic fibrosis. *Chest* 2003; 123: 37–41.

91. Blondeau K, Dupont LJ, Mertens V, *et al.* Gastro-oesophageal reflux and aspiration of gastric contents in adult patients with cystic fibrosis. *Gut* 2008; 57: 1049–1055.

92. Blondeau K, Pauwels A, Dupont L, *et al.* Characteristics of gastroesophageal reflux and potential risk of gastric content aspiration in children with cystic fibrosis. *J Pediatr Gastroenterol Nutr* 2010; 50: 161–166.

93. Ledson MJ, Tran J, Walshaw MJ. Prevalence and mechanisms of gastro-oesophageal reflux in adult cystic fibrosis patients. *J R Soc Med* 1998; 91: 7–9.

94. Cucchiara S, Santamaria F, Andreotti MR, *et al.* Mechanisms of gastro-oesophageal reflux in cystic fibrosis. *Arch Dis Child* 1991; 66: 617–622.

95. Pauwels A, Decraene A, Blondeau K, *et al.* Bile acids in sputum and increased airway inflammation in patients with cystic fibrosis. *Chest* 2012; 141: 1568–1574.

96. Palm K, Sawicki G, Rosen R. The impact of reflux burden on *Pseudomonas* positivity in children with cystic fibrosis. *Pediatr Pulmonol* 2012; 47: 582–587.

97. Sawyer SM, Tully M-AM, Dovey ME, *et al.* Reproductive health in males with cystic fibrosis: knowledge, attitudes, and experiences of patients and parents. *Pediatric Pulmonol* 1998; 25: 226–230.

98. Dreyfus DH, Bethel R, Gelfand EW. Cystic fibrosis 3849+10 kb C>T mutation associated with severe pulmonary disease and male fertility. *Am J Respir Crit Care Med* 1996; 153: 858–860.

99. Thickett KM, Stableforth DE, Davies RE, *et al.* Awareness of infertility in men with cystic fibrosis. *Fertil Steril* 2001; 76: 407–408.

100. Fair A, Griffiths K, Osman L. Attitudes to fertility issues among adults with cystic fibrosis in Scotland. *Thorax* 2000; 55: 672–677.

101. Siklosi KR, Gallagher CG, McKone EF. Development, validation, and implementation of a questionnaire assessing disease knowledge and understanding in adult cystic fibrosis patients. *J Cyst Fibros* 2010; 9: 400–405.

102. Sawyer S, Farrant B, Wilson J, *et al.* Sexual and reproductive health in men with cystic fibrosis: consistent preferences, inconsistent practices. *J Cystic Fibros* 2009; 8: 264–269.

103. Frayman KB, Cerritelli B, Wilson J, et al. Reproductive and sexual health in boys with cystic fibrosis: what do parents know and say? Pediatric Pulmonol 2008; 43: 1107–1116.

104. Sawyer S, Farrant B, Cerritelli B, et al. A survey of sexual and reproductive health in men with cystic fibrosis: new challenges for adolescent and adult services. Thorax 2005; 60: 326–330.

105. Rodgers HC, Baldwin DR, Knox AJ. Questionnaire survey of male infertility in cystic fibrosis. Respir Med 2000; 94: 1002–1003.

106. McCallum TJ, Milunsky JM, Cunningham DL, et al. Fertility in men with cystic fibrosis: an update on current surgical practices and outcomes. Chest 2000; 118: 1059–1062.

107. Hubert D, Patrat C, Guibert J, et al. Results of assisted reproductive technique in men with cystic fibrosis. Human Reprod 2006; 21: 1232–1236.

108. Moran F, Bradley JM, Boyle L, et al. Incontinence in adult females with cystic fibrosis: a Northern Ireland survey. Int J Clin Pract 2003; 57: 182–183.

109. Cornacchia M, Zenorini A, Perobelli S, et al. Prevalence of urinary incontinence in women with cystic fibrosis. BJU Int 2001; 88: 44–48.

110. Vella M, Cartwright R, Cardozo L, et al. Prevalence of incontinence and incontinence-specific quality of life impairment in women with cystic fibrosis. Neurourol Urodyn 2009; 28: 986–989.

111. Orr A, McVean RJ, Webb AK, et al. Questionnaire survey of urinary incontinence in women with cystic fibrosis. BMJ 2001; 322: 1521.

112. Nixon GM, Glazner JA, Martin JM, et al. Urinary incontinence in female adolescents with cystic fibrosis. Pediatrics 2002; 110: e22.

113. Buntain HM, Schluter PJ, Bell SC, et al. Controlled longitudinal study of bone mass accrual in children and adolescents with cystic fibrosis. Thorax 2006; 61: 146–154.

114. Gore AP, Kwon SH, Stenbit AE. A roadmap to the brittle bones of cystic fibrosis. J Osteoporos 2011; 2011: 926045.

115. Donovan DS, Papadopoulos A, Staron RB, et al. Bone mass and vitamin D deficiency in adults with advanced cystic fibrosis lung disease. Am J Respir Crit Care Med 1998; 157: 1892–1899.

116. Hardin DS, Leblanc A, Marshall G, et al. Mechanisms of insulin resistance in cystic fibrosis. Am J Physiol Endocrinol Metab 2001; 281: E1022–E1028.

117. Shead EF, Haworth CS, Condliffe AM, et al. Cystic fibrosis transmembrane conductance regulator (CFTR) is expressed in human bone. Thorax 2007; 62: 650–651.

118. King SJ, Topliss DJ, Kotsimbos T, et al. Reduced bone density in cystic fibrosis: ΔF508 mutation is an independent risk factor. Eur Respir J 2005; 25: 54–61.

119. Paccou J, Zeboulon N, Combescure C, et al. The prevalence of osteoporosis, osteopenia, and fractures among adults with cystic fibrosis: a systematic literature review with meta-analysis. Calcif Tissue Int 2010; 86: 1–7.

120. Conway SP, Morton AM, Oldroyd B, et al. Osteoporosis and osteopenia in adults and adolescents with cystic fibrosis: prevalence and associated factors. Thorax 2000; 55: 798–804.

121. Dwarakanath A, Etherington C, Daniels S, et al. WS13.3 reduction in prevalence of osteoporosis and osteopenia in adult patients attending a regional UK centre: 2011 vs. 1999. J Cyst Fibros 2012; 11: Suppl. 1, S29.

122. Aris RM, Merkel PA, Bachrach LK, et al. Guide to bone health and disease in cystic fibrosis. J Clin Endocrinol Metab 2005; 90: 1888–1896.

123. Thornton J, Rangaraj S. Anti-inflammatory Drugs and Analgesics for Managing Symptoms in People with Cystic Fibrosis-Related Arthritis. Hoboken, John Wiley and Sons, Ltd., 2008.

124. Merkel PA. Rheumatic disease and cystic fibrosis. Arthritis Rheum 1999; 42: 1563–1571.

125. Turner MA, Baildam E, Patel L, et al. Joint disorders in cystic fibrosis. J R Soc Med 1997; 90: Suppl. 31, 13–20.

126. Murphy L, Schwartz TA, Helmick CG, et al. Lifetime risk of symptomatic knee osteoarthritis. Arthritis Rheum 2008; 59: 1207–1213.

127. Bray F, Moller B. Predicting the future burden of cancer. Nat Rev Cancer 2006; 6: 63–74.

128. Miller RW. Digestive-tract cancer in cystic fibrosis. J Pediatr 1993; 123: 172.

129. Schoni MH, Maisonneuve P, Schoni-Affolter F, et al. Cancer risk in patients with cystic fibrosis: the European data. CF/CSG Group. J R Soc Med 1996; 89: Suppl. 27, 38–43.

130. Neglia JP, FitzSimmons SC, Maisonneuve P, et al. The risk of cancer among patients with cystic fibrosis. Cystic Fibrosis and Cancer Study Group. N Engl J Med 1995; 332: 494–499.

131. Maisonneuve P, FitzSimmons SC, Neglia JP, et al. Cancer risk in nontransplanted and transplanted cystic fibrosis patients: a 10-year study. J Natl Cancer Inst 2003; 95: 381–387.

132. Maisonneuve P, Marshall BC, Knapp EA, et al. Cancer risk in cystic fibrosis: a 20-year nationwide study from the United States. J Natl Cancer Inst 2013; 105: 122–129.

133. Meyer KC, Francois ML, Thomas HK, et al. Colon cancer in lung transplant recipients with CF: increased risk and results of screening. J Cyst Fibros 2011; 10: 366–369.

134. Reid DW, Withers NJ, Francis L, et al. Iron deficiency in cystic fibrosis: relationship to lung disease severity and chronic Pseudomonas aeruginosa infection. Chest 2002; 121: 48–54.

135. von Drygalski A, Biller J. Anemia in cystic fibrosis: incidence, mechanisms, and association with pulmonary function and vitamin deficiency. *Nutr Clin Pract* 2008; 23: 557–563.

136. Smith DJ, Anderson GJ, Lamont IL, *et al.* Accurate assessment of systemic iron status in cystic fibrosis will avoid the hazards of inappropriate iron supplementation: Letter to the editor. *J Cyst Fibros* 2013; 12: 303–304.

137. Johannesson M, Askling J, Montgomery SM, *et al.* Cancer risk among patients with cystic fibrosis and their first-degree relatives. *Int J Cancer* 2009; 125: 2953–2956.

138. Williams SJ, McGuckin MA, Gotley DC, *et al.* Two novel mucin genes down-regulated in colorectal cancer identified by differential display. *Cancer Res* 1999; 59: 4083–4089.

139. Freedman SD, Katz MH, Parker EM, *et al.* A membrane lipid imbalance plays a role in the phenotypic expression of cystic fibrosis in cftr(-/-) mice. *Proc Natl Acad Sci USA* 1999; 96: 13995–14000.

140. O'Connell OJ, McWilliams S, McGarrigle A, *et al.* Radiologic imaging in cystic fibrosis: cumulative effective dose and changing trends over 2 decades. *Chest* 2012; 141: 1575–1583.

141. O'Connell OJ, McGarrigle A, O'Connor OJ, *et al.* Response. *Chest* 2012; 142: 1078.

142. O'Connor OJ, Vandeleur M, McGarrigle AM, *et al.* Development of low-dose protocols for thin-section CT assessment of cystic fibrosis in pediatric patients. *Radiology* 2010; 257: 820–829.

143. Rhodes B, Nash EF, Tullis E, *et al.* Prevalence of dyslipidemia in adults with cystic fibrosis. *J Cyst Fibros* 2010; 9: 24–28.

144. Macnee W, Maclay J, McAllister D. Cardiovascular injury and repair in chronic obstructive pulmonary disease. *Proc Am Thorac Soc* 2008; 5: 824–833.

145. Mall MA, Boucher RC. Pathophysiology of cystic fibrosis lung disease. *In*: Mall MA, Elborn JS, eds. Cystic Fibrosis. *ERS Monogr* 2014; 64: 1–13.

146. Smith D, Reid D, Slaughter R, *et al.* Superior vena cava obstruction due to total implantable venous access devices in cystic fibrosis: case series and review. *Respir Med CME* 2011; 4: 99–104.

147. Ploessl C, Pettit RS, Donaldson J. Prevalence of depression and antidepressant therapy use in a pediatric cystic fibrosis population. *Ann Pharmacother* 2014; 48: 488–493.

148. Riekert KA, Bartlett SJ, Boyle MP, *et al.* The association between depression, lung function, and health-related quality of life among adults with cystic fibrosis. *Chest* 2007; 132: 231–237.

149. DiMatteo MR, Lepper HS, Croghan TW. Depression is a risk factor for noncompliance with medical treatment: meta-analysis of the effects of anxiety and depression on patient adherence. *Arch Intern Med* 2000; 160: 2101–2107.

150. Shearer JE, Bryon M. The nature and prevalence of eating disorders and eating disturbance in adolescents with cystic fibrosis. *J R Soc Med* 2004; 97: Suppl. 44, 36–42.

Disclosures: B.J. Plant reports personal fees for consultancy and speaker's honoraria from Novartis, Vertex, and Gilead outside the submitted work. M.D. Parkins reports receiving grants from Gilead Sciences and Cystic Fibrosis Canada outside of the submitted work. He also acknowledges being part of advisory boards for Novartis, Gilead and Roche outside the submitted work.

Chapter 16

Lung transplantation for cystic fibrosis

Jens Gottlieb and Mark Greer

The vast majority of adult cystic fibrosis (CF) patients will develop respiratory failure. Lung transplantation in CF represents an established treatment option in end-stage lung disease. Both adolescents and children can receive transplants successfully. Due to donor shortage and increasing waiting time, early referral of possible candidates to transplant centres is of critical importance. During the process of candidate selection, presumed improvements in quality of life and survival benefit should be weighed against contraindications. Lung transplantation in CF needs special consideration with regard to candidate selection, surgery and post-operative follow-up care. Centre-based follow-up and close cooperation with primary care providers are key factors for success.

L ung transplantation has become an established treatment option among patients with various end-stage lung diseases, with current international registry data reporting on approximately 3600 procedures annually [1]. Donor shortage remains the main limiting factor, resulting in every sixth patient on the waiting list dying before an organ becomes available. Due to donor shortages, appropriate candidate selection is of critical importance and centres upon certain disease-specific factors after excluding contraindications.

Lung transplantation may offer improved quality of life (QoL) and prolonged survival in selected cystic fibrosis (CF) candidates. Internationally, CF accounts for 17% of all listings for lung transplantation and 26% of patients awaiting sequential lung transplantation [1], and represents the third commonest indication for lung transplantation after emphysema and pulmonary fibrosis. Among adolescents and children, who represent around 3% of all lung transplant recipients worldwide, CF accounts for two-thirds of all lung transplantations performed [2]. When considering lung transplantation in CF, special selection criteria are needed, given the specific surgical considerations as well as complications in the early and long-term course post-transplant. In particular, the multiorgan nature of CF cannot be underestimated, and remaining organ morbidities (e.g. liver cirrhosis) remain following lung transplant and their management potentially can be more difficult.

Close cooperation between the transplant team and pulmonologists and/or paediatricians experienced in CF during the pre-, peri- and post-transplant phases is essential to ensure successful outcomes.

Dept of Respiratory Medicine, Hannover Medical School, Hannover, Germany.

Correspondence: Jens Gottlieb, Hannover Medical School, Dept of Respiratory Medicine OE6870, Carl-Neuberg-Str. 1, 30625 Hannover, Germany. E-mail: gottlieb.jens@mh-hannover.de

Copyright ERS 2014. Print ISBN: 978-1-84984-050-7. Online ISBN: 978-1-84984-051-4. Print ISSN: 2312-508X. Online ISSN: 2312-5098.

Selection criteria

Survival benefit should be considered the primary goal of transplant specialists. In assessing this, CF presents the clinician with numerous additional challenges. Airway colonisation increases the risk of serious post-operative infections in immunosuppressed patients. Extrapulmonary manifestations of CF, resulting in highly variable intestinal absorption and impaired hepatic metabolism of important drugs, can pose significant and serious risks to both graft survival and extrapulmonary end-organ damage. Conversely, CF patients represent comparatively young lung recipients, with a mean age of 25–30 years at the time of transplant, thus avoiding the typical cardiovascular comorbidities of more elderly patients transplanted due to other underlying diseases.

Absolute contraindications to lung transplant in CF exist and should be respected. The international guidelines on selection criteria consider the following to be absolute contraindications [3]: 1) malignancy with a <2-year disease-free interval (except cutaneous squamous and basal cell tumours); 2) untreatable advanced dysfunction of another major organ system (*e.g.* heart, liver or kidney); 3) incurable chronic extrapulmonary infection (*e.g.* overt sepsis, chronic active viral hepatitis B, hepatitis C and HIV); 4) documented nonadherence to recommended treatment; 5) untreatable psychiatric or psychological conditions associated with the inability to cooperate, or the absence of a consistent or reliable social support system; and 6) substance addiction (*e.g.* alcohol, tobacco or narcotics) that is either currently active or was active within the last 6 months.

Different specific guidelines relating to candidate selection in CF have been published [3, 4]. These recommendations, however, remain subject to constant change, due to changes in the course of the disease as a result of emerging treatment options. Among potential candidates, extensive work-up is necessary in preparation for lung transplantation (table 1). It is not uncommon, indeed it is preferable, that the results of this assessment may improve the candidate's baseline condition prior to lung transplantation. Examples include improved nutritional status, better physical fitness or effective treatment of potential foci of infection (*e.g.* paranasal sinuses and teeth).

The waiting time to transplantation following listing should be considered an important opportunity to actively prepare the candidate for the procedure and subsequent follow-up, as well as continually monitoring their clinical state. Vital aspects include the continuation of regular physical exercise, adequate psychological support, effective nutrition and comprehensive vaccination (including influenza, pneumococcal disease, diphtheria, poliomyelitis and tetanus).

While some variation in candidate assessment inevitably exists between transplant centres, certain core investigations are standard, including certain specific blood analyses (human leukocyte antigen antibodies, blood group, virus serology, *etc.*). Nonpulmonary complications frequently associated with CF, such as diabetes mellitus, osteoporosis, sinus disease and gastro-oesophageal reflux disease, should ideally be treated before or as soon as possible after surgery. If well controlled, these problems are not considered contraindications for transplant.

Certain resistant pathogens may predispose to poorer outcomes. Although specific data are currently lacking, pre-transplant colonisation with methicillin-resistant *Staphylococcus aureus*, multi- or pan-resistant nonfermenting Gram-negative pathogens such as

Table 1. Evaluation in potential lung transplant candidates with cystic fibrosis

History and physical examination
Sputum and nasal lavage microbiology
Echocardiography/evidence of pulmonary hypertension/right heart catheterisation
Abdominal ultrasound recording signs of portal hypertension
CT of paranasal sinuses
Thoracic CT
Dental evaluation and comprehensive treatment
Gynaecological assessment
Ultrasound evaluation of inguinal vessels/contraindication to ECMO
Patients ⩾45 years of age or smokers with >10 pack-years of exposure/coronary angiogram,
    ankle pressures

CT: computed tomography; ECMO: extracorporeal membrane oxygenation.

Achromobacter spp., *Stenotrophomonas maltophilia* and *Alcaligenes xylosoxidans*, as well as *Aspergillus fumigatus* require specific perioperative treatment regimens. Both single-centre reports and registry data indicate unacceptably high 1-year mortality rates among CF patients infected with *Burkholderia cenocepacia*. Although patients colonised with this organism have successfully received transplants at some centres, most currently refuse to offer transplantation to such patients. Antibiotic susceptibility testing should be repeated at regular intervals in such waiting-list candidates to ensure that an accurate and up-to-date antibiotic combination is administered at the time of transplant.

Existing guidelines on specific selection criteria have been primarily based on single-centre data from KEREM *et al.* [5], who identified a forced expiratory volume in 1 s (FEV1) of <30% predicted as a useful survival marker. Numerous authors have attempted to develop models incorporating several variables to predict long-term survival in larger CF cohorts. One model based on data from the US Cystic Fibrosis Foundation considered nine parameters (age, sex, FEV1 % predicted, weight, pancreatic function, diabetes, frequent exacerbations and colonisation with *Staphylococcus* or *Burkholderia cepacia*) to assess 5-year survival [6]. The ability of this model to predict mortality was, however, modest, and in the majority of patients, added little more insight than FEV1 <30% predicted alone. Defining predictors of mortality remains inevitably difficult, given the inherently variable course and prognosis between individuals, stemming from the multisystem nature of CF. In practical terms, the complex implications of transplantation should be discussed early with both the patient and their family, with early referral to a transplant centre being considered once the FEV1 approaches 30% predicted.

Implementation of current international recommendations on candidate selection into various national frameworks has been limited, mainly by differing allocation systems, donor organ availability and primary care delivery models. Current guidelines distinguish between two decision steps, namely timing of referral to the transplant centre and placement on the waiting list [3]. Referral to a lung transplant centre should follow when FEV1 is <30% predicted, or additionally in CF patients exhibiting a rapid loss in lung function, a history of frequent exacerbations requiring inpatient treatment (more than two per year), a complicated pneumothorax or history of repeated/severe pulmonary haemorrhage. Placement on the waiting list is advisable in patients demonstrating respiratory failure (oxygen dependency at rest or noninvasive ventilation) in whom no contraindication has been detected during comprehensive evaluation and who have provided informed consent.

Listing is also recommended in the absence of respiratory failure if two or more other negative prognostic factors (more than two hospitalisations annually, recent intensive care unit admission [7], recurrent/refractory pneumothorax [8] or pulmonary haemorrhage [9]) are present in an underweight CF patient exhibiting a FEV1 <30% predicted (fig. 1). In the absence of respiratory failure, individual risks and benefits must be weighted individually for the patient.

Comprehensive discussion of all aspects are necessary when consenting patients. This should include not only discussion of the pre- and perioperative risk and success rates, but also emphasise the life-long medical, social and psychological consequences of lung transplantation.

Preoperative ventilation and bridging with extracorporeal support

Proceeding to lung transplantation in CF patients currently requiring invasive mechanical ventilation is provocative and no consensus exists among transplant centres. Worldwide, only 3% of lung transplant recipients are preoperatively ventilated [1]. The patient's current neurological state is often unclear and complications relating to intensive care treatment lead to increased mortality both pre- and post-transplant. Pre-transplant invasive mechanical ventilation represents an accepted risk factor for mortality among lung transplant recipients as a whole. Mechanically ventilated patients with or without additional extracorporeal support demonstrate approximately 40% 1-year mortality after transplantation compared with 10–20% in nonintubated candidates [10].

The decision to proceed to intubation and mechanical ventilation introduces a difficult ethical dilemma that may interfere with appropriate initiation of terminal care. Lung

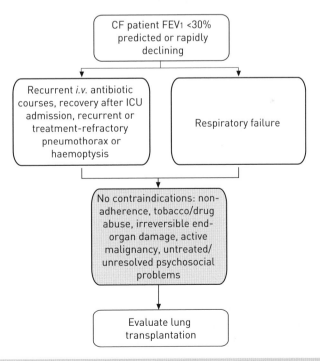

Figure 1. Decision-making algorithm for transplantation candidates with cystic fibrosis (CF). FEV1: forced expiratory volume in 1 s; ICU: intensive care unit.

transplantation in CF patients requiring invasive ventilation should only be considered in comprehensively evaluated patients listed prior to ventilatory assistance, neither exhibiting sepsis nor other significant organ dysfunction.

Extracorporeal life support systems enable direct oxygenation and/or carbon dioxide removal from blood. Such technologies, in particular venovenous and venoarterial extracorporeal membrane oxygenation have been successfully used in bridging to transplantation [11].

Liver disease

Lung transplantation without liver transplantation has been successfully performed in CF patients exhibiting portal hypertension with preserved hepatic function. About 25% of CF patients demonstrate liver dysfunction, which, in a subset of patients, may be so advanced that evidence of reduced liver synthesis or, more frequently, features associated with portal hypertension (splenomegaly, oesophageal varices and ascites) may arise. Combined liver–lung transplantation is limited, due to its complexity, to experienced centres in critically selected candidates with severe liver disease (model of end-stage liver disease score >15 and FEV1 <40% predicted) [12, 13]. For isolated liver transplantation, adequate pulmonary function (FEV1 >50% predicted) is essential.

Nutrition

Cachexia in advanced CF typically results from a combination of exocrine pancreatic insufficiency, diabetes mellitus, increased work of breathing and chronic infection. Studies have shown that a body mass index (BMI) <17 $kg \cdot m^{-2}$ increases perioperative risk [14]. Conversely, cachexia also reflects advanced disease and is a known indicator of poor prognosis among waiting-list candidates. In clinical practice, with the exception of extreme cachexia (BMI <14 $kg \cdot m^{-2}$), being underweight alone does not represent an absolute contraindication to lung transplantation but must be considered in the context of muscular condition and other comorbidities. Exhaustive efforts should be made to improve weight including optimal diabetes control, pancreatic supplements and supplementary enteral nutrition including feeding by percutaneous endoscopic gastrostomy tube.

Surgical considerations

Bilateral transplantation is mandatory in CF due to the presence of bronchiectasis. Unilateral lung transplantation is considered unacceptable, given inevitable re-infection of the graft from the remaining native lung. In recent years, most centres have adopted minimally invasive surgical procedures using an anterolateral thoracotomy without sternotomy [15], rather than the traditional clamshell incision incorporating a transverse thoracosternotomy previously used in CF recipients. In patients with a history of previous pleurodesis or indeed those frequent cases demonstrating dense pleural adhesions, special attention must be paid to avoid both phrenic and left recurrent laryngeal nerve injury while mobilising the native lung at the time of pneumectomy. Donor lung preparation is usually performed immediately prior to implantation. The donor bronchus is shortened so that only one cartilage ring remains proximal to the upper lobe bronchus. The peribronchial tissue must be preserved and denudation of the bronchus avoided under all circumstances to prevent bronchial healing complications.

Given that CF transplant recipients tend to be smaller than the average population, waiting list times may become unacceptably long. This has led to the development of several techniques to facilitate acceptance of oversized donor organs for urgent paediatric or adult recipients of small stature.

In cases of size mismatch, nonanatomical segmental resections have proven a straightforward technique to reduce donor lung size. Both the middle lobe and lingula are preferred targets for such resections. In cases of greater donor–recipient size discrepancy, lobar transplantation may be feasible in urgent cases.

Living-donor lobar lung transplantation was developed at the University of Southern California (Los Angeles, CA, USA) for patients awaiting cadaveric lung transplantation with a recognisably low probability of obtaining an available donor due to small stature. In this procedure, two compatible healthy donors donate their right or left lower lobes. To date, approximately 400 patients have undergone this procedure worldwide. Its popularity in the USA has decreased, mainly as a result of changes in their urgency/benefit allocation system for cadaveric donor lungs. In recent years, the vast majority of living lobar lung transplants have been performed in Japan [16]. Successful procedures have been performed there for a full spectrum of lung diseases, whereas most recipients in the USA and the few procedures in Europe (Newcastle upon Tyne, UK; Vienna, Austria; and Hannover, Germany) have been in CF.

Donor risk in this technique is attributable to lobectomy with an expected mortality rate of 1% and a complication rate of 20%. In general, donors exhibit a 15% reduction in vital capacity.

Allocation of donor lungs

Following evaluation, suitable patients are placed on the waiting list at their local transplant centre. In most European countries, all potential donor recipients are then registered with an organ procurement organisation that independently coordinates and assigns available donor lungs according to predetermined criteria. This distribution process is commonly referred to as organ allocation.

Various allocation criteria models exist, and may be based on geography (regional, national and international), urgency (e.g. by audit process, individual decision or objective scoring system) or waiting time. At the international level, combinations of these models are often used. The so-called "centre decision" with regional distribution is most common in Europe, as well as distribution by waiting time and considered urgency. Eurotransplant (www. eurotransplant.org) represents the largest transplant organisation in Europe, encompassing Austria, Belgium, Croatia, Hungary, Germany, Luxembourg, the Netherlands and Slovenia. Spain and Portugal have their own network, as do Scandinavia, France and the UK. Despite best efforts, only half of the lungs currently offered can successfully be transplanted.

In both Eurotransplant and the USA, lung allocation was historically based on waiting time. As a result of demonstrable high waiting-list mortality among pulmonary fibrosis patients in the USA, the lung allocation score (LAS) was developed [17]. Based on USA registry data, this score reflects the estimated 1-year survival benefit offered by lung transplantation as well as medical urgency. The LAS was subsequently introduced to guide donor lung allocation in the USA in 2005, with Germany following in December 2011 for candidates aged $\geqslant 12$ years.

Extension of this system within Eurotransplant is planned with the Netherlands commencing in May 2014. The major aim of the LAS system is to preferentially allocate lungs to recipients with the greatest estimated survival benefit from lung transplantation. It is a numerical value derived from various objective measures of patient health. The resulting score (between 0 and 100) can be calculated online (www.eurotransplant.org/cms/index.php?page=las_calculator).

Since the introduction of the LAS in the USA, there has been a ~25% increase in the number of CF transplant recipients, with 70% of listed CF patients being transplanted within 12 months of being listed [18]. 1-year waiting-list mortality for CF patients has also decreased from 15% to 10% [19]. It should be noted that the LAS is merely an allocation tool and is not suitable for decision making related to candidate selection. Individual patient assessment by an experienced medical specialist should remain the cornerstone of selection.

Follow-up reports based on data from the USA have shown a 69% reduction in the instantaneous risk of death for CF patients after lung transplantation since the introduction of LAS, with survival benefit being associated with the final LAS before transplant [20]. In Germany, early LAS experience corroborates findings from the USA, with disproportional increases in transplant activity among CF patients, as well as reduced waiting list mortality. The proportion of CF patients on respiratory support at the time of transplant more than doubled with LAS in Germany. The majority, however, had only been listed for very short periods, in a trend that cannot be directly attributed to the LAS.

Follow-up care

Patient follow-up after transplantation is a complex process, requiring both qualitatively and quantitatively high personnel and equipment costs. Immediate availability of numerous complex diagnostic tools as well as physicians with years of experience in both the fields of lung transplantation and CF are necessary. Successful follow-up is fundamentally based upon close cooperation between the patient (including their social environment), their primary care provider, the local hospital and the transplant centre. This cooperation applies equally to adults as children and adolescents. Several important aspects in the care of CF lung transplant recipients require special consideration.

Sinus problems

Pre-transplant, a CT scan of the sinuses along with nasal lavage to assess colonisation should be performed. Surgical management of CF sinus disease in the perioperative phase of lung transplantation is critically discussed at present. The aim of treatment centres is to reduce or eradicate upper airway colonisation to minimise allograft re-colonisation, which may increase subsequent risk of chronic lung allograft dysfunction and bronchiolitis obliterans syndrome (BOS) [21, 22]. Organisms recovered from the graft are frequently genotypically identical to those known to colonise the paranasal sinuses in the same patient.

It currently remains unclear whether conservative and/or surgical methods are superior in preventing graft re-colonisation. The Zürich group recently published their experience of routine early post-transplant sinus surgery (endoscopic frontosphenoethmoidectomy) in 82 CF patients. In combination with lifelong daily nasal douches, they demonstrated complete nasal and pulmonary eradication of pseudomonads in 35% subjects, while 27% had persistent nasal and 38% persistent nasal and pulmonary colonisation. Pseudomonad-free patients demonstrated better 5-year overall and BOS-free survival [23].

Mucous membranes of the upper airways and paranasal sinuses express the defective CF gene, meaning that the defective mucociliary clearance that generates the actual problem cannot be eliminated by surgery. Use of conservative therapy alone in sinonasal colonisation has not been sufficiently evaluated and is limited to case reports [24]. Conventional inhaled antibiotics generally do not reach the paranasal sinuses without prior surgical widening of the ostia. However, use of alternative pulsating aerosol devices has been shown to achieve antibiotic deposition in the paranasal sinuses, potentially avoiding the need for surgery. No reports have demonstrated statistically different survival rates for CF lung transplant recipients with and without prophylactic pre-transplant sinus surgery. This has led some centres to move away from surgical management, relying instead on conservative topical antibiotics for CF recipients exhibiting upper and lower airway colonisation with pseudomonads.

Infections

Atypical mycobacteria are present in approximately 4% of CF patients. It remains very challenging to assess whether the detection of most nontuberculous mycobacteria in an individual patient reflects insignificant airway colonisation or clinically evident infection. Solely, pre-transplant colonisation with *Mycobacterium abscessus* incurs a high risk of wound infection post-operatively. Most transplanted patients with such wound infections require long-term intravenous antibiotic combination regimes. Colonisation with *M. abscessus* must be considered a serious risk factor when profiling possible transplant candidates but, at present, is not usually considered an absolute contraindication to lung transplantation.

Aspergillus spp. may be transiently or permanently detectable in up to 50% of CF patients and, as such, should not be considered a contraindication to lung transplantation. Modern antifungal agents have significantly improved the treatment options for preventing or treating post-operative infections. Lung transplantation is performed as an aseptic procedure in CF patients and includes comprehensive perioperative prophylaxis, incorporating a modern azole, in colonised patients. Patients with demonstrable tracheobronchial aspergillosis should be considered for endoscopic application of topical therapy post-operatively.

Outcomes

According to international registry data, the unadjusted 3-month mortality following transplantation is lower in CF (9%) than for other major indications (16–25%) [1]. 5-year survival among all patients surviving at least 3 months is also significantly better among CF recipients (65%) than those with COPD and idiopathic pulmonary fibrosis (57% and 55%, respectively), reflecting younger age and comparatively fewer comorbidities. Long-term survival after lung transplantation remains limited by increased infection risk as well as chronic lung allograft dysfunction. Obliterative bronchiolitis is the pathological feature of chronic allograft dysfunction, which unfortunately remains the major limitation to long-term survival following lung transplantation, affecting approximately half of patients by 5 years. It is defined physiologically by the presence of progressive airflow obstruction and is clinically termed BOS.

Functional results in survivors measured in terms of both FEV1 and exercise performance remain impressive. Recipients can expect to attain their normal predicted FEV1 and vital capacity within the first year in the absence of complications. The diffusion capacity, however, usually remains reduced. It is reasonable for patients to expect restoration of normal lifestyle with little or no functional restriction during normal activities of daily living. Exercise data comparing the 6-min walking distances and peak oxygen uptake (V'_{O_2peak}) during an incremental symptom-limited exercise test show that recipients of successful transplants return to a normal 6-min walking distance with no evidence of desaturation on exercise. However, V'_{O_2peak} during a symptom-limited test remains at around 50% predicted for a given subject in the first year. This is partly due to long-term deconditioning inevitably resulting from the pre-transplant disability. The proportion of recipients returning to active working status has been shown to vary between 28% and 39% in large European single-centre cohorts [25, 26].

Advances in lung transplantation have allowed successful outcomes in adolescents and even children. Survival after paediatric lung transplantation is generally comparable to that reported in adults [2]. The provocative report by LIOU et al. [27] that suggested lung transplantation in CF patients <18 years of age rarely offers survival benefit has been critically discussed by other authors, and is no longer considered accurate due both to methodological weaknesses of the study and improved transplantation techniques in the modern era [28–30]. Paediatric lung transplantation in CF should, however, remain limited to centres with extensive experience in this field.

Conclusions

Lung transplantation now represents an effective treatment option for patients with end-stage CF lung disease. Comprehensive physical and psychosocial assessment in well-informed patients are essential elements of patient management prior to listing. Limited donor availability remains the major hurdle to achieving lung transplantation in suitable candidates, although this can be improved through refinements to allocation systems. In the long term, chronic lung allograft dysfunction and infections are the leading causes of death.

Patients who have received lung transplants and remain free of chronic lung allograft dysfunction enjoy an excellent standard of life with normal or near-normal restoration of activities and good prospects for prolonged survival.

References

1. Yusen RD, Christie JD, Edwards LB, et al. The Registry of the International Society for Heart and Lung Transplantation: thirtieth adult lung and heart-lung transplant report – 2013; focus theme: age. J Heart Lung Transplant 2013; 32: 965–978.
2. Benden C, Edwards LB, Kucheryavaya AY, et al. The Registry of the International Society for Heart and Lung Transplantation: sixteenth official pediatric lung and heart-lung transplantation report – 2013; focus theme: age. J Heart Lung Transplant 2013; 32: 989–997.
3. Orens JB, Estenne M, Arcasoy S, et al. International guidelines for the selection of lung transplant candidates: 2006 update – a consensus report from the Pulmonary Scientific Council of the International Society for Heart and Lung Transplantation. J Heart Lung Transplant 2006; 25: 745–755.
4. Yankaskas JR, Mallory GB Jr. Lung transplantation in cystic fibrosis: consensus conference statement. Chest 1998; 113: 217–226.
5. Kerem E, Reisman J, Corey M, et al. Prediction of mortality in patients with cystic fibrosis. N Engl J Med 1992; 326: 1187–1191.
6. Liou TG, Adler FR, FitzSimmons SC, et al. Predictive 5-year survivorship model of cystic fibrosis. Am J Epidemiol 2001; 153: 345–352.
7. Ellaffi M, Vinsonneau C, Coste J, et al. One-year outcome after severe pulmonary exacerbation in adults with cystic fibrosis. Am J Respir Crit Care Med 2005; 171: 158–164.
8. Flume PA, Strange C, Ye X, et al. Pneumothorax in cystic fibrosis. Chest 2005; 128: 720–728.
9. Flume PA, Yankaskas JR, Ebeling M, et al. Massive hemoptysis in cystic fibrosis. Chest 2005; 128: 729–738.

10. Gottlieb J, Warnecke G, Hadem J, *et al.* Outcome of critically ill lung transplant candidates on invasive respiratory support. *Intensive Care Med* 2012; 38: 968–975.

11. Fuehner T, Kuehn C, Hadem J, *et al.* Extracorporeal membrane oxygenation in awake patients as bridge to lung transplantation. *Am J Respir Crit Care Med* 2012; 185: 763–768.

12. Barshes NR, DiBardino DJ, McKenzie ED, *et al.* Combined lung and liver transplantation: the United States experience. *Transplantation* 2005; 80: 1161–1167.

13. Grannas G, Neipp M, Hoeper MM, *et al.* Indications for and outcomes after combined lung and liver transplantation: a single-center experience on 13 consecutive cases. *Transplantation* 2008; 85: 524–531.

14. Madill J, Gutierrez C, Grossman J, *et al.* Nutritional assessment of the lung transplant patient: body mass index as a predictor of 90-day mortality following transplantation. *J Heart Lung Transplant* 2001; 20: 288–296.

15. Fischer S, Strüber M, Simon AR, *et al.* Video-assisted minimally invasive approach in clinical bilateral lung transplantation. *J Cardiovasc Surg* 2001; 122: 1196–1198.

16. Date H. Update on living-donor lobar lung transplantation. *Curr Opin Organ Transplant* 2011; 16: 453–457.

17. Egan TM, Murray S, Bustami RT, *et al.* Development of the new lung allocation system in the United States. *Am J Transplant* 2006; 6: 1212–1227.

18. Valapour M, Paulson K, Smith JM, *et al.* OPTN/SRTR 2011 Annual Data Report: lung. *Am J Transplant* 2013; 13: Suppl. 1, 149–177.

19. Chen H, Shiboski SC, Golden JA, *et al.* Impact of the lung allocation score on lung transplantation for pulmonary arterial hypertension. *Am J Respir Crit Care Med* 2009; 180: 468–474.

20. Thabut G, Christie JD, Mal H, *et al.* Survival benefit of lung transplant for cystic fibrosis since lung allocation score implementation. *Am J Respir Crit Care Med* 2013; 187: 1335–1340.

21. Gottlieb J, Mattner F, Weissbrodt H, *et al.* Impact of graft colonization with Gram-negative bacteria after lung transplantation on the development of bronchiolitis obliterans syndrome in recipients with cystic fibrosis. *Respir Med* 2009; 103: 743–749.

22. Vos R, Vanaudenaerde BM, Dupont LJ, *et al.* Transient airway colonization is associated with airway inflammation after lung transplantation. *Am J Transplant* 2007; 7: 1278–1287.

23. Vital D, Hofer M, Benden C, *et al.* Impact of sinus surgery on pseudomonal airway colonization, bronchiolitis obliterans syndrome and survival in cystic fibrosis lung transplant recipients. *Respiration* 2013; 86: 25–31.

24. Mainz JG, Hentschel J, Schien C, *et al.* Sinonasal persistence of *Pseudomonas aeruginosa* after lung transplantation. *J Cyst Fibros* 2012; 11: 158–161.

25. De Baere C, Delva D, Kloeck A, *et al.* Return to work and social participation: does type of organ transplantation matter? *Transplantation* 2010; 89: 1009–1015.

26. Petrucci L, Ricotti S, Michelini I, *et al.* Return to work after thoracic organ transplantation in a clinically-stable population. *Eur J Heart Fail* 2007; 9: 1112–1119.

27. Liou TG, Adler FR, Cox DR, *et al.* Lung transplantation and survival in children with cystic fibrosis. *N Engl J Med* 2007; 357: 2143–2152.

28. Aurora P, Spencer H, Moreno-Galdo A. Lung transplantation in children with cystic fibrosis: a view from Europe. *Am J Respir Crit Care Med* 2008; 177: 935–936.

29. Egan TM. Solid benefit of lung transplantation for some children with cystic fibrosis. *Pediatr Transplant* 2008; 12: 125–128.

30. Sweet SC, Aurora P, Benden C, *et al.* Lung transplantation and survival in children with cystic fibrosis: solid statistics – flawed interpretation. *Pediatr Transplant* 2008; 12: 129–136.

Disclosures: J. Gottlieb has received fees for board membership from Novartis (€2000), Gilead (€1000) and MSD (€3000), fees for consultancy from Chiesi (€6000), fees for expert testimony from GLG Research (€6000), grants from Roche (€5000) and Astellas (€1000) (both paid to the author's institution), speaker's fees from Pfizer (€1000), AstraZeneca (€800), Boehringer (€800), Hexal (€2500 paid to the author's institution) and Novartis (€3000), and travel grants from Roche (€2000), Astellas (€4000), Nycomed (€2000), MSD (€2000), Novartis (€3000) and Biotest (€1000).

Chapter 17

Standards of care for patients with cystic fibrosis

Malena Cohen-Cymberknoh, David Shoseyov and Eitan Kerem

Standards of care define the optimal service provision necessary to deliver the best outcomes possible for patients. People with cystic fibrosis (CF) have complex care needs that demand extensive medical and allied healthcare expertise. Several guidelines have been written to assist CF caregivers in the evaluation and monitoring of patients, detection of complications and prevention of clinical deterioration. The better clinical status and improved survival of patients with CF is a result of understanding of the molecular mechanisms of CF and the development of therapeutic strategies that are based on insights into the natural course of the disease. Current CF treatments that target respiratory infections, inflammation, mucociliary clearance and nutritional status are associated with improved pulmonary function and reduced exacerbations. Patients benefit from treatment at specialised CF centres by a multidisciplinary dedicated team, with emphasis being placed on frequent visits, periodic testing and monitoring adherence to therapy. However, the current published standards of care in Europe and North America cannot be fully implemented in populations or countries with limited resources and where CF services are in the early stages of development.

The survival of patients with cystic fibrosis (CF) has progressively improved over the last four decades. Data from a number of patient registries show that length of survival is directly correlated to the decade the patient was born [1, 2]. Thus, for patients who were born in the last decade, the survival expectancy is significantly better than for those who were born earlier [1, 3]. Furthermore, according to the Cystic Fibrosis Foundation (CFF) Patient Registry database, in patients aged 18–19 years, forced expiratory volume in 1 s (FEV_1), the best predictor of survival in CF, increased from 67% in the year 2000 to 76% in the year 2006 [1]. The discovery and cloning of the cystic fibrosis transmembrane conductance regulator (*CFTR*) gene nearly 20 years ago led to the identification of the structure and function of the CFTR chloride channel. New therapies based on improved understanding of the function of CFTR are currently under development. However, the increased survival and improved clinical status of the patients is not a result of *CFTR* cloning, but is due to better understanding of the importance of nutrition and the natural course of infection and inflammation [4], and due to care in specialised CF centres by a multidisciplinary dedicated team [5]. Treatment opportunities vary depending on the country and sometimes even within the same country. The effect of socioeconomic status on health is well known. Patients with CF may experience deprivation-related health disparities in countries or populations with poor resources and treatment modalities need to be adapted accordingly. In this chapter,

Dept of Pediatrics and CF Center, Hadassah Hebrew University Medical Center, Jerusalem, Israel.

Correspondence: Eitan Kerem, Dept of Pediatrics and CF Center, Hadassah Hebrew University Medical Center, Jerusalem, 91240, Israel. E-mail: kerem@hadassah.org.il

Copyright ERS 2014. Print ISBN: 978-1-84984-050-7. Online ISBN: 978-1-84984-051-4. Print ISSN: 2312-508X. Online ISSN: 2312-5098.

we review the current CF modalities that are associated with the improved survival of patients with CF and that have become the standard of care in CF (table 1).

Care in specialised centres with regular and frequent routine evaluation

Care in dedicated centres by a team of trained and experienced health professionals is essential for optimal patient management and outcome. Specialist care in dedicated CF centres is associated with improved survival and quality of life (QoL) [5]. Care involves frequent clinical evaluations and monitoring for complications by physicians and other healthcare workers specifically trained in the management of CF. A retrospective multicentre study showed that earlier referral of children with CF to specialist care is associated with significantly better FEV1 and lower prevalence of *Pseudomonas aeruginosa* at the age of 13 years [6].

It was shown many years ago that survival of patients treated at the only CF centre in Denmark was significantly better than survival of patients treated by local physicians [7]. Subsequent reports from the UK showed that patients treated in CF clinics had better pulmonary function, better nutritional status and better chest radiography scores than those treated in nonspecialised CF clinics [8]. Data from the CFF database compared pulmonary function of patients treated in 194 centres in the USA, and showed that those treated in the top 25% of centres had significantly better nutritional status than those treated in the centres in the lowest 25% [9]. The upper quartile sites were characterised by more clinic visits and more routine tests, such as spirometry and sputum cultures. A similar study performed in the paediatric population showed comparable results, particularly in patients with mild CF lung disease [10]. Guidelines defining the necessary infrastructure for a CF centre, the standards

Table 1. Therapies for maintenance of lung function in patients with cystic fibrosis

Lung health maintenance	Available treatment	Effects
Avoiding *Pseudomonas aeruginosa* infection	Avoid cross-infection; frequent surveillance of sputum cultures; early eradication programme	Prevent, eradicate and postpone chronic *P. aeruginosa* infection
Enhancement of mucociliary clearance	Physiotherapy: manual and assisted; hypertonic saline; recombinant human DNase	Improve lung function; reduce exacerbation; accelerate mucus clearance; improve quality of life
Inhalation of antibiotics	Tobramycin; colistin; aztreonam	Improve lung function and reduce exacerbation; eradicate initial colonisation and postpone or suppress chronic *P. aeruginosa* infection
Anti-inflammatory treatment	Azithromycin; ibuprofen; corticosteroids (questionable)	Improve lung function and reduce exacerbation
Maintenance of good nutrition	Pancreatic enzymes; fat-soluble vitamins; supplementation with high-calorie/high-fat products; control of cystic fibrosis-related diabetes mellitus	Preserve lung function and reduce exacerbations

for routine evaluation and assessment of patients, documentation of results in a standard database and management of complications are available [4, 5, 8–10].

Correction of energy imbalance and maintenance of good nutrition

In CF, nutrition and survival are intimately related. In the past, growth failure and weight loss were seen as inevitable in the face of progressive lung disease in patients with CF. Under-nutrition in CF can be caused by pancreatic insufficiency, increased caloric needs and decrease in caloric intake. In the 1970s, the Toronto CF Clinic showed that a high-fat, high-calorie diet promoted a normal growth pattern that was associated with improved survival [11]. Longitudinal studies demonstrated that under-nutrition is closely related to the decline of lung function and early infection with *P. aeruginosa* [12–15]. Wasting was shown to be a significant predictor of survival in patients with CF, independent of lung function and arterial blood oxygen and carbon dioxide tensions [16]. Children who did not recover appropriate nutritional status by the age of 2 years had diminished lung function and more symptoms at 6 years compared with children who had better nutrition at 2 years of age [17]. In addition, correction of fat-soluble vitamin deficiency is essential. In this context, lower serum levels of vitamins A and E were associated with a higher rate of pulmonary exacerbations [18]. The energy needs of patients with CF vary widely and have been stated as 120–150% of those required by healthy individuals of the same age, sex and size. Techniques such as nasogastric feeding with bolus or overnight feeds should be considered as short-term solutions. Long-term supplementation *via* both gastrostomy and jejunostomy has also produced either acceleration in growth velocity or improved weight-for-height. Nutritional review is performed by a CF specialist dietician, and includes discussion of current diet, adequacy and knowledge of pancreatic enzyme replacement therapy, energy and vitamin supplements, oral nutritional supplements and enteral tube feeds (where appropriate). Weight profile and changes in nutritional status are monitored over time [19–21].

Enhancement of mucociliary clearance

CF is characterised by retained dry thick mucus, which becomes a focus for chronic infection. Current strategies to avoid progression of pulmonary disease in CF include augmentation of the mucociliary clearance by inhalation of hypertonic saline, by mucolitics such as Pulmozyme (dornase alfa, a DNase, manufactured by Genentech Inc. (San Francisco, CA, USA)), and by daily chest physiotherapy, to increase mucous drainage from the respiratory system.

Airway clearance

Airway clearance is an integral component of the management of CF. Several mechanical devices specifically tailored to the needs of patients with CF, such as positive expiratory pressure (PEP) masks, flutter and acapella devices, were developed to promote mucus transport and airway clearance [22]. In addition, techniques such as active cycle of breathing techniques and autogenic drainage were developed [22]. However, no airway clearance regime has been shown to be superior to others [23]. CF patients should start airway clearance treatment upon being diagnosed, even if there are no symptoms. Infants can be treated by their parents, using gentle percussions and chest vibrations in different positions. Older children and adults should receive at least 30 min of treatment daily, combining airway clearance techniques and physical activity [24]. Patients should adapt the regimen to suit them best and the regimen during each treatment session should be adapted according to the patient's needs, in order to improve efficacy and probably adherence [23]. Several mechanical airway clearance devices have been developed specifically for CF patients' needs. These devices include PEP masks, flutter and acapella, which cause positive pressure and vibrations during expiration to help transfer mucus from small and moderate airways to upper airways. Patients can use these devices independently. In the USA, high-frequency chest wall oscillation (HFCWO) is widely used. A long-term multicentre randomised controlled study in Canada showed better results with PEP use compared with HFCWO as the primary form of airway clearance in patients with CF [25].

Aerobic exercise is recommended for patients with CF as an adjunctive therapy for airway clearance and for its additional benefits to overall health, including improvement in the QoL and lowering anxiety and depression scores [26–29].

Hypertonic saline

Inhalation with hypertonic saline at 6% or 7% (4 mL twice daily, generally following pre-treatment with a bronchodilator) increases hydration of the airway surface [30, 31], mucociliary clearance and lung function, and reduces the frequency of exacerbations and absenteeism in patients with CF [32–35]. Hypertonic saline inhalation is also well tolerated in infants and young children [36]. It is an inexpensive, safe and effective therapy for patients with CF, producing sustained acceleration of mucus clearance and improved lung function [37].

Recombinant human DNase

Since the primary initiating event for airway obstruction in CF is the dry and thick mucus, mucolytics are a logical first-line therapy. The viscid nature of CF sputum is largely due to DNA from the vast numbers of degenerating neutrophils present in the airways. Airway obstruction by thickened secretions and cellular debris is the hallmark of CF lung disease. Inhalations of recombinant human DNase (dornase alfa, also known as Pulmozyme) degrade the large amount of free DNA that accumulates within CF mucus, thereby improving the viscoelastic properties of airway secretions and promoting airway clearance. Once-daily inhalation of dornase alfa has been associated with improved lung function and overall well-being and a reduction of CF exacerbations [38, 39], which may not be solely due to improved mucus clearance [40]. Several studies have suggested that dornase alfa prevents the progression of airway inflammation in patients with near-normal lung function [41]. In addition, this treatment was associated with an improvement in high-resolution chest computed tomography (CT) scores and in pulmonary function measurements [42, 43]. Therefore, it has been suggested that young asymptomatic patients in whom CF lung disease may not be apparent may benefit from early treatment with dornase alfa [39].

Infection with *P. aeruginosa*

Prevention of infection

Respiratory infection with *P. aeruginosa* is a leading cause of morbidity and mortality in patients with CF [44–48]. New acquisition of *P. aeruginosa* is frequently asymptomatic [49] and commonly occurs before the age of 3 years [50]. Early *P. aeruginosa* isolates have a phenotype distinct from usual isolates and are generally non-mucoid and antibiotic susceptible [50, 51]. Early infection by transmissible multiresistant strains is more difficult to eradicate [52]. A number of methods have been shown to be effective in reducing the rate of infection with *P. aeruginosa*, including strict adherence to infection control measures while avoiding cross-infection, and early and aggressive eradication of *P. aeruginosa* colonisation [53, 54]. In the absence of appropriate infection control measures, transmissible strains of *P. aeruginosa* pose a threat to *P. aeruginosa*-negative patients by creating an increased acquisition risk for infection [52, 55, 56]. Cross-infection with *P. aeruginosa* between patients occurs among siblings [57] or during social events, such as summer and winter camps [58, 59]. Despite a number of methods that are used to reduce the risk of cross-infection [60], it has not yet been determined whether patient segregation during clinic visits is superior to rigorous hygiene practices. Nevertheless, avoiding close social contacts or intimate contacts between patients is strongly recommended.

Eradication of new colonisation

The presence of *P. aeruginosa* in the lower airways may lead to increased airways inflammation (as measured by bronchoalveolar lavage (BAL), cytokine and neutrophil profiles, and poorer clinical status) [61]. Infection is also associated with lower respiratory function, decreased weight, height and body mass index (BMI), and more hospital admissions [62]. Therefore, it is critically important to offer all patients an early eradication regimen. There is increasing evidence that antibiotic therapy initiated early and close to the onset of *P. aeruginosa* infection is an effective strategy to eradicate the organism in the majority of cases and thereby postpone chronic *P. aeruginosa* infection [51, 63]. Since *P. aeruginosa* strains infecting CF airways at early stages are sensitive to antibiotics, their eradication is often achieved without the development of antibiotic resistance [64]. Although several protocols for eradication of *P. aeruginosa* after the first isolation are being used, at present no consensus exists regarding the optimal antibiotic protocol. It has been shown that treatment with inhaled tobramycin (300 mg twice a day) for 28 days is effective in eradication of early *P. aeruginosa* infection [65, 66].

Inhaled antibiotics for chronic infection

Chronic infection with *P. aeruginosa* is a major risk factor for loss of pulmonary function and decreased survival in CF [67, 68]. Therefore, anti-*Pseudomonas* antibiotics are extensively used for treatment in these patients [69]. Delivery of these antibiotics by aerosol inhalation has been widely studied as a route to suppress *P. aeruginosa*, and gives deposition in high concentrations in the airways without side-effects [70]. The following nebulised antibiotic preparations have been studied over the past three decades: gentamicin and carbenicillin combination [71], cephaloridine [72], gentamicin [73], colistin [74], ceftazidime [75], tobramycin [76–80] and aztreonam lysine [81–83].

Tobramycin is the most widely studied antibiotic for inhalation. Inhaled tobramycin was shown to produce sustained improvement in lung function, reduce pulmonary exacerbation and improve the nutritional status in patients with CF with chronic *P. aeruginosa* infections [77, 78]. Thus, chronic use of inhaled tobramycin is currently recommended by the CFF for CF patients with mild, moderate and severe lung disease and persistent colonisation with *P. aeruginosa* [84].

Colistin has been prescribed for more than 20 years for the treatment of CF patients with *P. aeruginosa* infections. At present, colistin is still one of the most commonly used drugs for inhalation in selected CF patients, and in many centres it is being used during the off-months of a standard tobramycin inhalation solution (TIS) regimen. In addition, recently, a new dry powder formulation of inhaled colistin was introduced and shown, in a randomised phase III open-label study, not to be inferior to TIS as measured by change in FEV1 % predicted at 24 weeks of treatment [85].

Aztreonam lysine for inhalation solution (Cayston, manufactured by Gilead Sciences, Inc., Foster City, CA, USA) was shown in recent years to improve lung function and health-related quality of life (HRQoL) in CF patients chronically infected with *P. aeruginosa* [81–83, 86] and, thus, is recommended by the CFF for chronic use in CF patients with mild, moderate or severe lung disease and persistent colonisation with *P. aeruginosa* [84].

Ceftazidime, cephaloridine and gentamicin, with or without carbenicillin, have all been used for inhalation therapy in CF patients with chronic *P. aeruginosa* infection. Unfortunately, these therapies have been studied only in small-scale trials [71–73, 75] and have not consistently been shown to improve outcome; thus, they are not recommended as standard therapy for CF patients. Despite the lack of evidence, we have recommended the use of inhalation of gentamicin intravenous solution in the CF patients from developing poorly resourced countries lacking tobramycin inhalation solution who consulted our CF centre.

Early and aggressive treatment of pulmonary exacerbations

Episodic respiratory exacerbations commonly occur in patients with CF, and are often related to reduced lung function and increased airways inflammation. LIOU *et al.* [87] showed that each acute pulmonary exacerbation had a negative impact on 5-year survival, equal to subtracting 12% of FEV1. A study using the CFF Patient Registry from 2003–2006 demonstrated that 25% of the patients failed to recover to baseline FEV1 within 3 months after treatment of exacerbation with *i.v.* antibiotics [88]. A higher risk of failing to recover to baseline was associated with female sex, pancreatic insufficiency, undernourishment, Medicaid insurance (in the USA), persistent infection with *P. aeruginosa*, *Burkholderia cepacia* complex or methicillin-resistant *Staphylococcus aureus* (MRSA), allergic broncho-pulmonary aspergillosis (ABPA), a longer time since baseline spirometric assessment, and a larger drop in FEV1 from baseline to treatment initiation. Early, aggressive treatment of CF lung disease may improve prognosis; therefore, identifying the presence of early airway disease in the young CF population is critical [89, 90]. Respiratory exacerbations in the first 2 years of life were shown to be markers for progressive CF lung disease, and were correlated with a lower FEV1 and higher exacerbations rates in later years. In addition, exacerbations were associated with bronchiectasis and lower weight-for-age z-scores at 5 years [91].

Currently, there is no consensus regarding the exact description of CF exacerbation. In most CF centres, current definitions of acute exacerbation are based on the subjective clinical assessment of physicians, and are classified as severe or mild and requiring *i.v.* or oral antibiotic therapy, based on "gut feeling". Furthermore, there are no clear guidelines regarding the time to start oral or *i.v.* antibiotic therapy and the optimal duration of antibiotic treatment. Currently, these parameters are based on the policies of each CF centre and the individual response to treatment. Several large clinical studies on new therapies for CF were published recently, with respiratory exacerbations being one of their end-points [78, 92, 93]. However, each study used different definitions for respiratory exacerbations. For the purpose of clinical trials, the simplest definition of pulmonary exacerbation is a physician-defined requirement to intervene with either oral or *i.v.* antibiotic therapy. The epidemiology, pathogenesis, prevention and management of acute exacerbations in CF were reviewed in the last few years [94, 95], emphasising the importance of prevention and early, immediate and aggressive treatment of pulmonary exacerbations.

Treatment of airway inflammation

Airway inflammation in patients with CF begins early in life, and results in increased airway obstruction and progressive damage. It is characterised by high concentrations of neutrophils and pro-inflammatory cytokines, and reduced concentrations of anti-inflammatory factors [96, 97]. However, monitoring airway inflammation in patients with CF continues to be a challenge [98], as the currently available sputum markers show considerable variability, and systemic markers of inflammation are often negative despite significant airway inflammation. Anti-inflammatory therapies have been shown to cause slight improvement in pulmonary function and to significantly reduce the rate of respiratory exacerbations [93, 99–101].

Azithromycin

Azithromycin is being used as an immunomodulating agent in the treatment of CF patients colonised and non-colonised with *P. aeruginosa* [93, 102], despite the fact that its exact mechanism is still unknown. Azithromycin was shown to significantly reduce the number of respiratory exacerbations and the rate in decline of lung function, and to improve QoL in patients colonised with *P. aeruginosa* and *S. aureus* [93, 103, 104]. It can reduce sputum viscosity and airway adhesion of *P. aeruginosa* and disrupt the ability of the bacteria to produce alginate [105]. Side-effects are mild and minimal with no increased *Pseudomonas* resistance [93]. Patients should be screened for nontuberculous mycobacteria (NTM) before initiating azithromycin, and reassessed periodically at 6- to 12-month intervals [84].

Ibuprofen

High-dose ibuprofen has been shown to slow the rate of deterioration of pulmonary function in CF [96, 106]. Despite its apparent benefit, ibuprofen is infrequently administered due to the need to measure plasma levels, and because of potential renal and gastrointestinal side-effects that are more common when it is administered together with aminoglycosides. Its maximal effect was observed in children younger than 13 years of age, emphasising the beneficial effect of early treatment.

Corticosteroids

Several studies have reported beneficial effects of systemic corticosteroids in the treatment of patients with CF, especially in children who have mild lung disease. However, the improvement was transient and was associated with significant adverse effects such as diabetes and cataract. Therefore, systemic corticosteroids are not recommended as a routine therapy [107]. The use of inhaled corticosteroids (ICS) in patients with CF is controversial. Short-term benefit was associated with a significant reduction in the rate of FEV_1 decline [108], particularly in patients with asthma [109]. However, the transient benefit of ICS was associated with decreased linear growth and increased insulin/oral hypoglycaemic agent use. Discontinuing treatment with ICS in patients with CF on chronic ICS therapy had no deleterious effect on lung function [110]. Therefore, oral or inhaled steroids are currently not the standard of care as a routine anti-inflammatory therapy in CF, but may be considered for a subgroup of patients, possibly those with concomitant asthma.

Early diagnosis and prevention of non-apparent lung damage

It is conceivable that early therapy, before lung disease is established, will provide the most significant long-term benefits for children with CF. Lung pathology in young children with CF is frequently underestimated; it was shown that 84% of infants [49] and 51% of children with *P. aeruginosa* [111] were asymptomatic. Children diagnosed early with CF, before developing symptoms, have better pulmonary function throughout early childhood [112], probably as a result of early and aggressive therapy that postpones the development and progression of the disease. A delay in diagnosis until the appearance of symptoms can lead to the development of malnutrition and/or irreversible lung disease [113]. Despite the wide availability of the sweat test, CF diagnosis can be missed in early childhood. Newborn screening for CF offers the opportunity for early intervention [114]. It has been shown that infants who were diagnosed by newborn screening or with a family history of CF showed fewer symptoms at diagnosis and had a better nutritional state [16, 17, 113, 115–118]. Lung function, measured by forced expiration, is normal in infants with CF at the time of diagnosis by newborn screening but is diminished in older infants [119]. However, it has not yet been proven that newborn screening causes decreased lung damage. A recent report from Australia demonstrated that a substantial number of infants diagnosed following newborn screening were asymptomatic, but many of them had active pulmonary inflammation and infection, with evidence of structural lung damage detected by chest CT at 3 months of age. Most of the infants with detectable lung disease were asymptomatic [49]. Several studies suggest that early intervention with physiotherapy, inhalations of hypertonic saline, dornase alfa or antibiotics and anti-inflammatory therapy are beneficial for asymptomatic children and for those with mild disease [120–122].

Early identification and treatment of complications

Prolonged survival exposes CF patients to secondary diseases that were previously rarely encountered. It is of utmost importance to diagnose these complications as early as possible and provide appropriate therapy.

Cystic fibrosis-related diabetes mellitus

Cystic fibrosis-related diabetes mellitus (CFRD) is the most frequent comorbidity diagnosed today [123], occurring in ~40% of adults, 25% of adolescents and 9% of children [124]. CFRD is associated with a rapid decline in lung function [125] and increased risk of death from respiratory failure, particularly in females [126]. Early identification and treatment of CFRD is associated with improved pulmonary function and survival. Common symptoms include weight loss or lack of weight gain, fatigue or loss of energy, worsening of pulmonary function and generally feeling unwell. The majority of patients with CFRD do not have fasting hyperglycaemia and, in the absence of classic symptoms, the diagnosis of CFRD frequently relies on the oral glucose tolerance test (OGTT), which has to be performed annually in patients older than 10 years of age (1.75 g·kg^{-1} glucose; maximal dose 75 g). Glycated haemoglobin (HbA1c) is not recommended as a tool for CFRD screening. Normal HbA1c does not exclude CFRD; however, an HbA1c $\geqslant 6.5\%$ is consistent with diabetes. The CFRD treatment of choice is insulin. The insulin regimen is tailored to fit the individual patient. Combinations of basal (long-acting) and bolus (rapid-acting) insulin are used in the setting of fasting hyperglycaemia. Pre-meal rapid-acting insulin is the primary approach to the treatment of CFRD without fasting hyperglycaemia. Treatment with insulin enhances the nutritional state and temporarily improves pulmonary function in CFRD patients, delaying the decline in FEV1 by 34 months [127]. Oral hypoglycaemic agents are not recommended for the treatment of CFRD. The nutritional recommendations for CFRD are to follow a high-fat/high-calorie regimen (calories 120–160% recommended dietary allowance (RDA), fat 35–40% of total caloric intake), with no deprivation of any food group and replacement of sweetened beverages and sugar with nutrient-dense calories. Patients should spread intake of carbohydrates throughout the day, match insulin to carbohydrates consumed and monitor weight and nutritional status.

Allergic bronchopulmonary aspergillosis

ABPA is a pulmonary hypersensitivity disease mediated by an allergic response to respiratory colonisation by *Aspergillus fumigatus* [128]. It is a complicating factor of CF that can result in clinical deterioration and worsening of lung disease. Early diagnosis and treatment of ABPA with systemic steroids and antifungal therapy is currently the treatment of choice and is of fundamental importance to ameliorate the progression of lung disease and prevent deterioration to a severe fibrotic stage, as well as permanent lung damage [129–131].

Gastro-oesophageal reflux

Gastro-oesophageal reflux (GOR) is relatively common in CF, with a reported incidence varying from 6.4% to 20% [132]. Pathologically increased GOR was demonstrated before radiological lung disease was established [133]. A significant correlation between oesophageal acid exposure and the number of coughs per 24 h has recently been reported. In addition, patients with GOR and cough had lower lung function than those who did not [134], which may lead to worsening of lung disease [135].

Distal intestinal obstruction syndrome

Distal intestinal obstruction syndrome (DIOS) is a common complication in patients with CF [136, 137]. It is characterised by the accumulation of viscid faecal material in the distal ileum and the first part of the colon, and may present acutely with intestinal obstruction or, more commonly, sub-acutely with intermittent abdominal pain generally in combination with abdominal distension and vomiting [136]. Characteristically, DIOS patients have a right lower quadrant mass that may be palpable and is usually seen on a plain abdominal radiograph. Rates for incomplete obstruction (impending DIOS) are likely to be higher. Risk factors include "severe" genotype, a previous episode of DIOS, previous history of meconium ileus and having had organ transplantation. Treatment of DIOS is still largely empirical. Patients with incomplete DIOS usually respond to oral rehydration combined with stool softeners like picosalax or osmotic laxative containing polyethylene glycol (PEG). The use of *N*-acetylcysteine (NAC) administered orally has been superseded by the above medication. When DIOS presents with more severe intestinal obstruction characterised by bilious vomiting, or when washout therapy has failed, hospitalisation should be recommended and *i.v.* rehydration and nasogastric aspiration commenced. Gastrografin can be used by enema (100 mL diluted four times with water). With early aggressive medical management, surgery is seldom required. As a previous episode of DIOS is a risk factor for recurrence, maintenance laxative therapy can be considered, with avoidance of dehydration and reassessment of adequate pancreatic enzyme dosage. These steps seem logical, although there is no evidence base. Oral PEG 0.5–1 g·kg^{-1}·day^{-1} is probably the best choice. The role of increasing dietary fibre in preventing a subsequent DIOS episode is unclear.

Anxiety, depression and other mental issues

Numerous studies have demonstrated that patients with chronic illnesses and with conditions that require a time-consuming treatment regimen and the potential for health to worsen, are at an increased risk for anxiety and depression [138, 139]. In these patients, depression and anxiety have been shown to have serious direct and indirect consequences on health outcomes. Depressed patients are less compliant with medical regimens, are more likely to miss clinic appointments, are more likely to engage in risky behaviours such as smoking and drinking, report worse HRQoL, and have higher healthcare utilisation and healthcare costs [140–143]. Rates of depression in adults with CF have ranged from 29% to 46% [144]. In school-age and adolescent children with CF, few studies of depression have been conducted, with prevalence in CF patients ranging from 11% to 14.5% in comparison to 2–6% in the general population [145]. Due to the importance of health issues that have an impact on the QoL of the patients, screening for anxiety/depression and addressing mental health issues is recommended as an element of routine healthcare for patients with chronic diseases and specifically in CF [146, 147].

Other complications

Other less common complications of CF, including cystic fibrosis liver disease (CFLD), spontaneous pneumothorax, haemoptysis, osteoporosis and depression, should be treated; however, their treatment has not been shown to be associated with improvement in lung function and prognosis.

Adherence to routine care

Adherence to these management procedures requires daily tiresome and time-consuming activities, including physiotherapy, inhalations, taking oral medicines and nutritional support. For many patients this is very difficult to perform. Poor adherence to medical advice and treatment is well documented in chronic illnesses in general. The consequences of poor adherence include increased symptoms, accelerated decline in lung function, more frequent hospitalisations, increased family stress and conflict, and higher healthcare costs [148]. Patients with no or only minor symptoms, who feel well, may be reluctant to adhere to tedious regimens in order to prevent the slow and non-apparent health decline. The feeling or appearance of well-being creates the false sense that the disease is not active and therefore reduces the motivation to adhere to the required daily care. In addition, therapy aimed at preventing complications is not associated with the direct perception of its efficacy, in contrast to treatments for symptoms. It has been shown that the greater the level of worry regarding the disease, the more likely that the patients will adhere to the physiotherapy, pancreatic enzyme and vitamin regimens [149]. People with strong beliefs in the necessity of taking medication to maintain their health were found to be more adherent to treatment, and those with higher levels of concern about the dangers of dependence and long-term side-effects of medication, were more likely to be non-adherent [150]. Increased adherence includes help, support, encouraging self-management, personal control, optimistic coping and individualised teaching [151]. Health information needs reiterating to ensure all parties approve the plan to ensure positive behaviour changes are covered. It is crucial that patients understand these types of treatments. A better understanding of the long-term benefits of complying with treatments will lead to improvement in health outcomes and the patient's QoL [152]. In order to improve adherence, partnership

Table 2. The "10 golden rules" of cystic fibrosis care

1	Maintain good nutrition and correct nutritional deficiencies
2	Daily chest physiotherapy
3	Enhance mucociliary clearance (inhaled hypertonic saline and dornase alfa)
4	Avoid and give early treatment for newly acquired *Pseudomonas aeruginosa* infection
5	Suppression of chronic *Pseudomonas aeruginosa* infection (inhaled antibiotics)
6	Early and aggressive treatment of pulmonary exacerbation
7	Anti-inflammatory therapy
8	Early identification and treatment of complications
9	Care in a specialised centre with frequent regular visits
10	Strict adherence to all the above therapies

with patients and families about the treatment plan might be important for improving adherence rate [153].

Conclusion

Since the cloning of the *CFTR* gene over 20 years ago, extensive research has provided understanding of the structure and function of the CFTR chloride channel. However, curative therapies are not yet available. Nevertheless, significant improvement in the survival and QoL of patients with CF has been achieved [4], which is mainly due to a better conception of the natural course of infection and inflammation in CF. The current strategies to increase the life expectancy of patients with CF are summarised in table 2 and include early diagnosis, early and aggressive nutritional support, early augmentation of mucociliary clearance and improved mucous drainage, early initiation of antimicrobial and anti-inflammatory therapy, early treatment of acute exacerbations, implementation of effective hygiene measures in and outside CF centres and early identification and treatment of complications. Treatment at a specialised CF centre by a multidisciplinary dedicated team, including frequent visits, periodic routine tests and review of adherence to therapy leading to more frequent early intervention, is mandatory for improved outcome in CF. Adherence to these therapies is challenging. Treatments to correct or modify the basic defect by gene replacement or pharmacological means are showing considerable promise. These new therapies are expected to further increase life expectancy of the patients. The best goal would be to conserve the maximal lung function by maximising current treatment regimens. Hopefully patients will benefit, in the near future, from a "personalised medicine" system, and therapies that could correct the basic CFTR defect could turn CF into a manageable disease.

References

1. Cystic Fibrosis Foundation Patient Registry. 2006 Annual Data Report. Bethesda, Cystic Fibrosis Foundation, 2008.
2. Elborn JS, Shale DJ, Britton JR. Cystic fibrosis: current survival and population estimates to the year 2000. *Thorax* 1991; 46: 881–885.
3. Stern M, Wiedemann B, Wenzlaff P. From registry to quality management: the German Cystic Fibrosis Quality Assessment project 1995–2006. *Eur Respir J* 2008; 31: 29–35.
4. Cohen-Cymberknoh M, Shoseyov D, Kerem E. Managing cystic fibrosis: strategies that increase life expectancy and improve quality of life. *Am J Respir Crit Care Med* 2011; 183: 1463–1471.
5. Kerem E, Conway S, Elborn S, *et al.* Standards of care for patients with cystic fibrosis: a European consensus. *J Cyst Fibros* 2005; 4: 7–26.
6. Lebecque P, Leonard A, De Boeck K, *et al.* Early referral to cystic fibrosis specialist centre impacts on respiratory outcome. *J Cyst Fibros* 2009; 8: 26–30.

7. Nielsen OH, Thomsen BL, Green A, *et al.* Cystic fibrosis in Denmark 1945 to 1985. An analysis of incidence, mortality and influence of centralized treatment on survival. *Acta Paediatr Scand* 1988; 77: 836–841.

8. Mahadeva R, Webb K, Westerbeek RC, *et al.* Clinical outcome in relation to care in centres specialising in cystic fibrosis: cross sectional study. *BMJ* 1998; 316: 1771–1775.

9. Johnson C, Butler SM, Konstan MW, *et al.* Factors influencing outcomes in cystic fibrosis: a center-based analysis. *Chest* 2003; 123: 20–27.

10. Padman R, McColley SA, Miller DP, *et al.* Infant care patterns at epidemiologic study of cystic fibrosis sites that achieve superior childhood lung function. *Pediatrics* 2007; 119: e531–e537.

11. Levy L, Durie P, Pencharz P, *et al.* Prognostic factors associated with patient survival during nutritional rehabilitation in malnourished children and adolescents with cystic fibrosis. *J Pediatr Gastroenterol Nutr* 1986; 5: 97–102.

12. Kerem E, Reisman J, Corey M, *et al.* Prediction of mortality in patients with cystic fibrosis. *N Engl J Med* 1992; 326: 1187–1191.

13. Nir M, Lanng S, Johansen HK, *et al.* Long-term survival and nutritional data in patients with cystic fibrosis treated in a Danish centre. *Thorax* 1996; 51: 1023–1027.

14. Steinkamp G, Wiedemann B. Relationship between nutritional status and lung function in cystic fibrosis: cross sectional and longitudinal analyses from the German CF quality assurance (CFQA) project. *Thorax* 2002; 57: 596–601.

15. Kerem E, Corey M, Stein R, *et al.* Risk factors for *Pseudomonas aeruginosa* colonization in cystic fibrosis patients. *Pediatr Infect Dis J* 1990; 9: 494–498.

16. Sharma R, Florea VG, Bolger AP, *et al.* Wasting as an independent predictor of mortality in patients with cystic fibrosis. *Thorax* 2001; 56: 746–750.

17. Lai HJ, Shoff SM, Farrell PM. Recovery of birth weight z score within 2 years of diagnosis is positively associated with pulmonary status at 6 years of age in children with cystic fibrosis. *Pediatrics* 2009; 123: 714–722.

18. Hakim F, Kerem E, Rivlin J, *et al.* Vitamins A and E and pulmonary exacerbations in patients with cystic fibrosis. *J Pediatr Gastroenterol Nutr* 2007; 45: 347–353.

19. Munck A, Duhamel JF, Lamireau T, *et al.* Pancreatic enzyme replacement therapy for young cystic fibrosis patients. *J Cyst Fibros* 2009; 8: 14–18.

20. Sinaasappel M, Stern M, Littlewood J, *et al.* Nutrition in patients with cystic fibrosis: a European Consensus. *J Cyst Fibros* 2002; 1: 51–75.

21. Borowitz D, Baker RD, Stallings V. Consensus report on nutrition for pediatric patients with cystic fibrosis. *J Pediatr Gastroenterol Nutr* 2002; 35: 246–259.

22. Hess DR. The evidence for secretion clearance techniques. *Respir Care* 2001; 46: 1276–1293.

23. Pryor JA, Tannenbaum E, Scott SF, *et al.* Beyond postural drainage and percussion: airway clearance in people with cystic fibrosis. *J Cyst Fibros* 2010; 9: 187–192.

24. Flume PA, Robinson KA, O'Sullivan BP, *et al.* Cystic fibrosis pulmonary guidelines: airway clearance therapies. *Respir Care* 2009; 54: 522–537.

25. McIlwaine MP, Alarie N, Davidson GF, *et al.* Long-term multicentre randomised controlled study of high frequency chest wall oscillation *versus* positive expiratory pressure mask in cystic fibrosis. *Thorax* 2013; 68: 746–751.

26. Schneiderman-Walker J, Pollock SL, Corey M, *et al.* A randomized controlled trial of a 3-year home exercise program in cystic fibrosis. *J Pediatr* 2000; 136: 304–310.

27. Selvadurai HC, Blimkie CJ, Meyers N, *et al.* Randomized controlled study of in-hospital exercise training programs in children with cystic fibrosis. *Pediatr Pulmonol* 2002; 33: 194–200.

28. Klijn PH, Oudshoorn A, van der Ent CK, *et al.* Effects of anaerobic training in children with cystic fibrosis: a randomized controlled study. *Chest* 2004; 125: 1299–1305.

29. Zigmond AS, Snaith RP. The hospital anxiety and depression scale. *Acta Psychiatr Scand* 1983; 67: 361–370.

30. Tarran R, Grubb BR, Parsons D, *et al.* The CF salt controversy: *in vivo* observations and therapeutic approaches. *Mol Cell* 2001; 8: 149–158.

31. Ratjen F. Restoring airway surface liquid in cystic fibrosis. *N Engl J Med* 2006; 354: 291–293.

32. Robinson M, Regnis JA, Bailey DL, *et al.* Effect of hypertonic saline, amiloride, and cough on mucociliary clearance in patients with cystic fibrosis. *Am J Respir Crit Care Med* 1996; 153: 1503–1509.

33. Robinson M, Hemming AL, Regnis JA, *et al.* Effect of increasing doses of hypertonic saline on mucociliary clearance in patients with cystic fibrosis. *Thorax* 1997; 52: 900–903.

34. Eng PA, Morton J, Douglass JA, *et al.* Short-term efficacy of ultrasonically nebulized hypertonic saline in cystic fibrosis. *Pediatr Pulmonol* 1996; 21: 77–83.

35. Ballmann M, von der Hardt H. Hypertonic saline and recombinant human DNase: a randomised cross-over pilot study in patients with cystic fibrosis. *J Cyst Fibros* 2002; 1: 35–37.

36. Dellon EP, Donaldson SH, Johnson R, *et al.* Safety and tolerability of inhaled hypertonic saline in young children with cystic fibrosis. *Pediatr Pulmonol* 2008; 43: 1100–1106.

37. Donaldson SH, Bennett WD, Zeman KL, *et al.* Mucus clearance and lung function in cystic fibrosis with hypertonic saline. *N Engl J Med* 2006; 354: 241–250.

38. Fuchs HJ, Borowitz DS, Christiansen DH, *et al.* Effect of aerosolized recombinant human DNase on exacerbations of respiratory symptoms and on pulmonary function in patients with cystic fibrosis. The Pulmozyme Study Group. *N Engl J Med* 1994; 331: 637–642.

39. Quan JM, Tiddens HA, Sy JP, *et al.* A two-year randomized, placebo-controlled trial of dornase alfa in young patients with cystic fibrosis with mild lung function abnormalities. *J Pediatr* 2001; 139: 813–820.

40. Laube BL, Auci RM, Shields DE, *et al.* Effect of rhDNase on airflow obstruction and mucociliary clearance in cystic fibrosis. *Am J Respir Crit Care Med* 1996; 153: 752–760.

41. Paul K, Rietschel E, Ballmann M, *et al.* Effect of treatment with dornase alpha on airway inflammation in patients with cystic fibrosis. *Am J Respir Crit Care Med* 2004; 169: 719–725.

42. Robinson TE, Leung AN, Northway WH, *et al.* Composite spirometric-computed tomography outcome measure in early cystic fibrosis lung disease. *Am J Respir Crit Care Med* 2003; 168: 588–593.

43. Geller DE, Eigen H, Fiel SB, *et al.* Effect of smaller droplet size of dornase alfa on lung function in mild cystic fibrosis. Dornase Alfa Nebulizer Group. *Pediatr Pulmonol* 1998; 25: 83–87.

44. Emerson J, Rosenfeld M, McNamara S, *et al.* *Pseudomonas aeruginosa* and other predictors of mortality and morbidity in young children with cystic fibrosis. *Pediatr Pulmonol* 2002; 34: 91–100.

45. Nixon GM, Armstrong DS, Carzino R, *et al.* Clinical outcome after early *Pseudomonas aeruginosa* infection in cystic fibrosis. *J Pediatr* 2001; 138: 699–704.

46. Kosorok MR, Zeng L, West SE, *et al.* Acceleration of lung disease in children with cystic fibrosis after *Pseudomonas aeruginosa* acquisition. *Pediatr Pulmonol* 2001; 32: 277–287.

47. Kerem E, Corey M, Gold R, *et al.* Pulmonary function and clinical course in patients with cystic fibrosis after pulmonary colonization with *Pseudomonas aeruginosa*. *J Pediatr* 1990; 116: 714–719.

48. Robinson TE, Leung AN, Chen X, *et al.* Cystic fibrosis HRCT scores correlate strongly with *Pseudomonas* infection. *Pediatr Pulmonol* 2009; 44: 1107–1117.

49. Sly PD, Brennan S, Gangell C, *et al.* Lung disease at diagnosis in infants with cystic fibrosis detected by newborn screening. *Am J Respir Crit Care Med* 2009; 180: 146–152.

50. Burns JL, Gibson RL, McNamara S, *et al.* Longitudinal assessment of *Pseudomonas aeruginosa* in young children with cystic fibrosis. *J Infect Dis* 2001; 183: 444–452.

51. Taccetti G, Campana S, Festini F, *et al.* Early eradication therapy against *Pseudomonas aeruginosa* in cystic fibrosis patients. *Eur Respir J* 2005; 26: 458–461.

52. Jones AM, Govan JR, Doherty CJ, *et al.* Spread of a multiresistant strain of *Pseudomonas aeruginosa* in an adult cystic fibrosis clinic. *Lancet* 2001; 358: 557–558.

53. Lee TW, Brownlee KG, Denton M, *et al.* Reduction in prevalence of chronic *Pseudomonas aeruginosa* infection at a regional pediatric cystic fibrosis center. *Pediatr Pulmonol* 2004; 37: 104–110.

54. Proesmans M, Balinska-Miskiewicz W, Dupont L, *et al.* Evaluating the "Leeds criteria" for *Pseudomonas aeruginosa* infection in a cystic fibrosis centre. *Eur Respir J* 2006; 27: 937–943.

55. Cheng K, Smyth RL, Govan JR, *et al.* Spread of beta-lactam-resistant *Pseudomonas aeruginosa* in a cystic fibrosis clinic. *Lancet* 1996; 348: 639–642.

56. Scott FW, Pitt TL. Identification and characterization of transmissible *Pseudomonas aeruginosa* strains in cystic fibrosis patients in England and Wales. *J Med Microbiol* 2004; 53: 609–615.

57. Picard E, Aviram M, Yahav Y, *et al.* Familial concordance of phenotype and microbial variation among siblings with CF. *Pediatr Pulmonol* 2004; 38: 292–297.

58. Jones AM, Dodd ME, Govan JR, *et al.* Prospective surveillance for *Pseudomonas aeruginosa* cross-infection at a cystic fibrosis center. *Am J Respir Crit Care Med* 2005; 171: 257–260.

59. Ojeniyi B, Frederiksen B, Hoiby N. *Pseudomonas aeruginosa* cross-infection among patients with cystic fibrosis during a winter camp. *Pediatr Pulmonol* 2000; 29: 177–181.

60. Saiman L, Siegel J. Infection control recommendations for patients with cystic fibrosis: microbiology, important pathogens, and infection control practices to prevent patient-to-patient transmission. *Am J Infect Control* 2003; 31: Suppl. 3, S1–S62.

61. Sagel SD, Gibson RL, Emerson J, *et al.* Impact of *Pseudomonas* and *Staphylococcus* infection on inflammation and clinical status in young children with cystic fibrosis. *J Pediatr* 2009; 154: 183–188.

62. Lee TW, Brownlee KG, Conway SP, *et al.* Evaluation of a new definition for chronic *Pseudomonas aeruginosa* infection in cystic fibrosis patients. *J Cyst Fibros* 2003; 2: 29–34.

63. Treggiari MM, Rosenfeld M, Retsch-Bogart G, *et al.* Approach to eradication of initial *Pseudomonas aeruginosa* infection in children with cystic fibrosis. *Pediatr Pulmonol* 2007; 42: 751–756.

64. Ho SA, Lee TW, Denton M, *et al.* Regimens for eradicating early *Pseudomonas aeruginosa* infection in children do not promote antibiotic resistance in this organism. *J Cyst Fibros* 2009; 8: 43–46.

65. Ratjen F, Munck A, Kho P, *et al.* Treatment of early *Pseudomonas aeruginosa* infection in patients with cystic fibrosis: the ELITE trial. *Thorax* 2010; 65: 286–291.

66. Treggiari MM, Rosenfeld M, Mayer-Hamblett N, *et al.* Early anti-pseudomonal acquisition in young patients with cystic fibrosis: rationale and design of the EPIC clinical trial and observational study. *Contemp Clin Trials* 2009; 30: 256–268.

67. Ratjen F, Döring G. Cystic fibrosis. *Lancet* 2003; 361: 681–689.
68. Kerem E, Viviani L, Zolin A, *et al.* Factors associated with FEV1 decline in cystic fibrosis: analysis of the ECFS Patient Registry. *Eur Respir J* 2014; 43: 125–133.
69. Gibson RL, Burns JL, Ramsey BW. Pathophysiology and management of pulmonary infections in cystic fibrosis. *Am J Respir Crit Care Med* 2003; 168: 918–951.
70. Ryan G, Singh M, Dwan K. Inhaled antibiotics for long-term therapy in cystic fibrosis. *Cochrane Database Syst Rev* 2011; 3: CD001021.
71. Hodson ME, Penketh AR, Batten JC. Aerosol carbenicillin and gentamicin treatment of *Pseudomonas aeruginosa* infection in patients with cystic fibrosis. *Lancet* 1981; 2: 1137–1139.
72. Nolan G, Moivor P, Levison H, *et al.* Antibiotic prophylaxis in cystic fibrosis: inhaled cephaloridine as an adjunct to oral cloxacillin. *J Pediatr* 1982; 101: 626–630.
73. Kun P, Landau LI, Phelan PD. Nebulized gentamicin in children and adolescents with cystic fibrosis. *Aust Paediatr J* 1984; 20: 43–45.
74. Jensen T, Pedersen SS, Garne S, *et al.* Colistin inhalation therapy in cystic fibrosis patients with chronic *Pseudomonas aeruginosa* lung infection. *J Antimicrob Chemother* 1987; 19: 831–838.
75. Stead RJ, Hodson ME, Batten JC. Inhaled ceftazidime compared with gentamicin and carbenicillin in older patients with cystic fibrosis infected with *Pseudomonas aeruginosa*. *Br J Dis Chest* 1987; 81: 272–279.
76. MacLusky IB, Gold R, Corey M, *et al.* Long-term effects of inhaled tobramycin in patients with cystic fibrosis colonized with *Pseudomonas aeruginosa*. *Pediatr Pulmonol* 1989; 7: 42–48.
77. Ramsey BW, Dorkin HL, Eisenberg JD, *et al.* Efficacy of aerosolized tobramycin in patients with cystic fibrosis. *N Engl J Med* 1993; 328: 1740–1746.
78. Ramsey BW, Pepe MS, Quan JM, *et al.* Intermittent administration of inhaled tobramycin in patients with cystic fibrosis. Cystic Fibrosis Inhaled Tobramycin Study Group. *N Engl J Med* 1999; 340: 23–30.
79. Hodson ME, Gallagher CG, Govan JR. A randomised clinical trial of nebulised tobramycin or colistin in cystic fibrosis. *Eur Respir J* 2002; 20: 658–664.
80. Wiesemann HG, Steinkamp G, Ratjen F, *et al.* Placebo-controlled, double-blind, randomized study of aerosolized tobramycin for early treatment of *Pseudomonas aeruginosa* colonization in cystic fibrosis. *Pediatr Pulmonol* 1998; 25: 88–92.
81. McCoy KS, Quittner AL, Oermann CM, *et al.* Inhaled aztreonam lysine for chronic airway *Pseudomonas aeruginosa* in cystic fibrosis. *Am J Respir Crit Care Med* 2008; 178: 921–928.
82. Retsch-Bogart GZ, Quittner AL, Gibson RL, *et al.* Efficacy and safety of inhaled aztreonam lysine for airway *Pseudomonas* in cystic fibrosis. *Chest* 2009; 135: 1223–1232.
83. Wainwright CE, Quittner AL, Geller DE, *et al.* Aztreonam for inhalation solution (AZLI) in patients with cystic fibrosis, mild lung impairment, and *P. aeruginosa*. *J Cyst Fibros* 2011; 10: 234–242.
84. Mogayzel PJ Jr, Naureckas ET, Robinson KA, *et al.* Cystic fibrosis pulmonary guidelines. Chronic medications for maintenance of lung health. *Am J Respir Crit Care Med* 2013; 187: 680–689.
85. Schuster A, Haliburn C, Döring G, *et al.* Safety, efficacy and convenience of colistimethate sodium dry powder for inhalation (Colobreathe DPI) in patients with cystic fibrosis: a randomised study. *Thorax* 2013; 68: 344–350.
86. Oermann CM, Retsch-Bogart GZ, Quittner AL, *et al.* An 18-month study of the safety and efficacy of repeated courses of inhaled aztreonam lysine in cystic fibrosis. *Pediatr Pulmonol* 2010; 45: 1121–1134.
87. Liou TG, Adler FR, Fitzsimmons SC, *et al.* Predictive 5-year survivorship model of cystic fibrosis. *Am J Epidemiol* 2001; 153: 345–352.
88. Sanders DB, Bittner RC, Rosenfeld M, *et al.* Failure to recover to baseline pulmonary function after cystic fibrosis pulmonary exacerbation. *Am J Respir Crit Care Med* 2010; 182: 627–632.
89. Davis SD, Fordham LA, Brody AS, *et al.* Computed tomography reflects lower airway inflammation and tracks changes in early cystic fibrosis. *Am J Respir Crit Care Med* 2007; 175: 943–950.
90. Fernandes B, Plummer A, Wildman M. Duration of intravenous antibiotic therapy in people with cystic fibrosis. *Cochrane Database Syst Rev* 2008; 2: CD006682.
91. Byrnes CA, Vidmar S, Cheney JL, *et al.* Prospective evaluation of respiratory exacerbations in children with cystic fibrosis from newborn screening to 5 years of age. *Thorax* 2013; 68: 643–651.
92. Elkins MR, Robinson M, Rose BR, *et al.* A controlled trial of long-term inhaled hypertonic saline in patients with cystic fibrosis. *N Engl J Med* 2006; 354: 229–240.
93. Saiman L, Marshall BC, Mayer-Hamblett N, *et al.* Azithromycin in patients with cystic fibrosis chronically infected with *Pseudomonas aeruginosa*: a randomized controlled trial. *JAMA* 2003; 290: 1749–1756.
94. Flume PA, Mogayzel PJ Jr, Robinson KA, *et al.* Cystic fibrosis pulmonary guidelines: treatment of pulmonary exacerbations. *Am J Respir Crit Care Med* 2009; 180: 802–808.
95. Anstead M, Saiman L, Mayer-Hamblett N, *et al.* Pulmonary exacerbations in CF patients with early lung disease. *J Cyst Fibros* 2014; 13: 74–79.
96. Elizur A, Cannon CL, Ferkol TW. Airway inflammation in cystic fibrosis. *Chest* 2008; 133: 489–495.

97. Bruscia EM, Zhang PX, Ferreira E, *et al.* Macrophages directly contribute to the exaggerated inflammatory response in cystic fibrosis transmembrane conductance regulator[-/-] mice. *Am J Respir Cell Mol Biol* 2009; 40: 295–304.

98. Cohen-Cymberknoh M, Kerem E, Ferkol T, *et al.* Airway inflammation in cystic fibrosis: molecular mechanisms and clinical implications. *Thorax* 2013; 68: 1157–1162.

99. Konstan MW, Schluchter MD, Xue W, *et al.* Clinical use of ibuprofen is associated with slower FEV1 decline in children with cystic fibrosis. *Am J Respir Crit Care Med* 2007; 176: 1084–1089.

100. Greally P, Hussain MJ, Vergani D, *et al.* Interleukin-1α, soluble interleukin-2 receptor, and IgG concentrations in cystic fibrosis treated with prednisolone. *Arch Dis Child* 1994; 71: 35–39.

101. Equi A, Balfour-Lynn IM, Bush A, *et al.* Long term azithromycin in children with cystic fibrosis: a randomised, placebo-controlled crossover trial. *Lancet* 2002; 360: 978–984.

102. Saiman L, Anstead M, Mayer-Hamblett N, *et al.* Effect of azithromycin on pulmonary function in patients with cystic fibrosis uninfected with *Pseudomonas aeruginosa*: a randomized controlled trial. *JAMA* 2010; 303: 1707–1715.

103. McCormack J, Bell S, Senini S, *et al.* Daily *versus* weekly azithromycin in cystic fibrosis patients. *Eur Respir J* 2007; 30: 487–495.

104. Wolter J, Seeney S, Bell S, *et al.* Effect of long term treatment with azithromycin on disease parameters in cystic fibrosis: a randomised trial. *Thorax* 2002; 57: 212–216.

105. Peckham DG. Macrolide antibiotics and cystic fibrosis. *Thorax* 2002; 57: 189–190.

106. Lands LC, Milner R, Cantin AM, *et al.* High-dose ibuprofen in cystic fibrosis: Canadian safety and effectiveness trial. *J Pediatr* 2007; 151: 249–254.

107. Flume PA, O'Sullivan BP, Robinson KA, *et al.* Cystic fibrosis pulmonary guidelines: chronic medications for maintenance of lung health. *Am J Respir Crit Care Med* 2007; 176: 957–969.

108. Ren CL, Pasta DJ, Rasouliyan L, *et al.* Relationship between inhaled corticosteroid therapy and rate of lung function decline in children with cystic fibrosis. *J Pediatr* 2008; 153: 746–751.

109. Bisgaard H, Pedersen SS, Nielsen KG, *et al.* Controlled trial of inhaled budesonide in patients with cystic fibrosis and chronic bronchopulmonary *Pseudomonas aeruginosa* infection. *Am J Respir Crit Care Med* 1997; 156: 1190–1196.

110. Balfour-Lynn IM, Lees B, Hall P, *et al.* Multicenter randomized controlled trial of withdrawal of inhaled corticosteroids in cystic fibrosis. *Am J Respir Crit Care Med* 2006; 173: 1356–1362.

111. Douglas TA, Brennan S, Gard S, *et al.* Acquisition and eradication of *P. aeruginosa* in young children with cystic fibrosis. *Eur Respir J* 2009; 33: 305–311.

112. Wang SS, O'Leary LA, Fitzsimmons SC, *et al.* The impact of early cystic fibrosis diagnosis on pulmonary function in children. *J Pediatr* 2002; 141: 804–810.

113. Farrell PM, Kosorok MR, Rock MJ, *et al.* Early diagnosis of cystic fibrosis through neonatal screening prevents severe malnutrition and improves long-term growth. Wisconsin Cystic Fibrosis Neonatal Screening Study Group. *Pediatrics* 2001; 107: 1–13.

114. Comeau AM, Accurso FJ, White TB, *et al.* Guidelines for implementation of cystic fibrosis newborn screening programs: Cystic Fibrosis Foundation workshop report. *Pediatrics* 2007; 119: e495–e518.

115. Parad RB, Comeau AM. Newborn screening for cystic fibrosis. *Pediatr Ann* 2003; 32: 528–535.

116. Castellani C. Evidence for newborn screening for cystic fibrosis. *Paediatr Respir Rev* 2003; 4: 278–284.

117. Merelle ME, Nagelkerke AF, Lees CM, *et al.* Newborn screening for cystic fibrosis. *Cochrane Database Syst Rev* 2001; 3: CD001402.

118. Farrell PM, Kosorok MR, Laxova A, *et al.* Nutritional benefits of neonatal screening for cystic fibrosis. Wisconsin Cystic Fibrosis Neonatal Screening Study Group. *N Engl J Med* 1997; 337: 963–969.

119. Linnane BM, Hall GL, Nolan G, *et al.* Lung function in infants with cystic fibrosis diagnosed by newborn screening. *Am J Respir Crit Care Med* 2008; 178: 1238–1244.

120. Nasr SZ, Kuhns LR, Brown RW, *et al.* Use of computerized tomography and chest X-rays in evaluating efficacy of aerosolized recombinant human DNase in cystic fibrosis patients younger than age 5 years: a preliminary study. *Pediatr Pulmonol* 2001; 31: 377–382.

121. Gibson RL, Emerson J, McNamara S, *et al.* Significant microbiological effect of inhaled tobramycin in young children with cystic fibrosis. *Am J Respir Crit Care Med* 2003; 167: 841–849.

122. Rosenfeld M, Gibson R, McNamara S, *et al.* Serum and lower respiratory tract drug concentrations after tobramycin inhalation in young children with cystic fibrosis. *J Pediatr* 2001; 139: 572–577.

123. Adler AI, Shine BS, Chamnan P, *et al.* Genetic determinants and epidemiology of cystic fibrosis-related diabetes: results from a British cohort of children and adults. *Diabetes Care* 2008; 31: 1789–1794.

124. Moran A, Doherty L, Wang X, *et al.* Abnormal glucose metabolism in cystic fibrosis. *J Pediatr* 1998; 133: 10–17.

125. Milla CE, Warwick WJ, Moran A. Trends in pulmonary function in patients with cystic fibrosis correlate with the degree of glucose intolerance at baseline. *Am J Respir Crit Care Med* 2000; 162: 891–895.

126. Milla CE, Billings J, Moran A. Diabetes is associated with dramatically decreased survival in female but not male subjects with cystic fibrosis. *Diabetes Care* 2005; 28: 2141–2144.

127. Mohan K, Israel KL, Miller H, *et al.* Long-term effect of insulin treatment in cystic fibrosis-related diabetes. *Respiration* 2008; 76: 181–186.

128. Hartl D, Latzin P, Zissel G, *et al.* Chemokines indicate allergic bronchopulmonary aspergillosis in patients with cystic fibrosis. *Am J Respir Crit Care Med* 2006; 173: 1370–1376.

129. Greenberger PA, Patterson R, Ghory A, *et al.* Late sequelae of allergic bronchopulmonary aspergillosis. *J Allergy Clin Immunol* 1980; 66: 327–335.

130. Kumar R. Mild, moderate, and severe forms of allergic bronchopulmonary aspergillosis: a clinical and serologic evaluation. *Chest* 2003; 124: 890–892.

131. Cohen-Cymberknoh M, Blau H, Shoseyov D, *et al.* Intravenous monthly pulse methylprednisolone treatment for ABPA in patients with cystic fibrosis. *J Cyst Fibros* 2009; 8: 253–257.

132. Vinocur CD, Marmon L, Schidlow DV, *et al.* Gastroesophageal reflux in the infant with cystic fibrosis. *Am J Surg* 1985; 149: 182–186.

133. Heine RG, Button BM, Olinsky A, *et al.* Gastro-oesophageal reflux in infants under 6 months with cystic fibrosis. *Arch Dis Child* 1998; 78: 44–48.

134. Blondeau K, Mertens V, Vanaudenaerde BA, *et al.* Gastro-oesophageal reflux and gastric aspiration in lung transplant patients with or without chronic rejection. *Eur Respir J* 2008; 31: 707–713.

135. Blondeau K, Dupont LJ, Mertens V, *et al.* Gastro-oesophageal reflux and aspiration of gastric contents in adult patients with cystic fibrosis. *Gut* 2008; 57: 1049–1055.

136. Houwen RH, van der Doef HP, Sermet I, *et al.* Defining DIOS and constipation in cystic fibrosis with a multicentre study on the incidence, characteristics, and treatment of DIOS. *J Pediatr Gastroenterol Nutr* 2010; 50: 38–42.

137. Colombo C, Ellemunter H, Houwen R, *et al.* Guidelines for the diagnosis and management of distal intestinal obstruction syndrome in cystic fibrosis patients. *J Cyst Fibros* 2011; 10: Suppl. 2, S24–S28.

138. Evans DL, Charney DS, Lewis L, *et al.* Mood disorders in the medically ill: scientific review and recommendations. *Biol Psychiatry* 2005; 58: 175–189.

139. Quittner AL, Barker DH, Snell C, *et al.* Prevalence and impact of depression in cystic fibrosis. *Curr Opin Pulm Med* 2008; 14: 582–588.

140. Whittemore R, Kanner S, Singleton S, *et al.* Correlates of depressive symptoms in adolescents with type 1 diabetes. *Pediatr Diabetes* 2002; 3: 135–143.

141. DiMatteo MR, Lepper HS, Croghan TW. Depression is a risk factor for noncompliance with medical treatment: meta-analysis of the effects of anxiety and depression on patient adherence. *Arch Intern Med* 2000; 160: 2101–2107.

142. Dowson CA, Kuijer RG, Mulder RT. Anxiety and self-management behaviour in chronic obstructive pulmonary disease: what has been learned? *Chron Respir Dis* 2004; 1: 213–220.

143. Bender BG. Risk taking, depression, adherence, and symptom control in adolescents and young adults with asthma. *Am J Respir Crit Care Med* 2006; 173: 953–957.

144. Pearson DA, Pumariega AJ, Seilheimer DK. The development of psychiatric symptomatology in patients with cystic fibrosis. *J Am Acad Child Adolesc Psychiatry* 1991; 30: 290–297.

145. Anderson DL, Flume PA, Hardy KK. Psychological functioning of adults with cystic fibrosis. *Chest* 2001; 119: 1079–1084.

146. Nici L, Donner C, Wouters E, *et al.* American Thoracic Society/European Respiratory Society statement on pulmonary rehabilitation. *Am J Respir Crit Care Med* 2006; 173: 1390–1413.

147. Besier T, Goldbeck L. Anxiety and depression in adolescents with CF and their caregivers. *J Cyst Fibros* 2011; 10: 435–442.

148. Modi AC, Quittner AL. Barriers to treatment adherence for children with cystic fibrosis and asthma: what gets in the way? *J Pediatr Psychol* 2006; 31: 846–858.

149. Abbott J, Dodd M, Webb AK. Health perceptions and treatment adherence in adults with cystic fibrosis. *Thorax* 1996; 51: 1233–1238.

150. Horne R, Weinman J. Patients' beliefs about prescribed medicines and their role in adherence to treatment in chronic physical illness. *J Psychosom Res* 1999; 47: 555–567.

151. Dodd ME, Webb AK. Understanding non-compliance with treatment in adults with cystic fibrosis. *J R Soc Med* 2000; 93: Suppl. 38, 2–8.

152. Kettler LJ, Sawyer SM, Winefield HR, *et al.* Determinants of adherence in adults with cystic fibrosis. *Thorax* 2002; 57: 459–464.

153. Zindani GN, Streetman DD, Streetman DS, *et al.* Adherence to treatment in children and adolescent patients with cystic fibrosis. *J Adolesc Health* 2006; 38: 13–17.

Disclosures: None declared.

Chapter 18

Using registries to improve cystic fibrosis care

Edward F. McKone[1] and Bruce C. Marshall[2]

Since their first introduction almost 50 years ago, cystic fibrosis (CF) registries have become an essential tool in improving our understanding of CF. More recently, CF registries have become important in the direct management of CF patients and have been developed to supply detailed information on how CF care is delivered throughout the world. This chapter will focus on the role of CF registries in improving quality of care for patients with CF. We will review the outcome variation and its interpretation in CF and the present and future role of CF patient registries in improving healthcare delivery through benchmarking, pharmaco-epidemiology and comparative effectiveness research.

Prognosis for patients with cystic fibrosis (CF) has improved dramatically over the recent decades, largely through the introduction of new therapies as well as the centralised delivery of CF care [1]. As more and more people are living with CF patient registries have become important tools in assessing the changes in CF care, and finding out how different interventions can lead to both improved survival rates and quality of life (QoL) for CF patients. CF patient registries now exist throughout Europe [2], North and South America [3–5] and Australasia [6, 7]. The registries collect information on patient demographics, measures of disease-related activity and the impact of current CF therapies on over 60 000 CF patients worldwide. Over the past 20 years CF registries have provided invaluable information about the changing epidemiology of CF, which has led to an improved understanding of the disease course of CF as well as an increased knowledge of factors that influence changes in CF outcomes, including survival [8–11]. While this knowledge has a practical use, for example predicting when to refer a patient for lung transplantation [12, 13], the influence of registries on delivering CF care is often not apparent to CF caregivers and patients [14–16]. This chapter will look at how CF patient registries have influenced CF care with a focus on the opportunities and challenges of international comparative studies and what they can offer us in the future.

Understanding the differences in outcomes to improve care

Outcomes for CF patients can vary from region to region. Measuring and understanding this variation may generate new hypotheses for improving the quality of care for people with

---

[1]National Referral Centre for Adult Cystic Fibrosis, School of Medical Sciences, University College Dublin, St. Vincent's University Hospital, Dublin, Ireland. [2]Cystic Fibrosis Foundation, Bethesda, MD, USA.

Correspondence: Edward F. McKone, National Referral Centre for Adult Cystic Fibrosis, School of Medical Sciences, University College Dublin, St. Vincent's University Hospital, Elm Park, Dublin 4, Ireland. E-mail: e.mckone@svuh.ie

CF [17]. Identifying CF centres with the best outcomes and how they differ from other centres can suggest targets for quality improvement that, if successful, would impact CF outcomes. This type of research is ideally suited to CF registries, which collect high-quality population-based longitudinal data from large numbers of CF patients over many years.

Despite the great promise of registries, comparing outcomes across countries or centres has a number of challenges including what is the best outcome to measure. Annual death rates in CF patients are generally less than 2% per year, so studies comparing survival differences between countries are difficult to undertake, as they require very large numbers of patients followed for many years. As a result very few studies directly compare survival outcomes between countries. This is especially true for registries from smaller countries, as the median annual survival is difficult to measure reliably due to: a low number of deaths per year, high variability in number of deaths from year to year, and limited patient follow-up time. This was seen in a series of recently published studies that compared survival between the US CF Foundation patient registry and the Irish CF patient registry. The widely used life-tables approach to estimating survival in the Irish CF population was unreliable [18], but worked well for large registries. The application of a parametric birth-cohort method of statistical modelling demonstrated similar survival outcomes between Irish and American CF patients. The authors concluded that this statistical approach may be a more reliable method of comparing survival outcomes for smaller countries [19].

With survival outcomes difficult to measure and compare, surrogates of survival are sought. In one of the largest registry studies from the European CF Demographics Registry Project, demographic data on 29 000 CF patients from 35 European Union (EU) countries and non-EU countries were compared. Analysis of the CF population age and genotype distribution across Europe demonstrated substantial variation in the age attained by CF patients between EU and non-EU countries [20]. Although survival was not specifically examined, it was clear that these results reflected poorer outcomes in the non-EU countries most likely due to differences in disease recognition and quality of care. Another registry study, using the USA, France, Australia and UK registries, looked at demographics as well as the more commonly used surrogates for survival; forced expiratory volume in 1 s (FEV1) and nutritional measures including height and weight. Differences in outcomes were seen between countries including median age attained, median height and weight and age at diagnosis [21]. The authors also highlighted the significant differences in the methodology used by each registry to collect information, which limits the certainty of their interpretation of the findings. A subsequent study comparing the Australian and US registries have also identified differences in outcomes after the introduction of a newborn screening programme, with the measured benefits of newborn screening being less in Australia than that observed in the USA [22].

Comparisons across single CF centres have also shown differences in outcome. In a pivotal publication in 1988, a comparison using centre registries based in Toronto (Canada) and Boston (MA, USA) demonstrated that a high-fat, high-calorie diet, which was routine practice in Toronto, was associated with better growth and survival [23]. This study led to a substantial change in CF practice that has now been adopted worldwide. In another registry-based study looking at differences in centre outcomes, data from the Epidemiologic Study of Cystic Fibrosis (ESCF) were used to examine differences between centres ranked according to their average age-adjusted lung function [24]. Centres with the highest lung function, monitored patients more closely and had a more aggressive approach to treating exacerbations. This more aggressive approach to exacerbation detection and treatment is likely to improve CF outcomes, especially given that significant centre-to-centre variation in exacerbation treatment has been recently reported [25].

These comparisons are good examples of how differences in outcome can be identified and measured using registries. One of the caveats is that these differences may not be entirely due the quality of care so they must be interpreted carefully.

Challenges in comparing outcomes using registries

Although differences in outcomes have been identified, caution is required when interpreting outcome variation found in registry studies. One of the main challenges in using registries to monitor and improve CF-care delivery is that significant variations exist in the type and quality of registry data being collected. Registry comparisons are influenced by: methods of data collection; rates of measure misclassification: statistical methods, including which reference equations are used; and how the final summary data is presented. Survival is one outcome that may be less prone to misclassification but, as noted earlier, comparisons can be difficult due to different statistical methods used. Comparison of lung function and nutritional measures as surrogates for survival are especially problematic. How measures of lung function and nutrition are collected varies with some registries collecting best FEV1 for the year, others reporting one FEV1 at annual review and others reporting average of the best quarterly FEV1 with multiple measures taken over the year [26, 27]. Another challenge is the use of different reference equations and values for predicted normal lung function, weight and height. The choice of reference equations should be specific to the population being studied, as different reference equations can lead to significant differences in average population values [28]. These different approaches to data collection and presentation make comparison of outcomes across registries very challenging. A consensus across registries on what should be collected and reported would be very valuable; although what "should be" collected *versus* what "can be" collected is often limited by registry personnel, time and financial resources.

These methodological considerations aside, real differences in outcomes between centres and/ or countries exist. Whether these differences are due to differences in clinical care is often not clear, and other factors unrelated to clinical care should be considered. While recognising that optimising delivery of care is an important part of improving CF outcomes, efforts focusing on identifying differences in outcomes need to ensure that these differences are due to modifiable factors. Identifying differences in outcomes due to factors that are not modifiable will result in costly and time consuming interventions, which may not benefit CF patients. To understand this, it is important to recognise the factors that influence the variability of CF severity.

Factors contributing to variability in disease severity

Variability in CF severity is due to a complex interaction between genetic, environmental and stochastic events. "Environmental influence" is a broad term that can refer to any non-genetic factor that influences the outcome of CF and can range from regional or local exposure to pollutants to something like the number of times a patient is seen in a CF clinic. As genetic and many environmental contributors to CF severity cannot be altered, identifying and quantifying the role of these differences is essential before embarking on a quality improvement programme, as care may be equal across centres and countries but outcomes very different due to non-modifiable factors.

CF patient registries have provided significant information on how genetic and environmental factors may influence CF outcomes. The cystic fibrosis transmembrane conductance regulator (*CFTR*) genotype influences survival with milder *CFTR* genotypes associated with more residual functions associated with milder disease [29, 30]. The distribution of *CFTR* genotypes in many larger countries is quite similar and effects of *CFTR* genetic variation may not be a big contributor to outcome, but for some smaller countries in Europe, the prevalence of *CFTR* genotypes can be quite different, which may impact outcomes when comparing to other countries [2]. This is currently being examined in detail in *CFTR2*, a large epidemiology study looking at how different *CFTR* genotypes affect CF disease severity, using clinical and genetic data on patients enrolled in CF patient registries around the world. In addition, modifier genes have a significant role to play in CF disease trajectory [31]. Variation in modifier gene frequencies in CF patients across countries is not known but could, in part, explain the variation in long-term outcomes.

Looking at the differences in environmental factors across continents, such as the USA and Europe, it is clear that environmental exposures associated with the worse disease outcome in CF are also highly variable from region to region [32, 33]. Epidemiological studies using CF-patient registries have identified factors such as exposure to pollutants [34], passive smoke [35], and sociodemographic [36, 37], as contributors to mortality and more rapid lung-function decline. Pollutant levels and smoking rates throughout Europe and the USA vary considerably; hence, regional differences in outcome due to these exposures could be falsely attributed to the delivery of care. Likewise, allergen levels [38] and temperature [39] have been associated with the development of allergic bronchopulmonary aspergillosis in CF patients and the acquisition of *Pseudomonas aeruginosa*, both of which are associated with a more rapid decline in lung function. Again, allergen levels and temperature show considerable variation throughout Europe and the USA.

These genetic and environmental considerations need to be factored in when comparisons are being made using registries, particularly when comparing countries or geographically distant centres. The strength of registries is that many of these factors can be incorporated into the analysis, ensuring that differences identified are more likely to be related to CF care variation.

These caveats aside, once differences are found that may be due to practice variation, how do we use registries to improve CF care?

Quality improvement and benchmarking using registries

The recognition of significant variations in care delivery and an association with poorer CF outcomes has prompted the development of strategies to assess and improve the delivery of care for CF patients [40]. In the USA, the Cystic Fibrosis Foundation has developed, through close collaboration with CF patients and caregivers, an extensive quality improvement programme throughout CF centres in the USA [27, 41]. Setting key centre-based performance indicators and providing feedback to centre directors using registry data on an annual basis, a transparent platform for quality improvement has evolved. The US registry, through a robust data quality programme, now contains accurate data on a high proportion of patients from each CF centre (fig. 1), thereby giving a reliable assessment of centre-level patient outcomes. This overcomes the frequent challenge of "poor data" that has occurred in the past. It also allows for case-mix adjustment to "level the playing field" for centres that care for more challenging CF patients, for example those centres with patients

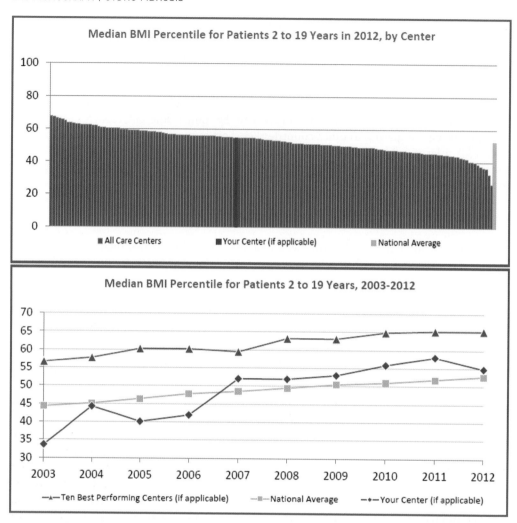

Figure 1. Centre-level feedback from the US registry showing how a participating centre compares with other cystic fibrosis centres and how this performance indicator has changed over time. BMI: body mass index. Reproduced from [3] with permission from the publisher.

from lower socioeconomic status. Examples of successful benchmarking using registry data includes improvements in diabetes screening rates in the North New England Cystic Fibrosis Consortium [40, 42], which saw rates of diabetic screening rise from 17% below the US national average to 4% above the national average after a 3-year quality improvement programme. Intensive behaviour and nutritional interventions in a study out of Cincinnati (OH, USA) resulted in a reduction in the decline in body mass index (BMI) z-scores compared to registry controls [43]. Reporting of the US centre-care data also led to the development of a strategic plan for quality improvement that highlighted seven attainable goals ("worthy goals") that would hopefully translate into increased CF survival [44].

In Europe, quality improvement programmes have generally been introduced at country level using country-specific patient registries to monitor outcomes. Germany has a very well developed CF quality improvement/benchmarking programme. In 1995, standardised clinical data on patients attending German CF centres were collected in 93 participating centres, creating a German registry [45]. Similar to the US registry, centre-based outcomes were collated and were available to each centre director. Over time, the German registry has evolved into a benchmark project where individual centres can assess their performance indicators in comparison with other centres [46]. Participating centres have agreed to the publication of comparisons between centres, within a framework that promotes audit and quality groups that facilitate interpretation and acting on the data [47]. As there are almost 7000 patients in the registry, mortality outcomes have been published, allowing comparison with survival data from other large registries and have shown broadly similar survival when compared to the French and US patient registries [45]. Similar centre-specific reports are also provided by the UK registry [48].

While the countries with larger registries are now extending beyond descriptive epidemiology, smaller countries may not have this capability as many do not have a registry or have a registry that is relatively new. For European countries that do not have their own country registry, the European Cystic Fibrosis Society Patient Registry (ECFSPR) offers software that can be used by European centres predominantly for data collection. The ECFSPR is now collecting data from over 30 000 patients, from 24 countries, with a view towards expanding its use to include quality improvement in the future. This is particularly relevant as the ECFS is developing standard of care programmes to promote consistent CF management throughout participating European countries [49].

Some registries can also be a very important tool in monitoring individual CF patient disease activity and/or for population management. These functions relate to their capability of collecting encounter-level patient data throughout the year. Individual patient summary reports can be generated, which include graphical displays of lung function and nutritional status, and can be very helpful in recognising patients with a more accelerated decline. Real-time presentation of patient data, including a list of CF complications such as diabetes or liver disease, can be reviewed by a CF team member at weekly team meetings, thereby promoting the development of a personalised multidisciplinary treatment plans for each patient (fig. 2). A copy of these graphical representations of serial registry data can then be given to the patient, which will hopefully lead to improved patient understanding of CF as well as more patient involvement in their own CF care. Population management tools can also be built into the registries. For example, reports that show patients overdue for a clinic visit or for diabetes screening can be easily generated by care centre staff. These reports can be very helpful to a care centre team focused on improving outcomes.

Where to next? Registries and pharmaco-epidemiology

One of the ways that disease-specific registries can have a major influence on patient care is through providing a "real-world" assessment of how CF therapies influence long-term outcomes [50]. Most approved CF therapies have been licensed based on relatively short clinical trials (often 6 or 12 month durations), which are carried out in a carefully selected patient group to maximise internal validity and exclude patients that may be at a greater risk of adverse events. As most approved CF drugs are prescribed in a broader population than the ones included in the original clinical trials, ongoing monitoring of effectiveness and safety is essential. CF registries are well designed to examine the long-term benefits of CF therapies as information on lung function, exacerbations and QoL. The outcomes of most clinical trials are collected at regular intervals. CF patient registries also contain data on large populations followed over many years and so the impact of new medicines on outcomes, such as survival,

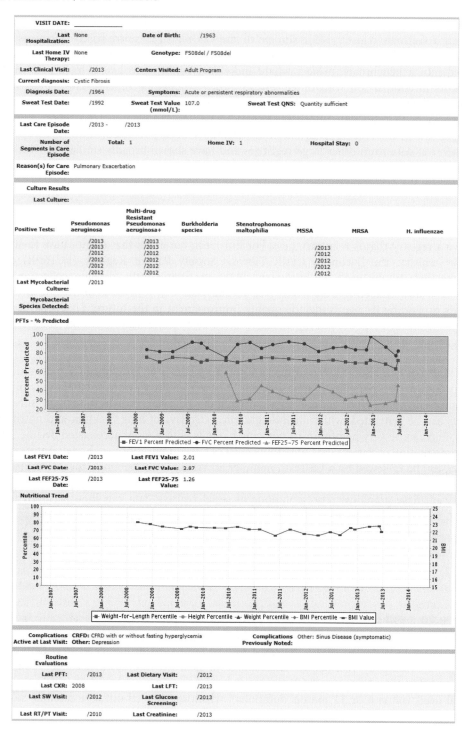

Figure 2. Examples of encounter-based data that is available from the US Cystic Fibrosis Patient Registry. The data came from the Cystic Fibrosis Foundation-accredited care centres in the USA who consented to have their data entered in 2012. Reproduced from [3] with permission from the publisher.

can be determined. Registry studies have shown survival benefits associated with long-term use of DNase [51] and inhaled tobramycin [52]. Survival benefits of CF therapies such as hypertonic saline and azithromycin are not known, as the widespread use of these drugs is still fairly recent. In addition to efficacy studies, CF registries can be adapted to collect specific information about the safety of newer drugs and are becoming an important tool in monitoring the safety profile of newly approved medications (pharmacovigilance). Registries can also provide a real-world assessment of drug prescribing patterns. A good example is ibuprofen, which has been shown to be associated with reduced lung function decline in long-term registry studies [53], yet still is relatively rarely prescribed in many CF centres [3, 54].

Demonstrating long-term benefits of CF medications is required to justify their use in the management of CF patients; however, with the increasing number of inhaled and oral therapies now available to treat CF, the burden of treatment for patients is increasing dramatically. As many of these medications target similar lung disease mechanisms, such as impaired mucus clearance (hypertonic saline, DNase) or chronic airway infection (inhaled tobramycin, aztreonam and colomicin), there is a need to determine which combinations of treatments work the best together. Repeating randomised clinical trials with combinations of CF therapies are too costly and are unlikely to fully determine the "real-world" effectiveness of multiple CF therapies. Understanding how these medications work together is an important goal and the American Thoracic Society's recent statement on comparative effectiveness research [55] has highlighted the role of disease-specific registries to address whether new medications or combination of older medications, outside of the clinical trial setting, continue to improve outcomes for patients. CF registries worldwide collect information on medications as well as outcomes, such as lung function, exacerbations and survival outcomes, making them ideal for comparing long-term treatment effectiveness research. This is essential as there is a need to rationalise and justify existing therapies for CF, especially in a setting of reduced healthcare spending and the emergence of newer high-priced targeted CFTR therapies. However, interpretation of registry studies requires caution as clinicians typically prescribe therapies more often for their "sickest patients". Adjusting for this indication bias can be very challenging [56]. Key findings of some retrospective registry studies will require confirmation in prospective clinical trials. Registries have been proposed as a means of conducting pragmatic comparative clinical trials of approved therapies [57].

Conclusion

In conclusion, CF patient registries play an important role in the care of patients with CF. Using registries to measure differences in outcomes across countries and between centres gives important information about approaches that might improve the delivery of care. Ongoing data collected in registries also provides a mechanism for monitoring the impact of interventions to improve care, such as benchmarking and quality improvement programmes. Also, as new medications are approved and CF care becomes more complex with a growing treatment burden on patients, data collected in registries can be used to determine which medications are continuing to work in CF and which of the many treatment options available to patients work best together.

References

1. Walters S, Mehta A. Epidemiology of cystic fibrosis. *In*: Hodson M, Geddes D, Bush A, eds. Cystic Fibrosis. Edward Arnold, London, 2007; pp. 21–45.
2. ECFS Patient Registry. 2008–2009 ECFS Patient Registry Annual Data Report. ECFSPR, Denmark, 2012.

3.   Cystic Fibrosis Foundation Patient Registry. 2011 Annual Data Report. Bethesda, Cystic Fibrosis Foundation, 2012.
4.   Cystic Fibrosis Canada. The Canadian Cystic Fibrosis Registry 2011 Annual Report. Toronto, Cystic Fibrosis Canada, 2012.
5.   Grupo Brasileiro De Estudos de Fibrose Cística. Fibrose Cística Registro Brasileiro de Ano 2011 [Brazilian Registry of Cystic Fibrosis Year 2011]. www.gbefc.org.br/gbefc/Registro2011_Portugues_site.pdf
6.   Cystic Fibrosis Network. Cystic Fibrosis Data. www.cysticfibrosisdata.org/ Date last accessed: March 2014.
7.   Cystic Fibrosis Australia. Cystic Fibrosis in Australia 2012: 15th Annual Report Australian Cystic Fibrosis Data Registry. Sydney, Cystic Fibrosis Australia, 2013.
8.   Buzzetti R, Salvatore D, Baldo E, et al. An overview of international literature from cystic fibrosis registries: 1. Mortality and survival studies in cystic fibrosis. J Cyst Fibros 2009; 8: 229–237.
9.   Salvatore D, Buzzetti R, Baldo E, et al. An overview of international literature from cystic fibrosis registries 2. Neonatal screening and nutrition/growth. J Cyst Fibros 2010; 9: 75–83.
10. Salvatore D, Buzzetti R, Baldo E, et al. An overview of international literature from cystic fibrosis registries. Part 3. Disease incidence, genotype/phenotype correlation, microbiology, pregnancy, clinical complications, lung transplantation, and miscellanea. J Cyst Fibros 2011; 10: 71–85.
11. Salvatore D, Buzzetti R, Baldo E, et al. An overview of international literature from cystic fibrosis registries. Part 4: update 2011. J Cyst Fibros 2012; 11: 480–493.
12. Liou TG, Adler FR, Fitzsimmons SC, et al. Predictive 5-year survivorship model of cystic fibrosis. Am J Epidemiol 2001; 153: 345–352.
13. Mayer-Hamblett N, Rosenfeld M, Emerson J, et al. Developing cystic fibrosis lung transplant referral criteria using predictors of 2-year mortality. Am J Respir Crit Care Med 2002; 166: 1550–1555.
14. Mehta G, Sims EJ, Culross F, et al. Potential benefits of the UK Cystic Fibrosis database. J R Soc Med 2004; 97: Suppl. 44, 60–71.
15. Mehta A. The how (and why) of disease registers. Early Hum Dev 2010; 86: 723–728.
16. Sheppard DN. The European cystic fibrosis patient registry: the power of sharing data. J Cyst Fibros 2010; 9: Suppl. 2, S1–S2.
17. Schechter MS, Margolis P. Improving subspecialty healthcare: lessons from cystic fibrosis. J Pediatr 2005; 147: 295–301.
18. Jackson AD, Daly L, Kelleher C, et al. The application of current lifetable methods to compare cystic fibrosis median survival internationally is limited. J Cyst Fibros 2011; 10: 62–65.
19. Jackson AD, Daly L, Jackson AL, et al. Validation and use of a parametric model for projecting cystic fibrosis survivorship beyond observed data: a birth cohort analysis. Thorax 2011; 66: 674–679.
20. McCormick J, Mehta G, Olesen HV, et al. Comparative demographics of the European cystic fibrosis population: a cross-sectional database analysis. Lancet 2010; 375: 1007–1013.
21. McCormick J, Sims EJ, Green MW, et al. Comparative analysis of Cystic Fibrosis Registry data from the UK with USA, France and Australasia. J Cyst Fibros 2005; 4: 115–122.
22. Martin B, Schechter MS, Jaffe A, et al. Comparison of the US and Australian cystic fibrosis registries: the impact of newborn screening. Pediatrics 2012; 129: e348–e355.
23. Corey M, McLaughlin FJ, Williams M, et al. A comparison of survival, growth, and pulmonary function in patients with cystic fibrosis in Boston and Toronto. J Clin Epidemiol 1988; 41: 583–591.
24. Johnson C, Butler SM, Konstan MW, et al. Factors influencing outcomes in cystic fibrosis: a center-based analysis. Chest 2003; 123: 20–27.
25. Kraynack NC, Gothard MD, Falletta LM, et al. Approach to treating cystic fibrosis pulmonary exacerbations varies widely across US CF care centers. Pediatr Pulmonol 2011; 46: 870–881.
26. Schechter MS. Patient registry analyses: seize the data, but caveat lector. J Pediatr 2008; 153: 733–735.
27. Schechter MS. Benchmarking to improve the quality of cystic fibrosis care. Curr Opin Pulm Med 2012; 18: 596–601.
28. Rosenfeld M, Pepe MS, Longton G, et al. Effect of choice of reference equation on analysis of pulmonary function in cystic fibrosis patients. Pediatr Pulmonol 2001; 31: 227–237.
29. McKone EF, Emerson SS, Edwards KL, et al. Effect of genotype on phenotype and mortality in cystic fibrosis: a retrospective cohort study. Lancet 2003; 361: 1671–1676.
30. McKone EF, Goss CH, Aitken ML. CFTR genotype as a predictor of prognosis in cystic fibrosis. Chest 2006; 130: 1441–1447.
31. Vanscoy LL, Blackman SM, Collaco JM, et al. Heritability of lung disease severity in cystic fibrosis. Am J Respir Crit Care Med 2007; 175: 1036–1043.
32. AirNow-International. www.airnow.gov/index.cfm?action=airnow.mapcenter&mapcenter=1#tabs-6 Date last accessed: March 2014.
33. European Environmental Protection Agency. Data And Maps. www.eea.europa.eu/data-and-maps#tab-maps Date last accessed: March 2014.
34. Goss CH, Newsom SA, Schildcrout JS, et al. Effect of ambient air pollution on pulmonary exacerbations and lung function in cystic fibrosis. Am J Respir Crit Care Med 2004; 169: 816–821.

35. Collaco JM, Vanscoy L, Bremer L, *et al.* Interactions between secondhand smoke and genes that affect cystic fibrosis lung disease. *JAMA* 2008; 299: 417–424.
36. Schechter MS, Shelton BJ, Margolis PA, *et al.* The association of socioeconomic status with outcomes in cystic fibrosis patients in the united states. *Am J Respir Crit Care Med* 2001; 163: 1331–1337.
37. O'Connor GT, Quinton HB, Kneeland T, *et al.* Median household income and mortality rate in cystic fibrosis. *Pediatrics* 2003; 111: e333–339.
38. Collaco JM, Morrow CB, Green DM, *et al.* Environmental allergies and respiratory morbidities in cystic fibrosis. *Pediatr Pulmonol* 2013; 48: 857–864.
39. Collaco JM, McGready J, Green DM, *et al.* Effect of temperature on cystic fibrosis lung disease and infections: a replicated cohort study. *PloS One* 2011; 6: e27784.
40. Quon BS, Goss CH. A story of success: continuous quality improvement in cystic fibrosis care in the USA. *Thorax* 2011; 66: 1106–1108.
41. Schechter MS, Gutierrez HH. Improving the quality of care for patients with cystic fibrosis. *Curr Opin Pediatr* 2010; 22: 296–301.
42. Quinton HB, O'Connor GT. Current issues in quality improvement in cystic fibrosis. *Clin Chest Med* 2007; 28: 459–472.
43. Stark LJ, Opipari-Arrigan L, Quittner AL, *et al.* The effects of an intensive behavior and nutrition intervention compared to standard of care on weight outcomes in CF. *Pediatr Pulmonol* 2011; 46: 31–35.
44. Cystic Fibrosis Foundation. Care Center Data. www.cff.org/LivingWithCF/CareCenterNetwork/CareCenterData/ Date last accessed: March 2014.
45. Stern M, Wiedemann B, Wenzlaff P. From registry to quality management: the German Cystic Fibrosis Quality Assessment project 1995–2006. *Eur Respir J* 2008; 31: 29–35.
46. Stern M, Niemann N, Wiedemann B, *et al.* Benchmarking improves quality in cystic fibrosis care: a pilot project involving 12 centres. *Int J Qual Health Care* 2011; 23: 349–356.
47. Stern M. The use of a cystic fibrosis patient registry to assess outcomes and improve cystic fibrosis care in Germany. *Curr Opin Pulm Med* 2011; 17: 473–477.
48. Cystic Fibrosis Trust. UK Cystic Fibrosis Registry Annual Data Report 2012. Bromley, Cystic Fibrosis Trust, 2013.
49. Colombo C, Littlewood J. The implementation of standards of care in Europe: state of the art. *J Cyst Fibros* 2011; 10: Suppl. 2, S7–S15.
50. Strobl J, Enzer I, Bagust A, *et al.* Using disease registries for pharmacoepidemiological research: a case study of data from a cystic fibrosis registry. *Pharmacoepidemiol Drug Saf* 2003; 12: 467–473.
51. Wagener JS, Kupfer O. Dornase alfa (pulmozyme). *Curr Opin Pulm Med* 2012; 18: 609–614.
52. Sawicki GS, Signorovitch JE, Zhang J, *et al.* Reduced mortality in cystic fibrosis patients treated with tobramycin inhalation solution. *Pediatr Pulmonol* 2012; 47: 44–52.
53. Konstan MW, Schluchter MD, Xue W, *et al.* Clinical use of ibuprofen is associated with slower FEV1 decline in children with cystic fibrosis. *Am J Respir Crit Care Med* 2007; 176: 1084–1089.
54. Konstan MW. Ibuprofen therapy for cystic fibrosis lung disease: Revisited. *Curr Opin Pulm Med* 2008; 14: 567–573.
55. Carson SS, Goss CH, Patel SR, *et al.* An official American Thoracic Society research statement: comparative effectiveness research in pulmonary, critical care, and sleep medicine. *Am J Respir Crit Care Med* 2013; 188: 1253–1261.
56. Bosco JL, Silliman RA, Thwin SS, *et al.* A most stubborn bias: no adjustment method fully resolves confounding by indication in observational studies. *J Clin Epidemiol* 2010; 63: 64–74.
57. Lauer MS, D'Agostino RB Sr. The randomized registry trial – the next disruptive technology in clinical research? *N Engl J Med* 2013; 369: 1579–1581.

Disclosures: E.F. McKone has received grants and personal fees from Vertex Pharmaceuticals Inc., personal fees from Novartis Pharmaceuticals, and personal fees from Gilead Pharmaceuticals outside of the submitted work.

Chapter 19

Transition from paediatric to adult cystic fibrosis care: a developmental framework

Anjana S. Madan, Adrianne N. Alpern and Alexandra L. Quittner

Currently, there are no consistent procedures for transitioning adolescents from paediatric to adult cystic fibrosis (CF) care, and little empirical evidence exists on the best practices for transition. Given increased survival among patients with CF, a more formalised transition process is necessary to ensure continuity of care across the lifespan. This chapter reviews current transition practices and makes specific recommendations for more gradual, developmentally appropriate procedures involving all members of the CF care team. To ensure successful transition, providers should be aware of the normative milestones of adolescence and emerging adulthood, and how CF disrupts youths' navigation of these milestones. Age-appropriate guidance should be given to adolescents and their families in gradual doses, beginning in early childhood and continuing until early adulthood. Importantly, the success of these recommendations depends on clear and active communication between paediatric and adult care teams, parents, and adolescents.

G iven the dramatic improvements in the diagnosis and treatment of cystic fibrosis (CF) over the past 20 years, increasing numbers of patients are living into adulthood. In fact, recent registry data indicates that approximately half of the USA, Canadian and Western European CF population is now above 18 years of age [1, 2]. Thus, CF is no longer a paediatric disease, but extends into adulthood, requiring a formalised process to facilitate transition from paediatric to adult care. However, many medical teams have not established a standardised age or set of procedures for transition, little evidence on best practices is available, and few established measures exist to assess readiness for transfer [3–7]. The transition process is complex and presents numerous challenges for patients, parents, and paediatric and adult healthcare providers. The purpose of this chapter is to outline normative processes for transition, the impact of CF on these tasks, current practices, and recommendations for ensuring successful transition.

Normative transitions during adolescence and emerging adulthood

To better facilitate adolescents' transition from paediatric to adult care, healthcare providers should be aware of the normative transitions of adolescence and emerging adulthood, and how

Dept of Psychology, University of Miami, Coral Gables, FL, USA.

Correspondence: Alexandra L. Quittner, Dept of Psychology, University of Miami, 5665 Ponce de Leon Blvd, Coral Gables, FL 33146, USA. E-mail: aquittner@miami.edu

Copyright ERS 2014. Print ISBN: 978-1-84984-050-7. Online ISBN: 978-1-84984-051-4. Print ISSN: 2312-508X. Online ISSN: 2312-5098.

CF potentially disrupts youths' navigation of these transitions. Normative development, defined as developmental changes identified in population-based samples [8, 9], is conceptualised in four domains: physical, cognitive, emotional and social/role development (fig. 1).

Physical transitions

In adolescence, major physical changes include growth spurts, organ growth, pubertal development and changes in brain structure. However, CF may complicate these normative physical transitions (fig. 1). First, adolescents with CF are often shorter in stature and experience pubertal delay more often than their peers [10–12], which may contribute to a negative body image among adolescents and young adults with CF [13]. Additionally, lung function decline accelerates in adolescents and young adults, which contributes to more frequent hospitalisations and infections [14]. An additional challenge for transition is the emergence of CF-related diabetes mellitus (CFRD), which requires management of a second chronic condition [15].

Simultaneously, biochemical changes in the brain increase adolescents' interest in risky behaviour, such as substance use, smoking and unprotected sex. In addition, the development of the frontal lobe, which governs inhibition of impulsive behaviour, is not yet complete [16]. As a result, adolescents are more likely to experiment with risky behaviours without considering the consequences. While some degree of experimentation is adaptive for adolescents, the consequences of risky behaviours can represent a serious threat to their health. For example, substance use and cigarette smoking, in particular, compromise lung function (fig. 1) [2]. Moreover, adolescents with chronic illnesses may engage in more risky behaviours than their healthy peers, perhaps in an effort to "fit in" and de-emphasise their chronic illness [17].

As adolescents enter emerging adulthood, they are more likely to have short- or long-term romantic relationships, many of which involve sexual activity. However, because adolescents and young adults with CF are aware of their infertility (males) or lower fertility (females), they may be less inclined to use contraception, including condoms [18, 19], which puts them at risk of sexually transmitted infections or pregnancy. To help patients avoid these risks, paediatric and adult healthcare providers should be comfortable discussing sexual health with their adolescent and young adult patients.

Cognitive transitions

A major cognitive development in adolescence is the expansion of formal operational thought, which encompasses higher-level cognitive processing and abstract reasoning [20]. Simultaneously, adolescents become more self-focused and egocentric, believing they are the centre of attention [21] and are invincible to common dangers [22]. Thus, adolescents with CF may not understand the long-term risks of poor adherence in relation to their lifespan. They may also be less adherent in front of peers to avoid drawing attention to their illness [23].

As teenagers transition to adulthood, they develop greater cognitive flexibility and openness to ideas, which may coincide with an interest in higher education (fig. 1) [24]. Simultaneously, emerging adults begin tailoring their education and work experiences to a specific career [25–27]. However, for young adults with CF, the challenges of managing their treatments and awareness of their deteriorating health may affect their educational or career

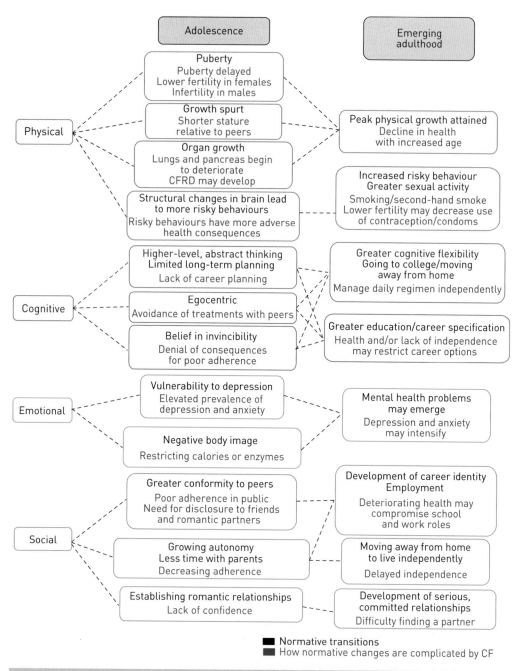

Figure 1. Normative physical, cognitive, emotional and social transitions of adolescence and emerging adulthood, and how they are disrupted by cystic fibrosis (CF). CFRD: CF-related diabetes mellitus.

planning. For example, worsening lung function and low energy, as well as lack of developmental maturity, may prevent them from attending school or work full-time.

Specifically, transitioning to higher education away from home may be more complicated for emerging adults with CF than for their healthy peers, especially if they depend on their parents for assistance with their treatments. Recently, an anonymous survey of 865 adults with CF across the USA [28] found that 38% of those surveyed lived with their parent or caregiver, and patients with severe lung disease were more likely to be living with their parents. The most significant predictor of achieving adult roles (*e.g.* employment and romantic relationships) was living independently, highlighting that gaining independence is a major goal during this period of transition.

Emotional transitions

Compared with younger children, adolescents are more susceptible to depression and suicidal behaviour [8]. Adolescents and adults with CF also report higher rates of depression and anxiety than healthy peers, with 29% of patients aged 7 to 17 years [29] and 30% of adults reporting clinically elevated levels of depression [30]. Furthermore, if adolescents feel dissatisfied with their bodies, they may restrict their caloric intake to lose weight [31], which can lead to nutritional deficiencies and declines in lung and immune function (fig. 1) [32]. Thus, both paediatric and adult care specialists should be aware of the emotional barriers that may impede optimal transition for CF patients.

As adolescents enter young adulthood, they may struggle to meet the demands of managing their illness while also finishing school, holding down a job, finding a partner and possibly starting a family [33]. Symptoms of depression and anxiety experienced by adolescents with CF may persist into adulthood [34], possibly intensifying with increased responsibilities and declining health [35, 36]. Recent evidence indicates that symptoms of depression and anxiety strongly affect adherence, attendance of school and work, and health-related quality of life (HRQoL) [29, 30].

Social transitions

As adolescents become more autonomous, they spend less time with parents and more time with peers, who become more influential in their decision-making [8]. However, for adolescents with CF, this shift in time spent with parents *versus* peers may impede their disease management (fig. 1) [37]. To facilitate their independence, young adolescents need successive approximations to complete their treatments on their own. For example, young teenagers should gradually take on some aspects of their regimen with parental assistance, such as turning on the compressor or mixing the medications (fig. 2). Problems with adherence may also be affected by adolescents' social interactions. In many cases, adolescents have not disclosed their illness to their friends, making it more difficult to complete their treatments in public [38]. The ADULT (Adult Data for Understanding Lifestyle and Transitions) study suggested that disclosure was an important process for adult independence; most adults reported that disclosure to friends, teachers and co-workers was greeted by neutral to positive responses [28]. Disclosure may also be important as adolescents begin dating and need to establish open and honest communication with their dating partners [39]. Difficulties with disclosure may play a role in the observed challenges they have in forming intimate relationships, which may contribute to a sense of isolation in daily life [40].

As adolescents enter adulthood, many leave the family home to attend university or live on their own [8, 29]. Establishment of a career and stable employment are essential tasks of young adulthood, which can be impeded by more frequent hospitalisations and deteriorating health, leading to absences from school or work (fig. 1). Poor school attendance and unsteady employment may, in turn, contribute to increased symptoms of depression and anxiety [41].

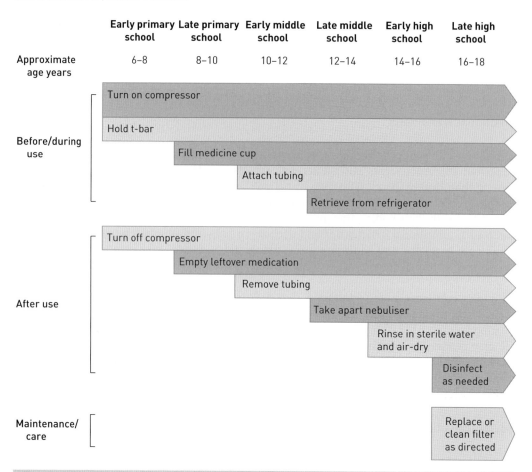

Figure 2. Behavioural analysis: transitioning responsibility for dornase alfa using successive approximation.

Thus, any transition model for CF must provide extra support for the normative changes complicated by CF. Support from family, peers and healthcare providers is essential for a successful transition from paediatric to adult care.

System-level challenges

Family-system level

At the family level, adolescents may struggle to "let go" of their paediatric providers and learn to trust a new healthcare team [42], and parents may also experience heightened anxiety about changing providers [43]. In a qualitative study of 22 adolescents with various chronic illnesses, including CF, four themes emerged during the transition process: 1) being unsure of the benefits of transfer; 2) fear of the unknown; 3) difficulty ending close relationships with the paediatric team; and 4) parents' reluctance to hand over control to the adolescent [44]. For some parents, their adolescent's transition from paediatric to adult care may signal an impending decline in health [45]; thus, they may wish to stay involved in their care. Moreover, many parents lack confidence in their adolescent's ability to manage their CF treatments independently [42, 43]. This degree of involvement may have an unintended consequence of leaving adolescents ill-prepared to manage their care effectively in adulthood

[46, 47]. This pattern of family involvement may negatively affect long-term adherence and clinic attendance [48].

Peer level

Peers provide valuable social support for young adults with chronic illnesses and their parents. However, because individuals with CF must be physically separated to prevent bacterial cross-infection, adolescents with CF and their parents lack the social support of families who are also undergoing transition [45, 49]. Importantly, this is the only chronic disease for which there is complete patient segregation. While efforts have been made to enable teenagers with CF to connect to one another *via* social media [50], these interventions have not been developed for adolescents and young adults who are transitioning their care.

It may also be important to encourage disclosure of the disease to healthy peers, who can provide much-needed support outside of the medical setting and normalise the shift toward independence [28]. A recent study examining peer support for adolescents with CF, aged 11 to 18 years (n=24), documented both helpful and unhelpful behaviours provided by healthy peers. The most frequently reported helpful behaviours were: 1) exercising together; 2) reminding and encouraging teenagers to perform their treatments; 3) helping manage the teenager's social network (updates on health status); 4) calling and visiting; and 5) providing distractions from illness [51]. The most frequently reported unhelpful behaviours included: 1) interfering with treatments by offering competing activities; 2) asking intrusive questions about CF; and 3) teasing or arguing with the teenager. Note that activating these helpful behaviours requires the adolescent to disclose their illness to healthy peers; thus, disclosure is a necessary step for accessing peer support.

Healthcare-system level

Several barriers to transition from paediatric to adult care have been documented, such as the proximity and expertise of adult providers, resources at the paediatric level to foster transition, reluctance of the paediatric team to let go of the adolescent patient, and lack of consensus on who is responsible for this process and when it should it occur [4, 6]. One major obstacle to facilitating this process is the lack of reliable and valid assessment tools to measure readiness of the patient, family and healthcare team for transfer. These measures should not simply be a guide to the timing of the transition, but should provide relevant targets for intervention that will facilitate the teenager and family's readiness [5]. Measures of disease management (including knowledge and skills), administered early in adolescence, could provide an important roadmap for intervention to remediate any gaps in knowledge or skills that are uncovered [52]. In addition, given the high rates of anxiety and depression observed in both patients and parent caregivers [29, 30, 53–56], annual screening of these symptoms is warranted, and may be especially important for anticipating challenges and planning appropriately for transition.

Timing of transfer: guidelines, current practices and future directions

Whereas the term "transition" refers to the gradual process of preparing for, completing and continuing engagement in adult care, "transfer" describes the act of shifting the patients' care from a paediatric to an adult CF centre or provider [2]. Guidelines for the timing of transfer typically rely on chronological age as the primary criterion [57], with built-in flexibility to consider the adolescent's self-management and self-advocacy skills, availability of adult care providers, and, occasionally, stage of illness [40]. The European consensus on standards of care recommends that transition to adult care occur between 16 and 18 years of age, and that timing should be flexible based on the adolescent's health status and maturity [58]. The CF Trust, based in the UK, advises that transfer of care occur between 14 and 18 years of age [59]. Similarly, consensus guidelines adopted in the USA recommend development of a timeline for transfer around the age of 14 years [40].

Data on the actual timing of this transition suggest that it highly variable. One study found that the median age of transfer across 170 CF centres in the USA was 19 years, with a range of 14–30 years [60]. Similarly, an international study of CF patients from the USA, UK, Australasia and mainland Europe found that the self-reported median age of transfer was 18 years, with a range of 14–58 years (n=344 CF patients) [2]. Thus, although the flexibility of the guidelines allows healthcare providers to delay transfer due to "developmental immaturity," this may distract the team from attempting to actively prepare the adolescent and family for the transition process. Instead, CF teams should routinely assess transition readiness at an early age and address the identified barriers so that the transition can be made in a timely fashion [5].

Transition readiness

Transition readiness is defined as "the capacity of the adolescent and those in his or her primary medical system of support (family and medical providers) to prepare for, begin, continue, and finish the transition process" [1]. Research has emphasised patient characteristics, such as knowledge and independent management skills, in evaluating transition readiness [61]. Importantly, systemic and contextual factors, such as relationships with and expectations of parents and providers, are often overlooked. For example, one study found that providers' plans to transfer paediatric cancer patients to adult care were related to patients' disease knowledge and skills, autonomy, psychosocial problems, parental involvement, patient–provider communication about transition, and availability/accessibility of an adult provider [61]. Thus, a model that places transition readiness in the healthcare context is essential to identify predictors of successful transitions. Unfortunately, most of this research has been conducted across chronic diseases, and we have no specific measures or models for this transition process in CF to date.

SCHWARTZ et al. [61] proposed a social–ecological model of adolescents' and young adults' readiness for transition (SMART) that incorporates systemic and interpersonal factors, along with patient characteristics (fig. 3). This model encompasses both factors that are amenable to change and those that are not. For example, it is not possible to modify sociodemographic characteristics, but effective interventions exist to improve knowledge, treatment skills and psychosocial functioning [52, 62, 63]. Given that CF patients attend clinics on a regular basis, this provides ample opportunity to prepare the adolescent and family for transition to adult care.

SMART is advantageous over more patient-focused models in several ways. First, it departs from the exclusive emphasis on patient characteristics and examines the reciprocal interactions between young adults, families, medical providers and outside factors (e.g. community and culture). Secondly, it was empirically developed and tested with primary stakeholders, including patients, families, and providers [64], thereby accounting for multiple perspectives. Finally, it highlights variables that can be improved with intervention (e.g. treatment skills and psychosocial functioning). To use this model, transition readiness should be assessed systematically.

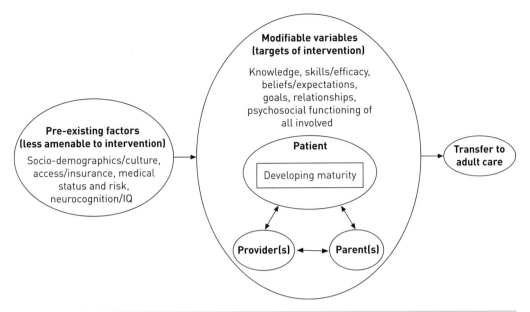

Figure 3. Social–ecological model of adolescents' and young adults' readiness for transition. IQ: intelligence quotient. Reproduced and modified from [61] with permission from the publisher.

Currently, a generic self-report transition readiness measure exists to assess self-management (*e.g.* taking medications) and self-advocacy (*e.g.* asking questions during medical visits) for youth with a variety of chronic conditions (TRAQ (Transition Readiness Assessment Questionnaire)) [65]. Importantly, some indicators of transition readiness are common across illness groups (*e.g.* knowing regimen, taking medications, making own appointments and calling pharmacy for refills) [66], whereas others are illness-specific (*e.g.* boosting calories and awareness of fertility issues). Accordingly, a modular measure with "core" items common across illnesses and "modules" for specific illness groups may be an efficient approach for measuring transition readiness. These measures should not only capture the frequency of self-management behaviours, but also the adolescent's ability to perform them competently and independently [67]. Furthermore, the measure should be completed by multiple respondents (parents and healthcare providers), since relying exclusively on adolescent self-report provides a limited perspective on self-management skills. Finally, longitudinal research is needed to examine the predictive validity of such a measure to determine its relationship to successful transfer, competent self-management and health outcomes once the transfer has occurred [67].

Current transition practices

Current practices suggest the need for greater uniformity and structure in patient–provider communication, assessment of transition readiness and plans for transition. Among nearly 2000 young adults (age 19–23 years) with a range of chronic health conditions, 55% reported that their providers discussed how their healthcare needs would change as they got older, 53% had discussions with their providers about how to secure health insurance as an adult and 62% indicated they had a transition plan in place [68]. Only 24% of those surveyed had received all three transition services. Given that this type of anticipatory guidance has been shown to improve clinic attendance and health outcomes for adolescents with juvenile arthritis and diabetes [69–71], current practices, as detailed above, lag behind what is recommended.

Similar to findings from other illness groups [43, 72–74], transition practices are inconsistent across CF centres. In a survey of 170 CF centres, representing the majority of those in the USA, the initial patient–provider discussion about transition did not occur until a median age of 17 years [60]. Fewer than half of the programmes had a transition timeline and less than 50% reported routinely providing transition-related materials. In terms of increasing transition readiness, a scant 18% employed interventions to improve self-management skills. A recent survey of 22 out of 25 Canadian CF centres found that nine (41%) used formalised transition programmes and more than half employed "informal transition practices" (*e.g.* discussing differences between paediatric and adult care, and having a nurse participate in the first adult clinic visit) [75]. Results indicated that, although efforts to establish transition practices are increasing, there is a need for greater uniformity across CF clinics.

Several transition programmes exist, but few have been evaluated empirically. At the University of Michigan CF centre (Ann Arbor, MI, USA), they have a two-stage process: preparing for transition and completing transition. Key preparation steps include encouraging independent visits for adolescents, monthly team meetings between the paediatric and adult centres (to review medical records), and re-education about CF and its treatments. To complete the transition, adolescents tour the adult clinic and meet with the adult pulmonologist in advance. Participants reported better health status and greater independence than nonparticipants [76]. Furthermore, patients stated that the most helpful component was meeting with the adult physician in the paediatric clinic, followed by having a social worker coordinate the transition process. This may reflect participants' concerns about establishing trust with their new CF team [42].

Anna Gravelle and colleagues (British Columbia Children's Hospital, Vancouver, Canada; personal communication) modified a generic transition programme (ON TRAC) for CF to facilitate transfer in an engaging and individualised manner. In addition to a readiness checklist, the intervention consists of a planning checklist and evidence record, which identify age-related needs and the specific team members who are responsible for addressing them (*e.g.* educational/career planning). Importantly, they begin this process at age 10 years and aim to complete it by age 18 years. This programme also addresses key developmental issues that are often neglected, using age-appropriate content and materials. For example, in the early transition phase (ages 10–12 years), topics such as pubertal changes and their impact on CF are discussed. In the middle transition (ages 13–15 years), the content shifts to basic fertility issues and contraception, followed by the late transition (ages 16–18 years), which outlines risky sexual behaviours, the need for genetic counselling and carrier testing of a future partner. We have highlighted sexual and reproductive health topics as they are so commonly ignored [18, 19]; however, this programme is much broader and more information about the ON TRAC generic model, including resources for adolescents, caregivers and providers, is available online [77]. Although these programmes incorporate evidence-based assessment and intervention strategies, patient outcomes have not been evaluated. Key outcomes should include consumer satisfaction with the programme (including patients, families and providers), knowledge and skills assessment, pulmonary and nutritional outcomes, and HRQoL.

Recommendations and conclusion

Awareness of normative developmental changes and how they are disrupted by CF is essential for designing the most effective transition process. Transition should begin early in life and requires envisioning a young child's future as a successful, independent adult. This

Table 1. Recommendations for transition to adult care using a developmental framework

Timing	Recommendation	Examples
Earliest steps (age 6–12 years)	Promote self-care "as early as possible" [1, 67]	Encourage children to participate in self-care in a graduated, developmentally appropriate way (e.g. teach young children to mix aerosols; fig. 2)
	Introduce transition to the family	Discuss the adult cystic fibrosis centre and possible timeline
Intermediate steps (age 12–16 years)	Anticipate developmental changes	Discuss family/peer relationships, increase shared decision making and responsibility for self-management
	Encourage independent clinic visits	Provider meets alone with adolescent and then jointly with parent(s) Encourage adolescent to come to the clinic with questions
	Conduct regular assessments of transition readiness	Measure self-management knowledge and skills, adherence to treatments [52, 65]; assess transition readiness with multi-informant tools [61] Identify areas to improve with intervention (e.g. improve adherence); plan the intervention [5]
	Make an individualised transition plan [65]	Discuss goals needed for transfer, specify timing
Preparing for transfer (ages 16–18 years)	Continue to assess transition readiness and identify areas for intervention	Monitor treatment adherence; intervene when necessary
	Familiarise adolescent with the adult care team and clinic procedures	Tour the hospital/treatment facility, meet the care team before first visit [40] Adolescent and family meet jointly with paediatric and adult physicians [4, 40, 76, 78, 79]
	Discuss differences between paediatric and adult care [40, 58]	Note differences in length of visit and clinic organisation; discuss insurance; new diagnostic procedures (e.g. echocardiogram)
	Discuss adolescent and parent concerns in clinic [80]	Ask about and address concerns about leaving paediatric care team, disease progression
	Establish communication between care teams [79]	Provide a written medical summary for adult team
	Paediatric and adult centres agree on a workable plan [80]	Hold monthly meetings with adult and paediatric teams present
Ongoing	Engage families and include parents in the process [79]	Provide parents with information, assess parents' readiness to facilitate adolescent independence; allow parent/caregiver to attend first appointment with adult team; help parents reconceptualise their role as an "ally" instead of "caregiver"
Centre specific	Evaluate transition policies and process regularly to update and modify [76]	

process should be broken down into small, manageable and measurable steps that provide a "scaffold" for the development of competent self-care. We have provided a detailed example of the transfer of responsibility for dornase alfa using successive approximations (fig. 2). This shift in responsibility from parent to child does not occur at a single moment in time, but represents a continuum of increasing independence for the child.

Expert consensus suggests that transition should be family-centred, coordinated and gradual [1, 5, 67]. Paediatric and adult teams should develop specific transition policies, including what should be accomplished, when, and by which member of the care team. Importantly, each team member should be accountable for specific tasks, given the complex and multifaceted nature of the process. Transition tasks should be documented in patients' medical charts to facilitate communication among different disciplines and to track the progress being made.

We have formulated specific recommendations for transition to adult care using a developmental framework (table 1). Recommendations are divided into developmental periods, which promote appropriately timed plans and goals. Underlying these recommendations is the need to begin early, communicate regularly with families, and systematically measure relevant goals and progress toward achieving them. Finally, ongoing communication between paediatric and adult providers, as well as within care teams, is essential to the success of this model.

References

1. Tuchman LK, Schwartz LA, Sawicki GS, *et al.* Cystic fibrosis and transition to adult medical care. *Pediatrics* 2010; 125: 566–573.
2. Cystic Fibrosis Foundation. Patient Registry Annual Data Report – 2012. www.cff.org/UploadedFiles/research/ClinicalResearch/PatientRegistryReport/2012-CFF-Patient-Registry.pdf Date last accessed: December 17, 2013. Date last updated: 2013.
3. Anderson DL, Flume PA, Hardy KK, *et al.* Transition programs in cystic fibrosis centers: perceptions of patients. *Pediatr Pulmonol* 2002; 33: 327–331.
4. Brumfield K, Lansbury G. Experiences of adolescents with cystic fibrosis during their transition from paediatric to adult health care: a qualitative study of young Australian adults. *Disabil Rehabil* 2004; 26: 223–234.
5. Flume PA. Smoothing the transition from pediatric to adult care: lessons learned. *Curr Opin Pulm Med* 2009; 15: 611–614.
6. Flume PA, Anderson DL, Hardy KK, *et al.* Transition programs in cystic fibrosis centers: perceptions of pediatric and adult program directors. *Pediatr Pulmonol* 2001; 31: 443–450.
7. Pai AL, Ostendorf HM. Treatment adherence in adolescents and young adults affected by chronic illness during the health care transition from pediatric to adult health care: a literature review. *Child Health Care* 2011; 40: 16–33.
8. Berk LE. Development through the Lifespan. Boston, Allyn & Bacon, 2010.
9. Ernst MM, Johnson MC, Stark LJ. Developmental and psychosocial issues in cystic fibrosis. *Pediatr Clin North Am* 2011; 58: 865–885.
10. Hardin DS, Adams-Huet B, Brown D, *et al.* Growth hormone treatment improves growth and clinical status in prepubertal children with cystic fibrosis: results of a multicenter randomized controlled trial. *J Clin Endocrinol Metab* 2006; 91: 4925–4929.
11. Sawyer S. Sexual and reproductive health. *In*: Hodson M, Bush A, Geddes D, eds. Cystic Fibrosis. 3rd Edn. Boca Raton, CRC Press, 2007; pp. 279–290.
12. Farrant B, Sawyer SM. Sexuality in young people with neurogenic bladder dysfunction. *In*: Esposito C, Guys JM, Gough D, *et al.*, eds. Pediatric Neurogenic Bladder Dysfunction. Berlin, Springer Berlin Heidelberg, 2006; pp. 317–323.
13. Pinquart M. Body image of children and adolescents with chronic illness: a meta-analytic comparison with healthy peers. *Body Image* 2013; 10: 141–148.
14. Welsh L, Robertson CF, Ranganathan SC. Increased rate of lung function decline in Australian adolescents with cystic fibrosis, *Pediatr Pulmonol* 2013 [In press DOI: 10.1002/ppul.22946].

15. Moran A, Hardin D, Rodman D, *et al.* Diagnosis, screening and management of cystic fibrosis related diabetes mellitus: a consensus conference report. *Diabetes Res Clin Pract* 1999; 45: 61–73.

16. Giedd JN. The teen brain: insights from neuroimaging. *J Adolesc Health* 2008; 42: 335–343.

17. Surís JC, Michaud PA, Akre C, *et al.* Health risk behaviors in adolescents with chronic conditions. *Pediatrics* 2008; 122: e1113–e1118.

18. Sawyer SM, Phelan PD, Bowes G. Reproductive health in young women with cystic fibrosis: knowledge, behavior and attitudes. *J Adolesc Health* 1995; 17: 46–50.

19. Sawyer SM, Farrant B, Cerritelli B, *et al.* A survey of sexual and reproductive health in men with cystic fibrosis: new challenges for adolescent and adult services. *Thorax* 2005; 60: 326–330.

20. Inhelder B, Piaget J. The Growth of Logical Thinking from Childhood to Adolescence: An Essay on the Construction of Formal Operational Structures. New York, Basic Books, 1958.

21. Elkind D, Bowen R. Imaginary audience behavior in children and adolescents. *Devel Psychol* 1979; 15: 38–44.

22. Elkind DA. Sympathetic Understanding of the Child: Birth to Sixteen. Boston, Allyn & Bacon, 1994.

23. Modi AC, Pai AL, Hommel KA, *et al.* Pediatric self-management: a framework for research, practice, and policy. *Pediatrics* 2001; 129: e473–e485.

24. Arnett JJ. Emerging adulthood: a theory of development from the late teens through the twenties. *Am Psychol* 2000; 55: 469–480.

25. Gottfredson LS. Applying Gottfredson's theory of circumscription and compromise in career guidance and counseling. *In*: Brown SD, Lent RW, eds. Career Development and Counseling. Hoboken, Wiley, 2005; pp. 71–100.

26. Super DE. A life span, life space approach to career development. *In*: Brown D, Brooks L, eds. Career Choice and Development. San Francisco, Jossey-Bass, 1990; pp. 197–261.

27. Super DE. A life span, life space perspective on convergence. *In*: Savikas ML, Lent RW, eds. Convergence in Career Development Theories. Palo Alto, Consulting Psychologists Press, 1994; pp. 62–71.

28. Modi AC, Quittner AL, Boyle MC. Assessing disease disclosure in adults with cystic fibrosis: the Adult Data for Understanding Lifestyle and Transitions (ADULT) survey Disclosure of disease in adults with cystic fibrosis. *BMC Pulm Med* 2010; 10: 46.

29. Smith BA, Modi AC, Quittner AL, *et al.* Depressive symptoms in children with cystic fibrosis and parents and its effects on adherence to airway clearance. *Pediatr Pulmonol* 2010; 45: 756–763.

30. Riekert KA, Bartlett SJ, Boyle MP, *et al.* The association between depression, lung function, and health-related quality of life among adults with cystic fibrosis. *Chest* 2007; 132: 231–237.

31. McCabe MP, Ricciardelli LA, Banfield S. Body image, strategies to change muscles and weight, and puberty: do they impact on positive and negative affect among adolescent boys and girls? *Eat Behav* 2001; 2: 129–149.

32. Berge JM, Patterson JM, Goetz D, *et al.* Gender differences in young adults' perceptions of living with cystic fibrosis during the transition to adulthood: a qualitative investigation. *Fam Syst Health* 2007; 25: 190–203.

33. Withers AL. Management issues for adolescents with cystic fibrosis. *Pulm Med* 2012; 2012: 134132.

34. Sawicki GS, Sellers DE, Robinson WM. Self-reported physical and psychological symptom burden in adults with cystic fibrosis. *J Pain Symptom Manage* 2008; 35: 372–380.

35. Gee L, Abbott J, Conway SP, *et al.* Quality of life in cystic fibrosis: the impact of gender, general health perceptions and disease severity. *J Cyst Fibros* 2003; 2: 206–213.

36. Pearson DA, Pumariega AJ, Seilheimer, DK. The development of psychiatric symptomatology in patients with cystic fibrosis. *J Am Acad Child Adolesc Psychiatry* 1991; 30: 290–297.

37. Graetz BW, Shute RH, Sawyer MG. An Australian study of adolescents with cystic fibrosis: perceived supportive and nonsupportive behaviors from families and friends and psychological adjustment. *J Adolesc Health* 2000; 26: 64–69.

38. Gjengedal E, Rustoen T, Wahl A, *et al.* Growing up and living with cystic fibrosis: everyday life and encounters with the health care and social services – a qualitative study. *ANS Adv Nurs Sci* 2003; 26: 149–159.

39. Carver K, Joyner K, Udry JR. National estimates of adolescent romantic relationships. *In*: Florsheim P, ed. Adolescent Romantic Relations and Sexual Behavior: Theory, Research, and Practical Implications. Mahwah, Erlbaum, 2003: pp. 23–56.

40. Yankaskas JR, Marshall BC, Sufian B, *et al.* Cystic fibrosis adult care: consensus conference report. *Chest* 2004; 125: Suppl., 1S–39S.

41. Axelsson L, Ejlertsson G. Self-reported health, self-esteem and social support among young unemployed people: a population-based study. *Int J Soc Welf* 2002; 11: 111–119.

42. Boyle MP, Farukhi Z, Nosky ML. Strategies for improving transition to adult cystic fibrosis care, based on patient and parent views. *Pediatr Pulmonol* 2001; 32: 428–436.

43. van Staa AL, Jedeloo S, van Meeteren J, *et al.* Crossing the transition chasm: Experiences and recommendations for improving transitional care of young adults, parents and providers. *Child Care Health Dev* 2011; 37: 821–832.

44. Tuchman LK, Slap GB, Britto MT. Transition to adult care: experience and expectations of adolescents with a chronic illness. *Child Care Health Dev* 2008; 34: 557–563.

45. Dupuis F, Duhamel F, Gendron S. Transitioning care of an adolescent with cystic fibrosis: Development of systemic hypothesis between parents, adolescents, and health care professionals. *J Fam Nurs* 2011; 17: 291–311.

46. Iles N, Lowton K. What is the perceived nature of parental care and support for young people with cystic fibrosis as they enter adult health services? *Health Soc Care Community* 2010; 18: 21–29.

47. Madge S, Bryon M. A model for transition from pediatric to adult care in cystic fibrosis. *J Pediatr Nurs* 2002; 17: 283–288.

48. Modi AC, Marciel KK, Slater SK, *et al.* The influence of parental supervision on medical adherence in adolescents with cystic fibrosis: developmental shifts from pre to late adolescence. *Child Health Care* 2008; 37: 78–82.

49. Saiman L, Siegel J. Infection control recommendations for patients with cystic fibrosis: microbiology, important pathogens, and infection control practices to prevent patient-to-patient transmission. *Infect Control Hosp Epidemiol* 2003; 24: Suppl. 5, S6–S52.

50. Marciel KK, Saiman L, Quittell LM, *et al.* Cell phone intervention to improve adherence: cystic fibrosis care team, patient, and parent perspectives. *Pediatr Pulmonol* 2010; 45: 157–164.

51. Barker D, Driscoll K, Modi A, *et al.* Supporting cystic fibrosis disease management during adolescence: the role of family and friends. *Child Care Health Dev* 2012; 38: 497–504.

52. Quittner AL, Alpern AN, Blackwell LS. Treatment adherence in adolescents with cystic fibrosis. *In*: Castellani C, Elborn S, Heijerman H, eds. Health Care Issues and Challenges in the Adolescent with Cystic Fibrosis. Oxford, Elsevier Inc., 2012; pp. 77–91.

53. Besier T, Born A, Henrich G, *et al.* Anxiety, depression, and life satisfaction in parents caring for children with cystic fibrosis. *Pediatr Pulmonol* 2011; 46: 672–682.

54. Havermans T, Colpaert K, Dupont LJ. Quality of life in patients with cystic fibrosis: association with anxiety and depression. *J Cyst Fibros* 2008; 7: 581–584.

55. Latchford G, Duff AJ. Screening for depression in a single CF centre. *J Cyst Fibros* 2013; 12: 794–796.

56. Driscoll KA, Johnson SB, Barker D, *et al.* Risk factors associated with depressive symptoms in caregivers of children with type 1 diabetes or cystic fibrosis. *J Pediatr Psychol* 2010; 35: 814–822.

57. Tuchman L, Slap G, Britto M. Transition to adult care: experiences and expectations of adolescents with a chronic illness. *J Adolesc Health* 2005; 36: 127–128.

58. Kerem E, Conway S, Elborn S, *et al.* Standards of care for patients with cystic fibrosis: a European consensus. *J Cyst Fibros* 2005; 4: 7–26.

59. Cystic Fibrosis Trust. Transition from paediatric to adult care: a guide for commissioners, hospital and clinical teams. https://cysticfibrosis.org.uk/media/151254/FS%20-%20Transition%20-%20commissioners_v2_Apr_2013.pdf Date last accessed: December 17, 2013. Date last updated: March 2013.

60. McLaughlin SE, Diener-West M, Indurkhya A, *et al.* Improving transition from pediatric to adult cystic fibrosis care: lessons from a national survey of current practices. *Pediatrics* 2008; 121: e1160–e1166.

61. Schwartz LA, Tuchman LK, Hobbie WL, *et al.* A social-ecological model of readiness for transition to adult-oriented care for adolescents and young adults with chronic health conditions. *Child Care Health Dev* 2011; 37: 883–895.

62. Quittner AL, Riekert KA. I change adherence and raise expectations: the iCARE study. *Pediatr Pulm* 2013; 48: Suppl. 36, 136.

63. Goldbeck L, Fidika A, Herle M, *et al.* Psychological interventions for individuals with cystic fibrosis and their families. *Cochrane Database Syst Rev* 2014 [In press].

64. Schwartz LA, Brumley LD, Tuchman LK, *et al.* Stakeholder validation of a model of readiness for transition to adult care. *JAMA Pediatr* 2013; 167: 939–946.

65. Sawicki GS, Lukens-Bull K, Yin X, *et al.* Measuring the transition readiness of youth with special healthcare needs: validation of the TRAQ – Transition Readiness Assessment Questionnaire. *J Pediatr Psychol* 2011; 36: 160–171.

66. Annunziato RA, Parkar S, Dugan CA, *et al.* Deficits in health care management skills among adolescent and young adult liver transplant recipients transitioning to adult care settings. *J Pediatr Psychol* 2011; 36: 155–159.

67. Pai AL, Schwartz LA. Introduction to the special section: health care transitions of adolescents and young adults with pediatric chronic conditions. *J Pediatr Psychol* 2011; 36: 129–133.

68. Sawicki GS, Whitworth R, Gunn L, *et al.* Receipt of health care transition counseling in the national Survey of Adult Transition and Health. *Pediatrics* 2011; 128: e521–e529.

69. Rettig P, Athreya BH. Adolescents with chronic disease. Transition to adult care. *Arthritis Care Res* 1991; 4: 174–180.

70. Orr DP, Fineberg NS, Gray DL. Glycemic control and transfer of health care among adolescents with insulin dependent diabetes mellitus. *J Adolesc Health* 1996; 18: 44–47.

71. Vanelli M, Caronna S, Adinolfi B, *et al.* Effectiveness of an uninterrupted procedure to transfer adolescents with Type 1 diabetes from the Paediatric to the Adult Clinic held in the same hospital: eight-year experience with the Parma protocol. *Diabetes Nutr Metab* 2004; 17: 304–308.

72. Allen D, Gregory J. The transition from children's to adult diabetes services: understanding the "problem". *Diabet Med* 2009; 26: 162–166.

73. McDonagh JE. Growing up and moving on: transition from pediatric to adult care. *Pediatr Transplant* 2005; 9: 364–372.

74. Rosen DS. Transition of young people with respiratory diseases to adult health care. *Paediatr Respir Rev* 2004; 5: 124–131.

75. Gravelle A, Davdison G, Chilvers M. Cystic fibrosis adolescent transition care in Canada: a snapshot of current practice. *Paediatr Child Health* 2012; 17: 553–556.

76. Chaudhry SR, Keaton M, Nasr SZ. Evaluation of a cystic fibrosis transition program from pediatric to adult care. *Pediatr Pulmonol* 2012; 48: 658–665.

77. Paone MC, Whitehouse SA. Developing a Transition Initiative for Youth and Young Adults with Chronic Health Conditions and/or Special Needs in BC. http://ontracbc.ca/wp-content/uploads/ON_TRACBackground2011.pdf Date last accessed: December 17, 2013. Date last updated: 2011.

78. Townshend J, Paquet F, Paolitto M, *et al.* Patient's perceptions of the transition from pediatric to adult care. *Pediatr Pulmonol*, 1999: Suppl. 17, 393–394.

79. Towns SJ, Bell SC. Transition of adolescents with cystic fibrosis from paediatric to adult care. *Clin Respir J* 2011; 5: 64–75.

80. Parker H. Transition and transfer of patients who have cystic fibrosis to adult care. *Clin Chest Med* 2007; 28: 423–432.

Disclosures: None declared.

Chapter 20

Challenges of providing care to adults with cystic fibrosis

Scott C. Bell[1,2,3] and David W. Reid[1,3,4]

The number of adults with cystic fibrosis (CF) equals or exceeds that of children in many parts of the world. Consequently the size and number of adult centres has grown. In association with these increased numbers, the complexity of care of the adult has also increased. Emerging complications are commonplace and include diabetes, drug allergy and toxicity, difficulties with venous access and multiresistant infections. Strategies to enhance self-management require further evaluation in the setting of therapy requirements, which are increasingly complex. Planning for the provision of facilities and resources for the care of adults with CF, including training of multidisciplinary healthcare members, has been variable within and between countries. Novel models for the delivery of adult CF care may provide the opportunity to continue to deliver effective management to a rapidly growing population.

The twenty-first century has seen a demographic shift in the cystic fibrosis (CF) population in countries with well-developed healthcare systems. Excellent paediatric care has been responsible for the majority of substantial improvements in survival well into adulthood and the onus now lies with adult CF teams to consolidate these successes and support adults with CF to lead a near-normal life. The spectrum of disease phenotypes that adult CF teams are likely to experience over the next 20–30 years will be different to that of yesteryear. "Generational waves" of adults are emerging. Inpatient wards are now predominantly filled with patients >30 years of age with the classic CF phenotype that grows ever more complex, accompanied by unexpected complications. The second generational wave consists of the adolescent or recently transitioned population with near-normal lung function, who do not have chronic *Pseudomonas aeruginosa* infection. This cohort of patients usually possesses a spectrum of more exotic lung pathogens, which are often antibiotic-resistant. The third future generational wave of adults may comprise adults from the gene-specific therapy era, a population cohort that may yet again possess a different disease phenotype to their predecessors.

In addition to the challenges of day-to-day CF management, strategic decisions need to be made on how best to provide care and support for a burgeoning population of adults with CF. New models need to: consider ceiling patient population numbers attending CF centres; optimise methods to increase the engagement of adults in self-management; take advantage

[1]Adult Cystic Fibrosis Centre, The Prince Charles Hospital, Chermside, Queensland, Australia. [2]Queensland Children's Medical Research Institute, Herston, Queensland, Australia. [3]School of Medicine, University of Queensland, Chermside, Queensland, Australia. [4]QIMR-Berghofer Institute of Medical Research, Herston, Queensland, Australia.

Correspondence: Scott C. Bell, Adult Cystic Fibrosis Centre, The Prince Charles Hospital, Chermside, Queensland, 4032, Australia. E-mail: scott.bell@health.qld.gov.au

Copyright ERS 2014. Print ISBN: 978-1-84984-050-7. Online ISBN: 978-1-84984-051-4. Print ISSN: 2312-508X. Online ISSN: 2312-5098.

of modern modes of communication, education and monitoring; and finally, encourage physicians, nurses and allied healthcare professionals to train and work in the field of adult CF care in a sustainable manner within a multidisciplinary healthcare team.

This chapter begins by describing the changing epidemiology of the CF population globally and highlights the growth in the proportion of adults with CF. We aim to show that the complexity of CF in adult life is increasing in parallel with numbers. The adult with CF is also experiencing increased complexity in terms of management regimens, which are long-term and time consuming. We discuss the evidence to support the facilitation of coping strategies and new approaches to self-management in adults with CF. Finally, we consider the challenges facing healthcare providers in delivering care in a sustainable and cost-effective way to a rapidly growing CF population, which is affected by an ever-increasing array of complications. Throughout this chapter, we challenge the reader to consider how CF care will be effectively delivered into the future and how disease progression may be shaped by new therapies.

A growing population

It is estimated that there are 70 000 people with CF globally, over 30 000 of which are from North America and Europe. Over the past 50 years there has been a dramatic change in the profile of the CF population in most parts of the world. CF has changed from a disease that was usually fatal in childhood to one in which childhood fatalities are much less common [1]. Consequently, the adult population in many nations outnumbers that of children [2–7]. In some countries (including Canada, Italy and Denmark), adult numbers approach or even exceed 60% of the total CF population [2, 3]. In the USA, median survival has increased from 31 years in 2002 to 41 years in 2012 [4]. A similar increase has been seen in the UK, where median survival has risen from 35 years in 2007 to 41.5 years in 2011 [5]. In some countries, median survival rates are even higher (e.g. 48 years in Canada in 2011) [3]. It is important to consider the methods used when comparing survival rates. Case ascertainment of the CF population (particularly completeness of entry into national data registries) and whether patients who have undergone lung transplantation are included in "mortality" estimates, are likely to have an impact on survival rates reported internationally.

Although median survival rates have increased dramatically over the past four decades, the median age at death is much lower (e.g. 26 years in the UK and 34 years in Canada) [3, 5]. The major contributor to the difference between median survival and median age of death is the influence of older patients with a milder disease phenotype (often characterised by a later diagnosis, i.e. after 2 years of age), pancreatic sufficiency, better nutritional status and, in many cases, better pulmonary function [8–11]. These studies suggest differences in the population characteristics of older patients compared with the adult CF population as a whole [8, 11]. The emerging cohort of older patients with CF is, therefore, made up of a heterogeneous population of long-term survivors, including those with "classic" CF, and those diagnosed at a later stage and who have atypical disease [11]. The explanation for long-term survival in individuals diagnosed early in life with classical features of CF is unknown, but may be influenced by non-CFTR (cystic fibrosis transmembrane conductance regulator) genetic, environmental (including access to care) and behavioural factors [12–16].

Centres providing care for adults with CF have developed rapidly in recent years. As an example, the first adult centre in the UK was established in the mid-1960s at the Royal Brompton Hospital in London. Initially, the Brompton team provided care for <10 patients but since then, numbers have increased to >600 patients [17]. Until the 1980s, most adults with CF in the UK either received their care at the Royal Brompton Hospital or continued to be managed by local paediatricians who had historically provided care since diagnosis. Beyond the Royal Brompton Hospital, the three largest adult centres in the UK cared for approximately 400 patients in 1993, increasing to >600 patients in 1998; they currently provide care for >1000 patients [18]. To cater for this incredible growth in the adult population, 28 new adult CF care centres were established by 2011, providing care for almost 4700 adults throughout the UK (centre population range 31–395) [5]. Similar growth has been seen in Europe, North America, Australia and New Zealand [2–7].

During this period of growth, the health of young adults has improved. The lung function and nutritional status of 18 year olds with CF in the USA has improved [4]. The median forced expiratory volume in 1 s (FEV1) was ~64% predicted in 1992 and increased to ~74% pred in 2002 and to ~84% pred in 2012 (fig. 1). Similarly, body mass index (BMI) percentiles in 18 year olds have increased during the same period, from below the 15th percentile to above the 30th percentile (fig. 2). In Canada, the proportion of adults with normal or mildly reduced lung function (FEV1 >70% pred) has risen from 35% to 42%, and the proportion of adults with severely impaired lung function (FEV1 <40% pred) has fallen from 30% to 19% [3]. *P. aeruginosa* remains the most common bacterial pathogen in the CF airways: it was previously reported to occur in >80% of adults, but in many parts of the world, adult prevalence has reduced to <50% [3–5]. Importantly, in the UK, younger adults (<36 years of age) with CF have *P. aeruginosa* infection rates of >60% and *P. aeruginosa* infection rates are significantly lower in the older adult population [5]. These changes in the microbiology and clinical features of the young adult CF population are highly likely to lead to further improvements in survival, even before considering the impact of further therapeutic advances in the coming years. It therefore remains unclear whether the growth of the CF population will plateau or continue to increase. Epidemiological studies suggest median survival will increase to beyond 50 years of age, although these estimates were made in the pre-CFTR modulator therapy era [19].

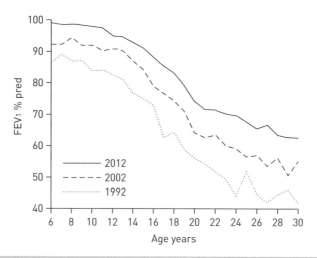

Figure 1. Median forced expiratory volume in 1 s (FEV1) % predicted according to age in three cohorts. The figure presents information from cystic fibrosis patients under care at Cystic Fibrosis Foundation-accredited care centres in the USA, who consented to have their data entered in 2012. Reproduced and modified from [4] with permission from the publisher.

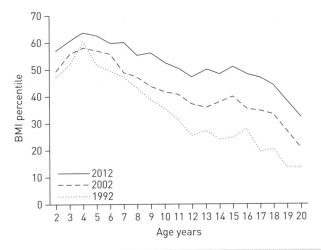

Figure 2. Median body mass index (BMI) percentile of children and teenagers in three cohorts. The figure presents information from cystic fibrosis patients under care at Cystic Fibrosis Foundation-accredited care centres in the USA, who consented to have their data entered in 2012. Reproduced and modified from [4] with permission from the publisher.

Despite dramatic increases in the numbers of adults with CF internationally, improvements in outcomes have not been uniform. In non-European Union (EU) countries, the median age of the CF population in 2003–2007 was 12.1 years (interquartile range (IQR) 6.0–19.2 years) and only 28% were ⩾18 years of age. In comparison, amongst those living in EU countries, the median age was 17.0 years (IQR 9.5–19.2 years) and 47% were ⩾18 years of age [20]. Lower proportions of adults with CF have also been reported in South America [21, 22].

Therefore, some healthcare systems face challenges that would allow the realisation of similar improvements in the outcomes of people with CF.

Complexity of care

Pulmonary complications

In parallel with the rising numbers of adults with CF, the complexity of care has also increased [4, 23]. This includes the emergence of complications that were not commonly seen in the past and difficulties that are faced by CF healthcare teams in most clinics and during most ward rounds on a daily basis *e.g.* massive haemoptysis, pneumothorax and difficult-to-treat infections [23, 24]. In an analysis of the patient registry data from the USA, pneumothorax was associated with increased morbidity (including an increased number of hospitalisations and days spent in the hospital) and a rise 2-year mortality rates [25]. Management of pneumothorax in CF can be complex, with recurrent episodes often occurring even when pleurodesis has been performed. Massive haemoptysis (>240 mL blood or blood transfusion requirement) is most common in the older patient (two out of three cases in adults >30 years of age), and in those with severe lung disease (~60% occurred in patients with FEV1 <30% pred). Massive haemoptysis is associated with high rates of 2-year mortality and is especially common in those with severe airflow obstruction [26]. Bronchial artery embolisation is frequently required to control and limit re-bleeding, although repeat embolisation procedures are often required [27].

Adults with CF have high rates of multidrug-resistant bacterial infections [4, 23, 28]. Many factors may contribute to increased antimicrobial resistance and treatment is often difficult in adults due to coexisting antibiotic allergy or toxicity issues, which may lead to limited treatment choices, particularly during acute exacerbations [29, 30]. A prime example of the changing microbiology in CF and limited treatment options is the increase in the prevalence of nontuberculous mycobacteria (NTM) infection, especially the difficult-to-treat *Mycobacterium abscessus* [31, 32]. Decisions on the timing and duration of treatment are very difficult due to the variable natural history of *M. abscessus*, its innate antibiotic resistance and the toxicity associated with combination antibiotic therapy [32]. Recent reports from the USA and UK have also suggested that there is a potential person-to-person spread of some strains of *M. abscessus*, further adding to the complexity of delivering care in adult CF centres, where growing patient numbers and cross-infection risks have resulted in the adoption of complex cohort segregation practices [33, 34].

Treatment regimens have inevitably become more complex over the past two decades, with the majority of patients taking long-term inhaled antibiotics combined with mucolytics, hydrator drugs and oral macrolides. The long-term consequences of such intensive therapies are not well understood. A recent study provides a timely reminder that add-on therapies may have undesired and potentially detrimental consequences [35]. In a clinical trial of inhaled antibiotics (tobramycin and aztreonam), NICK *et al.* [35] studied the impact on of these treatments on clinical and microbiological outcomes. Although there were significant limitations in the secondary analysis of this clinical trial, azithromycin was associated with an unexpected decline in absolute change in FEV1 in patients randomised to tobramycin, which was not seen in those patients randomised to aztreonam. In parallel, an *in vitro* culture model demonstrated reduced tobramycin killing of *P. aeruginosa* in the presence of azithromycin. These data suggest the potential for an unintended impact of two antibiotics used in combination, when in isolation both positively impact on clinical outcomes [36–38].

Non-pulmonary complications

As the adult population ages, the prevalence of established and well-characterised complications of CF increases (fig. 3); these complications are often difficult to manage (*e.g.* CF-related diabetes mellitus (CFRD) and multiresistant infection) [4–6, 39, 40]. CFRD is more common in older adults, with almost one-third of all CF patients >30 years of age requiring chronic insulin therapy [3, 39]. CFRD is associated with higher mortality rates and its management adds to the complexity of treatment for adults with CF. Intense education on the short- and long-terms goals of treatment and the beneficial impact of insulin therapy is required [41]. As the adult CF population ages further, it is likely that even more will develop CFRD [24, 39, 41].

Drug-related complications are increasingly seen in the adult CF clinic. Drug allergy (especially to β-lactam antibiotics) occurs in up to one-third of patients with CF [29, 30] and is more common in older patients who have higher cumulative exposure to antibiotics. In most cases, the allergic phenomenon is a delayed-type reaction that can be managed with anti-allergy approaches, including systemic corticosteroids and antihistamines [30]. This approach can be very effective but in some patients, it may be necessary to choose an alternative antibiotic class. Where the allergy is convincingly immediate-type, rechallenge following formal desensitisation may allow drug tolerance but this procedure needs to be repeated for each subsequent course of the same antibiotic [42, 43]. Drug toxicity is also increasingly recognised in adult CF patients [44, 45]. Recently, data from a large registry-based

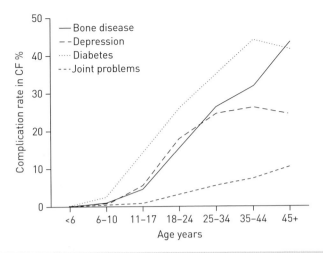

Figure 3. Common complications according to age in three cohorts. The figure presents information from cystic fibrosis (CF) patients under care at Cystic Fibrosis Foundation-accredited care centres in the USA, who consented to have their data entered in 2012. Reproduced and modified from [4] with permission from the publisher.

adult cohort study of ~12 000 CF patients demonstrated an overall annual prevalence of stage 3 chronic kidney disease (estimated glomerular filtration rate (EGFR) <60 mL·min⁻¹·1.73 m⁻²) of 2.3% [45]. Importantly, the prevalence of chronic kidney disease doubles with every additional 10 years of age, particularly in those with CFRD, following lung transplantation and in patients with a previous diagnosis of acute kidney failure. The role of aminoglycosides in the development of chronic kidney disease has been the subject of ongoing debate [46, 47]. A recent study demonstrated that cumulative exposure to aminoglycosides over 4 years was not associated with an increased prevalence of chronic kidney disease [45]. With long-term use of systemic aminoglycoside drugs, vestibulo-ototoxicity may occur, which may limit the choice of antibiotic used for acute exacerbations [48, 49].

Emerging medical complications

Other (as yet) less well-defined complications may be on the horizon, and these could well become commonplace amongst the young adults of today who are predicted to survive well beyond their fourth decade. These complications include bowel cancers, metabolic syndromes and the loss of practical vascular access for the safe and effective delivery of antibiotic therapy [24, 50–54]. Gastrointestinal cancers are more common in adults with CF, with the most prevalent being colorectal cancers [55, 56]. As median life expectancy and the number of adults >40 years of age increase further, the following issues relevant to risk of bowel cancer may require consideration by adult CF teams. 1) Should bowel cancer be screened for, and if so, at what age? 2) How should patients approaching lung transplantation be managed? 3) What is the optimal screening tool? At present, there are limited data available to answer any of these questions [50, 52].

Recent registry data have demonstrated improvements in nutritional status in adults with CF, yet adults >30 years of age (particularly males) now have median BMIs approaching the upper limit of the healthy weight range [6]. The metabolic consequences of being overweight or obese with CF are unclear; however, they may become important. Evidence of hyperlipidaemia in the adult CF population, particularly in older patients and those with a high BMI, has recently been found [54, 57]. Long-term systemic inflammation may be associated with vascular complications, as observed in other inflammatory lung conditions, such as chronic obstructive pulmonary disease (COPD) [58]. Indices of increased vascular wall stiffness have been reported in adults with CF and may herald the emergence of vascular diseases in long-term survivors [59, 60].

In summary, delivery of adult CF care is now complicated by new challenges, some of which are discussed in further detail later. These include: estimating the time of transplantation assessment, parenting in both mothers and now fathers with CF, eradication (of infection) therapy in adults and the implications of new therapies which for the first time address the basic CF defect.

Transplantation

The timing of lung transplantation assessment in patients with CF has added complexity to CF care, despite the development of sophisticated prediction methodologies [61, 62]. An early seminal study from Canada reported a median survival of 2 years in patients with FEV_1 <30% pred [63]. The study provided much of the basis for knowledge about indicators for lung transplantation timing. More recently, it was shown that the median survival of adults with established advanced lung disease (FEV_1 <30% pred) attending one large adult centre in the UK has dramatically increased over the past 20 years, from 13 months to 5.3 years [64]. CFRD and impaired renal function pre-transplant are important variables affecting renal function following transplantation [44, 45, 65, 66]. Intensive antibiotic therapy may be associated with increased antibiotic resistance of common bacterial pathogens [67]. *Burkholderia cenocepacia* has been associated with poorer post-transplant outcomes and, in many centres, it has been found to be a contraindication for listing for transplantation [68, 69]. To date, evidence would suggest that infection with other common bacterial pathogens (including *P. aeruginosa*, methicillin-resistant *Staphylococcus aureus* (MRSA) and *Achromobacter xylosoxidans*) does not adversely impact on post-transplant outcomes [70–73]. Donor availability remains a considerable obstacle in lung transplantation in most healthcare systems, and well-developed referral pathways are required between the CF centre and the lung transplant service [74]. Maintaining lung health (including the management of pulmonary complications, such as pneumothorax and massive haemoptysis) remains the key priority in the management of adults with CF, as most patients will still succumb to the consequences of advanced respiratory insufficiency [4]. Close communication between the patients, the CF team and the transplant service is vital in all patients with advanced lung disease where transplant is considered an option. An emerging dilemma for the patient and their treating team is the need to consider the potential impact of prolonging pre-transplant life (with intensive therapies) against the potential for aggravating complications of CF (*e.g.* renal insufficiency), which may impact on life following transplant.

Parenting

Parents with CF are now common in all adult CF centres. In Australia, one in seven adults is a parent [6], and the advent of methods that address male infertility (including intracytoplasmic sperm injection) means there are more fathers with CF [75]. Similarly, increasing numbers of mothers with CF are being reported internationally [76–78]. Whilst medium-term outcomes (⩽10 years) do not appear to be adversely affected by pregnancy and motherhood, the impact on day-to-day self-management can be challenging in the young female with CF [79–81]. Pregnancy itself requires careful interdisciplinary care and close teamwork between the obstetric and CF teams, especially when attempting to manage complications emerging during pregnancy, such as gestational diabetes [75]. A particular challenge arises when diabetes complicates pregnancy in CF and it becomes necessary to consider how best to sustain the nutritional requirements of the mother and fetus at the same time as maintaining glycaemic control. Pregnant females in the general population who develop gestational diabetes are encouraged to consume a low glycaemic-index diet and often need to reduce caloric intake [82], which is contrary to the high-fat, high-energy diet central to maintenance of nutrition in CF [83].

Care now and into the future

Aggressive eradication therapy in children with CF has resulted in a dramatic reduction in rates of chronic *P. aeruginosa* infection. There are a growing numbers of young adults transitioning from paediatric care who do not have *P. aeruginosa* infection. A recent European Cystic Fibrosis Society (ECFS) consensus statement on antibiotic therapy in CF supports eradication amongst older patients [72]. Several questions remain, including the following. 1) Should eradication be trialled? 2) Is it as effective in adults as it is children with CF? 3) How many times should it be trialled? From a practical perspective, many young adults are working and/or studying and may find the impact of such treatment demands difficult to accommodate in their already busy lives. Studies to support eradication approaches in older patients are urgently required.

Licensing of the first CF gene-specific therapy, ivacaftor, for patients with the Gly551Asp mutation is an exciting new development, which will have a potentially major impact on lung disease progression and quality of life in patients with this CF mutation [84–86]. The potential of such therapies is greatly anticipated within the CF community, particularly with regard to ongoing phase III clinical trials, which may be able to offer treatment advances for a greater proportion of the CF population. Unrealised expectations, the inability to access clinical trials, and anxiety about gene mutations for which therapies have yet to be developed to clinical trial stage, are all challenges for the patient, their families and CF care teams. At this point, we can only speculate how such CFTR modulator therapies will impact on the natural history of CF, particularly given the early administration to younger children with CF. Will ivacaftor use in patients with a Gly551Asp mutation impact on the development of bronchiectasis and reduce rates of chronic infection in children and adolescents with CF? And what about the potential of other combination CFTR modulators for patients with other CF gene mutations, if they are proven effective in the future? These new therapies may change the disease characteristics of the adolescent transitioning to adult care in the future. Similarly, CFTR modulators may lead to changes in disease progression in the adult with CF, although long-term observational studies will be required to address these theoretical outcomes.

Psychological issues

Mental health issues are a significant challenge to the delivery of adult CF care, particularly in terms of case finding, the patient's acceptance of diagnosis and the potential impact on disease progression. The International Depression/Anxiety Epidemiological Study (TIDES) (www.tides-cf.org) and a limited number of other studies demonstrate that anxiety and depression are relatively common in CF, affecting 17–46% of adults [87–92]. Both anxiety and depression are associated with a lower quality of life and reduced physical functioning, and depression is independently associated with longer hospitalisation for pulmonary exacerbations [92, 93]. Increased levels of self-reported anxiety and depression have been reported with increased age and a parallel reduction in "life satisfaction" [94]. Interestingly, when compared to the general population in Germany, the reported levels of anxiety (but not depression) were higher in adults with CF. This observation raises the possibility that the available screening tools for depression may not be sufficiently specific or sensitive to CF. In support of this possibility, a recent study found that 5.6% of adults attending a single centre were clinically depressed, according to the Hospital Anxiety and Depression Scale (HADS), whereas the Patient Health Questionnaire for Depression-9 (PHQ-9) showed that 33.4% were depressed and 10.4% expressed a worrying suicidal ideation [90]. The results of the ongoing TIDES study will hopefully support the need for more reliable screening tools for anxiety and depression in CF populations, which can be incorporated into usual clinical practice, perhaps as part of the annual review process. There are no prospective studies examining the impact of anxiety or depression on disease progression or how appropriate treatment leads to benefits in clinical outcome.

Coping strategies and self-management

There are very few published studies on health behaviours and coping strategies in adults with CF, but coping strategies and the ability to self-manage appear to be positively associated with lung function and nutritional status in CF [95, 96]. In contrast, failure of healthy coping strategies has been linked to poor adherence (discussed further later), risk-taking behaviour, anxiety and depression, and a reduced ability to self-manage. Coping is an active cognitive process that allows a person to tolerate their illness, but coping mechanisms may be disrupted by multiple factors, *i.e.* hospitalisation for an exacerbation, rapid disease progression, acute and chronic pain, new diagnoses (such as the onset of CFRD) or life-changes (including parenthood or the breakdown of a relationship) [97–99].

The extent to which the CF team can foster positive coping strategies has received limited attention to date, although one study developed the Eat Well for CF programme, an education intervention for nutrition that includes goal-setting and telephone-mentoring provided by dieticians [100]. Self-efficacy and knowledge increased, but there was no change in weight or lung function in the intervention arm compared with usual care, which may have reflected a lack of statistical power, as only 48 patients completed the study. These findings contrast with improvements in nutritional outcomes when behavioural interventions, including goal setting and education, are introduced in young children with CF [101]. A small number of other studies have demonstrated that behavioural therapy in adolescents and adults can improve self-management skills, but the longer-term benefits to disease outcomes and disease progression have not been assessed. It is also unclear which intervention may be most effective, with several strategies proposed including cognitive behavioural therapy, motivational interviews and mindfulness, each with its own proponents [102–105]. The adult CF population itself recognises the value of knowledge, and coping and self-management skills [106], and there is now a pressing need for adequately powered, large-scale randomised controlled trials involving educational self-management interventions to inform on the best method and duration of intervention. Careful consideration should also be given to outcome measures.

Adherence

As disease complexity increases with age and the number of therapies escalates, adherence to therapy may reduce at a time when the individual may also be struggling to maintain relationships, and family and work commitments, often in the setting of deteriorating health.

Adults with CF experience a treatment burden involving a median of seven different medications (range 0–20) and spend a mean ± SD duration of 108 ± 58 min per day engaged in treatment administration and physical therapies [107]. Perceived treatment burden appears to be greatest with inhaled medications and airway-clearance techniques, and there is evidence that adults make conscious choices on which treatments they will prioritise depending on other commitments in their daily lives, including family responsibilities and employment [107]. Importantly, poor adherence to prescribed drugs, as assessed by determining the medication possession ratio (MPR) (the sum of all the days for which medication is prescribed divided by the sum of all the days for which medication is supplied) [108], is associated with poor outcomes, including increased pulmonary exacerbations and hospitalisations, which are established predictors for accelerated lung function decline [109, 110]. Optimising adherence during adolescence is likely to be important in cementing future adult practices, and methods to consolidate adherence during the adult years need to be further explored. Reliable, easy-to-use and cost-effective tools are needed to accurately assess adherence, and whilst sophisticated electronic monitoring devices are being developed, validated tools such as the MPR should be further studied in combination with education and behavioural interventions [111–113].

Employment

The employment status of adults with CF reported in National CF data registries varies [4–6]. Approximately one-third of all adults are in full-time employment, but there is variation in the proportion that report being in part-time work or unemployed and receiving some form of disability support [4–6]. The importance of employment status has probably been under-appreciated in CF, although loss of employment or long-term unemployment has been associated with poorer health [114, 115]. Socioeconomic deprivation and poor lung function appear to have a multiplicative effect on employment potential. Despite significant interrelationships between socioeconomic status, lung disease severity and employment status, there is still substantial variability between individuals who have similar socio-economic status and lung disease characteristics in their clinical status. This suggests that other influences, including coping strategies and psychological factors, may also contribute to clinical status [114, 116]. A recent survey of 254 patients from three adult CF centres in the UK demonstrated that educational achievement and higher scores in the CF-specific health-related quality of life (HRQoL) domains of role and health perception were associated with employment status, but that disease severity was not [117]. The downsides of unemployment, including societal isolation and poverty, are understood for other chronic diseases, as is their impact on health outcomes [118–120]. In CF, these issues remain relatively unexplored but require further investigation [121].

Important work-related issues include decisions on whether to disclose the diagnosis to employers or work colleagues and what constitutes a safe work environment. Whilst most adults will disclose their diagnosis to relatives, close friends and those with whom they are in a close personal relationship, they are far less likely to disclose it to employers or work colleagues, although disclosure becomes more common as disease severity worsens [122–124]. Assistance from the CF team with regard to employment or vocational training decisions is probably suboptimal, and guidance on these issues varies between CF centres [117].

The impact of workload reduction on quality of life and disease progression has not been explored in CF. Approximately half of adults with CF who have worked will retire from the workforce and receive some form of disability support by 40 years of age [91]. CF-specific health issues are the most common reason for ceasing work [117]. Changing work practices or ceasing employment is a difficult decision for adults with CF, due to the impact this will have on financial status and the dynamics of relationships with families.

Given the overall benefits of employment, but the often difficult decisions regarding vocation choice and the impact of progressive disease on the ability to work, the role of occupational therapists in CF teams has perhaps been overlooked. Incorporating occupational therapists as a routine component of the adult CF team should receive greater emphasis.

Care in adult centres

The increasing size of existing adult CF centres and the establishment of many new services have placed pressure on hospitals in terms of available capacity, funding and the need for an adequately trained work force [18]. In some health jurisdictions, the lack of preparation and the limited capacity, resources and facilities have led to the ongoing care of many adults within paediatric hospitals; even today, co-located adult and paediatric services with shared staffing across all age groups exist. CF authorities in Europe and North America have advocated adult-specific facilities, with formalised planning for transition to adult centres commencing early in adolescence [125–128].

As a result of the increasing number of adult CF sufferers, the optimal population size that can attend an adult CF centre must be considered. There is a need for exposure to sufficient patient numbers in order to hone skills and to develop and maintain expertise. Yet an important question for healthcare planners is: when do the economies of scale in delivery of care get lost due to limited resources and the complexity of managing very large numbers of patients with limited out- and inpatient facilities? It may be that once an adult centre reaches a size where the facilities (including the out- and inpatient capacity), services and staffing numbers are near to capacity, healthcare planners should consider: enhanced resourcing; the establishment of a satellite service with governance remaining within the existing service; or the establishment of a completely new and independent CF centre. Even if funding is available, cooperation between an established adult centre and a newly established centre is required in order to train healthcare professionals new to CF care. Whichever of these options is deemed most appropriate at an individual site, significant time will be required with careful planning and sufficient funding to support current and future adult services.

Currently, a European Respiratory Society (ERS)/ECFS task force is developing a curriculum for training in adult CF care (due to be published in 2014). Similar challenges face the fields of nursing and allied health, as well as other specialities (*e.g.* genetics, microbiology/infectious diseases, obstetrics, endocrinology and gastroenterology). Publication of the updated European Cystic Fibrosis Society Standards of Care (also to be published in 2014) will provide a framework for discussions and negotiation, and be useful to funding authorities that are new to the rapidly changing face of CF.

Harnessing the internet and social media to improve communication and care

Considering new models of care requires consideration of new technologies, which may incorporate monitoring at home [105, 129–131], telehealth [132–134] and outreach services

[135–137]. All of these approaches may need to be adopted on a larger scale than previously undertaken, as it may not be practical to continue the current model in the future as adult patient numbers continue to increase.

The explosion of the internet's availability and social networking opportunities has led to a shift in communication strategies between people with CF and their healthcare team. To a certain extent, social media also overcomes the relative social isolation of people with CF (due to infection control policies) from peer support. CF lay organisations have been instrumental in establishing chat rooms so that patients may "safely" communicate with each other.

There are many opportunities for enhanced engagement with patients and for improved education, monitoring and encouragement of self-management through the use modern technology, *i.e.* smart phones (fig. 4) [105] such as the CFfone [129]. National data registries are also of greater importance in shaping healthcare delivery. These valuable "data warehouses" are now being used in a number of countries to provide "open" centre-to-centre comparisons, providing opportunities for individual CF centres to examine practices and institute change if the data registry identifies differences with other CF centres [135, 138–144]. "Real-time" reports that illustrate changes over time in lung function or weight in a graphical format can be generated from some registries, and these can be used as a focus point in discussions with the individual with CF. In parallel, use of validated tools to assess patient satisfaction with the care provided by their CF centre has recently been advocated as an important part of quality improvement initiatives, internationally [140, 145].

Patients living in remote regions may benefit from teleconferencing, which allows multidisciplinary input into management in collaboration with local healthcare professionals. High-speed broadband internet connections allow high-quality images to be sent and videoconferences to be held in suitable locations as close to home as possible, which may be the local hospital, general practitioner's surgery, community health centre or even the patient's home. In future, home monitoring devices may allow lung function, activity and blood sugar levels to be uploaded for review by the CF team [146]. There remain challenges in replicating all components of a clinical consultation when patients are seen remotely, including collection of sputum samples for microbial surveillance. And whilst these advances are very promising, the few studies that have been conducted to date have noted relatively low rates of adherence with lung function or symptom recording [133]. Telemedicine should function primarily as an adjunct to usual care and not as a replacement for face-to-face reviews by the multidisciplinary team, which should be performed at least annually either at outreach clinics or at the CF centre.

Social media is a relatively simple method of disseminating information from the CF Team to the patient population; it could be used to post guidelines, notices on changes in care arrangements (*e.g.* pharmacy protocols) and other important news items, such as the availability of influenza vaccines and imminent clinical trials (in lay terms so that entry into trials is as transparent as possible). There are potential disadvantages associated with the use of social media: the team and the hospital must give careful consideration to privacy issues and the maintenance of patient confidentiality, and they must monitor the use (and possible abuse) of such media. A strategy that may be effective in supporting such an initiative would be to invite adults with CF to establish a patient advisory committee, which acts as a patient advocate in discussions with CF health teams and hospitals.

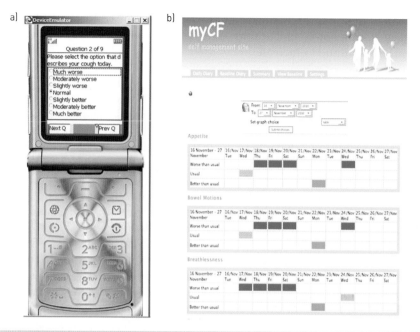

Figure 4. a) A smart phone that allows symptoms to be recorded, with immediate conversion to a graphical format (not shown) that provides feedback on progress for that individual when stable. b) Screenshot of an online symptom-recording system that provides feedback on clinical progress for that individual when stable using a traffic light colour coding system. Screenshot reproduced with the kind permission of Jenny Hauser (Adult CF Unit, Royal Hobart Hospital, Tasmania, Australia), Elizabeth Cummings and Paul Turner (both University of Tasmania, Australia) from the eHealth Services Research Group.

Conclusion

The number and complexity of complications in adult CF has grown rapidly, and this is likely to continue. Well-known CF complications are increasing in prevalence and newer ones will increasingly challenge the delivery of care in the coming decades. Many adult centres have grown to a size where coordination of care is difficult with available resources (including personnel), and many facilities are already at capacity. Coordinated planning for adult CF care is required internationally and requires close communication between healthcare professionals, healthcare planners and funders, and the lay community. Novel approaches to delivery of care will also be required to manage growth, including the establishment of outreach services and the use of internet technologies. Each of these requires careful assessment of their role and effectiveness to ensure that improvements in clinical outcomes are maintained into the future. Patient engagement remains vital in order to ensure strong support for new initiatives and to foster an effective approach to self-care in a management model that is likely to evolve ever more rapidly due to advances in therapies demonstrated to be effective and possibly disease-modifying in CF.

References

1. O'Sullivan BP, Freedman SD. Cystic fibrosis. *Lancet* 2009; 373: 1891–904.
2. European Cystic Fibrosis Patient Registry Annual Data Report 2008–2009. Karup, European Cystic Fibrosis Society, 2012.
3. Canadian Cystic Fibrosis Registry 2011 Annual Report. Toronto, Cystic Fibrosis Canada, 2012.
4. Cystic Fibrosis Foundation Patient Registry. 2012 Annual Data Report. Bethesda, Cystic Fibrosis Foundation, 2013.
5. UKCF Registry Annual Data Report 2011. London, Cystic Fibrosis Trust, 2013.
6. 15th Annual Report from the Cystic Fibrosis Data Registry. Sydney, Cystic Fibrosis Australia, 2013.

7.   Port CFNZ 2012 National Data Registry. Auckland, Cystic Fibrosis Association of New Zealand, 2013.

8.   Nick JA, Chacon CS, Brayshaw SJ, et al. Effects of gender and age at diagnosis on disease progression in long-term survivors of cystic fibrosis. Am J Respir Critical Care Med 2010; 182: 614–626.

9.   Nick JA, Rodman DM. Manifestations of cystic fibrosis diagnosed in adulthood. Curr Opin Pulm Med 2005; 11: 513–518.

10. Rodman DM, Reese K, Harral J, et al. Low-voltage-activated (T-type) calcium channels control proliferation of human pulmonary artery myocytes. Circ Res 2005; 96: 864–872.

11. Simmonds NJ, D'Souza L, Roughton M, et al. Cystic fibrosis and survival to 40 years: a study of cystic fibrosis transmembrane conductance regulator function. Eur Respir J 2011; 37: 1076–1082.

12. Collaco JM, McGready J, Green DM, et al. Effect of temperature on cystic fibrosis lung disease and infections: a replicated cohort study. PLoS One 2011; 6: e27784.

13. Collaco JM, Morrow CB, Green DM, et al. Environmental allergies and respiratory morbidities in cystic fibrosis. Pediatr Pulmonol 2013; 48: 857–864.

14. Green DM, Collaco JM, McDougal KE, et al. Heritability of respiratory infection with Pseudomonas aeruginosa in cystic fibrosis. J Pediatr 2012; 161: 290–295.

15. Schechter MS. Nongenetic influences on cystic fibrosis outcomes. Curr Opin Pulm Med 2011; 17: 448–454.

16. Schechter MS, McColley SA, Regelmann W, et al. Socioeconomic status and the likelihood of antibiotic treatment for signs and symptoms of pulmonary exacerbation in children with cystic fibrosis. J Pediatr 2011; 159: 819–824.

17. Batten J. Cystic fibrosis: a review. Br J Dis Chest 1965; 59: 1–9.

18. Conway SP, Stableforth DE, Webb AK. The failing health care system for adult patients with cystic fibrosis. Thorax 1998; 53: 3–4.

19. Dodge JA, Lewis PA, Stanton M, et al. Cystic fibrosis mortality and survival in the UK: 1947–2003. Eur Respir J 2007; 29: 522–526.

20. McCormick J, Mehta G, Olesen HV, et al. Comparative demographics of the European cystic fibrosis population: a cross-sectional database analysis. Lancet 2010; 375: 1007–1013.

21. Gutierrez HH, Sanchez I, Schidlow DV. Cystic fibrosis care in Chile. Curr Opin Pulm Med 2009; 15: 632–637.

22. Macri CN, de Gentile AS, Manterola A, et al. Epidemiology of cystic fibrosis in Latin America: preliminary communication. Pediatr Pulmonol 1991; 10: 249–253.

23. Simmonds NJ, Cullinan P, Hodson ME. Growing old with cystic fibrosis - the characteristics of long-term survivors of cystic fibrosis. Respir Med 2009; 103: 629–635.

24. Plant BJ, Goss CH, Plant WD, et al. Management of comorbidities in older patients with cystic fibrosis. Lancet Respir Med 2013; 1: 164–174.

25. Flume PA, Strange C, Ye X, et al. Pneumothorax in cystic fibrosis. Chest 2005; 128: 720–728.

26. Flume PA, Yankaskas JR, Ebeling M, et al. Massive hemoptysis in cystic fibrosis. Chest 2005; 128: 729–738.

27. Brinson GM, Noone PG, Mauro MA, et al. Bronchial artery embolization for the treatment of hemoptysis in patients with cystic fibrosis. Am J Respir Crit Care Med 1998; 157: 1951–1958.

28. Hodson ME, Simmonds NJ, Warwick WJ, et al. An international/multicentre report on patients with cystic fibrosis (CF) over the age of 40 years. J Cyst Fibros 2008; 7: 537–542.

29. Burrows JA, Nissen LM, Kirkpatrick CM, et al. Beta-lactam allergy in adults with cystic fibrosis. J Cyst Fibros 2007; 6: 297–303.

30. Whitaker P, Naisbitt D, Peckham D. Nonimmediate beta-lactam reactions in patients with cystic fibrosis. Curr Opin Allergy Clin Immunol 2012; 12: 369–375.

31. Catherinot E, Roux AL, Vibet MA, et al. Mycobacterium avium and Mycobacterium abscessus complex target distinct cystic fibrosis patient subpopulations. J Cyst Fibros 2013; 12: 74–80.

32. Leung JM, Olivier KN. Nontuberculous mycobacteria in patients with cystic fibrosis. Semin Respir Crit Care Med 2013; 34: 124–134.

33. Aitken ML, Limaye A, Pottinger P, et al. Respiratory outbreak of Mycobacterium abscessus subspecies massiliense in a lung transplant and cystic fibrosis center. Am J Respir Crit Care Med 2012; 185: 231–232.

34. Bryant JM, Grogono DM, Greaves D, et al. Whole-genome sequencing to identify transmission of Mycobacterium abscessus between patients with cystic fibrosis: a retrospective cohort study. Lancet 2013; 381: 1551–1560.

35. Nick JA, Moskowitz SM, Chmiel JF, et al. Azithromycin may antagonize inhaled tobramycin when targeting Pseudomonas aeruginosa in cystic fibrosis. Ann Am Thorac Soc 2014; 11: 342–350.

36. Ramsey BW, Pepe MS, Quan JM, et al. Intermittent administration of inhaled tobramycin in patients with cystic fibrosis. Cystic Fibrosis Inhaled Tobramycin Study Group. N Engl J Med 1999; 340: 23–30.

37. Saiman L, Marshall BC, Mayer-Hamblett N, et al. Azithromycin in patients with cystic fibrosis chronically infected with Pseudomonas aeruginosa: a randomized controlled trial. JAMA 2003; 290: 1749–1756.

38. Wolter J, Seeney S, Bell S, et al. Effect of long term treatment with azithromycin on disease parameters in cystic fibrosis: a randomised trial. Thorax 2002; 57: 212–216.

39. Moran A, Becker D, Casella SJ, et al. Epidemiology, pathophysiology, and prognostic implications of cystic fibrosis-related diabetes: a technical review. Diabetes Care 2010; 33: 2677–83.

40. Moran A, Dunitz J, Nathan B, et al. Cystic fibrosis-related diabetes: current trends in prevalence, incidence, and mortality. *Diabetes Care* 2009; 32: 1626–1631.

41. Kelly A, Moran A. Update on cystic fibrosis-related diabetes. *J Cyst Fibros* 2013; 12: 318–331.

42. Burrows JA, Toon M, Bell SC. Antibiotic desensitization in adults with cystic fibrosis. *Respirology* 2003; 8: 359–364.

43. Whitaker P, Shaw N, Gooi J, et al. Rapid desensitization for non-immediate reactions in patients with cystic fibrosis. *J Cyst Fibros* 2011; 10: 282–285.

44. Quon BS, Mayer-Hamblett N, Aitken ML, et al. Risk of post-lung transplant renal dysfunction in adults with cystic fibrosis. *Chest* 2012; 142: 185–189.

45. Quon BS, Mayer-Hamblett N, Aitken ML, et al. Risk factors for chronic kidney disease in adults with cystic fibrosis. *Am J Respir Crit Care Med* 2011; 184: 1147–1152.

46. Florescu MC, Lyden E, Murphy PJ, et al. Long-term effect of chronic intravenous and inhaled nephrotoxic antibiotic treatment on the renal function of patients with cystic fibrosis. *Hemodial Int* 2012; 16: 414–419.

47. O'Connell OJ, Harrison MJ, Murphy DM, et al. Peri-lung transplant renal issues in patients with cystic fibrosis. *Chest* 2013; 143: 271.

48. Mulrennan SA, Helm J, Thomas RB, et al. Aminoglycoside ototoxicity susceptibility in cystic fibrosis. *Thorax* 2009; 64: 271–272.

49. O'Donnell EP, Scarsi KK, Scheetz MH, et al. Risk factors for aminoglycoside ototoxicity in adult cystic fibrosis patients. *Int J Antimicrob Agents* 2010; 36: 94–95.

50. France MW, Bell SC. Gastrointestinal cancers in cystic fibrosis. *CML Cystic Fibrosis* 2014; 4: 1–14.

51. Garwood S, Flume PA, Ravenel J. Superior vena cava syndrome related to indwelling intravenous catheters in patients with cystic fibrosis. *Pediatr Pulmonol* 2006; 41: 683–687.

52. Meyer KC, Francois ML, Thomas HK, et al. Colon cancer in lung transplant recipients with CF: increased risk and results of screening. *J Cyst Fibros* 2011; 10: 366–369.

53. Nash EF, Helm EJ, Stephenson A, et al. Incidence of deep vein thrombosis associated with peripherally inserted central catheters in adults with cystic fibrosis. *J Vasc Interv Radiol* 2009; 20: 347–351.

54. Rhodes B, Nash EF, Tullis E, et al. Prevalence of dyslipidemia in adults with cystic fibrosis. *J Cyst Fibros* 2010; 9: 24–28.

55. Maisonneuve P, FitzSimmons SC, Neglia JP, et al. Cancer risk in nontransplanted and transplanted cystic fibrosis patients: a 10-year study. *J Natl Cancer Inst* 2003; 95: 381–387.

56. Maisonneuve P, Marshall BC, Knapp EA, et al. Cancer risk in cystic fibrosis: a 20-year nationwide study from the United States. *J Natl Cancer Inst* 2013; 105: 122–129.

57. Coderre L, Fadainia C, Belson L, et al. LDL-cholesterol and insulin are independently associated with body mass index in adult cystic fibrosis patients. *J Cyst Fibros* 2012; 11: 393–397.

58. Macnee W, Maclay J, McAllister D. Cardiovascular injury and repair in chronic obstructive pulmonary disease. *Proc Am Thorac Soc* 2008; 5: 824–833.

59. Hull JH, Garrod R, Ho TB, et al. Increased augmentation index in patients with cystic fibrosis. *Eur Respir J* 2009; 34: 1322–1328.

60. Hull JH, Garrod R, Ho TB, et al. Dynamic vascular changes following intravenous antibiotics in patients with cystic fibrosis. *J Cyst Fibros* 2013; 12: 125–129.

61. Liou TG, Adler FR, Huang D. Use of lung transplantation survival models to refine patient selection in cystic fibrosis. *Am J Respir Crit Care Med* 2005; 171: 1053–1059.

62. Mayer-Hamblett N, Rosenfeld M, Emerson J, et al. Developing cystic fibrosis lung transplant referral criteria using predictors of 2-year mortality. *Am J Respir Crit Care Med* 2002; 166: 1550–1555.

63. Kerem E, Reisman J, Corey M, et al. Prediction of mortality in patients with cystic fibrosis. *N Engl J Med* 1992; 326: 1187–1191.

64. George PM, Banya W, Pareek N, et al. Improved survival at low lung function in cystic fibrosis: cohort study from 1990 to 2007. *BMJ* 2011; 342: d1008.

65. Bradbury RA, Shirkhedkar D, Glanville AR, et al. Prior diabetes mellitus is associated with increased morbidity in cystic fibrosis patients undergoing bilateral lung transplantation: an "orphan" area? A retrospective case-control study. *Intern Med J* 2009; 39: 384–388.

66. Hofer M, Schmid C, Benden C, et al. Diabetes mellitus and survival in cystic fibrosis patients after lung transplantation. *J Cyst Fibros* 2012; 11: 131–136.

67. Emerson J, McNamara S, Buccat AM, et al. Changes in cystic fibrosis sputum microbiology in the United States between 1995 and 2008. *Pediatr Pulmonol* 2010; 45: 363–370.

68. Boussaud V, Guillemain R, Grenet D, et al. Clinical outcome following lung transplantation in patients with cystic fibrosis colonised with *Burkholderia cepacia* complex: results from two French centres. *Thorax* 2008; 63: 732–737.

69. De Soyza A, Meachery G, Hester KL, et al. Lung transplantation for patients with cystic fibrosis and *Burkholderia cepacia* complex infection: a single-center experience. *J Heart Lung Transplant* 2010; 29: 1395–1404.

70. Aris RM, Gilligan PH, Neuringer IP, et al. The effects of panresistant bacteria in cystic fibrosis patients on lung transplant outcome. *Am J Respir Crit Care Med* 1997; 155: 1699–1704.

71. Braun AT, Merlo CA. Cystic fibrosis lung transplantation. *Curr Opin Pulm Med* 2011; 17: 467–472.

72. Doring G, Flume P, Heijerman H, *et al.* Treatment of lung infection in patients with cystic fibrosis: current and future strategies. *J Cyst Fibros* 2012; 11: 461–479.

73. Hadjiliadis D, Steele MP, Chaparro C, *et al.* Survival of lung transplant patients with cystic fibrosis harboring panresistant bacteria other than *Burkholderia cepacia*, compared with patients harboring sensitive bacteria. *J Heart Lung Transplant* 2007; 26: 834–838.

74. Hirche TO, Knoop C, Hebestreit H, *et al.* Practical guidelines: lung transplantation in patients with cystic fibrosis. *Pulm Med* 2014; 2014: 621342.

75. Edenborough FP, Borgo G, Knoop C, *et al.* Guidelines for the management of pregnancy in women with cystic fibrosis. *J Cyst Fibros* 2008; 7: Suppl. 1, S2–S32.

76. Thorpe-Beeston JG, Madge S, Gyi K, *et al.* The outcome of pregnancies in women with cystic fibrosis–single centre experience 1998–2011. *BJOG* 2013; 120: 354–361.

77. Tonelli MR, Aitken ML. Pregnancy in cystic fibrosis. *Curr Opin Pulm Med* 2007; 13: 537–540.

78. Whitty JE. Cystic fibrosis in pregnancy. *Clin Obstet Gynecol* 2010; 53: 369–376.

79. Goss CH, Rubenfeld GD, Otto K, *et al.* The effect of pregnancy on survival in women with cystic fibrosis. *Chest* 2003; 124: 1460–1468.

80. McMullen AH, Pasta DJ, Frederick PD, *et al.* Impact of pregnancy on women with cystic fibrosis. *Chest* 2006; 129: 706–711.

81. Schechter MS, Quittner AL, Konstan MW, *et al.* Long-term effects of pregnancy and motherhood on disease outcomes of women with cystic fibrosis. *Ann Am Thorac Soc* 2013; 10: 213–219.

82. Landon MB, Spong CY, Thom E, *et al.* A multicenter, randomized trial of treatment for mild gestational diabetes. *N Engl J Med* 2009; 361: 1339–1348.

83. Corey M, McLaughlin FJ, Williams M, *et al.* A comparison of survival, growth, and pulmonary function in patients with cystic fibrosis in Boston and Toronto. *J Clin Epidemiol* 1988; 41: 583–591.

84. U.S. Food and Drug Administration. FDA approves Kalydeco to treat rare form of cystic fibrosis. www.fda.gov/NewsEvents/Newsroom/PressAnnouncements/ucm289633.htm Date last updated: January 31, 2012. Date last accessed: April 17, 2014.

85. Davies JC, Wainwright CE, Canny GJ, *et al.* Efficacy and safety of ivacaftor in patients aged 6 to 11 years with cystic fibrosis with a G551D mutation. *Am J Respir Crit Care Med* 2013; 187: 1219–1225.

86. Ramsey BW, Davies J, McElvaney NG, *et al.* A CFTR potentiator in patients with cystic fibrosis and the G551D mutation. *N Engl J Med* 2011; 365: 1663–1672.

87. Besier T, Born A, Henrich G, *et al.* Anxiety, depression, and life satisfaction in parents caring for children with cystic fibrosis. *Pediatr Pulmonol* 2011; 46: 672–682.

88. Cruz I, Marciel KK, Quittner AL, *et al.* Anxiety and depression in cystic fibrosis. *Semin Respir Crit Care Med* 2009; 30: 569–578.

89. Goldbeck L, Besier T, Hinz A, *et al.* Prevalence of symptoms of anxiety and depression in German patients with cystic fibrosis. *Chest* 2010; 138: 929–936.

90. Latchford G, Duff AJ. Screening for depression in a single CF centre. *J Cyst Fibros* 2013; 12: 794–796.

91. Riekert KA, Bartlett SJ, Boyle MP, *et al.* The association between depression, lung function, and health-related quality of life among adults with cystic fibrosis. *Chest* 2007; 132: 231–237.

92. Yohannes AM, Willgoss TG, Fatoye FA, *et al.* Relationship between anxiety, depression, and quality of life in adult patients with cystic fibrosis. *Respir Care* 2012; 57: 550–556.

93. Kopp BT, Wang W, Chisolm DJ, *et al.* Inpatient healthcare trends among adult cystic fibrosis patients in the U.S. *Pediatr Pulmonol* 2012; 47: 245–251.

94. Besier T, Goldbeck L. Growing up with cystic fibrosis: achievement, life satisfaction, and mental health. *Qual Life Res* 2012; 21: 1829–1835.

95. Abbott J, Dodd M, Gee L, *et al.* Ways of coping with cystic fibrosis: implications for treatment adherence. *Disabil Rehabil* 2001; 23: 315–324.

96. Segal TY. Adolescence: what the cystic fibrosis team needs to know. *J R Soc Med* 2008; 101: Suppl. 1, S15–S27.

97. Bury M. The sociology of chronic illness: a review and prospects. *Sociol Health Illn* 1991; 13: 451–468.

98. Collins S, Reynolds F. How do adults with cystic fibrosis cope following a diagnosis of diabetes? *J Adv Nurs* 2008; 64: 478–487.

99. Lowton K, Gaby J. Life on a slippery slope: perception of health in adults with cystic fibrosis. *Sociol Health Illn* 2003; 25: 289–319.

100. Watson H, Bilton D, Truby H. A randomized controlled trial of a new behavioral home-based nutrition education program, "Eat Well with CF," in adults with cystic fibrosis. *J Am Diet Assoc* 2008; 108: 847–852.

101. Stark LJ, Opipari-Arrigan L, Quittner AL, *et al.* The effects of an intensive behavior and nutrition intervention compared to standard of care on weight outcomes in CF. *Pediatr Pulmonol* 2011; 46: 31–35.

102. Duff AJ, Latchford GJ. Motivational interviewing for adherence problems in cystic fibrosis. *Pediatr Pulmonol* 2010; 45: 211–220.

103. Duff AJ, Latchford GJ. Motivational interviewing for adherence problems in cystic fibrosis; evaluation of training healthcare professionals. *J Clin Med Res* 2013; 5: 475–480.

104. Quinn J, Latchford G, Duff A, *et al.* Measuring, predicting and improving adherence to inhalation therapy in patients with CF: a randomised controlled study of motivational interviewing. *Pediatr Pulmonol* 2004; 38: S360.

105. Roehrer E, Cummings E, Turner P, *et al.* Supporting cystic fibrosis with ICT. *Stud Health Technol Inform* 2013; 183: 137–141.

106. Sawicki GS, Sellers DE, McGuffie K, *et al.* Adults with cystic fibrosis report important and unmet needs for disease information. *J Cyst Fibros* 2007; 6: 411–416.

107. Sawicki GS, Sellers DE, Robinson WM. High treatment burden in adults with cystic fibrosis: challenges to disease self-management. *J Cyst Fibros* 2009; 8: 91–96.

108. Steiner JF, Prochazka AV. The assessment of refill compliance using pharmacy records: methods, validity, and applications. *J Clin Epidemiol* 1997; 50: 105–116.

109. Eakin MN, Bilderback A, Boyle MP, *et al.* Longitudinal association between medication adherence and lung health in people with cystic fibrosis. *J Cyst Fibros* 2011; 10: 258–264.

110. Waters V, Stanojevic S, Atenafu EG, *et al.* Effect of pulmonary exacerbations on long-term lung function decline in cystic fibrosis. *Eur Respir J* 2012; 40: 61–66.

111. Daniels T, Goodacre L, Sutton C, *et al.* Accurate assessment of adherence: self-report and clinician report *vs* electronic monitoring of nebulizers. *Chest* 2011; 140: 425–432.

112. Eakin MN, Riekert KA. The impact of medication adherence on lung health outcomes in cystic fibrosis. *Curr Opin Pulm Med* 2013; 19: 687–691.

113. Finney JW, Hook RJ, Friman PC, *et al.* The overestimation of adherence to pediatric medical regimens. *Child Health Care* 1993; 22: 297–304.

114. Burker EJ, Sedway J, Carone S. Psychological and educational factors: better predictors of work status than FEV1 in adults with cystic fibrosis. *Pediatr Pulmonol* 2004; 38: 413–418.

115. Saldana PS, Pomeranz JL. Cystic fibrosis and the workplace: a review of the literature. *Work* 2012; 42: 185–193.

116. Taylor-Robinson DC, Smyth R, Diggle PJ, *et al.* A longitudinal study of the impact of social deprivation and disease severity on employment status in the UK cystic fibrosis population. *PLoS One* 2013; 8: e73322.

117. Targett K, Bourke S, Nash E, *et al.* Employment in adults with cystic fibrosis. *Occup Med (Lond)* 2014; 64: 87–94.

118. Bullough B. Poverty, ethnic identity and preventive health care. *J Health Soc Behav* 1972; 13: 347–359.

119. Duncan GJ, Brooks-Gunn J. Family poverty, welfare reform, and child development. *Child Dev* 2000; 71: 188–196.

120. Wagstaff A. Poverty and health sector inequalities. *Bull World Health Organ* 2002; 80: 97–105.

121. Ullrich G. Employment in CF adults deserves much more attention. *J Cyst Fibros* 2013; 12: 416.

122. Demars N, Uluer A, Sawicki GS. Employment experiences among adolescents and young adults with cystic fibrosis. *Disabil Rehabil* 2011; 33: 922–926.

123. Lowton K. Only when I cough? Adults' disclosure of cystic fibrosis. *Qual Health Res* 2004; 14: 167–186.

124. Modi AC, Quittner AL, Boyle MP. Assessing disease disclosure in adults with cystic fibrosis: the Adult Data for Understanding Lifestyle and Transitions (ADULT) survey Disclosure of disease in adults with cystic fibrosis. *BMC Pulm Med* 2010; 10: 46.

125. Standards for the Clinical Care of Children and Adults with Cystic Fibrosis in the UK (2nd edn). London, Cystic Fibrosis Trust, 2011.

126. Colombo C, Littlewood J. The implementation of standards of care in Europe: state of the art. *J Cyst Fibros* 2011; 10: Suppl. 2, S7–S15.

127. Kerem E, Conway S, Elborn S, *et al.* Standards of care for patients with cystic fibrosis: a European consensus. *J Cyst Fibros* 2005; 4: 7–26.

128. Yankaskas JR, Marshall BC, Sufian B, *et al.* Cystic fibrosis adult care: consensus conference report. *Chest* 2004; 125: 1S–39S.

129. Marciel KK, Saiman L, Quittell LM, *et al.* Cell phone intervention to improve adherence: cystic fibrosis care team, patient, and parent perspectives. *Pediatr Pulmonol* 2010; 45: 157–164.

130. Cummings E, Borycki EM, Roehrer E. Issues and considerations for healthcare consumers using mobile applications. *Stud Health Technol Inform* 2013; 183: 227–231.

131. Roehrer E, Cummings E, Beggs S, *et al.* Pilot evaluation of web enabled symptom monitoring in cystic fibrosis. *Inform Health Soc Care* 2013; 38: 354–365.

132. Bella S, Cotognini C, Alghisi F, *et al.* Program of home telemonitoring in patients with cystic fibrosis over a period of 2 years: a contribution to the rationalization of care. *Clin Ter* 2013; 164: e313–e317.

133. Cox NS, Alison JA, Rasekaba T, *et al.* Telehealth in cystic fibrosis: a systematic review. *J Telemed Telecare* 2012; 18: 72–78.

134. Murgia F, Cilli M, Renzetti E, *et al.* Remote telematic control in cystic fibrosis. *Clin Ter* 2011; 162: e121–e124.

135. Ledger SJ, Owen E, Prasad SA, *et al.* A pilot outreach physiotherapy and dietetic quality improvement initiative reduces IV antibiotic requirements in children with moderate-severe cystic fibrosis. *J Cyst Fibros* 2013; 12: 766–772.

136. Thomas C, Mitchell P, O'Rourke P, *et al.* Quality-of-life in children and adolescents with cystic fibrosis managed in both regional outreach and cystic fibrosis center settings in Queensland. *J Pediatr* 2006; 148: 508–516.

137. Thomas CL, O'Rourke PK, Wainwright CE. Clinical outcomes of Queensland children with cystic fibrosis: a comparison between tertiary centre and outreach services. *Med J Aust* 2008; 188: 135–139.

138. Britton LJ, Thrasher S, Gutierrez H. Creating a culture of improvement: experience of a pediatric cystic fibrosis center. *J Nurs Care Qual* 2008; 23: 115–120.

139. Chuang S, Doumit M, McDonald R, *et al.* Annual review clinic improves care in children with cystic fibrosis. *J Cyst Fibros* 2014; 13: 186–189.

140. Homa K, Sabadosa KA, Nelson EC, *et al.* Development and validation of a cystic fibrosis patient and family member experience of care survey. *Qual Manag Health Care* 2013; 22: 100–116.

141. Kern AS, Prestridge AL. Improving screening for cystic fibrosis-related diabetes at a pediatric cystic fibrosis program. *Pediatrics* 2013; 132: e512–e518.

142. Quon BS, Goss CH. A story of success: continuous quality improvement in cystic fibrosis care in the USA. *Thorax* 2011; 66: 1106–1108.

143. Schechter MS. Benchmarking to improve the quality of cystic fibrosis care. *Curr Opin Pulm Med* 2012; 18: 596–601.

144. Stern M, Niemann N, Wiedemann B, *et al.* Benchmarking improves quality in cystic fibrosis care: a pilot project involving 12 centres. *Int J Qual Health Care* 2011; 23: 349–356.

145. Steinkamp G, Stahl K, Ullrich G, *et al.* CF Care through the patients' eyes: development of a disease specific questionnaire measuring patient satisfaction with CF services. *J Cyst Fibros* 2010; 9: S100.

146. Cox NS, Alison JA, Button BM, *et al.* Assessing exercise capacity using telehealth: a feasibility study in adults with cystic fibrosis. *Respir Care* 2013; 58: 286–290.

Acknowledgements: The authors would like to thank Bruce C. Marshall and Mary Grimes (Cystic Fibrosis Foundation, Bethesda, MD, USA) for assistance with the figures from the Cystic Fibrosis Foundation Patient Registry 2011 Annual Data Report. We would also like to thank Jenny Hauser (Adult CF Unit, Royal Hobart Hospital, Tasmania, Australia), Elizabeth Cummings and Paul Turner (both University of Tasmania, Australia) from the eHealth Services Research Group for permitting the use of the smart phone image and webpage screenshots. Finally, we are also grateful for the support of all our dedicated colleagues in the Adult Cystic Fibrosis Centre at The Prince Charles Hospital (Chermside, Australia), who do an amazing job in providing care for an ever-increasing cohort of adults with CF.

Disclosures: S.C. Bell reports personal fees and non-financial support from Vertex Pharmaceuticals and Novartis, non-financial support from Rempex and non-financial support from Pharmaxis, outside the submitted work.

Chapter 21

Health-economic aspects of cystic fibrosis screening and therapy

Jiří Klimeš[1,2], Tomáš Doležal[1,3], Kateřina Kubáčková[4],
Marek Turnovec[5] and Milan Macek Jr[5]

There is an increasing need to manage cost-effectiveness issues of novel or relatively expensive technologies that are currently in use or being proposed for the treatment of cystic fibrosis (CF) (*e.g.* cystic fibrosis transmembrane conductance regulator (CFTR) modulation therapy). Health-economic evaluations of rising pharmacotherapeutic costs, as the major driver of overall cost, have to be part of the cost analysis of chronic and progressive (rare) diseases like CF that may require lifelong therapy. Total costs include not only direct healthcare costs but also the cost of lost productivity by both patients and family caregivers. When considering the results of cost-effectiveness analysis of new technologies associated with the management of CF, it is unreasonable to expect that the incremental cost-effectiveness ratio to be less than the generally applied thresholds (willingness to pay) for other common diseases. Therefore, when assessing CF and other rare diseases, such analyses should include complex health technology assessment approaches, which evaluate comparative treatment effectiveness (novel and established), as well as wider social benefits and ethical aspects.

Cystic fibrosis (CF) [1] is a life-limiting rare genetic disease with autosomal recessive inheritance associated with "CF-causing" mutations in the cystic fibrosis transmembrane conductance regulator (*CFTR*) gene [2]. CF is a chronic and progressive disease requiring lifelong care, which generally becomes increasingly complex and demanding with age. Therefore, CF represents a major medical and socioeconomic issue in Europe and North America [3], and could be used as an indicator of disparities in healthcare systems [4]. Recent estimates based on the available data from the European Cystic Fibrosis Registry [5], together with previous EuroCareCF project demographic surveys, indicate that there are more than 29 000 CF patients in Europe [6]. However, due to disparities in diagnosis and care, many CF patients, mainly in Eastern European countries, remain undiagnosed [7], highlighting the need to introduce nationwide CF newborn screening (CFNBS) programmes that assure equitable and early diagnosis of the disease [8].

The majority of healthcare system costs are associated with CF treatments such as bronchodilation, mucolytics and intensive anti-inflammatory therapy. In addition, acute

---

[1]Institute of Health Economics and Technology Assessment o.p.s, iHETA, Prague, Czech Republic. [2]Dept of Clinical and Social Pharmacy, Faculty of Pharmacy Hradec Králové, Charles University, Prague, Czech Republic. [3]Dept of Pharmacology, 2nd Faculty of Medicine, Charles University, Prague, Czech Republic. [4]Clinic of Oncology, 2nd Faculty of Medicine, Charles University and Faculty Hospital Motol, Prague, Czech Republic. [5]Dept of Biology and Medical Genetics, 2nd Faculty of Medicine, Charles University and Faculty Hospital Motol, Prague, Czech Republic.

Correspondence: Milan Macek Jr, Dept of Biology and Medical Genetics, 2nd Faculty of Medicine, Charles University, V Uvalu 84, Prague 5, CZ15006, Czech Republic. E-mail: Milan.Macek.Jr@LFmotol.Cuni.Cz

ERS Monogr 2014; 64: 304–319. DOI: 10.1183/1025448x.10010613

and/or long-term antibacterial and antifungal treatments are required to manage persistent or recurring infections, mainly caused by colonisation with *Pseudomonas aeruginosa* and/or *Burkholderia cepacia* complex [9]. Substitution therapy for pancreatic insufficiency and CF-related diabetes mellitus (CFRD), including use of secondary bile acids for CF liver disease, also contributes to increased costs of treatment. Lung transplantation is another costly option, which is available to eligible adolescent and adult CF patients [10].

The median life expectancy of CF patients has substantially improved from 5 years (in the early 1960s) to about 40 years today [11]. Much of the progress in extending life expectancy has been due to standardised multisystem treatment modalities comprising not only pharmacotherapy but also, for example, high-calorie nutrition and physiotherapy [9].

Following the ground-breaking introduction of CFTR-modulating therapies (CFTR-MTs) into clinical practice in 2012 [12], we can be hopeful of further increases in CF life expectancy. These novel orphan medicinal products (OMPs) are potentially clinically effective and promise to substantially alter the course of the disease [12]. As a result of ongoing and rapid advancements in CF care, it is now expected that children born with CF today will probably live into their fifties and beyond [13].

Ivacaftor (Kalydeco; Vertex Pharmaceuticals Inc., Boston, MA, USA) [14, 15] is an example of a recent CFTR-MT that carries a rather high price. Therefore, CF treatment costs require health-economic analyses, including other complex assessments, if an OMP of this kind is to receive lifelong reimbursement by a particular healthcare system [16]. As at the moment CFTR-MTs are targeted to small subsets of the overall CF population (*i.e.* less than 5% of the total number of CF patients), these medicines belong to the "ultra-OMP" category with specific reimbursement arrangements (see later) [17].

Health technology assessment

Presently, all healthcare systems in Europe and North America are faced with complex issues that have forced them to make difficult choices regarding prioritisation of investments for particular diagnostic methods, novel treatments, prevention programmes and surgical techniques, which represent essentially all medical advances that lead to improved health and quality of life (QoL). Medical successes have presented healthcare systems with an additional dilemma, that of a rapidly ageing population, which has started to strain available resources. Moreover, austerity measures affecting healthcare systems in many European Union (EU) countries [18] together with the ageing of the general population, which proportionally decreases the number of taxable citizens on which "solidarity-based" healthcare systems are built, further complicate these trends [19]. Additionally, those born with rare diseases now survive the historic infant mortality "barrier" and live quality lives well into adulthood due to intensive treatment. Thus, costs of treatment must be considered to last for the lifetime of an individual. Lastly, but by no means the least important, is easy access to information about novel medical technologies and treatments. Well-educated patients who are aware of cutting-edge treatments often specifically request (or even demand) access to them. Patient support groups are often at the forefront of such "lobbying" activities [20]. These organisations have increasing influence, which was recently emphasised by EU policy documents [21]. However, despite rapid progress in the medical domain, the ongoing economic crisis has generally produced limited political will to increase healthcare taxation and thus expenditures (the politics of this issue are beyond the scope of this chapter).

Generally speaking, European healthcare budgets are finite and taking resources from one treatment will inevitably shrink available resources for other treatments, both established and novel, in terms of individualised medicine [22]. The prioritisation [23] and selection of the novel approaches that offer the greatest benefits or fulfil the largest number of unmet needs is called health technology assessment (HTA). In many countries, there are agencies that systematically assess new medical technologies based on novel and/or available evidence; additionally, they regularly reassess existing technologies. In Europe, the most prominent HTA bodies are the UK National Institute for Health and Care Excellence (NICE) (www.nice. org.uk) and Scottish Medicines Consortium (www.scottishmedicines.org.uk), the Swedish Dental and Pharmaceutical Benefits Agency (TLV) (www.tlv.se), the French Haute Autorité de Santé (www.has-sante.fr), the Dutch College voor Zorgverzekeringen (http://vortal.htai. org), the German Institut für Qualität und Wirtschaftlichkeit im Gesundheitswesen (www. iqwig.de), and the Polish Agency for Health Technology Assessment (AHTAPol) (www. aotm.gov.pl). There is also a pan-EU initiative to develop a transnational HTA body that focuses on the relative (comparative) assessments of efficacy and safety of new technologies within the EUnetHTA European Union Joint Action project (www.eunethta.eu).

However, the ultimate decision regarding reimbursement of a particular technology should be made at the EU Member State level, as such decisions must address local needs, affordability and practice in relationship to the evaluated technology, including the economic situation (EU principle of "subsidiarity" of national healthcare systems) [24].

Within HTA, there are several key domains that are addressed and represent most parameters that are evaluated.

1) Efficacy, effectiveness and safety issues: in these terms, the greatest interest lies in comparative effectiveness/safety, which focusses on effectiveness in relation to current treatment practices. Meta-analyses, network meta-analyses and mixed treatment comparisons are always needed in order to address this issue for all relevant technologies/comparators [25–28].

2) Health-economic/pharmacoeconomic issues addressing questions such as: does a technology bring sufficient benefits (in terms of additional years gained/years of quality life) in relation to its cost, *i.e.* "is the new technology cost-effective?", and what will be the burden on the payers' budget, *i.e.* "is the launch of a novel technology affordable?"

3) Even if the technology is not cost-effective or represents a substantial burden to the budget, an effective and safe technology could still, under certain circumstances, be accepted by a healthcare system. This requires examining other circumstances of the technology that impact on its use, particularly the social aspects of the new technology and ethical issues. These issues are often stressed in technologies linked to treatments for infants and children, including rare genetic diseases. In this regard, the EU overarching rare genetic disease patient organisation (www.eurordis.org) is at the forefront of establishing criteria for the improvement of informed decisions based on the clinical added value of OMPs within the EU Committee of Experts on Rare Genetic Diseases (EUCERD) [29]. Importantly, CF meets the majority of the aforementioned criteria.

For instance, some HTA bodies primarily concentrate on health economics (in particular cost-effectiveness), *i.e.* England and Scotland (UK), Sweden, the Netherlands and Poland, while other HTA agencies are mainly interested in relative effectiveness and clinical added value, and are less concerned with health-economic/pharmacoeconomic issues, *e.g.* France and Germany. Currently, many HTA agencies are in the process of restructuring, and some that had been focused on results of cost-effectiveness analyses are starting to incorporated wider social benefit aspects and ethical issues into HTA processes, while others that were less interested in health-economic/pharmacoeconomic issues are starting to incorporate some degree of cost-effectiveness into their assessments.

Currently, there is a debate regarding the complex and systematic inclusion of all domains of HTA into one analysis that would support the assessment process as well as the final appraisal. This approach is represented by multicriterion analysis [30, 31], which is particularly useful for technologies associated with rare diseases [32]. Finally, there is an increasing trend for exchanging best practices and harmonising HTA approaches through the activities of the EUnetHTA consortium, including information exchange with the European Medicines Agency (EMA).

Health-economic/pharmacoeconomic studies

The principals of pharmacoeconomics are also applied to other fields of healthcare systems. In general, health economics is the application of theories, tools and concepts of the discipline of economics to the topics of healthcare and healthcare systems [33]. Economics as a science is concerned with the allocation of resources. Health economics is concerned with the allocation of (usually scarce) resources that improve health and QoL. This includes both resource allocation within the economy to healthcare systems, and within the healthcare systems themselves to different activities, programmes and individuals [34].

Generally, there are two major groups of health-economic studies. The first group is represented by studies that focus only on costs attributed to a particular health problem or disease (*e.g.* cost of illness, here as it relates to CF) or the cost/burden of a new technology (*e.g.* budget impacts of novel drugs or CFNBS) to be introduced into a healthcare system. The second group is represented by studies that, in addition to costs, also examine therapy-related outcomes (*e.g.* avoiding exacerbations or chronic infections, improvement in lung function, and longer and better QoL). These analyses are termed cost-effectiveness analysis or cost-utility analysis, while with regards to effectiveness, they are further divided into several subtypes (table 1).

Overview of health-economic studies

CF is a monogenic (autosomal recessive) disease with an overall clinical course that is, to a large degree, determined by the "milder" of the two *CFTR* mutations that the patient has inherited from their parents. Although genotype–phenotype correlations are more pronounced for pancreatic status rather than for the sinobronchial disease [38], *CFTR* mutation pathogenicity (or disease liability) has been objectively established within the CFTR2.org project [39].

Early diagnosis of the disease *via* CFNBS, which combines examination of a specific pancreatic dysfunction biomarker (immunoreactive trypsinogen (IRT)) with additional tiers (biochemical or DNA testing of population-specific *CFTR* genotypes), leads to improved prognosis in CF [40] by reducing the rate of avoidable complications. It is therefore not only possible to predict the general severity of the disease based on the *CFTR* genotype [41] (presence of specific CF-causing mutations or "pre-emptive *CFTR* genotype results") but also

Table 1. Health-economic studies

	Description of the analysis	Example of the analysis
Cost studies/ analysis		
COI	Total costs attributed to patient with particular disease, which can be expressed as an average cost per patient over 1 year or lifetime costs "from the diagnosis to demise"	The average cost of a CF patient for 1 year is related to disease severity (prevalence-based analysis) [35] The lifetime cost of CF from diagnosis (birth) to the end of life (average life-expectancy) (incidence-based analysis) [35]
BIA	Total costs added to a particular healthcare budget in relation to the introduction of a new technology [36]	The budget impact of introducing a new drug or treatment programme (i.e. CFNBS) e.g. 5 years after its launch; the impact on the HCS or other relevant budgets (i.e. social services), or on the entire society
Cost-effectiveness studies/analysis		
CMA	The outcomes (effectiveness) of new and current technology are the same; only costs matter	This analysis can be applied when comparing original and generic drugs, or "me-too" drugs with comparable efficacy and safety; however, the application of this type of analysis is scarce, as there is almost always a difference in the efficacy or safety profile of alternative technologies, and thus the impact on the patient's QoL is variable
CEA	Calculation of the total costs and outcomes (clinically relevant, i.e. exacerbations, hospitalisations, deterioration of lung function (FEV_1), sweat chloride concentration, nutrition assessed (BMI) or even LYG) for novel versus current technologies	Preferably performed with a lifetime horizon, i.e. from the first administration of a new and comparative technology; it provides incremental total costs per incremental benefit for the new and comparative technologies (ICER)
CUA	Calculation of total costs and outcomes that combine survival and QoL, i.e. QALY[#]) for new and current technologies This type of analysis is preferred and required in many countries that focus on cost-effectiveness within the HTA process As the outcome (QALYs) can be expressed for all diagnoses, this analysis enables the comparison of results across various technologies	The ICER is usually presented as cost per QALY gained; healthcare decision makers would ask questions such as what are the incremental costs in relation to incremental QALYs gained for e.g. CFTR-MT in relation to e.g. the current standards of care in CF?
CBA	Both costs and outcomes are expressed in monetary values, i.e. 1 LYG or 1 QALY is weighted against a particular monetary threshold; this arbitrary amount is called the WTP threshold and represents the amount of money a society is willing to pay for a unit of benefit	This analysis enables a comparison of investment in relation to outcomes not just within healthcare, but also within a broader perspective applied to other sectors (e.g. diminished use of social services, improved education, or employment of patients themselves or of family members caring for a chronically ill family member)

COI: cost of illness; BIA: budget impact analysis; CMA: cost-minimisation analysis; CEA: cost-effectiveness analysis; CUA: cost-utility analysis; CBA: cost-benefit analysis; CF: cystic fibrosis; CFNBS: cystic fibrosis newborn screening; HCS: healthcare system; QoL: quality of life; FEV_1: forced expiratory volume in 1 s; BMI: body mass index; LYG: life-years gained; ICER: incremental cost-effectiveness ratio; QALY: quality-adjusted life-year; HTA: health technology assessment; CFTR-MT: cystic fibrosis transmembrane conductance regulator-modulation therapy; WTP: willingness to pay. [#]: represents the number of years of life adjusted for patient utility (utility is QoL on a scale from 0 (death) to 1 ("perfect" health)); 1 QALY is 1 year of perfect health (patient utility of 1.0) [33, 34]. Although there is currently some criticism of the QALY concept [37], QALYs are still generally recommended and are mandatory outcomes within the CEAs of many HTA bodies.

to delay substantially the onset of specific disease features by targeting the specific CFTR protein defect associated with them [42]. In this regard, CFTR-MTs have not only ground-breaking medical consequences but also impact upon "genotype-independent" medical interventions, as recently reviewed elsewhere [43]. As a result of these generally promising medical developments and advances in harmonised, albeit predominantly symptomatic, therapies, according to the European Cystic Fibrosis Society (ECFS) Standards of Care [9] (currently under revision), an increasing number of CF patients reach adulthood [44]. As care for CF adults is increasingly demanding and costly [45], healthcare systems start to demand health-economic analyses in order to provide evidence for eventual reallocation of costs within healthcare systems and/or to prepare in advance "baseline cost data" for CFTR-MT reimbursement schemes. In addition, it needs to be stressed that currently it is not clear what the long-term impact of CFTR-MTs on current symptomatic medical care in CF will be, *i.e.* whether novel therapies will supersede many of the standard interventions, such as antimicrobial therapies [46], or continue to be used "on top" of them.

In this chapter, health-economic studies relevant to CF will be exemplified using CFNBS and CF pre-conception carrier screening (CFPCS), followed by an overview of cost-of-illness studies carried out on standard symptomatic therapies, which will be complemented by the discussion of issues related to the introduction of CFTR-MT and use of lung transplantation in patients with end-stage lung disease.

Cost of newborn and pre-conception carrier screening

An increasing number of countries now use CFNBS [47], as it leads to an early (and equitable) diagnosis, thereby enabling early onset of treatment (*i.e.* prior to the development of symptoms of multiorgan impairment). Additional positive benefits of early CF diagnosis are in the prevention of irreversible lung damage, which is often associated with a delayed clinical diagnosis of the disease [48], and in the early introduction of newly diagnosed infants with CF to standardised specialised care, *i.e.* in terms of public health by structuring "healthcare pathways" [49].

Moreover, *CFTR* genotype–phenotype correlations offer improved prognoses of disease severity (www.cftr2.org) [50] in IRT/DNA schemes. This offers greater potential for customisation of CF care based on the *CFTR* genotype. CFNBS reduces overall costs of therapy compared with clinically diagnosed cases by almost 40% [51, 52], even when longer therapy duration (*i.e.* CF is diagnosed earlier) is taken into account. A health-economic study performed in Canada [53] showed that CFNBS was a "cost-saving approach" when viewed over a 5-year time horizon compared with not screening at all. There are also health-economic studies that compare methods of CFNBS to each other, such as IRT *versus* DNA analysis [54]. The studies concluded that the IRT/IRT screening algorithm reduced laboratory costs and insurance costs, but produced more false positives, thereby increasing the overall burden of the scheme. The IRT/DNA method also offered additional advantages, including fewer delayed diagnoses and lower out-of-pocket costs for families. A cost-effectiveness analysis of CFNBS performed in Quebec, Canada [53] demonstrated that the IRT/pancreatitis-associated protein (PAP) scheme (IRT cut-off set at the 96th percentile) is cost-effective. However, it needs to be noted that the positive health-economic effects of CFNBS should always be considered within a local context, as data from other countries are not automatically "transferable" between individual healthcare systems [55].

In some regions, such as the USA or northern Italy, CFNBS is complemented by broadly offered CFPCS of a population-specific set of CF-causing mutations [56]. In contrast to CFNBS, the aim of CFPCS is to detect adult heterozygotes of reproductive age and offer information to assist in making informed reproductive choices prior to the birth of the first CF patient in a family with no *a priori* increased risk of the disease. Although CFPCS is restricted by law in some countries and poses various ethical questions, over time, it could lead to a decreased incidence of CF within specific populations [56]. An Australian health-economic study demonstrated that despite initial costs associated with introduction of a nationwide or regional CFPCS programme, the costs were offset by the long-term reduction in CF incidence, which allowed for reallocation of finite healthcare resources to CF patients born prior to the screening programme [57]. A recent report provided evidence that CFPCS and CFNBS are complementary [47].

Cost-of-illness studies

Several cost-of-illness studies have been published, most of which tended to be prevalence based, offering a cross-sectional view of the average cost per CF patient. The most valuable cost-of-illness studies are those that present the cost in relation to clinical or QoL outcomes, or special health states. These health statuses within CF are identified/structured according to patient age and the severity of the lung disease, indirectly assessed by pulmonary function testing (using forced expiratory volume in 1 s (FEV_1) % predicted) [58] and colonisation with pathognomonic bacterial strains (as described earlier).

Within cost-of-illness studies, results are highly dependent on which types of costs are considered relevant; therefore, this issue is a matter of the study's perspective [35]. Most studies focus on the healthcare system's perspective, which addresses only the costs attributed to therapy; for example, currently, the most expensive in CF are inhaled dornase alfa and antibiotics such as tobramycin, in-/outpatient care (*e.g.* treatment of exacerbations and oxygen therapy), surgical procedures (*e.g.* lung transplantation) and home care. Among the healthcare costs, pharmacotherapy usually represents the greatest percentage of total expenditures (up to 90%) [59]. Additionally, due the increasing availability of novel treatments, total medicine expenditures on CF are expected to increase substantially, as will the positive benefits these new treatments bring (expressed as quality-adjusted life-years (QALYs)) (see later). If CF patients undergo lung transplantation, then their healthcare costs usually double or even triple compared with those who do not undergo these costly, albeit lifesaving, procedures [60].

An overview of available cost-of-illness studies on CF and their results, presented from the healthcare system perspective, is shown in table 2 [60, 68, 71]. The mean annual cost per CF patient (excluding the USA) was about €20 000 (for 2013). Slightly higher costs were observed in the USA, which is in accordance with different healthcare financing, where generally higher consumption of care was documented [72].

Furthermore, there are other costs (or potential "economic losses") that could be attributed to CF. Thus, when taking such costs into account (*i.e.* when applying the societal perspective), such as loss of productivity, the financial burden of CF is far larger. Costs related to the deterioration of productivity are mainly due to absenteeism/ presenteeism, work limitations (disabilities) and/or premature mortality of the patient. Additionally, similar costs associated with family members or informal caregivers must also be evaluated [33, 73, 74].

Table 2. Cost of illness studies and healthcare costs

First author [ref.]	Study year	Study country	Patients n	Mean age years	Age range years	Mean annual cost# 2013 €
ROBSON [61]	1990	UK	119	21	16–44	15 461
WILDHAGEN [62]	1991	The Netherlands	81	14	0–37	16 325
IREYS [63]	1993	USA	204		0–18	14 466
BAUMANN [64]	1996	Germany	138		0–18	23 722
JOHNSON [65]	1996	Canada	303	18		5850
LIEU [66]	1996	USA	136	17	0–56	12 598
HORVAIS [67]	2001	France	65			15 674
HOUT [68]	2003	France	64	15.3	0–48	27 725
HEIMESHOFF [59]	2004	Germany	212	20	0–adult	36 419
EIDT-KOCH [69]	2006	Germany	301			20 103
OUYANG [60]	2006	USA	1250		0–64	38 293
DEWITT [70]	2008	USA	352	14.6	5–adult	28 747
VAN GOOL [71]	2009	Australia	2255	15.4		11 182

#: all originally reported national currencies converted to US dollars at 2009 prices applying Organisation for Economic Co-operation and Development (OECD) purchasing power parity conversion rates using the Campbell and Cochrane Economics Methods Group–Evidence for Policy and Practice Information and Co-ordinating Centre Cost Converter and then multiplied by nominal exchange rate from dollars to euros from the OECD for 2009 (blank: values not stated).

As CF is a progressive disease, it is highly valuable to describe the relationship between disease severity and lifetime costs, *i.e.* to adopt an incidence-based approach to cost-of-illness studies. Recently, this type of study was performed in Australia [71], in which patients were stratified according to their FEV1 into one of the three categories (mild disease: FEV1 ⩾70% predicted; moderate: FEV1 40% to <70% predicted; severe: FEV1 <40 predicted); an additional category represented patients who underwent a lung transplant. Healthcare costs were calculated for patients in each category for at least 2 years (data from 2003–2005). Subsequently, a Markov statistical model [75] was developed for disease progression based on the transition of patients to a more severe disease category with age. Based on this approach, a lifetime cost model was developed that simulated CF progression and estimated healthcare costs, *i.e.* costs from birth to demise in terms of their health status and based on the deterioration of lung function. The mean lifetime healthcare costs were calculated to be $306 332 (in 2009), with a 3.5% discount rate that represents correction of "future costs" based on current values [76].

Cost-effectiveness analysis

Essentially, cost-of-illness studies serve as prerequisites for subsequent cost-effectiveness analysis. Once we understand the costs of CF care relative to disease severity (usually based on FEV1), and as the severity of the lung disease is the main driver of costs as well as survival and QoL in CF [77, 78], we can compare different medical/health technologies used in CF care, using cost-effectiveness and/or cost-utility analysis.

Usually, clinical trials have short-term horizons and render outcomes in terms of "surrogates" and not in terms of patient survival [79]. Therefore, the most relevant way to present the cost-effectiveness of one technology compared to another (comparator) is to develop lifetime models [80], particularly for chronic and progressive diseases such as CF.

Based on this modelling approach, we could interpret results from clinical trials in terms of lifetime costs and outcomes (*i.e.* life-years gained and QALYs for current *versus* new technologies). There have been several parameters described for CF that can be used as data for regression analysis that predict survival probabilities, *i.e.* age, FEV1, body mass index (BMI) (which is indicative of the overall nutritional status) or its z-score, degree of pancreatic insufficiency, presence of CFRD, occurrence of acute disease exacerbations and bacterial lung colonisation [77, 78]. Once total costs and outcomes for current and new technologies are accounted for, the incremental cost-effectiveness ratio (ICER) (cost per QALY) can be evaluated using the following equation [34].

$$ICER = \frac{\text{total cost of new technology-total cost of current technology}}{\text{total QALYs of new technology-total QALYs of current technology}}$$

Basically, the ICER could occur in any one of the four quadrants shown in figure 1. When evaluating rare diseases, for new technologies that are usually more costly but simultaneously more effective from the "medical point of view" and in terms of the patient preferences (generating higher QALYs), ICERs fall into quadrant I. If the ICER is below the arbitrarily defined willingness to pay (WTP) threshold, then the respective technology is considered cost-effective by definition.

Importantly, some EU countries or healthcare systems (assuming that they use a HTA) have their own explicit or implicit WTP thresholds. Some EU countries have a fixed WTP threshold (*e.g.* for the UK National Health Service (NHS), the current WTP threshold is £30 000 per QALY), whereby technologies that exceed this monetary threshold do not receive healthcare system approval [81]. However, the UK HTA agency is already considering policy reforms that would allow them to take into account all other aspects of HTA (as discussed earlier), rather than merely using an isolated ICER outcome. Other countries (*e.g.* the Czech Republic, Poland and Hungary) currently use the World Health Organization CHOICE (Choosing Interventions that are Cost Effective) methodology, which defines the WTP threshold to be approximately three times the gross domestic product *per capita* per

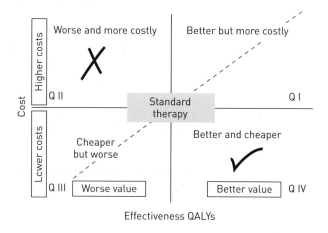

Figure 1. Results of a cost-effectiveness analysis. Presence of incremental cost-effectiveness ratio on the cost-effectiveness plane. Q: quadrant; WTP: willingness to pay; QALY: quality-adjusted life-year.

QALY [82]. Other EU countries, such as Sweden, assess nonmonetary benefits as part of the final HTA appraisal. This approach is generally referred to as value-based pricing [83]. Nonetheless, the current EU HTA landscape is undergoing a rapid transition as monitored by the EUnetHTA.

The small number of cost-effectiveness analyses, such as the recent study on dry-powder inhalation antibiotics in the treatment of *P. aeruginosa* [84], could probably be explained by the relatively limited number of new technologies introduced in the past several years for CF care, *i.e.* prior to the ground-breaking introduction of CFTR-MT.

Useful data for health-economic studies could be gathered from European CF registries. For example, the Irish registry provided data on the introduction of public health measures such as CFNBS in the country based on the high CF incidence and associated costs [85]. Additionally, the ECFS Registry provided aggregate data on factors associated with the decline in FEV_1 that is used as a crucial parameter in health-economic studies [86]. Nonetheless, it is important to coordinate efforts across EU CF registries [87], assuring, for example, their completeness and timeliness, representative CF population coverage, quality control of their datasets, broadly accepted definitions [88] and, lastly, that relevant health-economic data are introduced into their datasets [89], as recently elaborated for all rare diseases. Furthermore, long-term sustainability of registries is of paramount importance [90]. A successful example was reported in Australia where health-economic studies used data from the national CF registry [71]. Unfortunately, none of the current CF registries compile data on indirect costs, such as lost productivity or the cost of informal care.

Orphan medicinal products and CFTR-modifying therapies

CFTR-MT uses OMPs, which are rather expensive (both at the individual and healthcare-system levels) and require lifelong administration. It has been demonstrated in other rare diseases that the main driver of relative healthcare system expenditure increase is the number of new drugs obtaining OMP designation [91], which is offset by a decreasing success rate of new approvals or of their healthcare system reimbursement, and by the eventual loss of intellectual property protection for existing OMPs.

The total healthcare system budget impact of OMPs has been reviewed recently by two studies; however, several authors of these studies have declared competing interests. Disease-based epidemiological health-economic modelling has provided evidence that the costs of OMPs will probably peak in 2016 at a maximum of 6.6% of the total pharmacotherapy costs in the EU and that these will probably remain unchanged until the end of this decade [92]. Another study using a dynamic forecasting model was carried out to estimate the budget impact of OMPs in Sweden and France. Although there was uncertainty about the modelling parameters and sensitivity analysis, the conservative healthcare system budget impact was estimated to peak at 4.1% for Sweden and 4.9% for France by 2020. Naturally, such forecasts could be affected by the future (and to a large degree unpredictable) success rate of novel OMP approvals, variations in the average cost of OMPs (upwards or downwards based on regulatory pressures and/or "healthcare market reimbursement reality"), or by the number and character of pharmaceutical companies developing OMPs as their "niche busters" [93]. Finally, there have even been recent suggestions to revisit the special market access status of OMPs including revision of the US Orphan Drug Act [94], which, if applied, could markedly change the overall situation of OMPs.

Given such uncertainties, which also stem from the fact that HTA schemes devised to assess blockbuster drugs are not applicable to OMPs due to the small numbers of patients involved [95], many healthcare systems limit the initial time-frames of reimbursement schemes of OMPs and renewal of future reimbursement is conditional on monitoring of treatment outcomes by data drawn from dedicated registries, as reviewed elsewhere for other rare diseases [96]. Recently, multistakeholder and multicriterion decision algorithms for payers and HTA bodies were proposed [32]. Additionally, the multidisciplinary EU Committee of Experts on Rare Diseases is developing the much-awaited international guidelines on OMPs in rare diseases, whereby, due to its extraordinary advances in research, diagnosis and care, CF is commonly used as a model disorder [29].

Currently, the best available evidence for CFTR-MT is related to the approximately 2-year clinical experience with the CFTR potentiator ivacaftor [97]. In the UK, in 2013, the NHS Commission noted the views of specialist CF clinicians on the benefits of ivacaftor to eligible patients with the Gly551Asp (legacy name G551D) *CFTR* mutation (comprising approximately 4% of all CF patients in the country), and that the NHS is already funding similar ultra-OMPs for other rare diseases that have high opportunity cost and ICERs that probably fall in the same range as ivacaftor. Therefore, this OMP was excluded from the payment-by-results NHS tariffs [98] (and "QALY-based" HTA schemes) and will be funded through pass-through payment against invoices received from provider NHS Trusts subject to a patient access scheme. In Scotland, the Scottish Medical Council had rejected ivacaftor for NHS use twice based on its high ICER. However, since January 2013, ivacaftor has been covered through the new £21 million fund to help improve access to drugs for people with rare conditions; it should be noted that there had been no discount offered to NHS Scotland, hence the Council recommended against its use largely on cost grounds [99].

In general, managed introductions of OMPs (*i.e.* patient access scheme) associated with price adjustments, restrictions relative to patient subpopulations and funding of accompanying diagnostic tests, and many other introductory benefits from the OMP producers could/ should be the way to secure patient access to these therapies and simultaneously decrease the financial burden on healthcare systems [100].

Treatment outcomes for ivacaftor are being monitored by data drawn from the UK CF registry [101]. Experience gathered in ivacaftor will potentially also have an important role for other awaited OMPs in CF (*e.g.* the combined corrector/potentiator therapy for the most common Phe508del *CFTR* mutation) [102], including long-term demonstration of their added value.

A cost-effectiveness analysis and full HTA report of ivacaftor in CF patients over 6 years of age bearing the Gly551Asp channel-gating defect mutation has been published. The ICER varied between £335 000 and £1 274 000 per QALY gained [97]. When lifetime costs for all eligible CF patients residing in England, UK, were taken into account, they were more than six times higher than those of the current standardised symptomatic therapy. The authors concluded that clinical effectiveness of ivacaftor is very good but that "the high cost of ivacaftor may prove an obstacle in the uptake of this treatment" and that long-term effectiveness studies are still needed, using sweat chloride as a biomarker [103]. Compassionate use of ivacaftor therapy in patients with severe lung disease resulted in a statistically significant decrease in treatment requirements, contrary to what has been demonstrated in less severe cases [104]. This approach could also stabilise such patients before a suitable donor is found for lung transplantation.

Lung transplantation

Approximately a decade ago, lung transplantation in CF was subjected to cost-effectiveness/cost-utility analysis with regard to the type of end-stage lung disease [105, 106]. It has been documented that, in some patient groups, results from cost-effectiveness/cost-utility analysis were at "acceptable" levels. Variations in cost-effectiveness analysis (based on life-years gained) were higher than in cost-utility analysis based on QALYs (survival and QoL) in patients who received or did not receive lung transplants and the subsequent costly lifelong immune suppression therapy.

Conclusion

A proper understanding of the costs attributed to CF care and management is important for assuring introduction of novel therapeutic schemes, *i.e.* CFTR-MT, into EU healthcare systems that have finite resources limited by negative demographic trends and austerity measures. In general, the focus of health-economic studies should not only be on the direct consumption of healthcare resources but also on the overall loss of productivity of both patients and caregivers. Such analyses should primarily be performed with regards to the natural progression of the disease and taking lifelong costs into account. This can be accomplished by using pulmonary function tests (PFTs) as markers of CF lung disease progression and antibiotic treatment of chronic bacterial lung colonisation as key cost drivers. In addition, using the sweat chloride test as a biomarker in randomised controlled trials and long-term clinical effectiveness studies in CFTR-MT is important. Useful clinical data already exist in national and international CF patient registries but with lower health-economic utility and problematic quality. A well preformed cost-of-illness study is the basic prerequisite for a subsequent reliable cost-effectiveness/cost-utility analysis, which compares novel and established technologies against each other. As CF is a rare disease, novel technologies (and thus OMPs) are expected to be rather expensive. Therefore, the ICERs for OMPs are expected to be above the generally applied WTP threshold in the majority of EU countries that use this assessment strategy. Different countries will deal with this problem in different ways, as discussed earlier. Some countries do not perform any health-economic evaluation like cost-effectiveness/cost-utility analysis, while others attempt to use a flexible WTP threshold that is usually higher for technologies with real clinical added value addressing substantial unmet needs and/or those with complex social and ethical components, such as in the case of CF. Expensive novel technologies that offer substantial clinical and QoL benefits could still be reimbursed, *i.e.* receive a positive appraisal by a respective HTA body [107] and be introduced *via* managed healthcare market introductions, such as patient access schemes. Nonetheless, national political and policy decisions play a key role in healthcare system reimbursement schemes for all medical technologies, including OMPs. In this context, it is important that the rare disease-related EU policy documents [21] stipulate establishment of national plans or strategies [108] to prevent policy decisions that marginalise rare diseases relative to diseases with higher public awareness, such as cancer or diabetes. A positive step in this direction is the guidelines for the assessment of the clinical added value of OMPs, which have already been published by EUCERD. Initial data gathered on CFTR-MT provided clear evidence that ivacaftor is clinically effective but that long-term studies are needed, and that its high individual and lifelong pricing (approximately more than six times that of standard symptomatic therapies) may hinder its uptake by EU healthcare systems. Patient and professional advocacy for novel healthcare technologies (OMPs in the case of CF) should be evidence-based both in terms of clinical and health-economic data, and carefully balanced with regards to disease severity and unmet needs, and take into account broader ethical and social aspects of care for marginalised patient groups. However, transparent pricing and profit reinvestment policies from the OMP producers will also facilitate introduction of novel therapies into EU healthcare systems and beyond. Finally, *a priori* assessments of novel medical interventions that will establish their value from the point of view of a healthcare system will also be increasingly carried out.

References

1. Goss CH, Ratjen F. Update in cystic fibrosis 2012. *Am J Respir Crit Care Med* 2013; 187: 915–919.
2. Cystic Fibrosis Mutation Database. www.genet.sickkids.on.ca/app Date last accessed: January 12, 2014. Date last updated: April 25, 2011.
3. Stephenson A, Hux J, Tullis E, *et al.* Socioeconomic status and risk of hospitalization among individuals with cystic fibrosis in Ontario, Canada. *Pediatr Pulmonol* 2011; 46: 376–384.
4. Taylor-Robinson D, Schechter MS. Health inequalities and cystic fibrosis. *BMJ* 2011; 343: d4818.
5. De Boeck K, Zolin A, Cuppens H, *et al.* The relative frequency of *CFTR* mutation classes in European patients with cystic fibrosis. *J Cyst Fibros* 2014 [In press DOI: 10.1016/j.jcf.2013.12.003].
6. Mehta G, Macek M Jr, Mehta A, *et al.* Cystic fibrosis across Europe: EuroCareCF analysis of demographic data from 35 countries. *J Cyst Fibros* 2010; 9: Suppl. 2, S5–S21.
7. McCormick J, Mehta G, Olesen HV, *et al.* Comparative demographics of the European cystic fibrosis population: a cross-sectional database analysis. *Lancet* 2010; 375: 1007–1013.
8. Farrell PM. Is newborn screening for cystic fibrosis a basic human right? *J Cyst Fibros* 2008; 7: 262–265.
9. Kerem E, Conway S, Elborn S, *et al.* Standards of care for patients with cystic fibrosis: a European consensus. *J Cyst Fibros* 2005; 4: 7–26.
10. Thompson ML, Flynn JD, Clifford TM. Pharmacotherapy of lung transplantation: an overview. *J Pharm Pract* 2013; 26: 5–13.
11. Cohen-Cymberknoh M, Shoseyov D, Kerem E. Managing cystic fibrosis: strategies that increase life expectancy and improve quality of life. *Am J Respir Crit Care Med* 2011; 183: 1463–1471.
12. Ong T, Ramsey BW. Modifying disease in cystic fibrosis: current and future therapies on the horizon. *Curr Opin Pulm Med* 2013; 19: 645–651.
13. Deeks ED. Ivacaftor: a review of its use in patients with cystic fibrosis. *Drugs* 2013; 73: 1595–1604.
14. Ramsey BW, Davies J, McElvaney G, *et al.* A CFTR potentiator in patients with cystic fibrosis and the G551D mutation. *N Engl J Med* 2011; 365: 1663–1672.
15. Sermet-Gaudelus I. Ivacaftor treatment in patients with cystic fibrosis and the G551D-*CFTR* mutation. *Eur Respir Rev* 2013; 22: 66–71.
16. Kaiser J. Personalized medicine. New cystic fibrosis drug offers hope, at a price. *Science* 2012; 335: 645.
17. Hughes-Wilson W, Palma A, Schuurman A, *et al.* Paying for the Orphan Drug System: break or bend? Is it time for a new evaluation system for payers in Europe to take account of new rare disease treatments? *Orphanet J Rare Dis* 2012; 7: 74.
18. Richards T. European health systems must adapt to austerity, conference hears. *BMJ* 2013; 347: 6073.
19. Pammolli F, Riccaboni M, Magazzini L. The sustainability of European health care systems: beyond income and aging. *Eur J Health Econ* 2012; 13: 623–634.
20. Mavris M, La Cam Y. Involvement of patient organisations in research and development of orphan drugs for rare diseases in Europe. *Mol Syndromol* 2012; 3: 237–243.
21. Council recommendation of 8 June 2009 on an action in the field of rare diseases. *Off J Eur Union 2009; C,* 15102.
22. Hatz MH, Schremser K, Rogowski WH. Is individualized medicine more cost-effective? A systematic review. *Pharmacoeconomics* 2014 [In press DOI: 10.1007/s40273-014-0143-0].
23. Rogowski WH, Grosse SD, Schmidtke J, *et al.* Criteria for fairly allocating scarce health-care resources to genetic tests: which matter most? *Eur J Hum Genet* 2014; 22: 25–31.
24. Kanavos P, McKee M. Cross-border issues in the provision of health services: are we moving towards a European health care policy? *J Health Serv Res Policy* 2000; 5: 231–236.
25. Mills EJ, Thorlund K, Ioannidis JP. Demystifying trial networks and network meta-analysis. *BMJ* 2013; 346: f2914.
26. Egger M, Smith GD, Phillips AN. Meta-analysis: principles and procedures. *BMJ* 1997; 315: 1533–1537.
27. Jansen JP, Fleurence R, Devine B, *et al.* Interpreting indirect treatment comparisons and network meta-analysis for health-care decision making: report of the ISPOR Task Force on Indirect Treatment Comparisons Good Research Practices – part 1. *Value Health* 2011; 14: 417–428.
28. Hoaglin DC, Hawkins N, Jansen JP, *et al.* Interpreting indirect treatment comparisons and network meta-analysis for health-care decision making: report of the ISPOR Task Force on Indirect Treatment Comparisons Good Research Practices – part 2. *Value Health* 2011; 14: 429–437.

29. European Union Committee of Experts on Rare Diseases. EUCERD Recommendation for a CAVOMP Information Flow. www.eucerd.eu/?post_type=document&p=1446 Date last accessed: January 12, 2014. Date last updated: September 2012.

30. Thokala P, Duenas A. Multiple criteria decision analysis for health technology assessment. *Value Health* 2012; 15: 1172–1181.

31. Tony M, Wagner M, Khoury H, *et al.* Bridging health technology assessment (HTA) with multicriteria decision analyses (MCDA): field testing of the EVIDEM framework for coverage decisions by a public payer in Canada. *BMC Health Serv Res* 2011; 11: 329–341.

32. Sussex J, Rollet P, Garau M, *et al.* A pilot study of multicriteria decision analysis for valuing orphan medicines. *Value Health* 2013; 16: 1163–1169.

33. Drummond MF, Sculper MJ, Torrance GW, *et al.* Methods for the Economic Evaluation of Health Care Programmes. 3rd Edn. Oxford, Oxford University Press, 2005.

34. Kobelt G. Health Economics: an Introduction to Economic Evaluation. 3rd Edn. London, Office of Health Economics, 2013.

35. Largand A, Moss JR. Cost-of-illness studies: a guide to critical evaluation. *Pharmacoeconomics* 2011; 29: 653–671.

36. Mauskopf JA, Sullivan SD, Annemans L, *et al.* Principles of good practice for budget impact analysis: report of the ISPOR Task Force on Good Research Practices – budget impact analysis. *Value Health* 2007; 10: 336–347.

37. McGregor M, Caro JJ. QALYs: are they helpful to decision makers? *Pharmacoeconomics* 2006; 24: 947–952.

38. Green DM, McDougal KE, Blackman SM, *et al.* Mutations that permit residual CFTR function delay acquisition of multiple respiratory pathogens in CF patients. *Respir Res* 2010; 11: 140.

39. Sosnay PR, Siklosi KR, Van Goor F, *et al.* Defining the disease liability of variants in the cystic fibrosis transmembrane conductance regulator gene. *Nat Genet* 2013; 45: 1160–1167.

40. Lim MT, Wallis C, Price JF, *et al.* Diagnosis of cystic fibrosis in London and South East England before and after the introduction of newborn screening. *Arch Dis Child* 2014; 99: 197–202.

41. Clancy JP, Johnson SG, Yee SW, *et al.* Clinical Pharmacogenetics Implementation Consortium (CPIC) guidelines for ivacaftor therapy in the context of *CFTR* genotype. *Clin Pharmacol Ther* 2014 [In press DOI: 10.1038/clpt.2014.54].

42. Boyle MP, De Boeck K. A new era in the treatment of cystic fibrosis: correction of the underlying CFTR defect. *Lancet Respir Med* 2013; 1: 158–163.

43. Ong T, Ramsey BW. Modifying disease in cystic fibrosis: current and future therapies on the horizon. *Curr Opin Pulm Med* 2013; 19: 645–651.

44. Nazareth D, Walshaw M. Coming of age in cystic fibrosis – transition from paediatric to adult care. *Clin Med* 2013; 13: 482–486.

45. Briesacher BA, Quittner AL, Fouayzi H, *et al.* Nationwide trends in the medical care costs of privately insured patients with cystic fibrosis (CF), 2001–2007. *Pediatr Pulmonol* 2011; 46: 770–776.

46. Reznikov LR, Abou Alaiwa MH, Dohrn CL, *et al.* Antibacterial properties of the CFTR potentiator ivacaftor. *J Cyst Fibros* 2014 [In press DOI: 10.1016/j.jcf.2014.02.004].

47. Castellani C, Massie J. Newborn screening and carrier screening for cystic fibrosis: alternative or complementary? *Eur Respir J* 2014; 43: 20–23.

48. Walsh AC, Rault G, Li Z, *et al.* Pulmonary outcome differences in U.S. and French cystic fibrosis cohorts diagnosed through newborn screening. *J Cyst Fibros* 2010; 9: 44–50.

49. Dijk FN, Fitzgerald DA. The impact of newborn screening and earlier intervention on the clinical course of cystic fibrosis. *Paediatr Respir Rev* 2012; 13: 220–225.

50. Weiler CA, Drumm ML. Genetic influences on cystic fibrosis lung disease severity. *Front Pharmacol* 2013; 4: 40.

51. Sims EJ, Mugford M, Clark A, *et al.* Economic implications of newborn screening for cystic fibrosis: a cost of illness retrospective cohort study. *Lancet* 2007; 369: 1187–1195.

52. Sims EJ, McCormick J, Mehta G, *et al.* Neonatal screening for cystic fibrosis is beneficial even in the context of modern treatment. *J Pediatr* 2005; 147: Suppl., S42–S46.

53. Nshimyumukiza L, Bois A, Daigneault P, *et al.* Cost effectiveness of newborn screening for cystic fibrosis: a simulation study. *J Cyst Fibros* 2013; 13: 267–274.

54. Wells J, Rosenberg M, Hoffman G, *et al.* A decision-tree approach to cost comparison of newborn screening strategies for cystic fibrosis. *Pediatrics* 2012; 129: e339–e347.

55. Radhakrishnan M, van Gool K, Hall J, *et al.* Economic evaluation of cystic fibrosis screening: a review of the literature. *Health Policy* 2008; 85: 133–147.

56. Castellani C, Picci L, Tamanini A, *et al.* Association between carrier screening and incidence of cystic fibrosis. *JAMA* 2009; 302: 2573–2579.

57. Norman R, van Gool K, Hall J, *et al.* Cost-effectiveness of carrier screening for cystic fibrosis in Australia. *J Cyst Fibros* 2012; 11: 281–287.

58. Rosenfeld M, Allen J, Arets BH, *et al.* An official American Thoracic Society workshop report: optimal lung function tests for monitoring cystic fibrosis, bronchopulmonary dysplasia, and recurrent wheezing in children less than 6 years of age. *Ann Am Thorac Soc* 2013; 10: Suppl., S1–S11.

59. Heimeshoff M, Hollmeyer H, Schreyogg J, *et al.* Cost of illness of cystic fibrosis in Germany: results from a large cystic fibrosis centre. *Pharmacoeconomics* 2012; 30: 763–777.

60. Ouyang L, Grosse SD, Amendah DD, *et al.* Healthcare expenditures for privately insured people with cystic fibrosis. *Pediatr Pulmonol* 2009; 44: 989–996.

61. Robson M, Abbott J, Webb K, *et al.* A cost description of an adult cystic fibrosis unit and cost analyses of different categories of patients. *Thorax* 1992; 47: 684–689.

62. Wildhagen MF, Verheij JB, Verzijl JG, *et al.* Cost of care of patients with cystic fibrosis in the Netherlands in 1990–1. *Thorax* 1996; 51: 298–301.

63. Ireys HT, Anderson GF, Shaffer TJ, *et al.* Expenditures for care of children with chronic illnesses enrolled in the Washington State Medicaid program, fiscal year 1993. *Pediatrics* 1997; 100: 197–204.

64. Baumann U, Stocklossa C, Greiner W, *et al.* Cost of care and clinical condition in paediatric cystic fibrosis patients. *J Cyst Fibros* 2003; 2: 84–90.

65. Johnson JA, Connolly MA, Jacobs P, *et al.* Cost of care for individuals with cystic fibrosis: a regression approach to determining the impact of recombinant human dnase. *Pharmacotherapy* 1999; 19: 1159–1166.

66. Lieu T, Ray G, Farmer G, *et al.* The cost of medical care for patients with cystic fibrosis in a health maintenance organization. *Pediatrics* 1999; 103: e72.

67. Horvais V, Touzet S, Francois S, *et al.* Cost of home and hospital care for patients with cystic fibrosis followed up in two reference medical centers in France. *Int J Technol Assess Health Care* 2006; 22: 525–531.

68. Huot L, Durieu I, Bourdy S, *et al.* REMU study. Evolution of costs of care for cystic fibrosis patients after clinical guidelines implementation in a French network. *J Cyst Fibros* 2008; 7: 403–408.

69. Eidt-Koch D, Wagner TO, Mittendorf T, *et al.* Outpatient medication costs of patients with cystic fibrosis in Germany. *Appl Health Econ Health Policy* 2010; 8: 111–118.

70. DeWitt EM, Grussemeyer CA, Friedman JY, *et al.* Resource use, costs, and utility estimates for patients with cystic fibrosis with mild impairment in lung function: analysis of data collected alongside a 48-week multicenter clinical trial. *Value Health* 2012; 15: 277–283.

71. van Gool K, Norman R, Delatycki MB, *et al.* Understanding the costs of care for cystic fibrosis: an analysis by age and health state. *Value Health* 2013; 16: 345–355.

72. Blumenthal D, Dixon J. Health-care reforms in the USA and England: areas for useful learning. *Lancet* 2012; 380: 1352–1357.

73. Koopmanschap MA, Burdorf A, Jacob K, *et al.* Measuring productivity changes in economic evaluation, setting the research agenda. *Pharmacoeconomics* 2005; 23: 47–54.

74. Koopmanschap MA, van Exel JN, van den Berg B, *et al.* An overview of methods and applications to value informal care in economic evaluations of healthcare. *Pharmacoeconomics* 2008; 26: 269–280.

75. Siebert U, Alagoz O, Bayoum AM, *et al.* State-transition modeling: a report of the ISPOR-SMDM Modeling Good Research Practices Task Force-3. *Value Health* 2012; 15: 812–820.

76. Smith DH, Gravelle H. The practice of discounting in economic evaluations of healthcare interventions. *Int J Technol Assess Health Care* 2001; 17: 236–243.

77. Liou TG, Adler FR, FitzSimmons SC, *et al.* Predictive 5-year survivorship model of cystic fibrosis. *Am J Epidemiol* 2001; 153: 345–352.

78. Buzzetti R, Alicandro G, Minicucci L, *et al.* Validation of a predictive survival model in Italian patients with cystic fibrosis. *J Cyst Fibros* 2012; 11: 24–29.

79. Loeve M, Krestin GP, Rosenfeld M, *et al.* Chest computed tomography: a validated surrogate endpoint of cystic fibrosis lung disease? *Eur Respir J* 2013; 42: 844–857.

80. Caro JJ, Briggs AH, Siebert U, *et al.* Modeling good research practices – overview: a report of the ISPOR-SMDM Modeling Good Research Practices Task Force-1. *Value Health* 2012; 15: 796–803.

81. Rawlins MD, Culyer AJ. National Institute for Clinical Excellence and its value judgments. *BMJ* 2004; 329: 224–227.

82. World Health Organization. Cost effectiveness and strategic planning (WHO-CHOICE): cost effectiveness and strategic planning. www.who.int/choice/en/ Date last accessed: January 12, 2014.

83. Value based pricing in Sweden: lessons for design? http://news.ohe.org/2012/11/28/value-based-pricing-in-sweden-lessons-for-design/ Date last accessed: January 12, 2014. Date last updated: November 28, 2012.

84. Tappenden P, Harnan S, Uttley L, *et al.* Colistimethate sodium powder and tobramycin powder for inhalation for the treatment of chronic *Pseudomonas aeruginosa* lung infection in cystic fibrosis: systematic review and economic model. *Health Technol Assess* 2013; 17: 1–182.

85. Farrell P, Joffe S, Foley L, *et al.* Diagnosis of cystic fibrosis in the Republic of Ireland: epidemiology and costs. *Ir Med J* 2007; 100: 557–560.

86. Kerem E, Viviani L, Zolin A, *et al.* Factors associated with FEV1 decline in cystic fibrosis: analysis of the ECFS Patient Registry. *Eur Respir J* 2014; 43: 125–133.

87. Sheppard DN. The European cystic fibrosis patient registry: the power of sharing data. *J Cyst Fibros* 2010; 9: Suppl. 2, S1–S2.

88. Stern M. The use of a cystic fibrosis patient registry to assess outcomes and improve cystic fibrosis care in Germany. *Curr Opin Pulm Med* 2011; 17: 473–477.

89. Taruscio D, Gainotti S, Mollo E, *et al*. The current situation and needs of rare disease registries in europe. *Public Health Genomics* 2013; 16: 288–298.

90. Vittozzi L, Gainotti S, Mollo E, *et al*. A model for the European platform for rare disease registries. *Public Health Genomics* 2013; 16: 299–304.

91. European Medicines Agency. Committee for Orphan Medicinal Products (COMP). www.ema.europa.eu/ema/index.jsp?curl=pages/about_us/general/general_content_000263.jsp Date last accessed: April 1, 2014.

92. Schey C, Milanova T, Hutchings A. Estimating the budget impact of orphan medicines in Europe: 2010–2020. *Orphanet J Rare Dis* 2011; 6: 62.

93. Collier R. Bye, bye blockbusters, hello niche busters. *CMAJ* 2011; 183: E697–E698.

94. Simoens S, Cassiman D, Dooms M, *et al*. Orphan drugs for rare diseases: is it time to revisit their special market access status? *Drugs 2012; 30,* 72: 1437–1443.

95. Joppi R, Bertele' V, Garattini S. Orphan drugs, orphan diseases. The first decade of orphan drug legislation in the EU. *Eur J Clin Pharmacol* 2013; 69: 1009–1024.

96. Hollak CE, Aerts JM, Aymé S, *et al*. Limitations of drug registries to evaluate orphan medicinal products for the treatment of lysosomal storage disorders. *Orphanet J Rare Dis* 2011; 6: 16.

97. Whiting P, Al M, Burgers L, *et al*. Ivacaftor for the treatment of patients with cystic fibrosis and the G551D mutation: a systematic review and cost-effectiveness analysis. *Health Technol Assess* 2014; 18: 1–106.

98. Dept of Health. Guidance: Payment by results in the NHS: tariff for 2013 to 2014 www.gov.uk/government/publications/payment-by-results-pbr-operational-guidance-and-tariffs Date last accessed: April 1, 2014. Date last updated: March 25, 2013.

99. BBC News Scotland. Scottish "orphan drugs" fund launched. www.bbc.co.uk/news/uk-scotland-21016879 Date last updated: January 14, 2013.

100. Denis A, Mergaert L, Fostier Ch, *et al*. Critical assessment of Belgian reimbursement dossiers of orphan drugs. *Pharmacoeconomics* 2011; 29: 883–893.

101. Cystic Fibrosis Trust. UK Cystic Fibrosis Registry. www.cysticfibrosis.org.uk/registry Date last accessed: April 1, 2014.

102. Lane MA, Doe SJ. A new era in the treatment of cystic fibrosis. *Clin Med* 2014; 14: 76–78.

103. Accurso FJ, Van Goor F, Zha J, *et al*. Sweat chloride as a biomarker of CFTR activity: proof of concept and ivacaftor clinical trial data. *J Cyst Fibros* 2014; 13: 139–147.

104. Barry PJ, Plant BJ, Nair A, *et al*. Effects of Ivacaftor in cystic fibrosis patients carrying the G551D mutation with severe lung disease. *Chest* 2014 [In press DOI: 10.1378/chest.13-2397].

105. Vasiliadis HM, Collet JP, Penrod JR. A cost-effectiveness and cost-utility study of lung transplantation. *J Heart Lung Transplant* 2005; 24: 1275–1283.

106. Groen H, van der Bij W, Koëter GH, *et al*. Cost-effectiveness of lung transplantation in relation to type of end-stage pulmonary disease. *Am J Transplant* 2004; 4: 1155–1162.

107. Farrugia A, O'Mahony B, Cassar J. Health technology assessment and haemophilia. *Haemophilia* 2012; 18: 152–157.

108. European Commission. Public Health: Rare Diseases. http://ec.europa.eu/health/rare_diseases/national_plans/detailed/index_en.htm Date last accessed: January 12, 2014.

Support statement: J. Klimeš was supported by grant SVV 267 005 from Charles University (Prague). M. Macek Jr was supported by the Czech Ministry of Health Conceptual Development of Research Organization (University Hospital Motol, Prague, Czech Republic; grants 00064203, NT/13770-4 and CZ.2.16/3.1.00/24022OPPK).

Disclosures: None declared.

Other titles in the series

ERM 63 – Community-Acquired Pneumonia
James D. Chalmers, Mathias W. Pletz and Stefano Aliberti

ERM 62 – Outcomes in Clinical Trials
Martin Kolb and Claus F. Vogelmeier

ERM 61 – Complex Pleuropulmonary Infections
Gernot Rohde and Dragan Subotic

ERM 60 – The Spectrum of Bronchial Infection
Francesco Blasi and Marc Miravitlles

ERM 59 – COPD and Comorbidity
Klaus F. Rabe, Jadwiga A. Wedzicha and Emiel F.M. Wouters

ERM 58 – Tuberculosis
Christoph Lange and Giovanni Battista Migliori

ERM 57 – Pulmonary Hypertension
M.M. Hoeper and M. Humbert

ERM 56 – Paediatric Asthma
K-H. Carlsen and J. Gerritsen

ERM 55 – New Developments in Mechanical Ventilation
M. Ferrer and P. Pelosi

ERM 54 – Orphan Lung Diseases
J-F. Cordier

ERM 53 – Nosocomial and Ventilator-Associated Pneumonia
A. Torres and S. Ewig

ORDER INFORMATION

Monographs are individually priced.
Visit the European Respiratory Society bookshop
www.ersbookshop.com
For bulk purchases contact the Publications Office directly.
European Respiratory Society Publications Office,
442 Glossop Road, Sheffield, S10 2PX, UK.
Tel: 44 (0)114 267 2860; Fax: 44 (0)114 266 5064; E-mail: sales@ersj.org.uk